MYELOID LEUKEMIA – BASIC MECHANISMS OF LEUKEMOGENESIS

Edited by **Steffen Koschmieder** and **Utz Krug**

Myeloid Leukemia – Basic Mechanisms of Leukemogenesis
Edited by Steffen Koschmieder and Utz Krug

Published by InTech

Janeza Trdine 9, 51000 Rijeka, Croatia

Publishing Process Manager Ivana Zec

Technical Editor Teodora Smiljanic

Cover Designer InTech Design Team

Additional hard copies can be obtained from orders@intechopen.com

Myeloid Leukemia – Basic Mechanisms of Leukemogenesis,
Edited by Steffen Koschmieder and Utz Krug
p. cm.
ISBN 978-953-307-789-5

For EU product safety concerns:
IN TECH d.o.o., Prolaz Marije Krucifikse Kozulić 3, 51000 Rijeka, Croatia,
info@intechopen.com or visit our website at intechopen.com.

Meet the editors

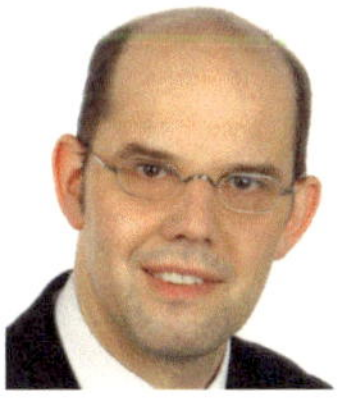

Professor Steffen Koschmieder is Professor of Translational Hematology and Oncology, Head of the Clinical Hematology Laboratory, and Attending Physician in the Department of Medicine (Oncology, Hematology, and Stem Cell Transplantation) at the University of Aachen, Germany. He is board-certified for Internal Medicine, Hematology and Medical Oncology, and Hemostaseology. He has received his medical training at the Universities of Bochum, Mainz, Dijon, Houston, Salt Lake City, Frankfurt, and Münster as well as the Harvard Institutes of Medicine in Boston where he was a postdoctoral fellow in Prof. Daniel Tenen´s group. His group has made significant contributions to the field of Myeloid Leukemias through basic and clinical research, including the elucidation of critical mechanisms of leukemia pathogenesis and progression, generation of tetracycline-inducible transgenic models of disease, characterization of leukemic stem cell populations as well as the development of novel treatment approaches.

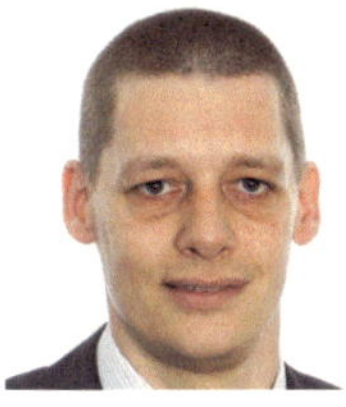

Dr. Utz Krug is Lecturer, Head of the Clinical Hematology Laboratory, Attending Physician, and Group Leader in the Department of Medicine (Hematology, Oncology, Hemostaseology, and Pulmonology) at the University of Münster, Germany. He is board-certified specialist in Internal Medicine, Hematology and Medical Oncology, Palliative Care, and Emergency Medicine. He attended Medical School at the University of Bochum and at Hannover Medical School, both in Germany. He completed his medical training at Hannover Medical School and at the University of Münster, Germany and was a postdoctoral fellow in Professor H. Phillipp Koeffler's Lab at the University of California, Los Angeles/USA. His group has identified and studied important novel targets in acute myeloid leukemia (AML) and has developed a new clinically relevant risk score for elderly patients with AML.

Contents

Preface

Myeloid leukemias have been studied for decades, and considerable progress has been made in the elucidation of critical pathogenetic factors including transcription factor networks and signaling pathways and in the diagnosis and treatment of these leukemias. However, while the prognosis of a fraction of patients (particularly those with chronic myeloid leukemia in chronic phase) has improved dramatically with the advent of novel rationally designed therapies, the prognosis of many other patients (i.e. with most subtypes of acute myeloid leukemia) has not improved to the same degree and have been compounded by the fact that molecular targeted therapies are expensive and are not readily available in all parts of the world.

The intention of this book is to provide a global scope on these issues. Following an open call, authors were invited to propose topics and send in an abstract of the chapter they wanted to contribute. After selection of appropriate abstracts, full chapters were provided and reviewed. Revised chapters were again reviewed and final chapters selected for publication.

The topics of the present book focus on basic mechanisms of leukemogenesis and cover the following:

- Chromosomal instability and DNA repair in CML and AML
- Novel BCR-ABL1 fusions
- Mechanisms of resistance to tyrosine kinase inhibitors and strategies how to overcome these
- Novel targets at the cellular and molecular level, including CML stem cells, proteasome inhibitors, and activators of phosphatases
- Genetic Alterations and new molecular markers in AML, including Acute Promyelocytic Leukemia
- The role of the bone marrow microenvironment and TGFß in the pathogenesis of AML
- Hematopoietic transcription factors and tumor suppressors, including the Id proteins, PU.1, Vav1, and p15INK4b
- Apoptosis and Apoptosis Modulators in Myeloid Leukemia
- Functional Analysis of Leukemogenic Gene Products in Hematopoietic Progenitor Cells

- Role of Signaling Pathways in Myeloid Leukemia, including BCR-ABL1 and mutant JAK2
- Epigenetic Changes Associated with Chromosomal Translocation in Leukemia
- Etiology and Risk factors of AML in Africa

Each chapter is a sole-standing publication that reflects each author´s interpretation of the data. However, the unifying theme is myeloid leukemia. Thus, the book displays a multi-facetted picture of our current understanding of myeloid leukemia pathogenesis. In addition, the open access structure of the book will guarantee wide-spread access even in cases where resources required for subscription to more expensive scientific journals or books are limited. We encourage the readers to send their comments. This is an exciting new way of discussing science and to support the effort of increasing the alertness and education of patients and physicians all around the globe.

Prof. Dr. Steffen Koschmieder
Department of Medicine (Oncology, Hematology,
and Stem Cell Transplantation) at the University of Aachen,
Germany

Dr. Utz Krug
Department of Medicine (Hematology, Oncology, Hemostaseology,
and Pulmonology) at the University of Münster,
Germany

1

BCR-ABL Hits at Mitosis; Implications for Chromosomal Instability, Aneuploidy and Therapeutic Strategy

Katarzyna Piwocka, Kamila Wolanin,
Monika Kusio-Kobialka and Paulina Podszywalow-Bartnicka
Nencki Institute of Experimental Biology, Polish Academy of Sciences
Poland

1. Introduction

1.1 Genomic and chromosomal instability in CML

An unstable genome is a common hallmark of nearly all solid tumors and most of leukemias in contrast to normal, healthy cells which are able to maintein genome integrity (Negrini et al., 2010). Genomic instability could result from changes in chromosome structure and number as well as changes on the DNA level. Chromosomal instability (CIN) arises from unproper chromosome segregation as well as division defects and leads to aneuploidy (Foijer, 2010), whereas accumulation of mutations and DNA alterations usually is an effect of the defective repair systems and DNA damage response in cancer cells (Economopoulou et al., 2011).

Chronic myeloid leukemia (CML) cells expressing the BCR-ABL tyrosine kinase have been found to accumulate mutations as well as chromosomal abnormalities. One of the first indications that CML correlates with additional chromosome changes has been presented in 1987 (Alimena et al., 1987). Moreover, authors showed that the rate of chromosomal anomalies increased during the blastic transformation. In the next years this has been also confirmed by other authors (Hagemeijer, 1987; Johansson et al., 2002; Su et al., 1999; Suzukawa et al., 1997). Later, random aneuploidy rate between chromosomes 9 and 18 has been reported in CML patients – both, untreated as well as upon imatinib therapy (Amiel et al., 2006). In broader analysis of CML patients it was found that chromosomal instability caused by centrosomal aberrations significantly correlated with the disease progression (Giehl et al., 2005). In the chronic phase only one sample out of 18 showed additional karyotypic alterations, in contrast to blast crisis where 73% patients (11/16) displayed additional karyotype alterations. The observation that CML patients have karyotype aberrations was confirmed in other studies where complex chromosomal rearrangements (CCR) were investigated (Babicka et al., 2006). By using cytogenetics, the FISH, and multicolor FISH (mFISH) methods, a very high level of the genomic instability at the chromosomal level, in cells obtained from chronic myeloid leukemia patients was observed.

Altogether, it was shown that the aberrations associated with the progression of BCR-ABL-positive CML chronic phase to the aggressive blast crisis include additional chromosomes (Ph^1, +8, +19), isochromosome 17q (associated with the loss of p53), reciprocal translocations, loss-of-heterozygosity at 14q32, homozygous mutations/deletions of pRb and p16/ARF, and mutations in p53 and RAS (Calabretta & Perrotti, 2004). The possible mechanisms participating in the BCR-ABL-mediated aneuploidy will be broadly described and discussed in the next paragraphs.

BCR-ABL has been also indicated as a promoter of secondary DNA mutations in CML (Burke & Carroll, 2010). This is the effect of the defective DNA damage response and DNA repair mechanisms found in CML cells. DNA damage can occur as single-nucleotide alterations, single-strand breaks (SSB), or double-strand breaks (DSB). Double-strand breaks are proposed to be the most mutagenic, as neither strand remains intact to serve as a template for repair. Single-nucleotide alterations are repaired by mismatch repair (MMR) or nucleotide excision repair (NER) mechanisms. Single or double-strand breaks are repaired by either high-fidelity homologous recombination repair (HRR) or non-homologous end-joining (NHEJ), when a sister chromatid is not available as a template. The last mechanism is error-prone and can lead to short deletions in the repaired strands.

Data from different laboratories collectively indicate that BCR-ABL promotes dysfunctions of nearly all mechanisms participating in the DNA repair. It is known that BCR-ABL cells treated with genotoxic agents present higher levels of DNA damage and aberrant repair systems, leading to the accumulation of DNA errors (Brady, 2003; Laurent et al., 2003; Slupianek et al., 2002). Studies from Skorski's group clearly showed that expression of BCR-ABL affects different mechanisms participating in the DNA repair. They found that BCR-ABL modifies the repair of DNA double-strand breaks (Koptyra et al., 2008; Nowicki et al., 2004; Slupianek et al., 2006). Briefly, CML cells produced increased rate of DSBs in S and G2/M phases of the cell cycle, as a result of oxidative DNA damage caused by BCR-ABL. These breaks were repaired, however with a high mutation rate and large deletions, as a result of defective HRR and NHEJ repair systems, respectively. Moreover, they found that BCR-ABL is able to inhibit both, mismatch repair (MMR) and inhibit apoptosis as well as to induce point mutations (Stoklosa et al., 2008). Upon this, CML cells were able to survive treatment leading to generation of the O(6)-methylguanine and O(4)-methylthymine recognized by the MMR system, however they displayed 15-fold higher mutation frequency than parental counterparts.

Deutsch et al indicated that DNA-PKcs, a protein involved in the NHEJ repair system, may be downregulated by BCR-ABL (Deutsch et al., 2001). This decrease was proteasome- and tyrosine kinase-dependent, as it was reversed by proteasome as well as tyrosime kinase inhibitors. Alternatively, the role of DNA-PKcs has been recently indicated to switch on the backup-NHEJ system, which is more error-prone (Poplawski & Blasiak, 2010). It was also shown that BCR-ABL upregulates the error-prone DSB repair pathways, particularly single-strand annealing and non-homologous end-joining due to an increased level of DNA-end-processing factor CtIP (Salles et al., 2011). Additionally, BCR-ABL also promotes the DNA DSB repair by using the highly mutagenic single-strand annealing (SSA) pathway which involves single repeats (Fernandes et al., 2009). This required the active Ras and PI3K pathways, acting downstream of the Y177 site of BCR-ABL, which is a major regulatory site for ROS induction and is necessary for the optimal activation of the PI3K and Ras pathways. Moreover, using stromal cell lines authors also showed that the stromal cell-conditioned media increased the SSA frequency, measured in K562 cells in the presence or absence of imatinib. This supported the hypothesis that microenvironment additionaly promotes mutagenesis in CML cells.

Altogether, there is no doubt, that defects in DNA repair mechanisms and genomic surveillance in CML cells are an effect of the expression of BCR-ABL itself. However, there was still an open question, whether occurrence of the genomic instability participates in the development of the blast crisis phase (Penserga & Skorski, 2007; Shet et al., 2002). This has been strongly indicated to play a significant role in the malignant progression of the disease by many authors (Burke & Carroll, 2010; Salleset al., 2011; Skorski, 2008; Skorski, 2011).
Till now, convincing data was presented and it seems clear, that genetic instability, accumulation of mutations and additional chromosomal alterations are the major factors involved in the CML progression and resistance to cell death. This leads to an accumulation of additional genetic aberrations and changes in gene expression, which result in the expansion of differentiation-arrested and increasingly malignant cell clones. Importantly, genetic instability of tyrosine kinase refractory cells, including leukemia stem cells (LSCs) has also recently been proposed as a reason for their fast transformation leading to the generation of additional resistant clones and transformation to a blast phase (Skorski, 2011). This mechanism could be responsible for clonal evolution and expansion causing finally relapse and malignant progression.
The current model of blastic transformation proposed recently by Perotti (Perrotti et al., 2010), indicates that acquiring of additional genetic and epigenetic changes by LSCs or their progeny causes leukemia transformation from the chronic phase to the advanced phases. This can explain the complexity of the disease progression and blast crisis as well as the inability to find common features of cells in blast crisis and specific secondary genetic aberrations. Most likely different mutations and aberrations are cumulated to obtain the critical point allowing the disease to progress. Thus, it will be very difficult to plan the therapeutic strategy against genetically unstable LSCs, resistant to tyrosine kinase inhibitors, with the already used agents and probably novel therapies need to be developed.

2. The role of aberrant divisions in CML cells

It has been known for more than a century that neoplastic cells could exhibit disturbances of the cell division process (Boveri, 1902, 1914). Boveri observed that sea urchin embryos manipulated to undergo mitosis in the presence of multipolar spindles produced aneuploid progeny and proposed that tumors arise from normal cells becoming aneuploid as a result of aberrant mitoses. Boveri's theory that division errors and aneuploidy could lead to cancer development has been revisited during the last decade (Duesberg et al., 2006; Holland & Cleveland, 2009; Weaver & Cleveland, 2006).
Today, it is commonly accepted that aberrant mitoses result in chromosomal instability (CIN), leading to the gain or loss of whole or large fragments of chromosomes, which are the main form of genomic instability in cancers. As it was mentioned in the previous chapter, it is fully convincing that expression of BCR-ABL leads to significant chromosomal aberrations. Moreover, these abnormalities increase along with the disease progression, participating in the blastic transformation. Below, we present current data concerning the role of BCR-ABL-mediated defects in the mechanisms controlling cell division as well as the role of BRCA1 in the development of aneuploidy in CML.

2.1 Centrosomal multiplication

Centrosomes are small organelles with a crucial role in the formation of bipolar mitotic spindle, which is necessary for the accurate segregation of chromosomes (Fukasawa, 2007;

Rusan & Rogers, 2009; Tanenbaum & Medema, 2010). Briefly, they are formed by paired centrioles surrounded by a protein matrix of pericentriolar material, including pericentrin. Their function is to nucleate and anchor microtubules to form an interphase cytoplasmic-microtubule network and mitotic spindle. During the cell division, each daughter cell receives one centrosome, thus the centrosome has to duplicate before the next mitosis. This takes place during the S phase and is driven at least partially by the Cdk2-cyclin E complex. Coordination of the DNA and centrosome replication is crucial to avoid their overduplication. Two mature centrosomes are generated at the late G2 phase and they become the spindle poles. It was shown that the DNA damage checkpoint proteins, such as ATM, ATR, Chk1 and Chk2 and others also localize at the centrosomes (Zhang et al., 2007). It seems that these proteins interact with gamma-tubulin and are involved in the controlling of microtubule kinetics during the DNA damage response. It was reported that DNA damage leads to centrosome amplification in the G2 phase as a result of cell cycle arrest (Inanc et al., 2010). Studies performed by Dodson and colleagues showed the involvement of ATM in the centrosome amplification in response to DNA damage, however gene targeting of *ATM* reduced, but did not abrogate completely centrosome amplification (Dodson et al., 2004). Alternatively, data from lymphoid gamma-irradiated cells showed that neither ATM nor ATR kinases are involved in this process, however Chk1-dependent signaling seems to be crucial (Bourke et al., 2007). This issue still needs to be clarified.

It is commonly accepted that the appearance of supernumerary centrosomes is associated with aberrant mitoses and chromosomal instability. Multipolar mitoses, lagging chromosomes or multinuclei are observed in cells with overduplicated centrosomes. Cells with three centrosomes usually undergo cytokinesis and some of the generated cells are viable, however aneuploid. Cells with multipolar (>3) spindles fail to undergo cytokinesis and can become polyploid if they are p53-deficient and are able to continue the cell cycle (Godinho et al., 2009).

Centrosome abnormalities are commonly observed in cancers and participate in the chromosomal instability and tumorigenesis (Carroll et al., 1999; Duensing & Duensing, 2010; Pihan et al., 2001). As mentioned before, mutlipolar mitosis as a result of centrosome overduplication can lead to gross chromosome missegregation and cell death. Thus cancer cells with supernumerary centrosomes possess the ability to suppress multipolar mitoses due to the inactivation, clustering or asymmetric segregation of extra centrosomes (Brinkley, 2001; Godinhoet al., 2009). This results in the formation of a bipolar, functional, however not symmetric mitotic spindle and so called mitotic stability of aneuploid cancer cells.

Abnormalities in the number of centrosomes were also found in leukemias. It was reported that defects in the number of centrosomes caused by the p53 mutation and cyclin E overexpression, detected in bladder cancers, led to centrosome amplification and chromosomal instability (Kawamura et al., 2004). Moreover, the centrosome aberrations were proposed as one of the main factors responsible for aneuploidy in acute myeloid leukemia (Kramer et al., 2003; Neben et al., 2003). Studies of CD34+ Ph+ cells isolated from chronic myeloid leukemia patients showed that centrosome aberrations correlate with the stage of the disease and aneuploidy (Giehl et al., 2005). In these studies freshly isolated cells from CML patients, in the chronic phase or blast crisis, were stained for pericentrin and gamma-tubulin to analyse the number as well as the structure of centrosomes. Moreover, they were studied for additional karyotypic abnormalities. Importantly, a strong correlation between the increase of centrosome aberrations, CML progression and blastic transformation was found. As centrosome defects were indicated as en early detectable feature of CML, they have been proposed as a cause of karyotype instability and aneuploidy in CML progenitor cells as well as a valuable prognostic factor. In the long-term *in vitro* studies, using a cellular model of the chronic phase of CML, authors confirmed, that expression of BCR-ABL leads to significant centrosomal hypertrophy visible already after 4 weeks of BCR-ABL expression (Giehl et al., 2007). This increased upon the next 10 weeks of propagation and correlated with the clonal expantion of aneuploid cells.

We also found, using a mouse cellular model of CML, that the stable expression of low or high level of BCR-ABL in mouse progenitor 32D cells leads to the generation of cells with supernumerary centrosomes (Wolanin et al., 2010). This was accompanied by increased percentage of cells with aberrant mitoses, particularly multipolar spindles, lagging chromosomes and multinuclei. The presence of aberrant cells correlated with the level of BCR-ABL expression, indicating that the BCR-ABL itself is responsible for these abnormalities. Interestingly, Patel and colleagues presented that CML cells have defects in the centrosome-centriole cycle (Patel & Gordon, 2009). They showed that p210 (BCR-ABL1) and p145 (ABL1) are both, centrosome-associated proteins and form a complex with the pericentriolar protein, pericentrin. Numerical and structural centrosomal abnormalities were found in CML cell lines and in primary CD34+ cells from CML patients as a result of an increased level of separase participating in the abnormalities in the centrosome-centriole cycle. They also confirmed the previous data that abnormal centrosome distribution, amplification and loss are more evident in the advanced stages of CML.

Although the tyrosine kinase inhibitors are very potent, selective and successful therapeutic agents for treatment of leukemia as well as some solid tumors it can not be neglected that some reports indicated that they can lead to centrosome aberrations in cancer as well as normal cells (Fabarius et al., 2005; Fabarius et al., 2008; Giehl et al., 2010). This was caused by blocking cells in the G1/S transition and the inhibition of cell growth which was followed by centrosomal aberrations. This should be taken into consideration with regards to the potential side-effects as well as a possible reason of dangerous clonal chromosomal abnormalities observed in BCR-ABL-negative progenitor cells under imatinib therapy.

2.2 Mitotic checkpoint failure

The spindle assembly checkpoint (SAC) plays a major role in the division control and segregation of sister chromatids, preventing occurence of aneuploidy (Chin & Yeong, 2010; Kops, 2008; Logarinho & Bousbaa, 2008; Nezi & Musacchio, 2009). SAC proteins, including Mad1 (mitotic arrest-deficient protein 1), Mad2, Bub1 (budding uninhibited by benzimidazoles 1), BubR1 (Bub1-related kinase 1) and Bub3 are recruited to unattached or tensionless kinetochores, forming mitotic checkpoint complex, which inhibits the anaphase promoting complex (APC). This protects cells from preearly anaphase entry and unproper segregation of chromatids. In physiological conditions the mitotic checkpoint is temporarily activated until the mitotic spindle is properly formed, whereas in anticancer therapy it is activated upon treatment with a group of microtubule damaging agents, such as taxanes and vinca alcaloids. Both interfere with tubulin organization and spindle formation, leading to the cell cycle arrest in mitosis and eventually cell death.

It is known that the complete loss of the mitotic checkpoint function results in embryonic lethality, what was shown in *Caenorhabditis elegans* (Kitagawa & Rose, 1999) as well as in mammalian cells (Michel et al., 2001; Schliekelman et al., 2009). Alternatively, partial loss of its function leads to chromosomes missegregation and chromosomal instability (Bharadwaj

& Yu, 2004; Ito & Matsumoto, 2010). This was due to the inability to activate the mitotic checkpoint and to arrest in mitosis in response to some disturbances. Instead - further progression of mitosis eventually leads to aberrant divisions and unproper chromosomes segregation.

Dysfunctions of the mitotic checkpoint were reported in different types of cancers (Baker et al., 2005; Bannon & Mc Gee, 2009; Tanaka & Hirota, 2009). They correlated with aneuploidy, disease progression and the increase of aggressiveness. Interestingly, similar effects were observed in case of the upregulation or decreased expression of mitotic checkpoint members. For example, the Mad2 protein has been recently proposed as a critical factor leading to aneuploidy in cancers with defects in the Rb and p53 pathways (Schvartzman et al., 2011). Authors found that Mad2 expression is repressed by p53 *via* the Rb pathway, thus the cancer cells lacking the Rb protein require Mad2 upregulation leading to chromosomal instability and tumor progression *in vivo*. On the other hand, also Mad2 haplo-insufficiency caused chromosomal instability in human cancer cells and murine primary embryonic fibroblasts (Michelet al., 2001).

BubR1 dysfunctions has also been found as a cause of cancer-susceptible disorder mosaic variegated aneuploidy (MVA) (Suijkerbuijk et al., 2010). Similarly to Mad2, BubR1 can be also overexpressed in cancer, what was shown in hepatocellular carcinoma (HCC) (Liu et al., 2009). Authors suggest that BubR1 overexpression, which was found in 45% of patients correlated with later stages and was associated with worse prognosis, thus it can be used as a potential prognostic factor for HCC.

There were indications that CML cells could have a dysfunctional mitotic checkpoint, as their resistance to spindle poisons was reported previously. In the K562 and Lama-84 CML cell lines, microtubule disruption caused either by paclitaxel, nocodazole or novel microtubule-targeting agent PBOX-6 led to polyploidization without the presence of significant apoptosis (Greene et al., 2007). Imatinib treatment minimized the formation of polyploid cells and enhanced the apoptotic index upon treatment of CML cells with spindle poisons. Resistance to paclitaxel was also shown in K562 cells (Blagosklonny, 2001), but mitotic checkpoint competence was not investigated. All these data suggested that BCR-ABL could somehow affect the response to microtubule disruption; however this issue was not discussed by the authors.

We have shown for the first time that the expression of BCR-ABL in mouse 32D cells decreases the expression of SAC proteins, such as Mad2, Bub1, Bub3 and BubR1, as well as their mRNA levels, what was estimated by real time RT-PCR (Wolanin et al., 2010). Decreased levels of the mitotic checkpoint proteins were associated with dysfunctions in the mitotic checkpoint competence observed upon nocodazole and paclitaxel treatment as well as resistance to cell death induced by these agents. We found that the inhibition of the BCR-ABL kinase activity by imatinib reversed the observed phenotype confirming the crucial role of BCR-ABL.

2.3 Aberrant expression of mitotic kinases

Mitotic kinases have also been implicated in the regulation of the centrosome cycle, spindle checkpoint and microtubule-kinetochore attachment, as well as spindle assembly and chromosome condensation. The family of Aurora kinases consists of the following proteins: Aurora A, B and C. The whole family has serine/threonine kinase activity which modifies microtubules during chromosome movement and segregation. Aurora kinases have been

found at the centrosomes of interphase cells, at the poles of the bipolar spindle and in the midbody of the mitotic apparatus. All three Aurora kinases members are overexpressed in many human cancers. This correlated with chromosomal instability and clinically aggressive forms of disease (Fu et al., 2007; Meraldi et al., 2004). Aurora A is localized in centrosomes and is important for maturation, spindle assembly and metaphase I spindle orientation. It has two independent functions in centrosome maturation and asymmetric protein localization during mitosis. Ectopic overexpression of Aurora A was shown to induce oncogenic transformation (Katayama et al., 2003). Moreover, overexpression of Aurora A and aneuploidy have been proposed as predictors of poor outcome in serous ovarian carcinoma (Lassus et al., 2011). Also a high level of Aurora B has been reported to promote tetraploidy and tumorigenesis in the mouse Xenograft model (Nguyen et al., 2009).
High expression of Aurora A in leukemia cell lines and freshly isolated leukemia CML cells has been presented by Ochi T et al (Ochi et al., 2009). We also showed that the expression of BCR-ABL leads to the mislocalization of Aurora A in the chromosomal passenger complex (Wolanin et al., 2006). The importance of Aurora A-dependent signaling in CML has been shown in studies indicating that Aurora inhibitors seem to be very effective therapeutics for CML treatment (Gontarewicz et al., 2008), what will be discussed by us later.
Another family of tubulin-associated serine/threonine kinases, Polo-like, has also received significant attention regarding its participation in tumorigenesis. As far, in mammalian cells four members of this family have been identified (PLK1-4), and each one of them has a distinct function. PLK1 is essentially involved in the control of mitotic steps, PLK2 and PLK3 have been described as potential regulators of the G1 and early S phases of the cell cycle, PLK4 as a major centrosome duplication regulator. Polo-like kinase 1 (PLK1) is a key regulator of mitosis and participates in regulating this process from its entry to cytokinesis (Yuan et al., 2011). Transcription and translation of PLK1 is highly coordinated with cell cycle progression. *Plk1* mRNA and protein levels begin to accumulate in the S-phase and reach a peak at the G2/M transition and then decline upon mitotic exit (Lee et al., 1995). At the G2/M phase, PLK1 regulates the Cdk1/Cyclin B1 complex promoting mitotic entry and regulating mitotic progression due to regulation of phosphorylation of Cyclin B1, Cdk1, Myt1 and Cdc25C. PLK1 also plays a role in centrosome maturation by promoting increased recruitment of microtubules to the spindle pole bodies. It also regulates the localization of Aurora A to the centrosomes for proper maturation. It is known today that all mitotic kinases interplay with each other and form an extensive functional network, thus targeting any of them has tremendous consequences for cell physiology (Lens et al., 2010). Additionally, it was shown that PLK1 catalysis survivin priming phosphorylation at Ser20, what is necessary for survivin-mediated Aurora B docking to the centromere and activation (Chu et al., 2010). Expression of the non-phosphorylable survivin mutant prevented Aurora B activation and corrected spindle microtubule attachment. We also observed that silencing of survivin in CML cells significantly affected CPC function and mitosis as well as proper completion of cytokinesis leading to the formation of giant polyploid cells (Wolanin et al., 2006). PLK1 also regulates the spindle assembly checkpoint (Nezi & Musacchio, 2009) probably by phosphorylation of BubR1 and finally, regulates chromosome segregation, cytokinesis and mitotic exit.
PLK1, similarly to other mitotic kinases has been shown to be upregulated in cancers, including lymphomas. Studies of a big group of non-Hodgkin's lymphoma (NHLs) patients presented that the level of PLK1 expression was significantly lower in low-grade NHLs than

in high-grade and intermediate-grade NHLs. Moreover, PLK1 has been proposed as a valuable marker of proliferating cells, even better than the commonly used Ki67 (Mito et al., 2005). It was also described that PLK1 is overexpressed in AML cell lines as well as in primary cells and its inhibition preferentially targeted lymphoid cells, indicating an important role of the PLK1-mediated signaling (Renner et al., 2009). Importantly, healthy hematopoietic progenitor CD34+ cells were much less sensitive to growth inhibition caused by PLK1 targeting, indicating a high potential of this therapeutic strategy. This observation was confirmed by studies performed by Ikezoe and colleagues, who also found PLK1 overexpressed in a number of human leukemia cell lines and freshly isolated leukemia cells from individuals with acute myelogenous leukemia as well as acute lymphoblastic leukemia, in comparison with normal bone marrow mononuclear cells (Ikezoe et al., 2009). As previously, they indicated PLK1 inhibition as a potent way to inhibit proliferation and induce cell death in leukemia cells. Moreover, the functional link between PLK1 and mTOR pathway has been shown in AML cells (Renner et al., 2010). Abnormal growth of cells overexpressing the active form of PLK1 was reversed by rapamycin, a specific inhibitor of the TORC1 complex. This showed a novel aspect of PLK1's role in leukemia and opened new therapeutic possibilities.

In chronic myeloid leukemia, PLK1was found to be expressed in the phosphorylated form in the CML cell line K562 as well as in primary CML cells from patients (Gleixner et al., 2010). Studies presenting the potential of the PLK1 inhibitors in therapy against CML were performed and indicate an important role of PLK1 in CML development and progression. They will be discussed in a detailed way in the chapter dedicated to anti-mitotic therapies against leukemia.

3. BCR-ABL-mediated downregulation of BRCA1

BRCA1, a tumor suppressor isolated in 1994 (Miki et al., 1994) has been implicated in a broad range of cellular processes, including DNA repair, cell cycle checkpoint control, cell division and gene transcription (Linger & Kruk, 2010; Thompson, 2010; Wu et al., 2010; Yang & Xia, 2010). It is a known familiar ovarian and breast cancer-specific tumor suppressor, however today it seems that it is involved in the development of other types of cancers as well. The protein contains two motifs: a RING domain at the N-terminus and two tandem copies of BRCT domain at the C-terminus (Baer, 2001). *In vivo* it exists in a heterodimeric complex with the BRCA1-associated RING domain (BARD1) protein, which resembles BRCA1 (Wu et al., 1996).

The first observation that BRCA1 protein is nearly undetectable in leukemia cells from chronic myeloid leukemia (CML) patients has been made by Deutsch et al (Deutsch et al., 2003). They found a significant downregulation of BRCA1 in primary CD34+ cells obtained from both, the chronic phase and the blast crisis patients as well as in cell lines expressing BCR-ABL. This was not accompanied by a decrease of the *BRCA1* mRNA, what was studied by real-time RT-PCR in one of the investigated cell lines.

Our group studied the direct influence of BCR-ABL on the BRCA1 expression, using the previously mentioned mouse progenitor 32D cell line stably expressing with BCR-ABL, particularly in clones, expressing low and high BCR-ABL levels (Fig.1A), (Wolanin et al., 2010). We found that BCR-ABL expression leads to a strong decrease of BRCA1 at the protein level. This was reversed by treatment with imatinib, a specific inhibitor of the BCR-ABL tyrosine kinase, confirming dependence on the tyrosine kinase activity (Fig. 1B). The lack of a significant decrease of mRNA confirmed the previous observation that BCR-ABL affects the posttranscriptional stages of protein expression. Incubation with the proteasome inhibitor MG132 did not lead to an increase at the BRCA1 protein level (Fig. 1C), thus excluding the possibility that increased degradation is responsible for the protein downregulation.

Recently, it was shown that BCR-ABL interferes with the Fanconi Anemia/BRCA1 pathway, thus increasing the predisposition to DNA repair errors and development of centrosomal and chromosomal aberrations (Valeri et al., 2010). The interference of BCR-ABL with the formation of BRCA1 and FANCD2 nuclear foci was observed in hematopoietic progenitors from CML patients. These authors also showed that the ectopic expression of BRCA1 reverted the generation of aberrant centrosomes induced by BCR-ABL. This suggests, however not directly studied, that overexpression of BRCA1 could antagonize also other effects of BCR-ABL expression, if they are mediated by BRCA1 downregulation, indeed.

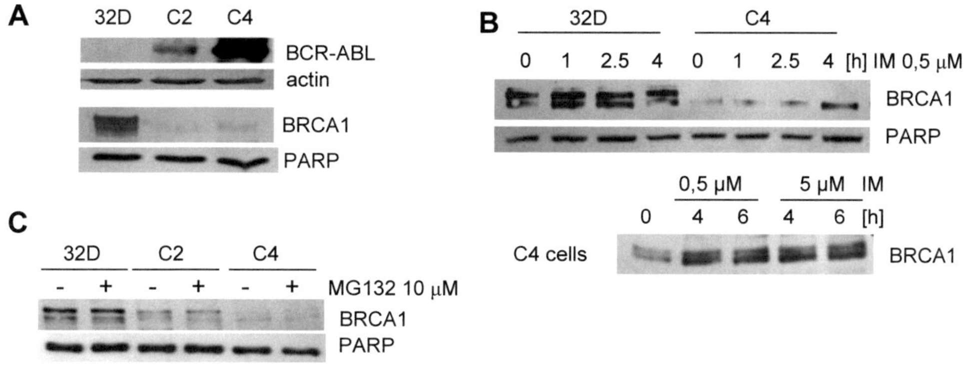

Fig. 1. The influence of BCR-ABL expression on the level of the BRCA1 Protein.
A. Expression of BCR-ABL leads to downregulation of the BRCA1 protein. The level of BRCA1 was determined by Western Blot in mouse progenitor 32D cells, control or stably expressing BCR-ABL at low (C2 cells) or high (C4 cells) level.
B. Imatinib treatment leads to upregulation of the BRCA1 protein level in cells expressing BCR-ABL. 32D and C4 cells were treated with 0.5 μM imatinib for 1, 2.5 or 4 hours (upper panel) or with 0.5 or 5 μM imatinib for 4 and 6 hours (lower panel) followed by estimation of the BRCA1 protein level.
C. BRCA1 downregulation caused by BCR-ABL is not a result of increased proteasomal degradation. 32D, C2 and C4 cells were treated with 10 μM proteasome inhibitor MG132 for 6 hours, followed by determination of the BRCA1 protein level by Western Blot.

Altogether, there are strong evidences indicating that the decrease of the BRCA1 protein and the BRCA1-dependent signaling is caused by BCR-ABL expression and is also specific for chronic myeloid leukemia, in addition to other types of tumors. There is a number of intracellular processes crucial for cell physiology controlled by BRCA1, including DNA damage response as well as activation of the cell cycle checkpoints, chromatin remodelling, apoptosis and mitosis. Aberrations in any of them, lead to the accumulation of mutations, genomic instability and finally an increased risk of cancerogenesis. Thus, we postulate that the decrease of BRCA1 caused by BCR-ABL could have tremendous consequences due to defective control of genomic stability. The role of BRCA1 in the regulation of the DNA damage response and cell cycle checkpoint control has been already well explained (Huen et al., 2010; Kim & Chen, 2008; Wuet al., 2010; Yang & Xia, 2010; Zhang & Powell, 2005). The detailed role of BRCA1 in the regulation of mechanisms participating in the occurence of genomic instability as a result of mitosis dysfunctions, referred as a CIN (chromosomal instability) will be discussed in the next paragraphs.

4. The role of BRCA1 in mitosis

4.1 BRCA1 in the transcriptional regulation

Currently, there is a lot of evidence suggesting that BRCA1 is involved in the transcriptional regulation. This opens a new list of possible interactions with intracellular processes (Murray et al., 2007). It has been shown that BRCA1 is a component of the RNA polymerase II (pol II) holoenzyme (Scully et al., 1997). Authors developed a purification strategy for the mammalian pol II holoenzyme to search for specific transcription factors and they found that the wild-type BRCA1 protein was copurified. Moreover, immunopurification of BRCA1 complexes also contained TFIIF, TFIIE and TFIIH transcription factors, which were previously reported to form a complex with the pol II holoenzyme (Maldonado et al., 1996). This strongly suggested that one of the BRCA1 functions is to regulate genes expression.

Unlike many enhancer-specific activators, BRCA1 does not appear to require the specific DNA binding domain to stimulate gene transcription, what was shown by investigation of the p53-responsive promoter *MDM2* (Nadeau et al., 2000). BRCA1 interacts rather with multiple transcription factors. Among them we can name ATF1, a member of the cAMP response element-binding protein/activating transcription factor (CREB/ATF) family. BRCA1 stimulates its transcription from a natural promoter as well as reporter systems (Houvras et al., 2000). Moreover, BRCA1 significantly enhanced the transcription of NF-kappaB target genes due to the binding to p65/RelA, one of the two subunits of the transcription factor NF-kappaB (Benezra et al., 2003). Authors suggested that BRCA1 acts as a coactivator and proposed a model in which BRCA1 interacts physically with p65/RelA, CBP as well as with RNA polymerase II and enhances transcriptional activation of the NF-kappaB target genes. Additionally, MacLachlan reported that p53 can be stabilized by BRCA1 in response to DNA damage and by this selectively transactivated towards genes involved in the growth arrest and DNA repair (MacLachlan et al., 2002). The role of BRCA1 in the regulation of p53-dependent gene expression has been also shown by other groups (Ouchi et al., 1998; Zhang et al., 1998).

BRCA1 is also able to interact with components of the histone deacetylase complex, particularly with HDAC1 and HDAC2 (Yarden & Brody, 1999). It was shown to interact *in vitro* and *in vivo* with the Rb protein as well as with the RB-binding proteins, RBAp46 and RBAp48, which are components of the histone deacetylase complexes and are involved in chromatin remodelling. Involvement of BRCA1 in chromatin remodelling suggests its important role in the regulation of transcription, replication, recombination and others. BRCA1-mediated activation of specific genes may result from sequestration of histone deacetylases from DNA promoters. It was also reported that BRCA1 interacts with the hGCN5/TRAP histone acetyltransferase complex (Oishi et al., 2006), which co-activates the transactivation function of BRCA1.

More recently, BRCA1 has also been shown to play a role in the transcriptional repression by ubiquitin-dependent mechanism (Horwitz et al., 2007). It leads to ubiquitination of the transcriptional preinitiation complex, thus preventing the stable association of TFIIE and

TFIIH transcription factors and blocking the initiation of mRNA synthesis. Amphiregulin (AREG) and early growth response-1 (EGR-1) are examples of genes repressed by BRCA1 in breast cancers. This phenomen could be broader and may contribute to the BRCA1-mediated tumor suppression.

4.2 BRCA1 in the regulation of the mitotic checkpoint

The role of BRCA1 in the regulation of the mitotic checkpoint has been indicated. BRCA1 was identified as a mitotic target of the Chk2 kinase in the absence of DNA damage (Stolz et al., 2010). Accordingly, loss of BRCA1 or its Chk2-mediated phosphorylation led to defects in the spindle formation and chromosomal instability (CIN) due to generation of lagging chromosomes and chromosome missegregation. It was shown that MCF-7 cells transfected with BRCA1 siRNA display a reduced mitotic index followed by premature cyclin B1 degradation upon paclitaxel treatment. This suggested that BRCA1 depletion results in the inactivation of the spindle checkpoint (Chabalier et al., 2006). They presented that BRCA1 up-regulates the expression of the protein kinase BubR1, an essential component of the functional spindle checkpoint. This indicated that BRCA1 directly influences the expression of the mitotic checkpoint components. It was also shown that BRCA1, due to an interaction with the transcription factor OCT-1, mediates the transactivation of Mad2 (mitotic arrest deficient protein 2) (Wang et al., 2004). The studies of BRCA1 knock-down in human prostate and breast cancer cell lines, by using the microarray technique, showed that BRCA1 depletion caused downregulation of many genes involved in mitosis progression (Bae et al., 2005). Specifically, mitotic checkpoint components (Bub1, STK6), proteins involved in the chromosome segregation and centrosome function as well as cytokinesis (including PLK) and finally proteins regulating mitosis entry and progression, such as cyclin B1, Cdc2 and Cdc20 were downregulated.

The influence of BRCA1 on the expression of components of the mitotic checkpoint was also confirmed in our studies (Wolanin et al., 2010). We showed that the downregulation of BRCA1, caused either by BCR-ABL expression or by gene silencing using siRNA, resulted in the downregulation of Mad2 as well as BubR1 and Bub3 gene expression, which all belong to the mitotic checkpoint complex and undergo common regulation. Decreased levels of these proteins finally led to dysfunctions of the mitotic checkpoint and increased occurence of aberrant mitoses and chromosomal instability. Moreover, we observed the increased rate of supernumerary centrosomes as well as aberrant divisions in cells expressing BCR-ABL. We propose that decrease of the BRCA1 protein caused by BCR-ABL could be an important factor participating in the development of genomic instability due to the generation of chromosomally unstable cells. We added the regulation of mitotic checkpoint to the repertoir of BRCA1-mediated mechanisms participating in the development of aneuploidy in CML cells.

Due to its function in the regulation of mitotic checkpoint competence, BRCA1 has been shown to correlate with the sensitivity to spindle poisons (Byrski et al., 2008; Quinn et al., 2007). As mentioned before, cells ability to activate the mitotic checkpoint is necessary for the sensitivity to spindle poisons. BRCA1 downregulation resulted in resistance to microtubule damage due to the inability to efficiently activate the mitotic checkpoint, block cells in mitosis and induce apoptosis. In our studies, cells expressing BCR-ABL with a significantly decreased BRCA1 level were resistant to cell death activated by nocodazole or paclitaxel (Wolanin et al., 2010). This was reversed by imatinib treatment, resulting in

BRCA1 upregulation. In ovarian cancer it was suggested that BRCA1 can act as a predictive marker of response to chemotherapy (Quinn et al., 2009) and dysfunctional BRCA1 resulted in resistance to taxanes and other chemotherapeutics. On the other hand, reconstitution of BRCA1 into ovarian cancer cells, carrying BRCA1 mutation, reversed the resistance and sensitized cells to paclitaxel (Zhou et al., 2003). BRCA1 was also proposed as a predicive marker of drug sensitivity in breast cancer treatment (Mullan et al., 2006). As resistance to spindle poisons has been reported for CML cells, this supports the previously proposed idea, that the overexpression of BRCA1 diminishes some effects of BCR-ABL expression. In our opinion, BRCA1 level could serve as a prognostic marker of sensitivity to different therapies also those used in leukemias.

4.3 BRCA1 in the regulation of centrosome number and function

The first observation that BRCA1 localizes to centrosomes has been made by Hsu et al (Hsu & White, 1998), who showed that BRCA1 is associated with centrosomes during mitosis in a cell cycle-dependent manner. Moreover, they found that BRCA1 forms a complex with gamma-tubulin, which is preferentially associated with the hypophosphorylated form of BRCA1. Gamma-tubulin is a crucial component of centrosomes and is responsible for nucleation of microtubules. Therefore, this confirmed the idea that BRCA1 could play a role in the regulation of centrosome amplification and function and led to the later findings that a BF3 domain of BRCA1 (BRCA1 fragment no. 3, amino acids 504-803) is responsible for the gamma-tubulin binding (Hsu et al., 2001). Overexpression of the BF3 domain in COS-7 cells resulted in the accumulation of mitotic cells with supernumerrary centrosomes and abnormal spindles, what is known to lead to aneuploidization.

The role of BRCA1 in the regulation of centrosome number has been indicated by experiments using the mutated forms of BRCA1. Centrosomal amplification was shown in mouse embryonic fibroblasts carrying a targeted deletion of exon 11 of BRCA1 (Xu et al., 1999) and in a BRCA1-mutant breast cancer cell line HCC1937 (Schlegel et al., 2003). What is important, Waever et al showed that mouse embryonic fibroblasts carrying different BRCA1 defects show supernumerary centrosomes and other features similar to human breast cancer cells, indicating that the mechanisms are conserved between mice and humans (Weaver et al., 2002).

Moreover, immunohistochemical analysis of 50 samples from breast cancer patients showed that numerical centrosome aberrations were signicantly associated with the negative BRCA1 expression as well as with the BRCA1 germline mutation, whereas there was no significant correlation with the centrosome aberrations in size (Shimomura et al., 2009). This suggests that BRCA1 plays a role rather in the regulation of centrosome duplication and defects in its expression or function result in numerical aberrations. Very recently, direct studies of 14 different missense mutations in the RING domain of BRCA1 and their influence on the control of centrosome number were performed (Kais et al., 2011). Authors showed that only 2 out of the 14 BRCA1 variant proteins were neutral in the centrosome duplication assay. The others were either very effective and resulted in mutated BRCA1 proteins that caused centrosome amplification (C24R, C27A, C39Y, H41F, C44F, C47G, M18T and I42V) or had an intermediate, however still significant effect on centrosome duplication (I21V, I31M, L52F and D67Y).

Interestingly, we also observed a correlation between the loss of BRCA1 expression and increased percentage of cells with supernumerary centrosomes in murine lymphoid cells

expressing BCR-ABL oncogene (Wolanin et al., 2010). This was in contrast with the hypothesis that BRCA1 defects lead to centrosome amplification in breast cells but not in other types of cells (Starita et al., 2004). This idea has been based on the data obtained using the transient expression of the BRCA1-inhibiting BIF peptide in nine different cell lines, where four non-breast cell lines - prostate (PC3), cervix (HeLa), colon (DLD-1) and osteosarcoma (U2OS), did not accumulate extra centrosomes. However, lymphoid cells were not included in these studies. To date, there were other indications, apart from ours, that the loss or mutation of BRCA1 could affect the centrosome number also in other types of cells. Recently, it was shown that BCR-ABL intereferes with the Fanconi Anemia (FA)/BRCA pathway and the ectopic expression of BRCA1 in CD34+ progenitor cells reversed the appearance of aberrant centrosomes, thus confirming our previous observations (Valeri et al., 2010).
The direct mechanism of BRCA1-mediated control of centrosome number is still not fully clear, although the BRCA1-dependent ubiquitination of gamma-tubulin is proposed to be involved in the regulation of centrosome function (Staritaet al., 2004). Gamma-tubulin is an important protein involved in the initiation of microtubule nucleation by centrosomes. Gamma-tubulin's lysines 48 and 344 have been indicated as crucial in the regulation of centrosome duplication and microtubule nucleation function, respectively (Sankaran et al., 2005). Cells with mutated lysines on gamma-tubulin, unable to be ubiquitinated, were characterized by centrosome amplification. On the other hand, the same phenotype was observed after inhibition of the enzymatic activity of BRCA1 by transfection of the BRCA1 (I26A) ligase-defective mutant (Sankaran et al., 2006). Additionally, *in vitro* experiments using *Xenopus* extracts, purified centrosomes and BRCA1 together with ubiquitination factors confirmed that BRCA1 is involved in the microtubule nucleation. It seems that BRCA1 controls the centrosome number by preventing reduplication due to ubiquitination of lysines of gamma-tubulin, which needs to be phosphorylated to prevent reduplication (Ko et al., 2006). Loss of BRCA1 did not affect centrosome duplication in the early S phase but rather caused a second round of duplication just prior to mitosis. The model has been proposed, in which BRCA1 marks centrosomes as already duplicated *via* the BRCA1-mediated ubiqutination of gamma-tubulin (Wong & Stearns, 2003). This issue is still not fully clarified, however there is no doubt about the significant role of the BRCA1-mediated ubiquitination of gamma-tubulin in this process (Kais & Parvin, 2008). Altogether, this led to the conclusion that the E3 ubiquitin ligase activity of BRCA1 is crucial for the effects on the biology of centrosomes, and controls centrosome duplication as well as microtubules nucleation.
Recently, it was demonstrated that BRCA1 interacts with centrosomal protein Nlp (ninein-like protein) (Jin et al., 2009), which is a fast turnover protein and plays a role in the centrosome maturation and spindle formation (Casenghi et al., 2005). Authors found that Nlp is a BRCA1-associated protein and colocalizes with BRCA1 in different types of cancer cells, including HeLa and U2OS cells. Moreover, Nlp expression and stability depends on normal cellular BRCA1 function. A variety of different types of cells expressing the mutated BRCA1 or silenced for BRCA1 exhibited disrupted Nlp colocalization to centrosomes as well as enhanced Nlp degradation. This data was consistent with our observations concerning the role of BRCA1 in different types of cancers. The lack of Nlp protein led to centrosome amplification, aberrant chromosome segregation, cytokinesis failure and appearance of miltinuclei, thus resembling the phenotype upon BRCA1 disruption. Recent studies showed that Nlp is recruited by the Aurora B protein and localizes at the midbody during

cytokinesis, thus its depletion or increased degradation triggers aborted division and subsequently leads to multinucleated phenotypes (Yan et al., 2010).
Altogether, this data strongly supported the idea that BRCA1 is one of the key elements controlling mitosis and the loss of BRCA1 could result in very severe dysfunctions of cell division. We propose that this can significantly participate in the generation of aneuploidy, CML progression and blastic transformation. A proposed model showing the influence of BCR-ABL-mediated downregulation of BRCA1 on the occurrence of genomic instability and aneuploidy in CML cells is presented in Figure 2.

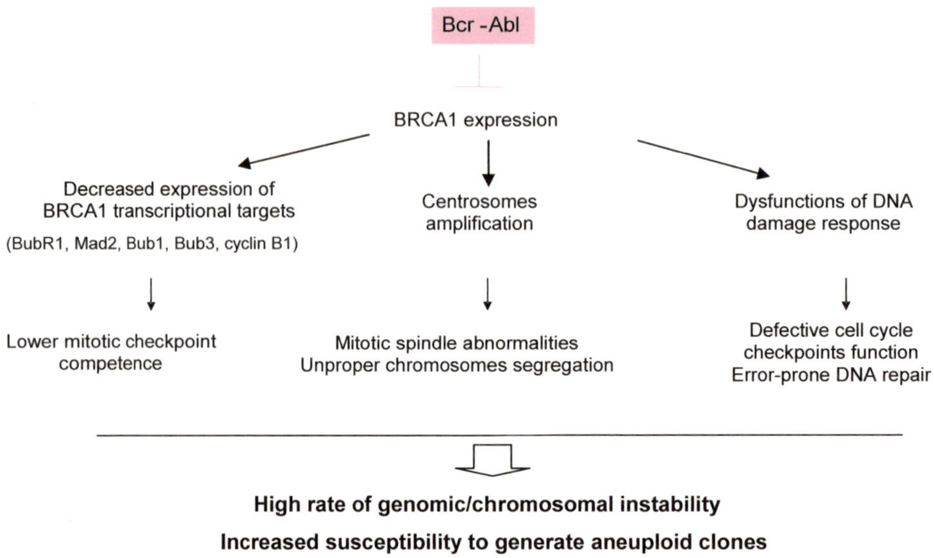

Fig. 2. Proposed scheme of the mechanisms influenced by BCR-ABL-mediated BRCA1 downregulation; role in the genomic instability and generation of aneuploid cells.

5. Therapeutic targeting of mitosis in CML cells

The effects of the improper control of mitosis in the development and progression of leukemias, including chronic myeloid leukemia has been already described above. The importance of these processes and their potential as targets for therapy is already obvious. In general, looking for new treatment options or combined therapies is still necessary to overcome the insensitivity or resistance to tyrosine kinase inhibitors, often developed in CML patients. In our opinion, targeting the chromosomal passenger complex and mitotic kinases is a very promising trend in the development of novel anti-leukemia therapeutic strategies. We will discuss the current data and implications for the future.

5.1 Chromosomal passenger complex and Aurora kinases

The chromosomal passenger complex (CPC) is a group of proteins, which are involved in the regulation of nearly all stages of mitosis (Vader et al., 2006; Vagnarelli & Earnshaw, 2004; Yanet al., 2010). In most organisms, the chromosomal passenger complex is formed by four main proteins: Aurora B kinase, INCENP, Survivin and Borealin/Dasra-B (Ruchaud et al., 2007). Other proteins, like telophase disk 60 kDa (TD-60) have been shown to interact with the CPC proteins and have a typical localization, however they are not members of the core complex. The complex undergoes a characteristic scenario of translocations during mitosis – they localize at the inner centromeres in prometaphase and metaphase then, at anaphase onset, they leave the chromosomes and transfer to the kinetochores at the central spindle to finally move to the midbody at cytokinesis. It plays a crucial role in the regulation of chromatin condensation, kinetochore function, mitotic checkpoint competence as well as cytokinesis (Terada, 2001; Vaderet al., 2006). Very recently it was presented that the chromosomal passenger complex is essential for correcting the non-bipolar chromosome attachments and for cytokinesis (Becker et al., 2010). To do this, Aurora B and INCENP have to be localized to centromeres. This is a very important finding as it indicates the supportive role of the CPC complex in case of mitotic checkpoint failure. Moreover, the translocation of Aurora B and other CPC proteins from centromeres to the spindle midzone in anaphase is necessary to prevent mitotic checkpoint engagement at anaphase (Vazquez-Novelle & Petronczki, 2010).

Members of the CPC complex have been proposed as very potent therapeutic targets. Treatment of imatinib-resistant CML cells carrying the T315I mutation with small molecule inhibitor, PHA-739358, which selectively targets BCR-ABL and Aurora kinases led to strong antiproliferative and apoptotic effects (Gontarewicz et al., 2008). Moreover, this has also been observed in CD34+ cells derived from untreated CML patients and from imatinib-resistant patients in the chronic phase or blast crisis, including those harbouring the T315I mutation. Similar effects were obtained by combined treatment of imatinib resistant CML cells with vorinostat together with Aurora kinase inhibitor MK-0457 (Dai et al., 2008). Effectivity of this combined treatment has been shown against primary CD34+ CML cells, murine Ba/F3 cells with various BCR-ABL mutations (T315I, E255K, and M351T), as well as in imatinib-resistant K562 cells with BCR-ABL-independent, Lyn-dependent resistance. The same combination of therapy was presented also in other studies by Fiskus et al (Fiskus et al., 2008). Authors studied different CML cell lines, murine cells expressing BCR-ABL as well as primary CML and AML cells and came to the same conclusions. Novel inhibitors of Aurora kinases are still investigated in the anti-leukemia therapy of imatinib-resistant cells (Fei et al., 2010; Kelly et al., 2010). Usually they are proposed to be used together with tyrosine kinase inhibitors, such as imatinib or dasatinib.

Survivin has been also proposed as a universal target for anticancer therapy (Andersen et al., 2007). Several trials are currently undergoing, using different methodologies, from small molecule antagonists to immunotherapy (Kanwar et al., 2010). However, the development of survivin inhibitors is not as advanced as other therapeutic small inhibitors. It is important to point that anti-survivin therapy should be probably combined with other treatments, as it is known that survivin depletion uncovers the function of the mitotic as well as post-mitotic p53-p21-dependent checkpoints, which protect from polyploidization upon mitosis disturbances (Beltrami et al., 2004). In case of cancers with the defective p53 function, survivin silencing led to reduced mitotic arrest and enhanced polyploidy, what is a very unwanted and dangerous side-effect. Also in our studies, specific depletion of survivin by siRNA approach in CML cells with checkpoints defects, resulted in strong polyploidization and chromosomal instability (Wolanin et al., 2006). However, when we used a natural compound – curcumin, which has been shown as a broadly acting, very potent anticancer agent, we found that it affects the CPC proteins and induces mitotic catastrophe, however without polyploidization. Curcumin decreased the level of survivin and caused unproper localization of Aurora B, leading to perturbances in mitosis and defective cytokinesis.

Thus, the status of the mitotic checkpoint competence as well as p53 should be taken into consideration when anti-survivin therapy is proposed. Another natural compound, 16-hydroxycleroda-3,13-dien-15,16-olide (PL3), one of the clerodane diterpenoid compounds isolated from *Polyalthia longifolia,* induced degradation of Aurora B, mitotic checkpoint dysfunctions and finally led to cell death of CML cells, including the T315I-mutated BCR-ABL+ BA/F3 cells (Lin et al., 2011). Additionally, it reversed the sensitivity to imatinib of T315I-mutated CML cells in comparizon to treatment only with imatinib.
Recently, Aurora inhibitors were indicated as promising agents for acute myeloid and chronic myeloid leukemias (Moore et al., 2010). The most promising data was obtained for FLT3-mutated AML and imatinib-resistant Ph+ CML, particularly with the T315I mutation. Clinical trials investigating these agents have been already initiated (Cheung et al., 2011).

5.2 Polo-like kinases

Polo-like kinases are of strong interest according to potential anticancer therapy, as similarly to Aurora kinases, they can be targeted with selective small molecule inhibitors (Warner et al., 2008). Additionally, many natural compounds with the ability to prevent cancerogenesis, such as wortmanin, quercetin, thymoquinone, genistein, indirubin and others, have been shown to modulate PLK1 level or activity. It is proposed that naturally occurring PLK1 inhibitors with low or no toxicity should be considered as interesting agents in prevention as well as treatment of cancer (Schmit et al., 2010).
As described before, PLK1 has been upregulated in different cancers, including leukemias. Its inhibition or silencing resulted in cell cycle arrest, decrease of cell viability and induction of apoptosis in various cancer cells. Inhibition of PLK1 by different small molecule compounds in acute myeloid leukemia (AML) cells led to mitotic accumulation and apoptosis (Didier et al., 2008). Comprehensive studies of PLK1 silencing and inhibition using the novel selective inhibitor GW843682X in a broad range of different leukemia cell lines and primary cells led to the conclusion that PLK1targeting can be a promising strategy (Ikezoeet al., 2009). This observation was confirmed by other studies of leukemia primary cells (Renneret al., 2009). The potential of PLK1 inhibition to improve the chemotherapy or irradiation of resistant leukemia cells has been also investigated in primary patient cells as well as *in vivo,* in mouse Xenograft models of B-lineage ALL studies, with the same conclusions (Uckun et al., 2010). Currently, several PLK1 inhibitors are in different phases of clinical development for anticancer therapy (Chopra et al., 2010; Schoffski, 2009). Data from one of the first clinical trials indicated that the PLK1 inhibitor BI 2536 was well tolerated and showed antitumor activity in patients with advanced solid tumors and refractory or relapsed AML (Wasch et al., 2010). According to CML, this scheme of therapy was not very intensively studied till now, however it also seems to be very potent and prospective. PLK1 inhibitor BI 2536 in a low, nanomolar concentration was able to induce growth inhibition and mitotic arrest followed by apoptosis in CML cells, including cell lines and primary cells from patients (Gleixneret al., 2010). Importantly, this agent was very effective not only against imatinib-sensitive CML cells, but also imatinib-resistant cells carrying the T315I mutation. Treatment with BI2536 together with imatinib or nilotinib showed synergistic effect, indicating possibility of a combined therapeutic application.

6. Final conclusions

Taken together, it is already clear that BRCA1 due to its multifunctional nature, is one of the key molecules controlling mitosis on the different levels of organization. There is no doubt that the decrease of BRCA1 caused by BCR-ABL in CML cells could be a critical factor determining the generation of supernumerary centrosomes, aberrant mitotic spindles, mitosis and cytokinesis failures, finally leading to aneuploidization. All data presented in this review convincingly show that activity of the BCR-ABL kinase is directly responsible for the promotion of chromosomally unstable phenotype. As chromosomal instability seems to play a crucial role in the disease progression, mitosis is a prospective target for treatment in CML. This opens new possibilities for therapeutical intervention based on the targeting processes involved in the control of mitosis. It can be an alternative strategy for alone or combined treatment of leukemia cells, which developed resistance to imatinib or second-generation tyrosine kinase inhibitors, such as dasatinib or nilotinib.

7. Acknowledgment

This work has been partially superted by grants from the Ministry of Science and Higher Education: 2P04A 05729 and N N301 425938 (for K.P.) and Iuventus Plus IP2010 032870 (for P.P-B.) Authors would like to thank Dr. Sharon McKenna from Cork Cancer Research Centre in Ireland for providing the 32D, C2 and C4 cell lines.

8. References

Alimena, G., De Cuia, M. R., Diverio, D., Gastaldi, R.&Nanni, M. (1987). The karyotype of blastic crisis. *Cancer Genet Cytogenet* 26(1): 39-50.

Amiel, A., Yukla, M., Gaber, E., Leopold, L., Josef, G., Fejgin, M.&Lishner, M. (2006). Random aneuploidy in CML patients at diagnosis and under imatinib treatment. *Cancer Genet Cytogenet* 168(2): 120-3.

Andersen, M. H., Svane, I. M., Becker, J. C.&Straten, P. T. (2007). The universal character of the tumor-associated antigen survivin. *Clin Cancer Res* 13(20): 5991-4.

Babicka, L., Zemanova, Z., Pavlistova, L., Brezinova, J., Ransdorfova, S., Houskova, L., Moravcova, J., Klamova, H.&Michalova, K. (2006). Complex chromosomal rearrangements in patients with chronic myeloid leukemia. *Cancer Genet Cytogenet* 168(1): 22-9.

Bae, I., Rih, J. K., Kim, H. J., Kang, H. J., Haddad, B., Kirilyuk, A., Fan, S., Avantaggiati, M. L.&Rosen, E. M. (2005). BRCA1 regulates gene expression for orderly mitotic progression. *Cell Cycle* 4(11): 1641-66.

Baer, R. (2001). With the ends in sight: images from the BRCA1 tumor suppressor. *Nat Struct Biol* 8(10): 822-4.

Baker, D. J., Chen, J.&van Deursen, J. M. (2005). The mitotic checkpoint in cancer and aging: what have mice taught us? *Curr Opin Cell Biol* 17(6): 583-9.

Bannon, J. H.&Mc Gee, M. M. (2009). Understanding the role of aneuploidy in tumorigenesis. *Biochem Soc Trans* 37(Pt 4): 910-3.

Becker, M., Stolz, A., Ertych, N.&Bastians, H. (2010). Centromere localization of INCENP-Aurora B is sufficient to support spindle checkpoint function. *Cell Cycle* 9(7): 1360-72.

Beltrami, E., Plescia, J., Wilkinson, J. C., Duckett, C. S.&Altieri, D. C. (2004). Acute ablation of survivin uncovers p53-dependent mitotic checkpoint functions and control of mitochondrial apoptosis. *J Biol Chem* 279(3): 2077-84.

Benezra, M., Chevallier, N., Morrison, D. J., MacLachlan, T. K., El-Deiry, W. S.&Licht, J. D. (2003). BRCA1 augments transcription by the NF-kappaB transcription factor by binding to the Rel domain of the p65/RelA subunit. *J Biol Chem* 278(29): 26333-41.

Bharadwaj, R.&Yu, H. (2004). The spindle checkpoint, aneuploidy, and cancer. *Oncogene* 23(11): 2016-27.

Blagosklonny, M. V. (2001). Treatment with inhibitors of caspases, that are substrates of drug transporters, selectively permits chemotherapy-induced apoptosis in multidrug-resistant cells but protects normal cells. *Leukemia* 15(6): 936-41.

Bourke, E., Dodson, H., Merdes, A., Cuffe, L., Zachos, G., Walker, M., Gillespie, D.&Morrison, C. G. (2007). DNA damage induces Chk1-dependent centrosome amplification. *EMBO Rep* 8(6): 603-9.

Boveri, T. (1902). Ueber mehrpolige Mitosen als Mittel zur Analyse des Zellkerns *Vehr. d. phys. med. Ges. zu Wurzburg NF* 35: 67–90.

Boveri T. (1914). Zur Frage der Entstehung maligner Tumoren (The Origin of Malignant Tumors), Gustav Fischer, Jena.

Brady, H. J. (2003). Apoptosis and leukaemia. *Br J Haematol* 123(4): 577-85.

Brinkley, B. R. (2001). Managing the centrosome numbers game: from chaos to stability in cancer cell division. *Trends Cell Biol* 11(1): 18-21.

Burke, B. A.&Carroll, M. (2010). BCR-ABL: a multi-faceted promoter of DNA mutation in chronic myelogeneous leukemia. *Leukemia* 24(6): 1105-12.

Byrski, T., Gronwald, J., Huzarski, T., Grzybowska, E., Budryk, M., Stawicka, M., Mierzwa, T., Szwiec, M., Wisniowski, R., Siolek, M., Narod, S. A.&Lubinski, J. (2008). Response to neo-adjuvant chemotherapy in women with BRCA1-positive breast cancers. *Breast Cancer Res Treat* 108(2): 289-96.

Calabretta, B.&Perrotti, D. (2004). The biology of CML blast crisis. *Blood* 103(11): 4010-22.

Carroll, P. E., Okuda, M., Horn, H. F., Biddinger, P., Stambrook, P. J., Gleich, L. L., Li, Y. Q., Tarapore, P.&Fukasawa, K. (1999). Centrosome hyperamplification in human cancer: chromosome instability induced by p53 mutation and/or Mdm2 overexpression. *Oncogene* 18(11): 1935-44.

Casenghi, M., Barr, F. A.&Nigg, E. A. (2005). Phosphorylation of Nlp by Plk1 negatively regulates its dynein-dynactin-dependent targeting to the centrosome. *J Cell Sci* 118(Pt 21): 5101-8.

Chabalier, C., Lamare, C., Racca, C., Privat, M., Valette, A.&Larminat, F. (2006). BRCA1 downregulation leads to premature inactivation of spindle checkpoint and confers paclitaxel resistance. *Cell Cycle* 5(9): 1001-7.

Cheung, C. H., Coumar, M. S., Chang, J. Y.&Hsieh, H. P. (2011). Aurora kinase inhibitor patents and agents in clinical testing: an update (2009-10). *Expert Opin Ther Pat* 21(6): 857-84.

Chin, C. F.&Yeong, F. M. (2010). Safeguarding entry into mitosis: the antephase checkpoint. *Mol Cell Biol* 30(1): 22-32.

Chopra, P., Sethi, G., Dastidar, S. G.&Ray, A. (2010). Polo-like kinase inhibitors: an emerging opportunity for cancer therapeutics. *Expert Opin Investig Drugs* 19(1): 27-43.

Chu, Y., Yao, P. Y., Wang, W., Wang, D., Wang, Z., Zhang, L., Huang, Y., Ke, Y., Ding, X.&Yao, X. (2010). Aurora B kinase activation requires survivin priming phosphorylation by PLK1. *J Mol Cell Biol*.

Dai, Y., Chen, S., Venditti, C. A., Pei, X. Y., Nguyen, T. K., Dent, P.&Grant, S. (2008). Vorinostat synergistically potentiates MK-0457 lethality in chronic myelogenous leukemia cells sensitive and resistant to imatinib mesylate. *Blood* 112(3): 793-804.

Deutsch, E., Dugray, A., AbdulKarim, B., Marangoni, E., Maggiorella, L., Vaganay, S., M'Kacher, R., Rasy, S. D., Eschwege, F., Vainchenker, W., Turhan, A. G.&Bourhis, J. (2001). BCR-ABL down-regulates the DNA repair protein DNA-PKcs. *Blood* 97(7): 2084-90.

Deutsch, E., Jarrousse, S., Buet, D., Dugray, A., Bonnet, M. L., Vozenin-Brotons, M. C., Guilhot, F., Turhan, A. G., Feunteun, J.&Bourhis, J. (2003). Down-regulation of BRCA1 in BCR-ABL-expressing hematopoietic cells. *Blood* 101(11): 4583-8.

Didier, C., Cavelier, C., Quaranta, M., Demur, C.&Ducommun, B. (2008). Evaluation of Polo-like Kinase 1 inhibition on the G2/M checkpoint in Acute Myelocytic Leukaemia. *Eur J Pharmacol* 591(1-3): 102-5.

Dodson, H., Bourke, E., Jeffers, L. J., Vagnarelli, P., Sonoda, E., Takeda, S., Earnshaw, W. C., Merdes, A.&Morrison, C. (2004). Centrosome amplification induced by DNA damage occurs during a prolonged G2 phase and involves ATM. *Embo J* 23(19): 3864-73.

Duensing, A.&Duensing, S. (2010). Centrosomes, polyploidy and cancer. *Adv Exp Med Biol* 676: 93-103.

Duesberg, P., Li, R., Fabarius, A.&Hehlmann, R. (2006). Aneuploidy and cancer: from correlation to causation. *Contrib Microbiol* 13: 16-44.

Economopoulou, P., Pappa, V., Papageorgiou, S., Dervenoulas, J.&Economopoulos, T. (2011). Abnormalities of DNA repair mechanisms in common hematological malignancies. *Leuk Lymphoma* 52(4): 567-82.

Fabarius, A., Giehl, M., Frank, O., Duesberg, P., Hochhaus, A., Hehlmann, R.&Seifarth, W. (2005). Induction of centrosome and chromosome aberrations by imatinib in vitro. *Leukemia* 19(9): 1573-8.

Fabarius, A., Giehl, M., Rebacz, B., Kramer, A., Frank, O., Haferlach, C., Duesberg, P., Hehlmann, R., Seifarth, W.&Hochhaus, A. (2008). Centrosome aberrations and G1 phase arrest after in vitro and in vivo treatment with the SRC/ABL inhibitor dasatinib. *Haematologica* 93(8): 1145-54.

Fei, F., Stoddart, S., Groffen, J.&Heisterkamp, N. (2010). Activity of the Aurora kinase inhibitor VX-680 against Bcr/Abl-positive acute lymphoblastic leukemias. *Mol Cancer Ther* 9(5): 1318-27.

Fernandes, M. S., Reddy, M. M., Gonneville, J. R., DeRoo, S. C., Podar, K., Griffin, J. D., Weinstock, D. M.&Sattler, M. (2009). BCR-ABL promotes the frequency of mutagenic single-strand annealing DNA repair. *Blood* 114(9): 1813-9.

Fiskus, W., Wang, Y., Joshi, R., Rao, R., Yang, Y., Chen, J., Kolhe, R., Balusu, R., Eaton, K., Lee, P., Ustun, C., Jillella, A., Buser, C. A., Peiper, S.&Bhalla, K. (2008). Cotreatment with vorinostat enhances activity of MK-0457 (VX-680) against acute and chronic myelogenous leukemia cells. *Clin Cancer Res* 14(19): 6106-15.

Foijer, F. (2010). CINister thoughts. *Biochem Soc Trans* 38(6): 1715-21.

Fu, J., Bian, M., Jiang, Q.&Zhang, C. (2007). Roles of Aurora kinases in mitosis and tumorigenesis. *Mol Cancer Res* 5(1): 1-10.

Fukasawa, K. (2007). Oncogenes and tumour suppressors take on centrosomes. *Nat Rev Cancer* 7(12): 911-24.

Giehl, M., Fabarius, A., Frank, O., Erben, P., Zheng, C., Hafner, M., Hochhaus, A., Hehlmann, R.&Seifarth, W. (2007). Expression of the p210BCR-ABL oncoprotein drives centrosomal hypertrophy and clonal evolution in human U937 cells. *Leukemia* 21(9): 1971-6.

Giehl, M., Fabarius, A., Frank, O., Hochhaus, A., Hafner, M., Hehlmann, R.&Seifarth, W. (2005). Centrosome aberrations in chronic myeloid leukemia correlate with stage of disease and chromosomal instability. *Leukemia* 19(7): 1192-7.

Giehl, M., Leitner, A., Haferlach, C., Duesberg, P., Hofmann, W. K., Hofheinz, R., Seifarth, W., Hochhaus, A.&Fabarius, A. (2010). Detection of centrosome aberrations in disease-unrelated cells from patients with tumor treated with tyrosine kinase inhibitors. *Eur J Haematol* 85(2): 139-48.

Gleixner, K. V., Ferenc, V., Peter, B., Gruze, A., Meyer, R. A., Hadzijusufovic, E., Cerny-Reiterer, S., Mayerhofer, M., Pickl, W. F., Sillaber, C.&Valent, P. (2010). Polo-like kinase 1 (Plk1) as a novel drug target in chronic myeloid leukemia: overriding imatinib resistance with the Plk1 inhibitor BI 2536. *Cancer Res* 70(4): 1513-23.

Godinho, S. A., Kwon, M.&Pellman, D. (2009). Centrosomes and cancer: how cancer cells divide with too many centrosomes. *Cancer Metastasis Rev* 28(1-2): 85-98.

Gontarewicz, A., Balabanov, S., Keller, G., Colombo, R., Graziano, A., Pesenti, E., Benten, D., Bokemeyer, C., Fiedler, W., Moll, J.&Brummendorf, T. H. (2008). Simultaneous targeting of Aurora kinases and Bcr-Abl kinase by the small molecule inhibitor PHA-739358 is effective against imatinib-resistant BCR-ABL mutations including T315I. *Blood* 111(8): 4355-64.

Greene, L. M., Kelly, L., Onnis, V., Campiani, G., Lawler, M., Williams, D. C.&Zisterer, D. M. (2007). STI-571 (imatinib mesylate) enhances the apoptotic efficacy of pyrrolo-1,5-benzoxazepine-6, a novel microtubule-targeting agent, in both STI-571-sensitive and -resistant Bcr-Abl-positive human chronic myeloid leukemia cells. *J Pharmacol Exp Ther* 321(1): 288-97.

Hagemeijer, A. (1987). Chromosome abnormalities in CML. *Baillieres Clin Haematol* 1(4): 963-81.

Holland, A. J.&Cleveland, D. W. (2009). Boveri revisited: chromosomal instability, aneuploidy and tumorigenesis. *Nat Rev Mol Cell Biol* 10(7): 478-87.

Horwitz, A. A., Affar el, B., Heine, G. F., Shi, Y.&Parvin, J. D. (2007). A mechanism for transcriptional repression dependent on the BRCA1 E3 ubiquitin ligase. *Proc Natl Acad Sci U S A* 104(16): 6614-9.

Houvras, Y., Benezra, M., Zhang, H., Manfredi, J. J., Weber, B. L.&Licht, J. D. (2000). BRCA1 physically and functionally interacts with ATF1. *J Biol Chem* 275(46): 36230-7.

Hsu, L. C., Doan, T. P.&White, R. L. (2001). Identification of a gamma-tubulin-binding domain in BRCA1. *Cancer Res* 61(21): 7713-8.

Hsu, L. C.&White, R. L. (1998). BRCA1 is associated with the centrosome during mitosis. *Proc Natl Acad Sci U S A* 95(22): 12983-8.

Huen, M. S., Sy, S. M.&Chen, J. (2010). BRCA1 and its toolbox for the maintenance of genome integrity. *Nat Rev Mol Cell Biol* 11(2): 138-48.

Ikezoe, T., Yang, J., Nishioka, C., Takezaki, Y., Tasaka, T., Togitani, K., Koeffler, H. P.&Yokoyama, A. (2009). A novel treatment strategy targeting polo-like kinase 1 in hematological malignancies. *Leukemia* 23(9): 1564-76.

Inanc, B., Dodson, H.&Morrison, C. G. (2010). A centrosome-autonomous signal that involves centriole disengagement permits centrosome duplication in G2 phase after DNA damage. *Mol Biol Cell* 21(22): 3866-77.

Ito, D.&Matsumoto, T. (2010). Molecular mechanisms and function of the spindle checkpoint, a guardian of the chromosome stability. *Adv Exp Med Biol* 676: 15-26.

Jin, S., Gao, H., Mazzacurati, L., Wang, Y., Fan, W., Chen, Q., Yu, W., Wang, M., Zhu, X., Zhang, C.&Zhan, Q. (2009). BRCA1 interaction of centrosomal protein Nlp is required for successful mitotic progression. *J Biol Chem* 284(34): 22970-7.

Johansson, B., Fioretos, T.&Mitelman, F. (2002). Cytogenetic and molecular genetic evolution of chronic myeloid leukemia. *Acta Haematol* 107(2): 76-94.

Kais, Z., Chiba, N., Ishioka, C.&Parvin, J. D. (2011). Functional differences among BRCA1 missense mutations in the control of centrosome duplication. *Oncogene*.

Kais, Z.&Parvin, J. D. (2008). Regulation of centrosomes by the BRCA1-dependent ubiquitin ligase. *Cancer Biol Ther* 7(10): 1540-3.

Kanwar, R. K., Cheung, C. H., Chang, J. Y.&Kanwar, J. R. (2010). Recent advances in anti-survivin treatments for cancer. *Curr Med Chem* 17(15): 1509-15.

Katayama, H., Brinkley, W. R.&Sen, S. (2003). The Aurora kinases: role in cell transformation and tumorigenesis. *Cancer Metastasis Rev* 22(4): 451-64.

Kawamura, K., Izumi, H., Ma, Z., Ikeda, R., Moriyama, M., Tanaka, T., Nojima, T., Levin, L. S., Fujikawa-Yamamoto, K., Suzuki, K.&Fukasawa, K. (2004). Induction of centrosome amplification and chromosome instability in human bladder cancer cells by p53 mutation and cyclin E overexpression. *Cancer Res* 64(14): 4800-9.

Kelly, K. R., Ecsedy, J., Medina, E., Mahalingam, D., Padmanabhan, S., Nawrocki, S. T., Giles, F. J.&Carew, J. S. (2010). The novel Aurora A kinase inhibitor MLN8237 is active in resistant chronic myeloid leukemia and significantly increases the efficacy of nilotinib. *J Cell Mol Med*.

Kim, H.&Chen, J. (2008). New players in the BRCA1-mediated DNA damage responsive pathway. *Mol Cells* 25(4): 457-61.

Kitagawa, R.&Rose, A. M. (1999). Components of the spindle-assembly checkpoint are essential in Caenorhabditis elegans. *Nat Cell Biol* 1(8): 514-21.

Ko, M. J., Murata, K., Hwang, D. S.&Parvin, J. D. (2006). Inhibition of BRCA1 in breast cell lines causes the centrosome duplication cycle to be disconnected from the cell cycle. *Oncogene* 25(2): 298-303.

Kops, G. J. (2008). The kinetochore and spindle checkpoint in mammals. *Front Biosci* 13: 3606-20.

Koptyra, M., Cramer, K., Slupianek, A., Richardson, C.&Skorski, T. (2008). BCR/ABL promotes accumulation of chromosomal aberrations induced by oxidative and genotoxic stress. *Leukemia* 22(10): 1969-72.

Kramer, A., Schweizer, S., Neben, K., Giesecke, C., Kalla, J., Katzenberger, T., Benner, A., Muller-Hermelink, H. K., Ho, A. D.&Ott, G. (2003). Centrosome aberrations as a possible mechanism for chromosomal instability in non-Hodgkin's lymphoma. *Leukemia* 17(11): 2207-13.

Lassus, H., Staff, S., Leminen, A., Isola, J.&Butzow, R. (2011). Aurora-A overexpression and aneuploidy predict poor outcome in serous ovarian carcinoma. *Gynecol Oncol* 120(1): 11-7.

Laurent, E., Mitchell, D. L., Estrov, Z., Lowery, M., Tucker, S. L., Talpaz, M.&Kurzrock, R. (2003). Impact of p210(Bcr-Abl) on ultraviolet C wavelength-induced DNA damage and repair. *Clin Cancer Res* 9(10 Pt 1): 3722-30.

Lee, K. S., Yuan, Y. L., Kuriyama, R.&Erikson, R. L. (1995). Plk is an M-phase-specific protein kinase and interacts with a kinesin-like protein, CHO1/MKLP-1. *Mol Cell Biol* 15(12): 7143-51.

Lens, S. M., Voest, E. E.&Medema, R. H. (2010). Shared and separate functions of polo-like kinases and aurora kinases in cancer. *Nat Rev Cancer* 10(12): 825-41.

Lin, Y. H., Lee, C. C., Chan, W. L., Chang, W. H., Wu, Y. C.&Chang, J. G. (2011). 16-Hydroxycleroda-3,13-dien-15,16-olide deregulates PI3K and Aurora B activities that involve in cancer cell apoptosis. *Toxicology* 285(1-2): 72-80.
Linger, R. J.&Kruk, P. A. (2010). BRCA1 16 years later: risk-associated BRCA1 mutations and their functional implications. *Febs J* 277(15): 3086-96.
Liu, A. W., Cai, J., Zhao, X. L., Xu, A. M., Fu, H. Q., Nian, H.&Zhang, S. H. (2009). The clinicopathological significance of BUBR1 overexpression in hepatocellular carcinoma. *J Clin Pathol* 62(11): 1003-8.
Logarinho, E.&Bousbaa, H. (2008). Kinetochore-microtubule interactions "in check" by Bub1, Bub3 and BubR1: The dual task of attaching and signalling. *Cell Cycle* 7(12): 1763-8.
MacLachlan, T. K., Takimoto, R.&El-Deiry, W. S. (2002). BRCA1 directs a selective p53-dependent transcriptional response towards growth arrest and DNA repair targets. *Mol Cell Biol* 22(12): 4280-92.
Maldonado, E., Shiekhattar, R., Sheldon, M., Cho, H., Drapkin, R., Rickert, P., Lees, E., Anderson, C. W., Linn, S.&Reinberg, D. (1996). A human RNA polymerase II complex associated with SRB and DNA-repair proteins. *Nature* 381(6577): 86-9.
Meraldi, P., Honda, R.&Nigg, E. A. (2004). Aurora kinases link chromosome segregation and cell division to cancer susceptibility. *Curr Opin Genet Dev* 14(1): 29-36.
Michel, L. S., Liberal, V., Chatterjee, A., Kirchwegger, R., Pasche, B., Gerald, W., Dobles, M., Sorger, P. K., Murty, V. V.&Benezra, R. (2001). MAD2 haplo-insufficiency causes premature anaphase and chromosome instability in mammalian cells. *Nature* 409(6818): 355-9.
Miki, Y., Swensen, J., Shattuck-Eidens, D., Futreal, P. A., Harshman, K., Tavtigian, S., Liu, Q., Cochran, C., Bennett, L. M., Ding, W.&et al. (1994). A strong candidate for the breast and ovarian cancer susceptibility gene BRCA1. *Science* 266(5182): 66-71.
Mito, K., Kashima, K., Kikuchi, H., Daa, T., Nakayama, I.&Yokoyama, S. (2005). Expression of Polo-Like Kinase (PLK1) in non-Hodgkin's lymphomas. *Leuk Lymphoma* 46(2): 225-31.
Moore, A. S., Blagg, J., Linardopoulos, S.&Pearson, A. D. (2010). Aurora kinase inhibitors: novel small molecules with promising activity in acute myeloid and Philadelphia-positive leukemias. *Leukemia* 24(4): 671-8.
Mullan, P. B., Gorski, J. J.&Harkin, D. P. (2006). BRCA1--a good predictive marker of drug sensitivity in breast cancer treatment? *Biochim Biophys Acta* 1766(2): 205-16.
Murray, M. M., Mullan, P. B.&Harkin, D. P. (2007). Role played by BRCA1 in transcriptional regulation in response to therapy. *Biochem Soc Trans* 35(Pt 5): 1342-6.
Nadeau, G., Boufaied, N., Moisan, A., Lemieux, K. M., Cayanan, C., Monteiro, A. N.&Gaudreau, L. (2000). BRCA1 can stimulate gene transcription by a unique mechanism. *EMBO Rep* 1(3): 260-5.
Neben, K., Giesecke, C., Schweizer, S., Ho, A. D.&Kramer, A. (2003). Centrosome aberrations in acute myeloid leukemia are correlated with cytogenetic risk profile. *Blood* 101(1): 289-91.
Negrini, S., Gorgoulis, V. G.&Halazonetis, T. D. (2010). Genomic instability--an evolving hallmark of cancer. *Nat Rev Mol Cell Biol* 11(3): 220-8.
Nezi, L.&Musacchio, A. (2009). Sister chromatid tension and the spindle assembly checkpoint. *Curr Opin Cell Biol* 21(6): 785-95.
Nguyen, H. G., Makitalo, M., Yang, D., Chinnappan, D., St Hilaire, C.&Ravid, K. (2009). Deregulated Aurora-B induced tetraploidy promotes tumorigenesis. *Faseb J* 23(8): 2741-8.

Nowicki, M. O., Falinski, R., Koptyra, M., Slupianek, A., Stoklosa, T., Gloc, E., Nieborowska-Skorska, M., Blasiak, J.&Skorski, T. (2004). BCR/ABL oncogenic kinase promotes unfaithful repair of the reactive oxygen species-dependent DNA double-strand breaks. *Blood* 104(12): 3746-53.

Ochi, T., Fujiwara, H., Suemori, K., Azuma, T., Yakushijin, Y., Hato, T., Kuzushima, K.&Yasukawa, M. (2009). Aurora-A kinase: a novel target of cellular immunotherapy for leukemia. *Blood* 113(1): 66-74.

Oishi, H., Kitagawa, H., Wada, O., Takezawa, S., Tora, L., Kouzu-Fujita, M., Takada, I., Yano, T., Yanagisawa, J.&Kato, S. (2006). An hGCN5/TRRAP histone acetyltransferase complex co-activates BRCA1 transactivation function through histone modification. *J Biol Chem* 281(1): 20-6.

Ouchi, T., Monteiro, A. N., August, A., Aaronson, S. A.&Hanafusa, H. (1998). BRCA1 regulates p53-dependent gene expression. *Proc Natl Acad Sci U S A* 95(5): 2302-6.

Patel, H.&Gordon, M. Y. (2009). Abnormal centrosome-centriole cycle in chronic myeloid leukaemia? *Br J Haematol* 146(4): 408-17.

Penserga, E. T.&Skorski, T. (2007). Fusion tyrosine kinases: a result and cause of genomic instability. *Oncogene* 26(1): 11-20.

Perrotti, D., Jamieson, C., Goldman, J.&Skorski, T. (2010). Chronic myeloid leukemia: mechanisms of blastic transformation. *J Clin Invest* 120(7): 2254-64.

Pihan, G. A., Purohit, A., Wallace, J., Malhotra, R., Liotta, L.&Doxsey, S. J. (2001). Centrosome defects can account for cellular and genetic changes that characterize prostate cancer progression. *Cancer Res* 61(5): 2212-9.

Poplawski, T.&Blasiak, J. (2010). BCR/ABL downregulates DNA-PK(CS)-dependent and upregulates backup non-homologous end joining in leukemic cells. *Mol Biol Rep* 37(5): 2309-15.

Quinn, J. E., Carser, J. E., James, C. R., Kennedy, R. D.&Harkin, D. P. (2009). BRCA1 and implications for response to chemotherapy in ovarian cancer. *Gynecol Oncol* 113(1): 134-42.

Quinn, J. E., James, C. R., Stewart, G. E., Mulligan, J. M., White, P., Chang, G. K., Mullan, P. B., Johnston, P. G., Wilson, R. H.&Harkin, D. P. (2007). BRCA1 mRNA expression levels predict for overall survival in ovarian cancer after chemotherapy. *Clin Cancer Res* 13(24): 7413-20.

Renner, A. G., Creancier, L., Dos Santos, C., Fialin, C., Recher, C., Bailly, C., Kruczynski, A., Payrastre, B.&Manenti, S. (2010). A functional link between polo-like kinase 1 and the mammalian target-of-rapamycin pathway? *Cell Cycle* 9(9): 1690-6.

Renner, A. G., Dos Santos, C., Recher, C., Bailly, C., Creancier, L., Kruczynski, A., Payrastre, B.&Manenti, S. (2009). Polo-like kinase 1 is overexpressed in acute myeloid leukemia and its inhibition preferentially targets the proliferation of leukemic cells. *Blood* 114(3): 659-62.

Ruchaud, S., Carmena, M.&Earnshaw, W. C. (2007). Chromosomal passengers: conducting cell division. *Nat Rev Mol Cell Biol* 8(10): 798-812.

Rusan, N. M.&Rogers, G. C. (2009). Centrosome function: sometimes less is more. *Traffic* 10(5): 472-81.

Salles, D., Mencalha, A. L., Ireno, I. C., Wiesmuller, L.&Abdelhay, E. (2011). BCR-ABL stimulates mutagenic homologous DNA double-strand break repair via the DNA-end-processing factor CtIP. *Carcinogenesis* 32(1): 27-34.

Sankaran, S., Starita, L. M., Groen, A. C., Ko, M. J.&Parvin, J. D. (2005). Centrosomal microtubule nucleation activity is inhibited by BRCA1-dependent ubiquitination. *Mol Cell Biol* 25(19): 8656-68.

Sankaran, S., Starita, L. M., Simons, A. M.&Parvin, J. D. (2006). Identification of domains of BRCA1 critical for the ubiquitin-dependent inhibition of centrosome function. *Cancer Res* 66(8): 4100-7.

Schlegel, B. P., Starita, L. M.&Parvin, J. D. (2003). Overexpression of a protein fragment of RNA helicase A causes inhibition of endogenous BRCA1 function and defects in ploidy and cytokinesis in mammary epithelial cells. *Oncogene* 22(7): 983-91.

Schliekelman, M., Cowley, D. O., O'Quinn, R., Oliver, T. G., Lu, L., Salmon, E. D.&Van Dyke, T. (2009). Impaired Bub1 function in vivo compromises tension-dependent checkpoint function leading to aneuploidy and tumorigenesis. *Cancer Res* 69(1): 45-54.

Schmit, T. L., Ledesma, M. C.&Ahmad, N. (2010). Modulating polo-like kinase 1 as a means for cancer chemoprevention. *Pharm Res* 27(6): 989-98.

Schoffski, P. (2009). Polo-like kinase (PLK) inhibitors in preclinical and early clinical development in oncology. *Oncologist* 14(6): 559-70.

Schvartzman, J. M., Duijf, P. H., Sotillo, R., Coker, C.&Benezra, R. (2011). Mad2 Is a Critical Mediator of the Chromosome Instability Observed upon Rb and p53 Pathway Inhibition. *Cancer Cell* 19(6): 701-14.

Scully, R., Anderson, S. F., Chao, D. M., Wei, W., Ye, L., Young, R. A., Livingston, D. M.&Parvin, J. D. (1997). BRCA1 is a component of the RNA polymerase II holoenzyme. *Proc Natl Acad Sci U S A* 94(11): 5605-10.

Shet, A. S., Jahagirdar, B. N.&Verfaillie, C. M. (2002). Chronic myelogenous leukemia: mechanisms underlying disease progression. *Leukemia* 16(8): 1402-11.

Shimomura, A., Miyoshi, Y., Taguchi, T., Tamaki, Y.&Noguchi, S. (2009). Association of loss of BRCA1 expression with centrosome aberration in human breast cancer. *J Cancer Res Clin Oncol* 135(3): 421-30.

Skorski, T. (2008). BCR/ABL, DNA damage and DNA repair: implications for new treatment concepts. *Leuk Lymphoma* 49(4): 610-4.

Skorski, T. (2011). Chronic myeloid leukemia cells refractory/resistant to tyrosine kinase inhibitors are genetically unstable and may cause relapse and malignant progression to the terminal disease state. *Leuk Lymphoma* 52 Suppl 1: 23-9.

Slupianek, A., Hoser, G., Majsterek, I., Bronisz, A., Malecki, M., Blasiak, J., Fishel, R.&Skorski, T. (2002). Fusion tyrosine kinases induce drug resistance by stimulation of homology-dependent recombination repair, prolongation of G(2)/M phase, and protection from apoptosis. *Mol Cell Biol* 22(12): 4189-201.

Slupianek, A., Nowicki, M. O., Koptyra, M.&Skorski, T. (2006). BCR/ABL modifies the kinetics and fidelity of DNA double-strand breaks repair in hematopoietic cells. *DNA Repair (Amst)* 5(2): 243-50.

Starita, L. M., Machida, Y., Sankaran, S., Elias, J. E., Griffin, K., Schlegel, B. P., Gygi, S. P.&Parvin, J. D. (2004). BRCA1-dependent ubiquitination of gamma-tubulin regulates centrosome number. *Mol Cell Biol* 24(19): 8457-66.

Stoklosa, T., Poplawski, T., Koptyra, M., Nieborowska-Skorska, M., Basak, G., Slupianek, A., Rayevskaya, M., Seferynska, I., Herrera, L., Blasiak, J.&Skorski, T. (2008). BCR/ABL inhibits mismatch repair to protect from apoptosis and induce point mutations. *Cancer Res* 68(8): 2576-80.

Stolz, A., Ertych, N., Kienitz, A., Vogel, C., Schneider, V., Fritz, B., Jacob, R., Dittmar, G., Weichert, W., Petersen, I.&Bastians, H. (2010). The CHK2-BRCA1 tumour suppressor pathway ensures chromosomal stability in human somatic cells. *Nat Cell Biol* 12(5): 492-9.

Su, X. Y., Wong, N., Cao, Q., Yu, L. Z., Niu, C., Wickham, N., Johnson, P. J., Chen, Z.&Chen, S. J. (1999). Chromosomal aberrations during progression of chronic myeloid leukemia identified by cytogenetic and molecular cytogenetic tools: implication of 1q12-21. *Cancer Genet Cytogenet* 108(1): 6-12.

Suijkerbuijk, S. J., van Osch, M. H., Bos, F. L., Hanks, S., Rahman, N.&Kops, G. J. (2010). Molecular causes for BUBR1 dysfunction in the human cancer predisposition syndrome mosaic variegated aneuploidy. *Cancer Res* 70(12): 4891-900.

Suzukawa, K., Taki, T., Abe, T., Asoh, H., Kamada, N., Yokota, J.&Morishita, K. (1997). Identification of translocational breakpoints within the intron region before the last coding exon (exon 12) of the EVI1 gene in two cases of CML-BC with inv(3)(q21q26). *Genomics* 42(2): 356-60.

Tanaka, K.&Hirota, T. (2009). Chromosome segregation machinery and cancer. *Cancer Sci* 100(7): 1158-65.

Tanenbaum, M. E.&Medema, R. H. (2010). Mechanisms of centrosome separation and bipolar spindle assembly. *Dev Cell* 19(6): 797-806.

Terada, Y. (2001). Role of chromosomal passenger complex in chromosome segregation and cytokinesis. *Cell Struct Funct* 26(6): 653-7.

Thompson, M. E. (2010). BRCA1 16 years later: nuclear import and export processes. *Febs J* 277(15): 3072-8.

Uckun, F. M., Ozer, Z., Qazi, S., Tuel-Ahlgren, L.&Mao, C. (2010). Polo-like-kinase 1 (PLK1) as a molecular target to overcome SYK-mediated resistance of B-lineage acute lymphoblastic leukaemia cells to oxidative stress. *Br J Haematol* 148(5): 714-25.

Vader, G., Medema, R. H.&Lens, S. M. (2006). The chromosomal passenger complex: guiding Aurora-B through mitosis. *J Cell Biol* 173(6): 833-7.

Vagnarelli, P.&Earnshaw, W. C. (2004). Chromosomal passengers: the four-dimensional regulation of mitotic events. *Chromosoma* 113(5): 211-22.

Valeri, A., Alonso-Ferrero, M. E., Rio, P., Pujol, M. R., Casado, J. A., Perez, L., Jacome, A., Agirre, X., Calasanz, M. J., Hanenberg, H., Surralles, J., Prosper, F., Albella, B.&Bueren, J. A. (2010). Bcr/Abl interferes with the Fanconi anemia/BRCA pathway: implications in the chromosomal instability of chronic myeloid leukemia cells. *PLoS One* 5(12): e15525.

Vazquez-Novelle, M. D.&Petronczki, M. (2010). Relocation of the chromosomal passenger complex prevents mitotic checkpoint engagement at anaphase. *Curr Biol* 20(15): 1402-7.

Wang, R. H., Yu, H.&Deng, C. X. (2004). A requirement for breast-cancer-associated gene 1 (BRCA1) in the spindle checkpoint. *Proc Natl Acad Sci U S A* 101(49): 17108-13.

Warner, S. L., Stephens, B. J.&Von Hoff, D. D. (2008). Tubulin-associated proteins: Aurora and Polo-like kinases as therapeutic targets in cancer. *Curr Oncol Rep* 10(2): 122-9.

Wasch, R., Hasskarl, J., Schnerch, D.&Lubbert, M. (2010). BI_2536--targeting the mitotic kinase Polo-like kinase 1 (Plk1). *Recent Results Cancer Res* 184: 215-8.

Weaver, B. A.&Cleveland, D. W. (2006). Does aneuploidy cause cancer? *Curr Opin Cell Biol* 18(6): 658-67.

Weaver, Z., Montagna, C., Xu, X., Howard, T., Gadina, M., Brodie, S. G., Deng, C. X.&Ried, T. (2002). Mammary tumors in mice conditionally mutant for Brca1 exhibit gross genomic instability and centrosome amplification yet display a recurring distribution of genomic imbalances that is similar to human breast cancer. *Oncogene* 21(33): 5097-107.

Wolanin, K., Magalska, A., Kusio-Kobialka, M., Podszywalow-Bartnicka, P., Vejda, S., McKenna, S. L., Mosieniak, G., Sikora, E.&Piwocka, K. (2010). Expression of oncogenic kinase Bcr-Abl impairs mitotic checkpoint and promotes aberrant divisions and resistance to microtubule-targeting agents. *Mol Cancer Ther* 9(5): 1328-38.

Wolanin, K., Magalska, A., Mosieniak, G., Klinger, R., McKenna, S., Vejda, S., Sikora, E.&Piwocka, K. (2006). Curcumin affects components of the chromosomal passenger complex and induces mitotic catastrophe in apoptosis-resistant Bcr-Abl-expressing cells. *Mol Cancer Res* 4(7): 457-69.

Wong, C.&Stearns, T. (2003). Centrosome number is controlled by a centrosome-intrinsic block to reduplication. *Nat Cell Biol* 5(6): 539-44.

Wu, J., Lu, L. Y.&Yu, X. (2010). The role of BRCA1 in DNA damage response. *Protein Cell* 1(2): 117-23.

Wu, L. C., Wang, Z. W., Tsan, J. T., Spillman, M. A., Phung, A., Xu, X. L., Yang, M. C., Hwang, L. Y., Bowcock, A. M.&Baer, R. (1996). Identification of a RING protein that can interact in vivo with the BRCA1 gene product. *Nat Genet* 14(4): 430-40.

Xu, X., Weaver, Z., Linke, S. P., Li, C., Gotay, J., Wang, X. W., Harris, C. C., Ried, T.&Deng, C. X. (1999). Centrosome amplification and a defective G2-M cell cycle checkpoint induce genetic instability in BRCA1 exon 11 isoform-deficient cells. *Mol Cell* 3(3): 389-95.

Yan, J., Jin, S., Li, J.&Zhan, Q. (2010). Aurora B interaction of centrosomal Nlp regulates cytokinesis. *J Biol Chem* 285(51): 40230-9.

Yang, E. S.&Xia, F. (2010). BRCA1 16 years later: DNA damage-induced BRCA1 shuttling. *Febs J* 277(15): 3079-85.

Yarden, R. I.&Brody, L. C. (1999). BRCA1 interacts with components of the histone deacetylase complex. *Proc Natl Acad Sci U S A* 96(9): 4983-8.

Yuan, K., Huang, Y.&Yao, X. (2011). Illumination of mitotic orchestra during cell division: a Polo view. *Cell Signal* 23(1): 1-5.

Zhang, H., Somasundaram, K., Peng, Y., Tian, H., Zhang, H., Bi, D., Weber, B. L.&El-Deiry, W. S. (1998). BRCA1 physically associates with p53 and stimulates its transcriptional activity. *Oncogene* 16(13): 1713-21.

Zhang, J.&Powell, S. N. (2005). The role of the BRCA1 tumor suppressor in DNA double-strand break repair. *Mol Cancer Res* 3(10): 531-9.

Zhang, S., Hemmerich, P.&Grosse, F. (2007). Centrosomal localization of DNA damage checkpoint proteins. *J Cell Biochem* 101(2): 451-65.

Zhou, C., Smith, J. L.&Liu, J. (2003). Role of BRCA1 in cellular resistance to paclitaxel and ionizing radiation in an ovarian cancer cell line carrying a defective BRCA1. *Oncogene* 22(16): 2396-404.

2

BCR/ABL1 Extra Fusions in Patients with Chronic Myeloid Leukaemia (CML)

Maria Teresa Vargas
Division of Genetics, Department of Pathology, Virgen Macarena University Hospital, Seville, Spain

1. Introduction

Chronic myelogenous leukemia (CML) is characterized by the Philadelphia chromosome (Ph), which is originated by a balanced translocation between chromosomes 9 and 22, that is, t(9;22)(q34;q11) results in production of a BCR-ABL1 fusion protein with constitutive Abl kinase activity. In experimental models, the expression of said activity causes expansion of pluripotent stem cells, preferentially favours myeloid lineage differentiation, and inhibits erythroid differentiation [1,2].

The BCR/ABL1 fusion in 22q11 is observed in ~95% of patients with chronic myeloid leukemia (CML). The BCR/ABL1 fusion signal on the derivative chromosome 22 is present in most CML patients.

In 5-10% of cases, this signal is generated by variant rearrangements (variant Ph) that involve other genomic regions [3-7]. More than 600 CML cases with variant rearrangements have been reported. The breakpoint distribution clearly exhibits a non-random pattern, with marked clustering to some chromosome bands, such as 1p36, 3p21, 5q13, 6p21, 9q22, 11q13, 12p13, 17p13, 17q21, 17q25, 19q13, 21q22, 22q12, and 22q13, which suggests that these regions may be particularly prone to breakage. In addition, some specific variants are also known to be more frecuent, with the two translocations t(3;9;22)(p21;q34;q11) and t(17;22)(q25;q11) both having been reported in more than 10 cases [8].

The occurrence of additional chromosomal aberrations (ACA) in Ph-positive CML is strongly associated with disease progression and has been interpreted as a sign of clonal evolution as well as chromosomal instability. Mitelman et al. [9] identified +Ph, +8, and i(17q) as the most common secondary changes that occur in nearly 90% of the cases with additional abnormalities. These three abnormalities were proposed to follow the 'major route' of clonal evolution, whereas other changes, which evolved more rarely, were suggested to follow the 'minor route' [9]; the terms 'major' and 'minor' refer to frequencies of the aberrations but not to the pathogenetic impact. Thus the three major route changes, followed by +19, were the most common ACA. Other additional chromosomal abnormalities take place in less than 10% of the cases, the most frequent being –Y, +21, +17, –7, and –17. On the other hand, no apparent differences in ACA between CML with standard Ph and CML cases with Ph variants are observed. The most common additional chromosomal changes are +8 (34%), +Ph (30%), i(17q) (20%), +19 (13%), –Y (8% of anomalies), +21 (7%), +17 (5%), and -7 (5%), when these two CML groups are combined (Table 1).

Chronic Phase (in order of appearance)	Accelerated and Blastic Phase (in order of appearance)
+Ph classical	+Ph classical
+Ph variant	+ Ph variant
+ Ph, +8	+Ph, +8
+Ph, -Y	+Ph, -Y
+Ph, -21	+Ph, i(17q)
+8	+19/ +17 /-7
Complex Karyotype	Complex karyotype

Table 1. Secondary chromosome abnormality patterns in CML patients.

The chromosome bands frequently involved in secondary structural changes are similar in both groups. It is apparent that some chromosome segments are particularly 'breakprone': 1q, 3q21, 3q26, 7p, 9p, 11q23, 12p13, 13q11–14, 17p11, 17q10, 21q22, and 22q10 when breakpoint distribution is observed in CML with standard Ph.

The ACA are found in various combinations and it has been suggested that i(17q) followed by +8 are rather early changes, whereas trisomy 19 is a relatively late one [10,11]. Although this temporal order of ACA seems common, exceptions clearly exist. There are several examples of Ph-positive CML cases with +8 in all metaphases but i(17q) may also occur in only subclones, and Ph-positive CML cases with a trisomy 19 [12]. Moreover, some combinations are more frequent than others. While +8, +Ph, and i(17q) often occur together, the combination i(17q),+19 (without +8/+Ph) has only been reported in 2 cases; +8,i(17q),+19 (without +Ph) in 16 cases; and i(17q),+19,+Ph (without +8) in 2 cases[12]. Some combinations (+8, i(17q); +8,+19; +19,+Ph) are positively associated, while i(17q),+19 and i(17q),+Ph are negatively associated according to Hashimoto et al. [13].

Thus, the selective ACA appearance seems to vary, depending on other aberrations present in the combination. Furthermore, available data indicate that the most common secondary abnormalities occur in a step-wise, well-ordered manner, with a putative frequent pathway which starts with i(17q), then followed by +8 and +Ph, and lastly +19. Since three out of the four most frequent ACA involve gains, i.e. +8, +19, and +Ph, thus hyperdiploidy is the most common modal number in CML with ACA [14,15]; nearly 50% of the cases have 47–50 chromosomes. Pseudodiploidy (46 chromosomes with structural abnormalities) is observed in almost 40% of the cases, while other modal numbers are uncommon. It is worth bearing in mind that the distributions of ploidy levels are not different between CML cases with standard Ph and those with variant Ph translocations, which confirms a strong indication that there are not any major differences between these two groups when related to cytogenetic evolution patterns. Most of the ACA in CML are genomically unbalanced, such as trisomies, monosomies, and deletions. In fact, this is common in hematologic malignancies, therefore while the primary changes have been proposed as balanced, the secondary changes are said to be unbalanced [16]. However, there are some notable exceptions in CML, in 10 cases the presence of t(15;17)(q22;q12–21) has been reported [12]. Other balanced rearrangements which are characteristically found in acute myeloid leukemia (AML) or myelodysplastic syndromes (MDS) and occasionally also found in CML

BC include: inv(3)(q21q26)/t(3;3)(q21;q26), t(3;21)(q26;q22), t(7;11)(p15;p15), t(8;21)(q22;q22), and inv(16) (p13q22) [12, 18-22].

Although secondary by definition, these ACA do not behave as ordinary secondary changes. Firstly, they are strongly related to quite specific phenotypic features as the i(17q) have been associated with marked basophilia and the presence of pseudo Pelger-Huët neutrophils [4], while other secondary aberrations are not. Secondly, they do not normally take place at the same time as other common additional changes, such as +8, i(17q), and +Ph, which clearly indicates that they follow a different evolutionary pathway. Rather than being secondary changes, they may be seen as second primary changes. It is worth noting that the fact that balanced aberrations characteristic of acute lymphoblastic leukemia (ALL), such as t(4;11)(q21;q23) and t(8;14)(q24;q32), have, to date, never been reported in CML blastic phase [12]. The idea that ALL-associated translocations cannot originate during the particular differentiation stage that characterizes the Ph-positive stem cell population is a possibility. On the other hand, and equally possible, ALL-associated translocations may not provide any selective advantage for cells expressing the BCR/ABL1 chimeric protein.

In 60–80% of the cases, ACA precede or accompany blastic phase [14, 15, 23-33], thus there is undoubtedly a strong association between secondary changes and transformation. Furthermore, early studies of splenic CML transformations give rise to strong support for the clinical importance of additional changes, showing that the secondary aberrations appeared in the spleen before bone marrow [34-36]. However, the prognostic impact of ACA has turned out to be difficult to assess. First, although most studies have reported that lack of ACA during blastic phase give rise to a better prognosis [32, 33, 37-41], some investigators have not found any prognostic differences between CML blastic phase cases with and without secondary changes [23, 30]. Second, it has been debated whether additional changes found during chronic phase constitute a dismal prognostic sign, announcing transformation. On one hand, as has been repeatedly highlighted, the emergence of new clones does not necessarily lead to disease progression and some clones appear only transiently [23, 42, 43]. On the other hand, the appearance of new ACA or increment of the clone with additional abnormalities has been shown to be generally associated with clinical deterioration [28, 37, 44].

Moreover, Sokal et al. [45] reported that patients' survival with secondary changes already present at the time of diagnosis had a shorter survival rate, but with survival curves for those with and without additional changes not diverging until after the 2-year point. Third, the number and types of aberrations present during chronic phase and blastic phase may also play a role. Quite often the karyotypic changes observed in the chronic phase are single events, particularly the loss of the Y chromosome, +8, +Ph, and i(17q) [47], while they are multiple and complex in blastic phase [15,31,37,42,46]. The aberrations in i(17q), or other changes that result in loss of 17p seem particularly ominous [15,23,25,37,42.47-49]. Furthermore, trisomy 8 and +Ph that take place in the blastic phase have been associated with poor prognosis [15, 50-52] (table 1). Thus, the prognostic impact of secondary abnormalities in CML is complex, heterogeneous, and is probably related to several parameters such as time of appearance and specific abnormalities [52].

Therefore, response to imatinib on the one hand, and resistance on the other, may also be conditioned by different types of ACAs. Enhanced response or resistance to treatment may be associated with the occurrence of different cytogenetic or molecular changes which are capable of activating the metabolic pathways with different outcomes [53,54]. Several studies have assessed the impact of ACA on the clinical efficacy of imatinib by assuming that these abnormalities may confer BCR/ABL1-independent proliferation and decrease sensitivity to imatinib [50-55].

However, the presence of additional copies of the BCR/ABL1 fusion onto structurally abnormal chromosomes has rarely been reported in the chronic or blastic phase of CML patients.

We present two CML patients with additional copies of BCR/ABL1 fusions: the first patient with +Ph and BCR/ABL1 extra fusion in chromosome 18 in the blastic phase, and the second patient with four BCR/ABL1 fusion signals at diagnosis .

2. Case report nº 1

A 34-year-old patient was diagnosed with CML. The hematologic features were: Hb, 96 g; WBC, 354x10^9/L with 2% blasts, 4% basophils; platelets, 716x10^9/L. Neutrophil alkaline phosphatase (NAF) activity was absent. The bone marrow aspirate was hypercellular with 1% blast cells.

A cytogenetic study was performed on bone marrow cells and revealed a 46,XY,t(9;22)(q34;q11) karyotype in all cells analyzed. FISH was performed on chromosome preparations using commercially available probe sets (LSI BCR/ABL-ES probe; Vysis, Downers Grove, IL) and based on a count of 100 cells (metaphases and interphases). The existence of the classic BCR/ABL1 fusion was proved. The patient was treated with hydroxyurea and *a*-interferon, with a satisfactory clinical, but unsatisfactory cytogenetic and FISH response , the maximum response reached, based on a count of 120 cells, was 27/120 cells with the BCR/ABL1 rearrangement during the 4 year follow-up . A bone marrow transplantation could not be performed because no compatible HLA-matched donor was available.

After the aforementioned, 4 years after the initial diagnosis, a decrease of Hb, hematocrit, and platelets took place in the peripheral blood: WBC was 4.8x10^9/L with 38% blasts. Bone marrow was hypercellular, with 30% of cells representing the erythroid lineage at all the maturation stages, and with intense dyserythropoietic changes: 21% in the myeloid series (myeloid/erythroid ratio 5:1.5); 9% in the lymphoplasmocytoid series; and 40% as large blasts with fine chromatin in the nucleus, with two nucleoli, and irregularly shaped nongranular cytoplasms. Blast cells gave positive histochemical reactions for peroxidise and naphthol AS-D chloracetate esterase (inhibited by fluoride) and were periodic acid Schiff (PAS) positive as granules. Analysis in bone marrow of more than 100 cells at this time revealed that 94% of the cells had two fused BCR/ABL signals: one on the Ph chromosome and the other on the short arm of a derivative chromosome 18, detected by metaphase FISH analysis with Vysis LSI-BCR/ABL-ES and Cytocell mBCR/ABL probes (Fig. 1). Karyotype in bone marrow samples showed one Ph chromosome and one normal chromosome 22, and one normal chromosome 18 and another with a deletion of part of its short arm. The remaining 6% of cells only had the usual BCR/ABL1 fusion, without any other abnormalities.

The patient was then treated with mitoxantrone and cytarabine without clinical response, and later with splenic radiotherapy, which led to an intense pancytopenia; the patient then died 4 years 8 months after the initial diagnosis.

The occurrence of additional chromosome changes is an ominous sign, indicating that illness progression is imminent; however, the etiology of blastic transformation is still not completely clear. Erythroblastic transformation of CML has been reported in 10% of patients in blastic crisis; nonetheless, this has not been clearly associated to specific chromosome aberrations [3-7, 61-66].

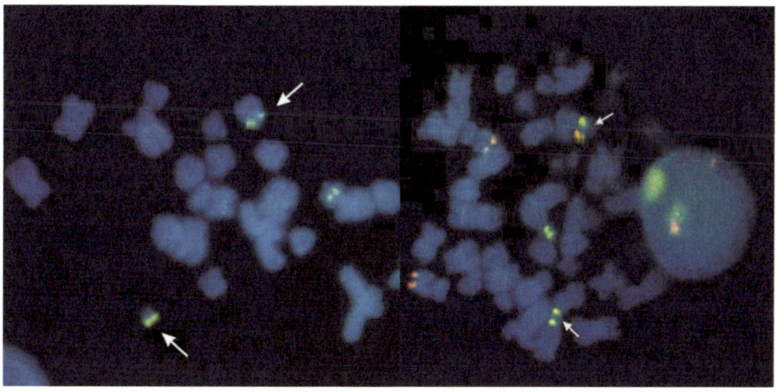

(a) (b)

Fig. 1. (a) Metaphase cell FISH showing two fusions (a classic one in the Ph chromosome and another BCR/ABL fusion in 18p) (arrows), two orange signals (normal and residual ABL probe in 9q34), and one green signal (BCR in the normal 22 chromosome) (94% of cells). (b) Partial FISH metaphase with DAPI/ FITC showing the three copies of the BCR gene (in the Ph chromosome; in 18p, indicated by arrows; and in the normal chromosome 22) (94% of more than 100 cells).

Three cases have been described with additional BCR/ABL1 fusions onto 18p accompanied by other chromosome alterations [67, 68], two of which have been reported by the same authors [68]. In the case described by Tanaka et al. [67], the blast morphology was not specified. Khac et al. [68], however, described two patients with CML in blastic transformation with a duplication and transposition of BCR/ABL1 to 18p that presented loss of part of its short arm; both patients had erythroblastic transformations, which the authors believed to be associated with this particular cytological subtype of disease progression in CML. The present case supports the relationship suggested by Khac et al. [68] between a tendency for erythroblastic transformation and the presence of extra fused BCR/ABL1 onto 18p, as in the patient we described, with a duplication and transposition of BCR/ABL1 onto 18p in the majority line (95%) in blastic phase, with no other chromosome alterations, together with an increase of red cells, intense dyserythropoietic features and PAS in granules leading to a fatal outcome.

3. Case report nº 2

A 31-year-old caucasian man, a smoker (10 cigarettes/day) and with a past appendectomy, presented with a history of abdominal pain with diarrhea and an abscess in the jawbone; he was attended at the Department of Hematology. Clinical examination revealed hepatosplenomegaly. Complementary tests revealed leukocytosis in a peripheral blood examination. His white blood cell count was $52x10^9/L$, with a peripheral monocytosis of $18x10^9/L$ and a left shift. The number of platelets was $94x10^9/L$; hemoglobin was normal; leukocyte alkaline phosphatase was reduced. In the biochemical study (which included lipids and thyroid hormones) increased HDL, vitamin B12 and uric acid were observed; findings of the remaining studies were normal. The thoracoabdominal computed tomography scan revealed mild bilateral axillary adenopathy, right pleural effusion, hepatomegaly, and periaortic adenopathy; the gastroduodenal endoscopy was unremarkable. The patient's bone marrow was described as hypercellular, without visible fat spaces; megakaryocytes were present, normal in both number and morphology. The myeloid/erythroid ratio was 20:1. Myeloid precursors were high in number and left-shifted, with a relative increase in promyelocytes (7%) and eosinophils (6%). The blast percentage was 4%. Erythroid precursors were present in normal numbers.

Cytogenetic analysis with G-banding was performed on chromosomes obtained from 24-hour bone-marrow cell cultures following the standard procedures. Fluorescence in situ hybridization (FISH) was performed on chromosome preparations using a commercially available dual-color LSI BCR/ABL-ES probe (Abbott Molecular, Des Plaines, IL) labelled in SpectrumGreen and SpectrumOrange, respectively, to detect the BCR/ABL1 rearrangements in interphase and metaphase nuclei. To identify the chromosomes 9 correctly, a Vysis whole chromosome paint (WCP 9) was used, labeled in Spectrum- Orange. The hybridization was performed according to the manufacturer's protocols.

Molecular studies using real-time polymerase chain reaction (RT-PCR) from peripheral blood were performed. One microgram of the total RNA was used for cDNA synthesis, and later PCR was performed based on a Biomed protocol and using a LightCycler 2.0 [69] (Roche Diagnostics, Indianapolis, IN; Mannheim, Germany). A RT-PCR study with a fluorescence resonance energy transfer (FRET) probe quantification kit t(9;22) (Roche) that detected BCR/ABL1 fusion transcripts resulting from the major and minor breakpoint cluster regions (M-BCR and m-BCR) was also performed. The primers used in this kit were specifically designed to detect b3a2, b2a2, and e1a2 fusion transcripts, thereby covering >95% of the described t(9;22) translocations.

At diagnosis, cytogenetic studies indicated the following karyotype:
46,XY,der(22)t(9;22)(q34;q11.2)[3]/48,XY,+9,t(9;22)(q34;q11.2)x2,+22[40] (figure 2A).

FISH studies on 167 metaphase and interphase cells revealed the presence of a mosaicism formed by three distinct cellular clones at diagnosis. In the major clone, 150/167 cells (90%) presented four BCR/ABL1 fusion signals, with two signals on the two chromosomes der(9) and the other two signals on the two Ph chromosomes (Fig. 2B and 3). Three chromosomes 9 were observed with a WCP-9 probe. A sole BCR/ABL1 fusion signal, on chromosome 22, was observed in 5/167 cells (3%), and there were no rearrangements in the remaining cells analyzed (12/167, or 7%). The FISH technique was performed twice, confirming the results. The RT-PCR demonstrated a p210, b3a2 fusion transcript.

Once the patient was diagnosed as CML, treatment with imatinib was initiated at a dose of 400 mg/day. Two months later the patient was asymptomatic and in hematological remission. The b3a2 transcripts detected by RT-PCR were at 59%. The patient continued with the same imatinib treatment of 400 mg/day. Ten months after beginning therapy, a FISH follow-up study performed on a bone marrow sample revealed a cellular mosaicism, with partial remission. The initial majority line with four fusions was present in only 20/300 cells, only one BCR/ABL1 rearrangement was seen, on chromosome 22, in 25/300 cells; the remaining 255/300 cells were normal, without any fusion signals. The p210 BCR-ABL1 fusion transcript, identified using RT-PCR (Biomed protocol), decreased to 1.66%.

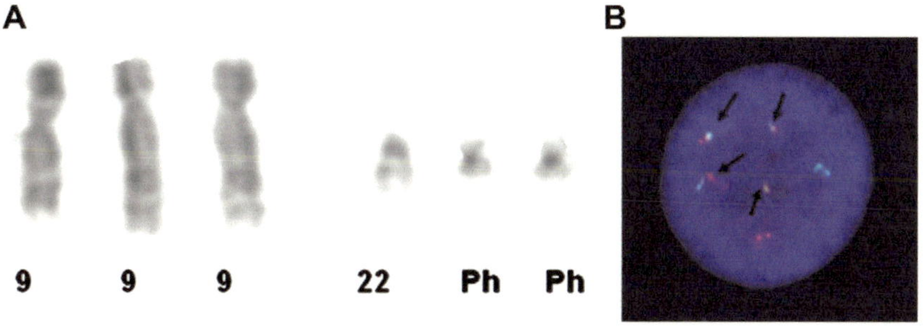

Fig. 2. (A) Partial metaphase karyogram shows two derivative chromosomes 9 and two derivative chromosomes 22, along with one each of normal chromosomes 9 and 22 in case report nº 2 of chronic myeloid leukemia in chronic phase. (B) For the same patient, interphase FISH with LSI BCR/ABL-ES probes (Vysis; Abbott Molecular, Des Plaines, IL) shows four BCR/ABL1 fusion genes (arrows). Filter: 4', 6-diamidino-2-phenylindole-rhodamine-fluoresceinisothiocyanate

A year after diagnosis, in a routine evaluation, the patient was still asymptomatic and in hematological remission. The RT-PCR study performed using FRET probes detected BCR/ABL1 transcripts. A quantification analysis (Biomed protocol) performed then was negative for p210 (b3a2), but p190 (e1a2) was found at 23.3%. Thus, the original sample was analyzed again, in which p190 was also positive. The original imatinib treatment was changed to dasatinib at 100 mg/day due to the disappearance of p210 and the presence of p190 in 23.3%.

At diagnosis, the patient in the present case had a karyotype with 48 chromosomes and four BCR/ABL1 fusion signals distributed between the two Ph chromosomes and two out of the three chromosomes 9 in 90% of all the cells analyzed by FISH. One possible explanation could be that the classical BCR/ABL1 fusion occurs initially, followed first by the duplication and translocation of the fusion to a derivative 9 chromosome and then by a duplication of both Ph chromosomes and 9q+ (the remaining chromosomes were unaltered). The possible poor prognostic effect of a BCR/ABL1 fusion located on chromosome 9 has been described [4, 5, 61, 70]. Nevertheless, other researchers have reported cases of patients with a chimerical BCR/ABL1 fusion gene on chromosome 9 in ~80% of CML samples [62] and a double fusion on both chromosomes 9 [71, 72], and the clinical course of the disease seemed unaffected by the positional regulation. In the present case, there was only hematologic remission after treatment. With regard to treatment with imatinib, additional copies of the Ph chromosome have been reported [73, 74]. The development of additional chromosomal aberrations (ACA) in Ph negative or Ph+ cells during treatment is a sign of clonal evolution and of treatment failure. Patients with ACA more frequently tended to have BCR/ABL1 mutations (53% *versus* 29%) and more resistant mutations (60% *versus* 38%) [75]. The acquisition of ACAs may confer resistance to imatinib mesylate a mechanism for imatinib resistance. Therefore, response to imatinib on one hand and resistance on the other may also be conditioned by different types of ACAs. Enhanced response or resistance to treatment may be associated with the occurrence of different cytogenetic or molecular changes that are able to activate metabolic pathways with different outcomes [76-77].

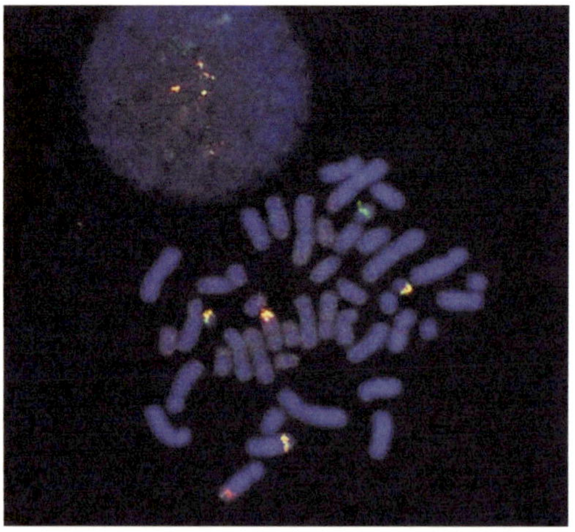

Fig. 3. Metaphase FISH with Vysis LSI BCR/ABLeES probes shows four BCR/ABL fusion signals (yellow): two signals on the two der(9) chromosomes and two signals on the two der(22) chromosomes. The green and orange signals indicate, respectively, the BCR gene on the normal chromosome 22 and the ABL gene on the normal chromosome 9.

In the present case, all the cytogenetic aberrations began to decrease with imatinib treatment, and only a small percentage of cells maintained the initial karyotype.

At the molecular level, the patient showed a p210 and p190 fusion. A p210 decrease coincided with an important partial cytogenetical remission of the four BCR/ABL1 fusions. During evolution of the disease, the p210 protein disappeared with imatinib as first-line treatment, but p190 increased until treatment with dasatinib was started.

Five months after the start of treatment with dasatinib, RT-PCR showed that p210 remained negative and p190 had decreased to 1%. Two years after diagnosis, the patient was still clinically asymptomatic and hematologically in remission. New FISH studies, with 200 cells analyzed, also showed complete cytogenetic remission. Molecular studies remained negative for p210 and positive for p190 in only 0.09%.

Although interphase FISH is increasingly used for BCR/ABL1 gene rearrangement identification in CML, we believe, in agreement with Lim et al. [72] and Primo et al. [79] and supported by the present case, that the exact interpretation of any atypical interphase FISH pattern is dependent on FISH metaphase studies and molecular breakpoint definition of BCR/ABL1 fusion.

4. References

[1] Deininger MWN, Goldman JM, Melo JV. The molecular biology of chronic myeloid leukemia. Blood. 2000; 96: 3343-3356.

[2] Era T, Witte ON. Regulated expression of p210 Bcr-Abl during embryonic stem cell differentiation stimulates multipotential progenitor expansion and myeloid cell fate. Proc Natl Acad Sci U S A. 2000; 97: 1737-1742.

[3] Sandberg AA. The chromosomes in human cancer and leukemia. 2nd ed. New York: Elsevier, 1990.

[4] Mitelman F. The cytogenetic scenario of chronic myeloid leukemia. Leuk Lymphoma 1993; 11(Suppl. 1):11-5.

[5] Saglio G, Pane F, Gottardi E, Frigeri F, Buonaiuto MR, Guerrasio Ade Micheli D, Parziale A, Fornaci MN, Martinelli G, Salvatore F. Consistent amounts of acute leukemia-associated p190 BCR/ABL transcripts are expressed by chronic myelogenous leukemia patients at diagnosis. Blood 1996; 87: 1075-80.

[6] Van Rhee F, Hochhaus A, Lin F, Melo JV, Goldman JM, Cross NC. p190 BCR/ABL mRNA is expressed at low levels in p210-positive chronic myeloid and acute lymphoblastic leukemias. Blood 1996; 87: 5213-7.

[7] Brunel V, Sainty D, Costello R, Mozziconacci MJ, Simonetti J, Arnoulet C, Coignet L, Bouabdallah R, Gastaut JA, Gabert J, Lafage- Pochitaloff M. Translocation of BCR to chromosome 9 in a Philadelphia- negative chronic myeloid leukemia. Cancer Genet Cytogenet 1995; 85: 82-4.

[8] Mitelman F, Johansson B, Mertens F: Recurrent Chromosome Aberrations in Cancer (2001). http://cgap.nci.nih.gov/Chromosomes/ RecurrentAberrations.

[9] Mitelman F, Levan G, Nilsson PG, Brandt L: Non-random karyotypic evolution in chronic myeloid leukemia. Int J Cancer 1976; 18: 24- 30.

[10] Heim S, Mitelman F: Cancer Cytogenetics, ed 2. New York, Wiley-Liss, 1995.

[11] Prigogina EL, Fleischman EW, Volkova MA, Frenkel MA: Chromosome abnormalities and clinical and morphologic manifestations of chronic myeloid leukemia. Hum Genet 1978; 41:143–156.

[12] Mitelman F, Johansson B, Mertens F: Database of Chromosome Aberrations in Cancer (2001). http://cgap.nci.nih.gov/Chromosomes/ Mitelman.

[13] Hashimoto T, Ohtaki M, Kamada N, Yamamoto H, Munaka M: Application of log-linear model in inference on karyotypic evolution in chronic myelocytic leukemia. Environ Health Perspect 1990; 87: 135–141.

[14] First International Workshop on Chromosomes in Leukaemia: Chromosomes in Ph1-positive chronic granulocytic leukaemia. Br J Haematol 1978; 39: 305–309.

[15] Ishihara T, Sasaki M, Oshimura M, Kamada N, Yamada K, Okada M, Sakurai M, Sugiyama T, Shiraishi Y, Kohno S-I: A summary of cytogenetic studies on 534 cases of chronic myelocytic leukemia in Japan. Cancer Genet Cytogenet 1983; 9: 81–92.

[16] Johansson B, Mertens F, Mitelman F: Primary vs. secondary neoplasia-associated chromosomal abnormalities - Balanced rearrangements vs. genomic imbalances? Genes Chromosomes Cancer 1996; 16: 155–163.

[18] Pintado T, Ferro MT, San Roman C, Mayayo M, Larana JG: Clinical correlations of the 3q21;q26 cytogenetic anomaly. A leukemic or myelodysplastic syndrome with preserved or increased platelet production and lack of response to cytotoxic drug therapy. Cancer 1985; 55: 535–541.

[19] Rubin CM, Larson RA, Bitter MA, Carrino JJ, Le Beau MM, Diaz MO, Rowley JD: Association of a chromosomal 3;21 translocation with the blast phase of chronic myelogenous leukemia. Blood 1987; 70: 1338–1342.

[20] Sato Y, Abe S, Mise K, Sasaki M, Kamada N, Kouda K, Musashi M, Saburi Y, Horikoshi A, Minami Y, Miyakuni T, Yokoyama Y, Ishihara Y, Miura Y: Reciprocal translocation involving the short arms of chromosomes 7 and 11, t(7p-;11p+), associated with myeloid leukaemia with maturation. Blood 1987; 70: 1654–1658.

[21] Ferro MT, Steegman JL, Escribano L, Heiurichs B, Parada L, Garcia-Sagredo JM, Resino M, Cabello P, San Roman C: Ph-positive chronic myeloid leukemia with t(8;21)(q22;q22) in blastic crisis. Cancer Genet Cytogenet 1992; 58: 96–99.

[22] Heim S, Egelund Christensen B, Fioretos T, Sörensen A-G, Tinggaard Pedersen N: Acute myelomonocytic leukemia with inv(16)(p13q22) complicating Philadelphia chromosome positive chronic myeloid leukemia. Cancer Genet Cytogenet 1992; 59: 35–38.

[23] Bernstein R, Morcom G, Pinto MR, Mendelow B, Dukes I, Penfold G, Bezwoda W: Cytogenetic findings in chronic myeloid leukaemia (CML); evaluation of karyotype, blast morphology, and survival in the acute phase. Cancer Genet Cytogenet 1980; 2: 23–37.

[24] Tomiyasu T, Sasaki M, Kondo K, Okada M: Chromosome banding studies in 106 cases of chronic myelogenous leukemia. Jpn J Hum Genet 1982; 27: 243–258.

[25] Bernstein R: Cytogenetics of chronic myelogenous leukemia. Semin Hematol 1988; 25: 20–34.

[26] Stoll C, Oberling F: Non-random clonal evolution in 45 cases of chronic myeloid leukemia. Leuk Res 1978; 3: 61–66.

[27] Carbonell F, Benitez J, Prieto F, Badia L, Sanchez- Fayos J: Chromosome banding patterns in patients with chronic myelocytic leukemia. Cancer Genet Cytogenet 1982; 7: 287–297.

[28] Swolin B, Weinfeld A, Westin J, Waldenström J, Magnusson B: Karyotypic evolution in Ph-positive chronic myeloid leukemia in relation to management and disease progression. Cancer Genet Cytogenet 1985; 18: 65– 79.

[29] Löwenberg B, Hagemeijer A, Abels J: Detection of the blastic crisis cell clone in chronic myeloid leukaemia. Br J Haematol 1985; 59: 27–36.

[30] Cervantes F, Ballesta F, Mila M, Rozman C: Cytogenetic studies in blast crisis of Ph-positive chronic granulocytic leukemia: Results and prognostic evaluation in 52 patients. Cancer Genet Cytogenet 1986; 21: 239–246.

[31] Krulik M, Smadja N, de Gramont A, Gonzalez- Canali G, Audebert AA, Dray C, Brissaud P, Debray J: Sequential karyotype study onPh-positive chronic myelocytic leukemia. Significance of additional chromosomal abnormalities during disease evolution. Cancer 1987; 60: 974–979.

[32] 4 Kantarjian HM, Keating MJ, Talpaz M, Walters RS, Smith TL, Cork A, McCredie KB, Freireich EJ: Chronic myelogenous leukaemia in blast crisis. Analysis of 242 patients. Am J Med 1987; 83: 445–454.

[33] Przepiorka D, Thomas ED: Prognostic significance of cytogenetic abnormalities in patients with chronic myelogenous leukemia. Bone Marrow Transplant 1988; 3: 113–119.

[34] Mitelman F, Brandt L, Nilsson PG: Cytogenetic evidence for splenic origin of blastic transformation in chronic myeloid leukaemia. Scand J Haematol 1974;13:87–92.

[35] Gomez G, Hossfeld DK, Sokal JE: Removal of abnormal clone of leukaemic cells by splenectomy. Br Med J 1975; ii: 421–423.

[36] Mitelman F, Nilsson PG, Brandt L: Abnormal clones resembling those seen in blast crisis arising in the spleen in chronic myelocytic leukemia. J Natl Cancer Inst 1975; 54: 1319- 1321.

[37] Fleischman EW, Prigogina EL, Volkova MA, Frenkel MA, Zakhartchenko NA, Konstantinova LN, Puchkova GP, Balakirev SA: Correlations between the clinical course, characteristics of blast cells, and karyotype patterns in chronic myeloid leukemia. Hum Genet 1981; 58: 285–293.

[38] Swolin B, Weinfeld A, Waldenström J, Westin J: Cytogenetic studies of bone marrow and extramedullary tissues and clinical course during metamorphosis of chronic myelocytic leukemia. Cancer Genet Cytogenet 1983 ; 9: 197– 209.

[39] Alimena G, Dallapiccola B, Gastaldi R, Mandelli F, Brandt L, Mitelman F, Nilsson PG: Chromosomal, morphological and clinical correlations in blastic crisis of chronic myeloid leukaemia. A study of 69 cases. Scand J Haematol 1982; 28: 103–117.

[40] 199 Sadamori N, Gomez GA, Sandberg AA: Therapeutic and prognostic value of initial chromosomal findings at the blastic phase of Ph1-positive chronic myeloid leukemia. Blood 1983; 61: 935–939.

[41] Muehleck SD, McKenna RW, Arthur DC, Parkin JL, Brunning RD: Transformation of chronic myelogenous leukemia: Clinical, morphologic, and cytogenetic features. Am J Clin Pathol 1984; 82: 1–14.

[42] Hagemeijer A, Stenfert Kroeze WF, Abels J: Cytogenetic follow-up of patients with nonlymphocytic leukemia I. Philadelphia chromosome- positive chronic myeloid leukemia. Cancer Genet Cytogenet 1980; 2: 317–326.

[43] Watmore AE, Potter AM, Sokol RJ, Wood JK: Value of cytogenetic studies in prediction of acute phase CML. Cancer Genet Cytogenet 1985; 14: 293–301.

[44] Lilleyman JS, Potter AM, Watmore AE, Cooke P, Sokol RJ, Wood JK: Myeloid karyotype and the malignant phase of chronic granulocytic leukaemia. Br J Haematol 1978; 39: 317–323.

[45] Sokal JE, Gomez GA, Baccarani M, Tura S, Clarkson BD, Cervantes F, Rozman C, Carbonell F, Anger B, Heimpel H, Nissen NI, Robertson JE: Prognostic significance of additional cytogenetic abnormalities at diagnosis of Philadelphia chromosome-positive chronic granulocytic leukemia. Blood 1988; 72: 294–298.

[46] Gödde-Salz E, Schmitz N, Bruhn H-D: Philadelphia chromosome (Ph) positive chronic myelocytic leukemia (CML): Frequency of additional findings. Cancer Genet Cytogenet 1985; 14: 313–323.

[47] Lawler SD, O'Malley F, Lobb DS: Chromosome banding studies in Philadelphia chromosome positive myeloid leukaemia. Scand J Haematol 1976; 17: 17–28.

[48] Majlis A, Smith TL, Talpaz M, O'Brien S, Rios MB, Kantarjian HM: Significance of cytogenetic clonal evolution in chronic myelogenous leukemia. J Clin Oncol 1996; 14: 196–203.

[49] Borgström GH, Vuopio P, de la Chapelle A: Abnormalities of chromosome No. 17 in myeloproliferative disorders. Cancer Genet Cytogenet 1982; 5: 123–135.

[50] Olah E, Rak K: Prognostic value of chromosomal findings in the blast phase of Ph1-positive chronic myeloid leukaemia (CML). Int J Cancer 1981; 27: 287–295.

[51] Cervantes F, Rozman M, Rosell J, Urbano- Ispizua A, Montserrat E, Rozman C: A study of prognostic factors in blast crisis of Philadelphia chromosome-positive chronic myelogenous leukaemia. Br J Haematol 1990; 76: 27–32.

[51] Griesshammer M, Heinze B, Hellmann A, Popp C, Anger B, Heil G, Bangerter M, Heimpel H: Chronic myelogenous leukaemia in blast crisis: Retrospective analysis of prognostic factors in 90 patients. Ann Hematol 1996; 73: 225–230.

[52] Cytogenetic and molecular genetic evolution of chronic myeloid leukemia. Johansson B, Fioretos T, Mitelman F. Acta Haematol. 2002; 107(2): 76-94.

[53] Hochhaus A, Kreil S, Corbin AS, La Rose´e P, Mu¨ller MC, Lahaye T, Hanfstein B, Schoch C, Cross NC, Berger U, Gschaidmeier H, Druker BJ, Hehlmann R.

Molecular and chromosomal mechanisms of resistance to imatinib (STI571) therapy. Leukemia 2002; 16: 2190-6.
[54] Ossard- Receveur A, Bernheim A, Clausse B, Danglot G, Fauvet D, Leon B, Lozach F. Duplication of the Ph-chromosome as a possible mechanism of resistance to imatinib mesylate in patients with chronic myelogenous leukemia. Cancer Genet Cytogenet 2005; 163: 189-90.
[55] Cortes JE, Talpaz M, Giles F, O'Brien S, Rios MB, Shan J, et al. Prognostic significance of cytogenetic clonal evolution in patients with chronic myelogenous leukemia on imatinib mesylate therapy. Blood. 2003; 101(10): 3794-800.
[56] Mohamed AN, Pemberton P, Zonder J, Schiffer CA. The effect of imatinib mesylate on patients with Philadelphia chromosome- positive chronic myeloid leukemia with secondary chromosomal aberrations. Clin Cancer Res. 2003; 9(4): 1333-7.
[57] O'Dwyer ME, Mauro MJ, Blasdel C, Farnsworth M, Kurilik G, Hsieh YC, et al. Clonal evolution and lack of cytogenetic response are adverse prognostic factors for hematologic relapse of chronic phase CML patients treated with imatinib mesylate. Blood. 2004; 103(2): 451-5.
[58] O'Dwyer ME, Mauro MJ, Kurilik G, Mori M, Balleisen S, Olson S, et al. The impact of clonal evolution on response to imatinib mesylate (STI571) in accelerated phase CML. Blood. 2002; 100 (5): 1628-33.
[59] Schoch C, Haferlach T, Kern W, Schnittger S, Berger U, Hehlmann R, et al. Occurrence of additional chromosome aberrations in chronic myeloid leukemia patients treated with imatinib mesylate. Leukemia. 2003; 17(2): 461-3.
[60] Palandri F, Testoni N, Luatti S, Marzocchi G, Baldazzi C, Stacchini M, et al. Influence of additional cytogenetic abnormalities on the response and survival in late chronic phase chronic myeloid leukemia patients treated with imatinib: long-term results. Leuk Lymphoma. 2009; 50(1): 114-8.
[61] Aurich J, Dastugue N, Duchayne E, Schlaifer D, Rigal-Huguet F, Caballin MR. Location of the BCR-ABL fusion gene on the 9q34 band in two cases of Ph-positive chronic myeloid leukemia. Genes Chromosomes Cancer 1997; 20: 148-54.
[62] Macera MJ, Smith LJ, Frankel E, Szabo P, Verma RS. A Philadelphia negative chronic myelogenous leukemia with the chimeric BCR/ABL gene on chromosome 9 and b3-a2 splice junction. Cancer Genet Cytogenet 1998; 101:143-7.
[63] Mitelman F, Johansson B, Mertens F (Eds.). Mitelman database of chromosome aberrations and gene fusions in cancer. Updated February 2011. Available from http://cgap.nci.nih.gov/Chromosomes/Mitelman
[64] Johansson B, Fioretos T, Mitelman F. Cytogenetic and molecular genetic evolution of chronic myeloid leukemia. Cytogenetic and molecular genetic evolution of chronic myeloid leukemia. Acta Haematol. 2002; 107(2): 76-94.
[65] Jiang DZ, Chen ZM, Lou JY, Wang YG, Liang Y, Jin J. Cytogenetic and molecular analysis of 1193 cases with chronic myeloid leukaemia. Zhonghua Xue Ye Xue Za Zhi. 2007 Jan; 28(1): 1-5.
[66] Qiu HR, Miao KR, Qian SX, Wang R, Hong M, Qiao C, Zhang JF, Fan L, Wu HX, Lu H, Qiu HX, Chen LJ, Liu P, Zhang SJ, Xu W, Li JY. Cytogenetic analysis of 362 cases of chronic myeloid leukaemia. Zhongguo Shi Yan Xue Ye Xue Za Zhi. 2009 Feb; 17(1): 27-30.

[67] Tanaka K, Arif M, Kyo T, Dohy H, Kamada N. Transposition of duplicated chromosomal segment involving fused BCR/ABL gene or ABL oncogene alone in chronic myelocytic leukemia and Ph chromosomepositive acute leukemia with complex karyotypes. Cancer Genet Cytogenet 2000; 119: 8–14.

[68] Khac FN, Waill MC, Romana SP, Radford-Weiss I, Busson M, Collonge-Rame MA, Ribadeau-Dumas A, Piffaut MC, Daniel MT, Davi F, Merle-Be´ral H, Berger R, Arock M. Identical abnormality of the short arm of chromosome 18 in two Philadelphia-positive chronic myelocytic leukemia patients with erythroblastic transformation, resulting in duplication of BCR/ABL1 fusion. Cancer Genet Cytogenet 2002; 138: 22–6.

[69] Gabert J, Beillard E, Van der Velden VH, Bi W, Grimwade D, Pallisgaard N, Barbany G, Cazzaniga G, Cayuela JM, Cave´ H, Pane F, Aerts JL, De Micheli D, Thirion X, Pradel V, Gonza´lez M, Viehmann S, Malec M, Saglio G, van Dongen JJ. Standardization and quality control studies of 'real-time' quantitative reverse transcriptase polymerase chain reaction of fusion gene transcripts for residual disease detection in leukemia: a Europe Against Cancer Program. Leukemia 2003; 17: 2318-57.

[70] Aurer I, Canaani E, Gale RP. Hypothesis: additional cytogenetic abnormalities and progression to acute phase in chronic myelogenous leukemia. Leukemia 1991; 5:1012e3.

[71] Michalova´ K, Zemanova´ Z, Bkezinova´ J, Moravcova´ J, Oltova´ A, Sobotka J, Kuglı´k P, Kozak T, Sindelarova´ L, Jankovska´ M, Obomilova´ A, Sieglova´ Z, Pola´k J, Na´dvornı´kova´ S, Haskovec C. Location of the BCR/ABL fusion genes on both chromosomes 9q34 in Ph negative chronic myeloid leukemia. Leuk Lymphoma 2002; 43: 1695-700.

[72] Lim TH, Tien SL, Lim P, Lim AS. The incidence and patterns of BCR/ABL rearrangements in chronic myeloid leukaemia (CML) using fluorescence in situ hybridisation (FISH). Ann Acad Med Singapore 2005; 34: 533-8.

[73] Gambacorti-PasseriniCB,GunbyRH, Piazza R,GaliettaA, Rostagno R, Scapozza L. Molecular mechanisms of resistance to imatinib in Philadelphia- chromosome-positive leukaemias. Lancet Oncol 2003; 4: 75-85.

[74] Melo JV, Hughes TP, Apperley JF. Chronic myeloid leukemia. Hematology Am Soc Hematol Educ Program 2003; 2003: 132-52.

[75] Hochhaus A, Kreil S, Corbin AS, La Rose´e P, Mu¨ller MC, Lahaye T, Hanfstein B, Schoch C, Cross NC, Berger U, Gschaidmeier H, Druker BJ, Hehlmann R. Molecular and chromosomal mechanisms of resistance to imatinib (STI571) therapy. Leukemia 2002; 16: 2190-6.

[76] Ossard- Receveur A, Bernheim A, Clausse B, Danglot G, Fauvet D, Leon B, Lozach F. Duplication of the Ph-chromosome as a possible mechanism of resistance to imatinib mesylate in patients with chronic myelogenous leukemia. Cancer Genet Cytogenet 2005; 163: 189-90.

[77] Zaccaria A, Testoni N, Valenti AM, Luatti S, Tonelli M, Marzocchi G, Cipriani R, Baldazzi C, Giannini B, Stacchini M, Gamberini C, Castagnetti F, Rosti G, Azzena A, Cavazzini F, Cianciulli AM, Dalsass A, Donti E, Giugliano E, Gozzetti A, Grimoldi MG, Ronconi S, Santoro A, Spedicato F, Zanatta L, Baccarani M; GIMEMA Working Party on CML. Chromosome abnormalities additional to the

Philadelphia chromosome at the diagnosis of chronic myelogenous leukemia: pathogenetic and prognostic implications. Cancer Genet Cytogenet. 2010 Jun; 199 (2): 76-80.

[78] Kim TD, Türkmen S, Schwarz M, Koca G, Nogai H, Bommer C, Dörken B, Daniel P, le Coutre P Impact of additional chromosomal aberrations and BCR-ABL kinase domain mutations on the response to nilotinib in Philadelphia chromosome-positive chronic myeloid leukemia. Haematologica. 2010; 95 (4): 582-8.

[79] Primo D, Tabernero MD, Rasillo A, Sayague´s JM, Espinosa AB, Chillon MC, Garcia-Sanz R, Gutierrez N, Giralt M, Hagemeijer A, San Miguel JF, Orfao A. Patterns of BCR/ABL gene rearrangements by interphase fluorescence in situ hybridization (FISH) in BCR/ABL+ leukemias: incidence and underlying genetic abnormalities. Leukemia 2003; 17:1124-9.

3

Causative Factors Involved in Development of Resistance to Tyrosine Kinase Inhibition and Novel Strategies Designed to Override This Resistance

Ellen Weisberg and James D. Griffin
Dana Farber Cancer Institute
USA

1. Introduction

This article describes original work performed in our laboratory related to the characterization of kinase inhibitors developed to treat myeloid leukemia, as well as identified mechanisms that likely contribute to resistance to kinase inhibition. Specifically, we provide detailed overviews of the kinase inhibitors nilotinib, used in the treatment of chronic myeloid leukemia (CML) and midostaurin, which is currently under investigation in late stage clinical trials for the treatment of mutant FLT3-positive acute myeloid leukemia (AML). Presented as well is a description of studies investigating strategies that leukemic cells employ to escape killing through kinase inhibition, including alterations in the expression and composition of targeted proteins and chemoresistance conferred by the bone marrow microenvironment. We provide a general overview of kinase inhibitors in preclinical and clinical development for CML and AML, and also discuss the use of combination therapy as an approach to enhancing the efficacy of tyrosine kinase inhibition and reducing the incidence of residual disease.

2. Development of BCR-ABL inhibitors and combination therapy studies geared toward overriding resistance to BCR-ABL inhibition

Imatinib resistance: Introduction

The development of resistance in leukemia patients to treatment with targeted tyrosine kinase inhibitors is a growing area of concern. For instance, the ABL inhibitor imatinib (STI571) (Druker et al., 1996; Buchdunger et al., 2001), which also inhibits KIT and platelet-derived growth factor receptor (PDGFR), has proven to be a highly effective, front line therapy for CML, a hematopoietic malignancy caused by the product of a reciprocal t(9;22) chromosomal translocation, *BCR-ABL* (Deininger et al., 2000). This targeted therapy has changed how newly diagnosed CML patients are treated and has substantially improved their prognosis. However, patients in the more advance phases of CML (namely, accelerated or blast crisis phase CML patients) often relapse due to drug resistance resulting from the emergence of imatinib-resistant point mutations within the BCR-ABL tyrosine kinase domain that reduce sensitivity towards imatinib (Gorre et al., 2001) or amplification of the target gene (Weisberg and Griffin, 2000).

Imatinib resistance and disease relapse in some patients can also be due to BCR-ABL-independent mechanisms, as exemplified by the small residual pool of BCR-ABL-positive quiescent leukemic stem cells existing in CML patients that have achieved complete responses after imatinib treatment. This inability of imatinib to completely eradicate quiescent leukaemic stem cells occurs despite the high expression of BCR-ABL mRNA and protein in these cells (Michor et al., 2005; Roeder et al., 2006; Copland et al., 2006), which suggests that these leukemic stem cells are not dependent on BCR-ABL for viability. Therefore, a population of BCR-ABL-positive, quiescent stem cells continues to exist after imatinib therapy even in patients who have achieved complete responses, and the insensitivity of these cells to imatinib is believed to contribute to relapse observed in some patients following termination of imatinib treatment. The existence of this quiescent cell population is important to consider when attempting development of effective therapies for overriding intrinsic kinase inhibitor resistance and resistance due to stromal-mediated mechanisms. Such novel treatment approaches must be able to eradicate this cell population if maximum clinical benefit and complete disease-free survival is to be achieved.

Among strategies to override imatinib resistance are the direct targeting of the BCR-ABL protein and the targeting of mediators of signaling pathways downstream of BCR-ABL that are needed for transformation. Biorational drug design has led to the development of novel agents that overcome some forms of imatinib resistance, and impressive results obtained in clinical trials have led to rapid FDA approval of second generation compounds that are presently used to treat newly diagnosed CML patients.

BCR-ABL point mutations as a mechanism of imatinib resistance

Although early studies based on cell line models pointed toward *BCR-ABL* gene amplification and over-expression of BCR-ABL mRNA and protein as contributing to imatinib resistance (Weisberg and Griffin, 2000; Mahon et al., 2000; le Coutre et al., 2000), the most common mechanism of imatinib resistance was later discovered to be point mutations in the *BCR-ABL* gene that lead to changes in amino acids in the BCR-ABL protein catalytic domain. Of the mechanisms considered to be of major importance in the development of drug resistance, gene amplification accounts for approximately 10% of relapse in patients, whereas mutations in the kinase domain account for 40-90% of relapse in patients. Other important mechanisms include mutations or activation of other genes (i.e. Lyn) (Wu et al., 2008) and the contribution of organic cation transporter 1 or other related drug pumps (Engler et al., 2010). Mechanisms of minor importance or uncertain significance include the influence of multidrug resistance 1 gene (Gambacorti-Passerini et al., 2000) and alpha1 acidic glycoprotein (Mahon et al., 2000).

BCR-ABL point mutations, which diminish the binding of imatinib to its target, are often those that directly or indirectly impair the binding of imatinib to the BCR-ABL protein without compromising the function of the ABL tyrosine kinase domain. Point mutations that reduce imatinib binding through a direct mechanism are generally positioned around the imatinib binding site, and diminish imatinib binding through alterations in amino acid side chains or topographical changes that sterically hinder the binding of imatinib. Phe317 and Thr315 are examples of this type of BCR-ABL point mutation (Cowan-Jacob et al., 2004). Point mutations that reduce imatinib binding through an indirect mechanism utilize the distinct binding mode of a drug to BCR-ABL. Generally, there are three primary kinase inhibitor binding modes that represent main mechanisms for pharmacological inhibition of kinase activity (Liu and Gray et al., 2006):

1. Kinase inhibitor directly competes with ATP in the ATP binding site. Inhibitors of this type are known as "Type I" and bind to the "Asp-Phe-Gly (DFG)-in" conformation (the "DFG" motif is highly conserved in protein kinases and sits near the beginning, or N-terminus, of the activation loop) .
2. Kinase inhibitor engages an adjacent allosteric binding site, typically accessible when the activation loop and/or alpha-c helix is folded away from the binding site, which leads to kinase inactivation. Inhibitors of this type are known as "Type II" and bind to the "DFG-out" conformation.
3. Kinase inhibitor binds at sites distal from the ATP binding site.

Imatinib, a "Type II" inhibitor, binds to the catalytically inactive conformation of the ABL kinase domain. BCR-ABL point mutations that destabilize the inactive conformations of the DFG motif diminish the binding capacity of imatinib, and therefore work through an indirect mechanism.

Over fifty different BCR-ABL point mutations have been identified (Rourmiantsev et al., 2002; Von Bubnoff et al., 2002; Shah et al., 2002; Hochhaus et al., 2002) and generally fall into different categorical regions that include the hinge region (which bridges the C- and N-terminal lobes of the kinase domain to develop the ATP-binding cleft), A-loop, and P-loop (or "nucleotide-binding loop"). The position of the A-loop, which includes amino acids 381-402, regulates ABL kinase activity. Mutations in the A-loop typically confer moderate resistance. In contrast, P-loop mutations, which occur at the binding site for phosphates of ATP, include amino acids 244-255 of ABL, are highly imatinib-resistant, and confer a worse prognosis than other mutations (Soverini et al., 2005). Point mutations in the ABL kinase domain that destabilize the inactive conformations of the P-loop increase the free energy of the imatinib-ABL drug-protein complex, and in effect diminish imatinib binding. Gly250, Tyr 253, and Glu255 in the P-loop are examples of mutations that reduce imatinib binding through an indirect mechanism.

The vast majority of the BCR-ABL point mutations identified occur infrequently. Mutations such as those occurring at residues Thr315, Phe359, Met351, Gly250, Glu255, and Tyr253 comprise up to 70% of all existing mutations. It is possible that extremely rare levels of BCR-ABL point mutations pre-exist treatment with imatinib and increase in frequency during imatinib therapy (Roche-Lestienne et al., 2002; Hofmann et al., 2003).

In addition to detection of BCR-ABL point mutations in patients, BCR-ABL point mutations characterized as conferring imatinib resistance have been identified through *in vitro* random mutagenesis of BCR-ABL (Shah et al., 2002; Hochhaus et al., 2002). Some identified mutations were found to exist distal to the kinase domain, including the Src homology 2 (SH2) and SH3 domains and N-terminal cap region (Hochhaus et al., 2002; Azam et al., 2003; Pluk et al., 2002).

The detection of a point mutation in the BCR-ABL kinase domain was first reported in imatinib-resistant CML patients: three out of nine patients were characterized by *BCR-ABL* gene amplification, while six out of nine patients were characterized by an isoleucine substitution in the Thr315 residue located at the periphery of the nucleotide-binding site of ABL (also referred to as the "gatekeeper position") (Gorre et al., 2001). The Thr315 residue, located in the hinge region, participates through a hydroxymethylene side chain in a critical H-bond interaction between imatinib and its protein target (Schindler et al., 2000; Manley et al., 2002; Nagar et al., 2002). Mutation of threonine to isoleucine confers resistance to imatinib because of direct steric intrusion of the bulky isoleucine side chain, as well as loss of the hydrogen-bonding interaction in the ATP-cleft. An independent study of the crystal structure of an imatinib analog bound to ABL had shown Thr315 to be critical for the binding of imatinib to ABL, and the mutation of threonine to valine at this residue (T315V) was observed to confer imatinib resistance (Schindler et al., 2000; Corbin et al., 2002).

Development of second generation BCR-ABL inhibitors designed to override imatinib resistance

Nilotinib

As an approach to overriding imatinib resistance, we characterized and developed the phenylaminopyrimidine-based Type II ATP competitive inhibitor, nilotinib (NVP-AMN107-NX; 4-methyl-N-[3-(4-methyl-1H-imidazol-1-yl)-5-(trifluoromethyl)phenyl]-3-[[4-3-pyridinyl)-2-pyrimidinyl]amino]benzamide), based on the crystal structures of inhibitors complexed with ABL (Cowan-Jacob et al., 2004). As with imatinib, another Type II ATP competitive inhibitor, part of nilotinib's structure binds the ATP binding site, while part of its structure binds adjacent to the ATP binding site. Nilotinib was designed to fit into the ATP-binding site of BCR-ABL with higher affinity than imatinib, and demonstrates significantly higher potency than imatinib in inducing apoptosis of BCR-ABL-expressing cells (IC50≤10 nM) by directly inhibiting ABL tyrosine kinase (Weisberg et al., 2005). Nilotinib also shows activity against a panel of imatinib-resistant BCR-ABL mutants, with the exception of T315I, and is effective in preventing the onset of leukemia in a BCR-ABL+ leukemic mouse model, and in prolonging the survival of mice harboring imatinib-resistant BCR-ABL-expressing cells (Weisberg et al., 2005; O'Hare et al., 2005). Crystallographic analysis of nilotinib complexed with ABL shows that, like imatinib, nilotinib binds to the inactive conformation of ABL. This suggests that the superior topographical fit to the ABL protein, as well as differences in the binding nature of nilotinib to ABL, contribute to the higher potency of nilotinib versus imatinib.

Clinical trial results with nilotinib in imatinib-resistant patients were favorable (Kantarjian et al., 2006; le Coutre et al., 2006; Ottmann et al., 2006). A phase III randomized, open-label multicenter study was conducted as a direct comparison of imatinib and nilotinib in CML patients. Results showed nilotinib to be superior to imatinib in patients with newly diagnosed chronic phase CML (Saglio et al., 2010). On October 29, 2007, the FDA granted accelerated approval to nilotinib for use in the treatment of chronic phase and accelerated phase Philadelphia chromosome positive (Ph+) CML in adult patients resistant or intolerant to prior therapy that included imatinib. On June 17, 2010, the FDA granted accelerated approval to nilotinib for treatment of adult patients with newly diagnosed Ph+ CML in chronic phase.

Dasatinib

Dasatinib (BMS-354825) is a second generation Type I ATP competitive inhibitor of BCR-ABL that is both a potent ABL inhibitor and a potent Src family kinase inhibitor (Shah et al., 2004; O'Hare et al., 2005; Burgess et al., 2005; Das et al, 2006; Melnick et al., 2006). Over-expression and activation of Src family kinases, such as LYN and HCK, have been shown to be associated with imatinib resistance (Donato et al., 2003), which suggests that the simultaneous targeting of BCR-ABL and Src family kinases may be effective in overriding resistance to imatinib. Unlike imatinib and nilotinib, which bind to the inactive conformation of BCR-ABL, dasatinib binds to the active conformation (Tokarski et al., 2006). Similar to nilotinib, dasatinib is effective against a number of imatinib-resistant BCR-ABL point mutants, with the notable exception of the T315I gatekeeper mutant (Shah et al., 2004; O'Hare et al., 2005; Burgess et al., 2005).

Dasatinib received accelerated approval by the FDA in June 2006 and the European Medicines Agency (EMEA) in November 2006 for treatment of adults in all phase of CML with resistance or intolerance to imatinib treatment. This approval was based on positive results in early (Phase I and II) clinical trials (Talpaz et al., 2006; Cortes et al., 2007). Dasatinib was also approved for treatment of drug-resistant Ph+ acute lymphoblastic leukemia (ALL) patients, in which a 190 kDa BCR-ABL protein is expressed resulting from an alternative breakpoint in the *BCR* gene. As with nilotinib, dasatinib has been granted FDA approval for therapy of newly diagnosed CML patients (Kantarjian et al, 2010).

Other BCR-ABL inhibitors

Dual ABL and Src inhibitors, bosutinib (SKI-606) (Puttini et al., 2006; Golas et al., 2003), which is a Type I ATP competitive inhibitor that only occupies the region normally occupied by ATP, and INNO-406 (first developed as NS-187) (Kimura et al., 2005), are active against a panel of imatinib-resistant BCR-ABL point mutants with the exception of the T315I gatekeeper mutant. AZD0530 is another dual ABL and Src inhibitor and Type I ATP competitive inhibitor that only weakly inhibits BCR-ABL (Lockton et al., 2005; Hennequin et al., 2006).

Aurora kinase inhibitors, which work through inhibition of the Aurora family of serine/threonine kinases, members of which are important for mitotic progression, represent another class of second generation inhibitors of BCR-ABL. Examples include PHA-739358 (Nerviano Medical Sciences) (Fancelli et al., 2006), which has been tested in early clinical trials in patients that relapsed after treatment with imatinib. PHA-739358 is a Type I inhibitor that binds the ATP binding site directly. Another example of an Aurora kinase inhibitor is MK-0457 (first developed as VX-680), which inhibits the proliferation of cells expressing the T315I-BCR-ABL gatekeeper mutant at submicromolar concentrations (Carter et al., 2005). MK-0457 has shown activity in some patients harboring the T315I mutation (Giles et al., 2007).

Non-ATP-competitive BCR-ABL inhibitors represent another class of second generation BCR-ABL inhibitors that work either via a non-ATP competitive allosteric mechanism or by prevention of substrate binding. Examples include ON012380, which shows potent activity against BCR-ABL-positive cells (Gumireddy et al., 2005). Compounds of this class make a covalent bond to the kinase and act as irreversible inhibitors. One complication is the fact that these compounds bind the substrate binding sites of multiple kinases, and therefore are very cytotoxic. Consequently, no clinical compound has been derived from this series. Non-ATP competitive inhibitors are also exemplified by the GNF2 and GNF5 family of inhibitors, which bind to the myristate binding site of BCR-ABL and inhibit its activity by stabilizing a catalytically less competent conformation of the protein (Adrian et al., 2006; Zhang et al., 2010). In addition, a type II inhibitor, GNF-7, has been shown to inhibit the T315I mutant *in vitro* and *in vivo* (Choi et al., 2010).

As an approach to overriding imatinib resistance, we developed and characterized HG-7-85-01, which is a Type II ATP competitive inhibitor that opens up a new chemical space in the field of kinase inhibitor development (Weisberg et al., 2010a). The structural inspiration for HG-7-85-01 is an amalgam of dasatinib and nilotinib, and is mostly utilization of the Type II nilotinib binding mode. Part of the structure of HG-7-85-01 binds to the ATP binding site, while the other part of its structure binds adjacent to the ATP binding site. In addition to inhibiting T315I-BCR-ABL in CML, HG-7-85-01 was observed to inhibit gatekeeper mutants of multiple kinases of therapeutic interest including T670I c-Kit and T674I-PDGFRalpha, which are clinically observed in gastrointestinal stromal tumor (GIST) and hypereosinophilic syndrome (HEL). Despite this broad profile with respect to 'gatekeeper' mutant kinases, HG-7-85-01 is not a promiscuous inhibitor, and no other inhibitor has been reported to possess this biological profile. Demonstration that this multi-gatekeeper mutant profile can be achieved is very important to the field because many pharmaceutical companies are reluctant to develop inhibitors for drug-resistant mutant kinases as they do not believe a sufficient number of patients are likely to benefit. The biological profile of HG-7-85-01 demonstrates that a single compound could be developed that is capable of simultaneously targeting drug-resistant target kinases relevant across a range of malignancies.

Progress is being made toward development of pan-BCR-ABL inhibitors that target all identified BCR-ABL point mutants, including T315I-BCR-ABL gatekeeper mutation (the so-called "third generation" of BCR-ABL inhibitors). However, as the potential for emergence of new drug-resistant BCR-ABL point mutations still exists, benefit is likely to be gained from further development of BCR-ABL inhibitors displaying higher potency and distinct mutagenicity profiles, as well as therapeutic approaches involving administration of more than one BCR-ABL inhibitor or combined use of signal transduction inhibitors and BCR-ABL inhibitors.

Combination therapy as an approach to overriding resistance to BCR-ABL inhibition

As it was anticipated that, similar to imatinib, resistance to nilotinib and dasatinib would likely also emerge due to arising BCR-ABL point mutations in CML and Ph+ ALL, mutagenesis screens were performed to identify nilotinib- and dasatinib-resistant BCR-ABL point mutations and showed overlapping but distinct mutagenicity profiles (Von Bubnoff et al., 2006; Bradeen et al., 2006; Ray et al., 2007). There has been substantial interest in testing the notion that simultaneous or sequential administration of more than one ABL inhibitor might delay the onset of emergence of drug-resistant BCR-ABL point mutations. For instance, we have shown beneficial paired combinations of imatinib and nilotinib against imatinib-resistant CML (Weisberg et al., 2007a). Specifically, we demonstrate the synergistic interaction between nilotinib and imatinib against both non-mutated BCR-ABL and imatinib-resistant BCR-ABL point mutants. It has been suggested that the differential uptake mechanisms for imatinib and nilotinib may contribute to the observed synergy between the two agents (White et al., 2006). Alternatively, synergy may be explained by the ability of imatinib to increase the intracellular uptake and retention of nilotinib (and therefore its overall concentration), possibly through imatinib inhibition of ABCB1-mediated efflux of nilotinib (White et al., 2007). The demonstrated synergy between imatinib and nilotinib complements other published reports showing synergistic interaction between imatinib and the dual Src/Abl inhibitors, dasatinib and AP23848 (O'Hare et al., 2005), as well as synergistic interactions between imatinib and a panel of standard chemotherapeutic agents (Liu et al., 2002). In addition, combinations of dasatinib and imatinib have proven to be effective in diminishing the frequency of occurrence of drug-resistant BCR-ABL mutants, with the exception of T315I (Shah et al., 2004; Burgess et al., 2005; Bradeen et al., 2006; Talpaz et al., 2006). As improvement of disease-free survival could potentially be achieved from combination therapy involving inhibitors from the same or diverse structural classes, these studies could serve as a guide for further clinical investigation.

Since clonal resistance could potentially be overcome by combining two agents with different resistance profiles, we investigated the ability of HG-7-85-01 to positively combine with GNF-5, which is unable to potently inhibit T315I as a single agent (Zhang et al., 2010; Weisberg et al., 2010c). We demonstrated that combinations of HG-7-85-01 with GNF-5 have at least additive effects against both non-mutated BCR-ABL and BCR-ABL T315I *in vitro* and *in vivo* (Weisberg et al., 2010c). GNF-5 was also shown to enhance the activity of nilotinib against both non-mutated BCR-ABL and T315I-BCR-ABL *in vitro* and *in vivo* (Zhang et al., 2010).

An important characteristic of leukemia that confers survival advantages is the common deregulation of one or more of the three signaling pathways: PI3K/PTEN/Akt/mTOR, RAS/Raf/MEK/ERK, and Jak/STAT, each frequently activated by mutations in upstream genes. The redundancy and simultaneous/cross-activation between the three pathways warrants consideration of the use of a multi-targeted therapeutic strategy, or the use of more than one type of signaling inhibitor. We have shown that the dual PI3K/PDK-1 inhibitor, BAG956, has the ability to enhance the inhibitory effects of imatinib and nilotinib, respectively, to effectively kill BCR-ABL-expressing cells both *in vitro* and *in vivo* (Weisberg et al., 2008a). Similarly, enhanced apoptosis of BCR-ABL-positive cells has been found to result from treatment with a STAT5 inhibitor and imatinib or nilotinib (Nelson et al., 2011). In addition, inhibitors of MAPK and PI3K/Akt signaling have been implicated in up-regulation of proapoptotic BIM expression (Strasser et al., 2005). This is of potential importance with respect to imatinib resistance, as the proapoptotic BH3 domain-only protein, BIM, as well as proapoptotic BAD, mediate imatinib-induced apoptosis (Kuroda et al., 2006). Of relevance, the BH3 mimetic, ABT-737, overrides imatinib resistance due to loss of BIM and BAD (Kuroda et al., 2006). Inhibition of PI3K/Akt signaling also may be of potential benefit insofar as stromal-mediated chemoresistance is concerned, as Akt has been shown to be involved in leukemic cell survival in the bone marrow microenvironment (Tabe et al., 2007).

3. Development of inhibitors of FLT3, and combination therapy studies geared toward overriding resistance to FLT3 inhibition

Mutant FLT3 as a therapeutic target for AML

The hematological malignancy, AML, is generally characterized by a block in cellular differentiation at different stages and aberrant proliferation of myeloid precursor cells. Early models have indicated that two types of mutations are responsible for the development of AML: One type of mutation is responsible for blocking terminal differentiation and the other type of mutation is responsible for promotion of growth and viability. However, full genome sequencing results suggest that up to 20 different mutations initiate AML, and disease development is thus likely more complicated than what the two mutation model proposes.

Approximately 30% of AML patients, as well as a portion of ALL patients, express a mutated form of the class III receptor tyrosine kinase, FLT3 (*F*ms-*L*ike *T*yrosine kinase-3; STK-1, human *S*tem Cell *T*yrosine *K*inase-1; FLK-2, *F*etal *L*iver *K*inase-2) (Stirewalt and Radich, 2003). The existence of a FLT3 mutation generally translates into a poorer prognosis in terms of overall survival and disease-free survival (Mattison et al., 2007). The fact that FLT3 mutations are only found in a portion of AML cells suggests that FLT3 mutations may be involved in promotion of disease rather than initiation of disease.

The most prevalent form of constitutively activated FLT3, found in approximately 20-25% of AML patients (although in less than 5% of myelodysplastic syndrome patients), occurs as internal tandem duplications (ITDs) that are located within the juxtamembrane domain (Nakao et al., 1996; Horiike et al., 1997; Kiyoi et al., 1998; Kondo et al., 1999; Rombouts et al., 2000). This mutation has been shown to cause a rapidly lethal myeloproliferative disorder in mice in the absence of a block in differentiation, suggesting that its main role may be to cause hyper-proliferation of primitive myeloid cells (Kelly et al., 2002a). Mutant FLT3 is believed to interact with additional oncogenes that block differentiation, such as AML1/ETO (t(8;21)) PML/RARalpha (t(15;17).) to cause full leukemia development.

Occurring in approximately 7% of AML cases are gain-of-function FLT3 kinase domain point mutations, frequently at position 835 (Yamamoto et al., 2001). Also identified have been other kinase domain point mutations, including Y842C (Kindler et al., 2005) and N841I (Jiang et al., 2004). An activating point mutation with comparatively weaker transforming potential has also been discovered in a stretch of the FLT3 juxtamembrane domain (Reindl et al., 2006).

Inhibitors of mutant FLT3

There are several FLT3 inhibitors presently in clinical trials, and a number of novel agents under preclinical investigation. Unfortunately, the FLT3 inhibitors tested thus far clinically induce only partial and transient responses in patients- at best- when used as single agents.

We identified and developed a small molecule inhibitor, the *N*-indolo-carbazole midostaurin (PKC412; N-benzoylstaurosporin), (Weisberg et al., 2002), a broad-spectrum first generation inhibitor that targets constitutively activated mutant FLT3. Other targets of midostaurin include (PDGFRbeta), c-KIT and c-FMS (Weisberg et al., 2002). Midostaurin showed high potency against mutant FLT3 as a target *in vitro*, and progressive leukemia was prevented in mice transplanted with marrow transduced with a FLT3-ITD-expressing retrovirus (Weisberg et al., 2002).

In early clinical trials, midostaurin administered in sequential and simultaneous combinations with standard chemotherapeutic agents such as daunorubicin and cytarabine induction and high-dose cytarabine consolidation yielded clinical responses with transient and/or reversible side effects (Stone et al., 2004). Midostaurin is one of several FLT3 inhibitors presently undergoing clinical testing, and it is currently under investigation in late stage clinical trials for AML.

We have demonstrated the activity of midostaurin against imatinib-resistant GIST (Weisberg et al., 2006). Specifically, we demonstrated the potent activity of midostaurin against cells expressing two PDGFRalpha mutants associated GIST: the V561D juxtamembrane domain mutation and the less imatinib-sensitive D842V kinase domain mutation. We also demonstrated the ability of nilotinib to positively combine with either imatinib or midostaurin against cells expressing the D842V-PDGFRalpha mutant. Findings reported introduce midostaurin as a potential treatment option for mutant PDGFRalpha-positive GIST and warrant its clinical testing for this disease target.

Additional multi-targeted inhibitors, such as dasatinib and the biaryl urea compound and first-generation inhibitor, sorafenib (BAY 43-9006), have been shown to have activity against mutant FLT3 and are under clinical investigation for AML (Auclair et al., 2007; Kancha et al., 2007; Lierman et al., 2007; Zhang et al., 2008; Metzelder et al., 2009; Guerrouahen et al., 2010). Other FLT3 inhibitors that have been clinically investigated and which elicited transient responses in early phase trials include the indolocarbazole alkaloid and first-generation inhibitor, CEP-701 (lestaurtinib) (Levis et al., 2002; Smith et al., 2004; Knapper et al., 2006), KW-2449 (Pratz and Levis, 2008; Pratz et al., 2009; Shiotsu et al., 2009), 3-substituted indolinones SU5416 (Semaxanib) and SU5614 (Yee et al., 2002; Fielder et al., 2003; Giles et al., 2003; O'Farrell et al., 2004), the indolinone derivative and first-generation inhibitor, SU11248 (SU011248, sunitinib) (Fielder et al., 2005; Kancha et al., 2007; O'Farrell et al., 2003a,b), and the piperazinyl quinazoline and first-generation inhibitor, MLN518 (tandutinib; CT53518) (Kelly et al., 2002b; Cheng and Paz, 2008). Among FLT3 inhibitors in early development are the *N*-(4-(3-amino-1H-indazol-4yl)phenyl-*N*1(2-fluoro-5-methylphenyl) urea ABT-869 (Albert et al., 2006; Shankar et al., 2007; Zhou et al., 2008), the benzimidalzole-quinoline CHIR-258 (TKI258) (Lopes de Menezes et al., 2005), the hydroxystyryl-acrylonitrile LS104 (Kasper et al., 2008) and AP24534 (Gozgit et al., 2011).

AC220 (Chao et al., 2009; Zarrinkar et al., 2009) is a second-generation FLT3 inhibitor that exhibits significantly higher potency and selectivity than first-generation inhibitors, and is under clinical investigation for mutant FLT3-expressing AML and wild-type FLT3-harboring AML. A study by Pratz and colleagues suggested, however, that the potency and selectivity of agents targeting mutant FLT3 may not, in fact, be the best predictor of clinical efficacy (Pratz et al., 2010). In their study, AC220 was found to be the most potent inhibitor of several common FLT3 inhibitors tested (including lestaurtinib, midostaurin, sorafenib, and sunitinib) and had the highest index of selectivity. However, lestaurtinib- which had the lowest index of selectivity- was found to be the most effective when tested against FLT3-ITD-positive patient samples. Results shown in this study suggested that inhibition of FLT3 autophosphorylation in a FLT3-ITD specimen does not always induce death. For example, a side-by-side comparison of AC220 and lestaurtinib showed that while both compounds fully inhibited FLT3 autophosphorylation and suppressed downstream STAT5 activation in one patient sample, only lestaurtinib induced apoptosis. Relapsed AML samples were observed to be more sensitive to FLT3 inhibition than diagnostic AML, suggesting that some FLT3-ITD AML (i.e. diagnostic) may not be addicted to FLT3 signaling. This study suggested that more selective inhibitors, like AC220 may be less effective in the diagnostic setting while less selective inhibitors- like lestaurtinib or midostaurin- may be more effective at diagnosis.

Resistance to FLT3 inhibition

Thus far, none of the FLT3 inhibitors under clinical investigation has elicited a sustained clinical response when used as a single agent. As an example, a phase I clinical trial for KW-2449 showed that FLT3 inhibition in patients occurred only transiently to less than 20% of baseline levels (Pratz et al., 2009). It has been suggested that partial and transient FLT3 inhibition such as this applies to other FLT3 inhibitors in clinical development and may be responsible for their limited efficacy (Chu and Small, 2009).

One putative resistance mechanism related to FLT3 inhibition is dysregulation of signaling molecules, such as those associated with the PI3K/Akt and Ras/MEK/MAPK pathways (Piloto et al., 2007). Also implicated in drug resistance are aberrant STAT signaling (Zhou et al., 2009), the aberrant expression of the STAT5 target gene, PIM (Kim et al., 2005; Kim et al., 2006), and high levels of phosphoprotein expression of the forkhead transcription factor, FOXO3A (Kornblau et al., 2010). Additional mechanisms include up-regulation of anti-apoptotic proteins (Kohl et al., 2007; Brietenbuecher et al., 2009; Stolzel et al., 2010), up-regulation of inhibitors of apoptosis proteins, and elevated FLT3 ligand levels (Zhou et al., 2009). The concentration of FLT3 ligand has been observed to be significantly higher in patients treated with chemotherapy or radiotherapy (Lyman et al., 1995; Wodnar-Filipowicz et al., 1996; Zwierzina et al., 1999; Bojko et al., 2002), and this is predicted to impede the action of FLT3 inhibitors administered after chemotherapy.

Another possible resistance mechanism is cytoprotection conferred by the bone marrow microenvironment. Indeed, FLT3 inhibition was found to actually enhance the survival of CD34+CD38-CD123+ leukemic stem cells and progenitor cells in a "niche-like" *in vitro* microenvironment that was comprised of factors including IL-6, IL-3, stem cell factor (SCF), and immobilized fibronectin (Mony et al., 2008). Small molecule CXCR4 inhibitors may be effective in enhancing kinase inhibitor-induced apoptosis of stromal-protected leukemic cells, implicating a causal relationship between the chemokine receptor CXCR4 and stroma-derived factor 1alpha (SDF-1a) interaction and drug-resistant leukemia (Zeng et al., 2006).

Pre-existing or acquired point mutations in the FLT3 kinase domain that interfere with drug binding may also contribute to drug resistance in patients (Cools et al., 2004; Heidel et al., 2006).

Point mutations in the FLT3 receptor are generally analogous to point mutations in BCR-ABL, the most prevalent mechanism of resistance to imatinib. However, there is little evidence for the existence of overlapping resistance profiles for FLT3 inhibitors, such as those demonstrated for imatinib, dasatinib, and nilotinib with respect to the T315I gatekeeper mutation (Von Bubnoff et al., 2006; Bradeen et al., 2006; Ray et al., 2007). Instead, non-overlapping mechanisms of resistance between PKC412, sorafenib, and SU5614 were found in a screening assay designed to study drug resistance profiles (Von Bubnoff et al., 2009). For example, SU5614 resistance was characterized predominantly as mutations in the D835 residue, while sorafenib resistance was characterized by unique mutations such as F691L and point mutations in the Y842 residue (Von Bubnoff et al., 2009). Another study confirmed the involvement of acquired mutations, D835N and Y842H, in resistance to SU5614 (Bagrintseva et al., 2004). In contrast, PKC412 resistance was characterized by mutations in the N676 residue, which was previously identified and characterized in a PKC412-resistant AML patient as the sole determinant of drug resistance (Heidel et al., 2006).

In addition to non-overlapping mutagenicity profiles between existing FLT3 inhibitors, each shows variable activity toward different mutations, for example activation loop mutants versus ITD mutations. As an example, sunitinib inhibits ITD and activation loop mutants with equal potency, whereas sorafenib is less efficacious toward activation loop mutants than ITD (Kancha et al., 2007). PKC412 shows comparable activity against different FLT3 activation loop mutants, whereas MLN518 shows variable activity (Clark et al., 2004; Barry et al., 2007).

Combination therapy as an approach to treating mutant FLT3-positive disease

As responses of patients to FLT3 inhibition is generally only partial and transient, there is a need for development of novel agents that can either be used effectively alone or combined with FLT3 inhibitors to suppress disease progression and prolong lifespan. FLT3 inhibitors have been tested in combination with standard chemotherapy agents as an approach to assessing the overall efficacy of combined therapies. For example, SU11248, combined with cytarabine or daunorubicin, exhibited additive-to-synergistic inhibitory effects on cells expressing mutant FLT3 (Yee et al., 2004). Similarly, CEP-701 showed synergy when combined with etoposide, mitoxantrone, daunorubicin, and cytarabine (Levis et al., 2004). PKC412 demonstrated synergy when combined with vincristine, 4-hydroperoxycyclophosphamide, etoposide, mitoxantrone, cytarabine, doxorubicin, and idarubicin (Mollgard et al., 2008; Furukawa et al., 2007). The sequence of administration of FLT3 inhibitors and standard chemotherapy appears to often, depending on the FLT3 inhibitor, be sequence-dependent, resulting in antagonism when the FLT3 inhibitor is administered prior to chemotherapy and resulting in synergy when the FLT3 inhibitor is administered after chemotherapy (Pratz and Levis, 2008).

One strategy geared toward overriding resistance to FLT3 inhibition includes the combined use of more than one FLT3 inhibitor, providing their interaction with the FLT3 protein target or FLT3 signaling pathway components is distinct enough for the two inhibitors to synergize. We demonstrated the potent and selective activity of the novel type II ATP competitive inhibitors, HG-7-85-01 and HG-7-86-01, against mutant FLT3, as well as their ability to synergize well with standard chemotherapeutic agents or midostaurin (Weisberg et al., 2010b). The ability of HG-7-85-01 and HG-7-86-01 to inhibit mutant FLT3, in addition to a number of gatekeeper mutants of multiple kinases of therapeutic interest, highlights their unique versatility and potential widespread clinical usefulness. Other potent FLT3 inhibitors, such as NVP-AST487, have the ability to effectively combine with midostaurin to kill drug-sensitive and insensitive mutant FLT3-expressing cells (Weisberg et al., 2008b). The ability of two targeted FLT3 inhibitors to synergize may translate into clinical benefit in terms of reducing toxicity, as clinical responses achieved with late-stage FLT3 inhibitors like midostaurin and CEP-701 depend on combined administration with standard chemotherapeutic agents.

Alternatively, FLT3 inhibitors can be combined with small molecule inhibitors that interact with key mediators of major signaling pathways that play a significant role in AML. Cross-talk between the three main pathways activated by mutant FLT3 (RAS/Raf/MEK/ERK, Jak/STAT, and PI3K/PTEN/Akt/mTOR) warrants the development of multi-targeted approaches for treatment of mutant FLT3-positive AML (Brandts et al., 2005; Recher et al., 2005; Kornblau et al., 2006; Rocnik et al., 2006; Al Shaer et al., 2008). We have shown that signaling pathway inhibitors, such as the dual PI3K/PDK-1 inhibitor, BAG956, can positively combine with midostaurin against mutant FLT3-positive cells (Weisberg et al., 2008a). Of relevance, PKC412 and the mTOR inhibitor, rapamycin, synergize against PKC412-sensitive and –resistant mutant FLT3-expressing cells (Mohi et al., 2004). The rapamycin derivative, RAD001, enhances the anti-leukemic effects of sunitinib (Ikezoe et al., 2006), as does the MEK1/2 kinase inhibitor, AZD6244 (ARRY-142886) (Nishioka et al., 2008b). Other agents effective in killing mutant FLT3-expressing cells are heat shock protein 90 (Hsp90) inhibitors and histone deacetylase inhibitors, which disrupt the major signaling pathways (Al Shaer et al., 2008; Nishioka et al., 2008a), and drugs that inhibit farnesyl-transferase (Mollgard et al., 2008).

4. Characterization of underlying mechanisms of stroma-mediated chemoresistance to tyrosine kinase inhibition

In addition to identifying and developing potent kinase inhibitors representative of novel and unique structural classes with the ability to override drug resistance due to changes in the target protein, there is a push toward gaining a better understanding of the mechanisms underlying drug resistance in CML and AML as they relate to the leukemic cell microenvironment. Bone marrow is comprised of hematopoietic and stromal cells, in addition to other factors including extracellular matrix and blood vessels; growth factors and cell:cell interactions (Charbord et al. 1996). Bone marrow stroma and factors derived from stroma have been suggested to play a role in the long-term survival and proliferation of normal and leukemia cells (Ashley et al., 1994; Bradstock et al., 1996; Rafii et al., 1997; Lagneaux et al., 1998, Lagneaux et al., 1999; Konopleva et al., 2002; Litwin et al., 2002). Specifically, bone marrow stroma provides signals, such as granulocyte colony-stimulating factor (G-CSF), granulocyte macrophage colony-stimulating factor (GM-CSF), and terminal differentiation of hematopoietic stem cells or mediate/support their proliferation (Verfaillie et al., 1993; Liesveld et al., 1996; Harrison et al., 1997; Breems et al., 1997; O'Prey et al., 1998; Leslie et al., 1998; Shih et al., 1999). SSpenic stroma, as well, has been implicated in enhanced survival of both normal and leukemic cells (Shaked et al., 2005; Despars and O'Neill, 2006).

Clinical trial data with tyrosine kinase inhibitors show that while the peripheral blood of patients responds well, bone marrow responds less well. It appears possible that small numbers of leukemic CD34+ cells can persist in the marrow microenvironment of leukemia patients after years of therapy with kinase inhibitors. Stromal cells have been implicated, as they provide viability signals to leukemic cells that protect them from inhibitor effects. Indeed, the quantity of leukemic stem cells that rely on stroma to survive is predictive of disease outcome (Kumagai et al., 1996).

We revealed highest tumor burden and residual disease to occur *in vivo* in stroma-associated tissues in imatinib/nilotinib-treated NCr nude mice, suggesting that significant reservoirs for tumor growth appear to be tissues that are able to support normal hematopoietic and malignant stem cell development (Weisberg et al., 2008c). These studies, which showed a pattern of leukemia distribution consistent with what is observed in imatinib- and nilotinib-treated chronic myeloid leukemia patients, were followed by a more in-depth analysis of stroma-leukemia cell interactions that lead to protection of leukemia cells from nilotinib-induced cytotoxicity. For the latter, we used the human BCR-ABL-positive cell line, KU812F, and the human bone marrow stroma cell line, HS-5, to more closely approximate the bone marrow-associated cytoprotection observed in drug-treated leukemia patients. Partial stromal-mediated protection of BCR-ABL-positive leukemic cells from nilotinib treatment involved the cooperative interaction of members of a select panel of stromal-secreted viability factors, including IL-6 and GM-CSF (Weisberg et al., 2008c). Similar results were observed with mutant FLT3-positive leukemia cells treated with midostaurin in the presence of HS-5-stromal-conditioned media versus the same panel of stromal-secreted viability factors (Weisberg et al., 2009).

5. Potentiation of anti-leukemic effects of tyrosine kinase inhibitors by IAP inhibition: Implications for use of IAP inhibition to prevent or reduce residual disease following tyrosine kinase inhibition

Deregulated signaling molecules associated with viability/apoptotic signaling represent attractive targets for therapeutic intervention, and several strategies have emerged that may be effective in preventing drug resistance due to this. One approach involves combining targeted inhibitors with small molecule inhibitors of key components of major signaling pathways affecting the viability/expansion of leukemic cells. Accordingly, we have developed effective inhibitors of the inhibitor of apoptosis (IAP) family of proteins (Liu et al., 2000; Wu et al., 2000), such as LBW242 (Weisberg et al., 2007b), and its structural analog, LCL161, which bind to and inhibit multiple IAPs (i.e. XIAP, c-IAP) to enhance the activity of different proapoptotic signaling pathways. We have demonstrated the ability of LBW242 to synergize with midostaurin *in vivo* against progressive mutant FLT3-positive leukemia and to override stromal-mediated chemoresistance *in vitro* (Weisberg et al., 2007b).

Clinical trial data with midostaurin show that while good responses are achievable in mutant FLT3-positive AML patient peripheral blood, patient bone marrow responses are more modest. This suggests that stromal cells provide viability signals to AML cells that protect the cells from the effects of the selective inhibitor being used. We investigated the responsiveness of Ba/F3-FLT3-ITD cells cultured in the presence and absence of WEHI (used as a source of IL-3) to the cytotoxic effects of midostaurin, and we found that the presence of IL-3 completely protected cells from midostaurin-inhibition of cellular proliferation (Weisberg et al., 2007b). In contrast to midostaurin, the IAP inhibitor, LBW242, inhibited Ba/F3-FLT3-ITD proliferation in both the absence and the presence of IL-3 (Weisberg et al., 2007b). Interestingly, LBW242 plus midostaurin inhibited the growth of Ba/F3-FLT3-ITD cells cultured in the presence of IL-3 to a greater extent than either agent alone; this inhibition was similar to that achieved with co-administration of both agents in the absence of IL-3, suggesting that an IAP inhibitor is able to enhance the effects of a FLT3 inhibitor and override chemoresistance due to provision of viability signals (Weisberg et al., 2007b).

In an attempt to more closely model putative stromal-AML cell interactions and stromal-mediated viability signaling effects on the cytotoxic effects of midostaurin, we tested the human stroma cell line, HS-5, in combination with the mutant FLT3 AML line, MOLM-13-luc+ (luciferase was used to specifically quantify only the leukemia component in the assay using light emission). A confluent layer of HS-5 stromal cells enhanced the growth of MOLM13-luc+ cells and was partially protective against the inhibitory effects of midostaurin (Weisberg et al., 2007b). LBW242 enhanced the cytotoxic effects of midostaurin against MOLM13-luc+ cells in the presence of HS-5 human stromal cells, supporting the notion that stromal-mediated viability signals may contribute to chemoresistance to FLT3 inhibitors (such as midostaurin) observed in marrow, as well as the idea that such resistance may be overcome by inclusion of IAP inhibitor treatment (Weisberg et al., 2007b).

We have also shown the ability of LCL161 to significantly delay disease recurrence in mice injected with BCR-ABL-expressing cells and treated for several weeks with a moderate dose of nilotinib (Weisberg et al., 2010d). Specifically, using *in vitro* models of intrinsic drug resistance and stromal-mediated chemoresistance, as well as functional mouse models of progressive and residual disease, we showed the ability of the novel IAP inhibitor, LCL161, to enhance the cytotoxic effects of tyrosine kinase inhibitors against leukemic disease. Importantly, we observed LCL161 to synergize *in vivo* with nilotinib to reduce leukemia burden significantly below the baseline level suppression exhibited by a moderate-to-high dose of nilotinib. Our results support the idea of using IAP inhibitors in conjunction with targeted tyrosine kinase inhibition to suppress or eradicate progressive and drug-resistant or residual disease. Phase I studies in advanced solid tumors are currently ongoing, and LCL161 is being considered for testing in clinical trials for leukemia.

6. Conclusion

Elucidation of mechanisms of resistance to tyrosine kinase inhibition is critical for the optimization of existing therapies and prolongation of patient survival via delaying or eradicating the recurrence of disease. For CML, the discovery and characterization of BCR-ABL point mutations in the kinase target of a number of inhibitors in clinical use has been a tremendous step forward in understanding an important underlying mechanism of drug resistance. While second generation BCR-ABL inhibitors, such as nilotinib and dasatinib, have proven to be highly effective in the clinic and override imatinib resistance to an extent, the existence of highly imatinib-resistant mutants, such as the T315I gatekeeper mutant, is a limiting factor. Even for third generation BCR-ABL inhibitors that are able to override T315I, the potential exists for the evolution of novel drug-resistant point mutations that impede the binding of drug to its target. Thus, there continues to be a need for development of BCR-ABL inhibitors with high potency and unique mutagenicity profiles, as well as a continued need for combination therapy approaches to overriding drug resistance.

For mutant FLT3-positive AML, due to the only transient and partial effects observed clinically with FLT3 inhibitors in late-stage development, there is an urgent need for the development of new treatment approaches that could potentially lead to improved clinical effectiveness. As with CML, the key to improved patient responsiveness may lie in continued development of compounds conferring a higher degree of potency, as well as novel combination therapy strategies.

For both CML and mutant FLT3-positive AML, elucidation of mechanisms of resistance that are associated with leukemic cell survival, such as stromal-mediated chemoresistance and up-regulation of viability signaling molecules, warrants the investigation of single agent activity of pro-apoptotic agents. It also warrants the development of treatment approaches that rely on administration of kinase inhibitors combined with other agents targeting components of leukemia:stromal cell interactions and stromal-derived viability factors.

7. References

Adrian, F.J., Ding, Q., Sim, T., Velentza, A., Sloan, C., Liu, Y., Zhang, G., Hur, W., Ding, S., Manley, P., Mestan, J., Fabbro, D., & Gray, N.S. (2006). Allosteric inhibitors of Bcr-abl-dependent cell proliferation. *Nat Chem Biol*, Feb;2 (2), pp. 95-102.

Albert, D.H., Tapang, P., Magoc, T.J., Pease, L.J., Reuter, D.R., Wei, R.Q., Li, J., Guo, J., Bousquet, P.F., Ghoreishi-Haack, N.S., Wang, B., Bukofzer, G.T., Wang, Y.C., Stavropoulos, J.A., Hartandi, K., Niquette, A.L., Soni, N., Johnson, E.F., McCall, J.O., Bouska, J.J., Luo, Y., Donawho, C.K., Dai, Y., Marcotte, P.A., Glaser, K.B., Michaelides, M.R., & Davidsen, S.K. (2006). Preclinical activity of ABT-869: a multitargeted receptor tyrosine kinase inhibitor. *Mol Cancer Ther,* Apr;5(4), pp. 995–1006.

Al Shaer, L., Walsby, E., Gilkes, A., Tonks, A., Walsh, V., Mills, K., Burnett, A., & Rowntree, C. (2008). Heat shock protein 90 inhibition is cytotoxic to primary AML cells expressing mutant FLT3 and results in altered downstream signaling. *Br J Haematol,* May;141(4), pp. 483–493.

Ashley, D.M., Bol, S.J., & Kannourakis G. (1994). Human bone marrow stromal cell contact and soluble factors have different effects on the survival and proliferation of paediatric B-lineage acute lymphoblastic leukaemic blasts. *Leuk Res,* May;18(5), pp. 337–346.

Auclair, D., Miller, D., Yatsula, V., Pickett, W., Carter, C., Chang, Y., Zhang, X., Wilkie, D., Burd, A., Shi, H., Rocks, S., Gedrich, R., Abriola, L., Vasavada, H., Lynch, M., Dumas, J., Trail, P.A., & Wilhelm, S.M. (2007). Antitumor activity of sorafenib in FLT3-driven leukemic cells. *Leukemia,* Mar;21(3), pp. 439–445.

Azam, M., Latek, R. R. & Daley, G. Q. (2003). Mechanism of autoinhibition and STI-571/imatinib resistance revealed by mutagenesis of BCR-ABL. *Cell,* Mar 21;112(6), pp. 831–843.

Bagrintseva, K., Schwab, R., Kohl, T.M., Schnittger, S., Eichenlaub, S., Ellwart, J.W., Hiddemann, W., & Spiekermann, K. (2004). Mutations in the tyrosine kinase domain of FLT3 define a new molecular mechanism of acquired drug resistance to PTK inhibitors in FLT3-ITD-transformed hematopoietic cells. *Blood,* Mar 15;103(6), pp. 2266–2275.

Barry, E.V., Clark, J.J., Cools, J., Roesel, J., & Gilliland, D.G. (2007). Uniform sensitivity of FLT3 activation loop mutants to the tyrosine kinase inhibitor midostaurin. *Blood,* Dec 15;110(13), pp. 4476–4479.

Bojko, P., Pawloski, D., Stellberg, W., Schroder, J.K., & Seeber, S. (2002). Flt3 ligand and thrombopoietin serum levels during peripheral blood stem cell mobilization with chemotherapy and recombinant human glycosylated granulocyte colony-stimulating factor (rhu-G-CSF, lenograstim) and after high-dose chemotherapy. *Ann Hematol,* Sep;81(9), pp. 522–528.

Bradeen, H.A., Eide, C.A., O'Hare, T., Johnson, K.J., Willis, S.G., Lee, F.Y., Druker, B.J., & Deininger, M.W. (2006). Comparison of imatinib mesylate, dasatinib (BMS-354825), and nilotinib (AMN107) in an N-ethyl-N-nitrosourea (ENU)-based mutagenesis screen: high efficacy of drug combinations. *Blood,* 108(7), pp. 2332-8.

Bradstock, K., Bianchi, A., Makrynikola, V., Filshie, R., & Gottlieb, D. (1996). Long-term survival and proliferation of precursor B acute lymphoblastic leukemia cells on human bone marrow stroma. *Leukemia,* May;10(5), pp. 813–820.

Brandts, C.H., Sargin, B., Rode, M., Biermann, C., Lindtner, B., Schwable, J., Buerger, H., Muller-Tidow, C., Choudhary, C., McMahon, M., Berdel, W.E., & Serve, H. (2005). Constitutive activation of Akt by Flt3 internal tandem duplications is necessary for increased survival, proliferation, and myeloid transformation. *Cancer Res,* Nov 1;65(21), pp. 9643–9650.

Breems, D.A., Blokland, E.A., & Ploemacher, R.E. (1997). Stroma-conditioned media improve expansion of human primitive hematopoietic stem cells and progenitor cells. *Leukemia,* Jan;11(1), pp. 142-50.

Breitenbuecher, F., Markova, B., Kasper, S., Carius, B., Stauder, T., Bohmer, F.D., Masson, K., Ronnstrand, L., Huber, C., Kindler, T., & Fischer, T. (2009). A novel molecular mechanism of primary resistance to FLT3-kinase inhibitors in acute myeloid leukemia. *Blood,* Apr 23;113(17), pp. 4063-73.

Burgess, M.R., Skaggs, B.J., Shah, N.P., Lee, F.Y., & Sawyers, C.L. (2005). Comparative analysis of two clinically active BCR-ABL kinase inhibitors reveals the role of conformation-specific binding in resistance. *Proc Natl Acad Sci USA,* Mar 1;102(9), pp. 3395-3400.

Buchdunger, E., Matter, A., & Druker, B.J. (2001). Bcr-Abl inhibition as a modality of CML therapeutics. *Biochim Biophys Acta,* Aug 31;1551(1), pp. M11-M18.

Carter, T. A., Wodicka, L.M., Shah, N.P., Velasco, A.M., Fabian, M.A., Treiber, D.K., Milanov, Z.V., Atteridge, C.E., Biggs, W.H. 3rd, Edeen, P.T., Floyd, M., Ford, J.M., Grotzfeld, R.M., Herrgard, S., Insko, D.E., Mehta, S.A., Patel, H.K., Pao, W., Sawyers, C.L., Varmus, H., Zarrinkar, P.P., & Lockhart, D.J. (2005). Inhibition of drug-resistant mutants of ABL, KIT, and EGF receptor kinases. *Proc. Natl Acad. Sci, USA* Aug 2;102(31), pp. 11011–11016.

Chao, Q., Sprankle, K.G., Grotzfeld, R.M., Lai, A.G., Carter, T.A., Velasco, A.M., Gunawardane, R.N., Cramer, M.D., Gardner, M.F., James, J., Zarrinkar, P.P., Patel, H.K., & Bhagwat, S.S. (2009). Identification of N-(5-tert-butyl-isoxazol-3-yl)-N'{4-[7-(2-morpholin-4-yl-ethoxy)imidazo[2,1-b][1,3]benzothiazol-2-yl]phenyl}urea dihydrochloride (AC220), a uniquely potent, selective, and efficacious FMS-like tyrosine kianse-3 (FLT3) inhibitor. *J Med Chem,* Dec 10;52(23), pp. 7808–7816.

Charbord, P., Tavian, M., Humeau, L., & Peault, B. (1996). Early ontogeny of the human marrow from long bones: an immunohistochemical study of hematopoiesis and its microenvironment. *Blood,* May 15;87(10), pp. 4109-4119.

Cheng Y. & Paz K. (2008). Tandutinib, an oral, small molecule inhibitor of FLT3 for the treatment of AML and other cancer indications. *IDrugs,* Jan;11(1), pp. 46–56.

Choi, H.G., Ren, P., Adrian, F., Sun, F., Lee, H.S., Wang, X., Ding, Q., Zhang, G., Xie, Y., Zhang, J., Liu, Y., Tuntland, T., Warmuth, M., Manley, P.W., Mestan J., Gray N.S., & Sim T. (2010). A type-II kinase inhibitor capable of inhibiting the T315I "gatekeeper" mutant of Bcr-Abl. *J Med Chem,* Aug 12;53(15), pp. 5439-48.

Chu, S.H. & Small, D. (2009). Mechanisms of resistance to FLT3 inhibitors. *Drug Resist Updates,* Apr;12(1-2), pp. 8-16.

Clark, J.J., Cools, J., Curley, D.P., Yu, J.C., Lokker, N.A., Giese, N.A., & Gilliland, D.G. (2004). Variable sensitivity of FLT3 activation loop mutations to the small molecule tyrosine kinase inhibitor MLN518. *Blood,* Nov 1;104(9), pp. 2867–2872.

Cools, J., Mentens, N., Furet, P., Fabbro, D., Clark, J.J., Griffin, J.D., Marynen, P., & Gilliland, D.G. (2004). Prediction of resistance to small molecule FLT3 inhibitors: Implications for molecularly targeted therapy of acute leukemia. *Cancer Res,* Sept 15;64(18), pp. 6385-6389.

Copland, M., Hamilton, A., Elrick, L.J., Baird, J.W., Allan, E.K., Jordanides, N., Barow, M., Mountford, J.C., & Holyoake, T.L. (2006). Dasatinib (BMS-354825) targets an earlier progenitor population than imatinib in primary CML but does not eliminate the quiescent fraction. *Blood,* Jun 1;107(11), pp. 4532–4539.

Corbin, A. S., Buchdunger, E., Pascal, F. & Druker, B. J. (2002). Analysis of the structural basis of specificity of inhibition of the ABL kinase by STI-571. *J. Biol. Chem,* Aug 30;277(35), pp. 32214–32219.

Cowan-Jacob, S. W., Guez, V., Fendrich, G., Griffin, J.D., Fabbro, D., Furet, P., Liebetanz, J., Mestan, J., & Manley, P.W. (2004). Imatinib (STI571) resistance in chronic myelogenous leukemia: molecular basis of the underlying mechanisms and potential strategies for treatment. *Mini Rev. Med. Chem,* Mar;4(3), pp. 285–299.

Deininger, M.W., Goldman, J.M., & Melo, JV. (2000). The molecular biology of chronic myeloid leukemia. *Blood,* Nov 15;96(10), pp. 3343-3356. PMID: 11071626.

Druker, B.J., Tamura, S., Buchdunger, E., Ohno, S., Segal, G.M., Fanning, S., Zimmermann, J., & Lydon, N.B. Effects of a selective inhibitor of the Abl tyrosine kinase on the growth of Bcr-Abl positive cells. (1996). *Nat Med,* May;2(5), pp. 561-566.

Despars, G. & O'Neill, H.C. (2006). Splenic endothelial cell lines support development of dendritic cells from bone marrow. *Stem Cells,* Jun;24(6), pp. 1496–1504.

Donato, N. J., Wu, J.Y., Stapley, J., Gallick, G., Lin, H., Arlinghaus, R., & Talpaz, M. (2003). BCR-ABL independence and LYN kinase overexpression in chronic myelogenous leukemia cells selected for resistance to STI571. *Blood,* Jan 15;101(2), pp. 690–698.

Engler, J.R., Frede, A., Saunders, V.A., Zannettino, A.C., Hughes, T.P., & White, D.L. (2010). Chronic myeloid leukemia CD34+ cells have reduced uptake of imatinib due to low OCT-1 activity. *Leukemia,* Apr;24(4), pp. 765-70.

Fancelli, D., Moll J., Varasi, M., Bravo, R., Artico, R., Berta, D., Bindi, S., Cameron, A., Candiani, I., Cappella, P., Carpinelli, P., Croci, W., Forte, B., Giorgini, M.L., Klapwijk, J., Marsiglio, A., Pesenti, E., Rocchetti, M., Roletto, F., Severino, D., Soncini, C., Storici, P., Tonani, R., Zugnoni, P., & Vianello, P. (2006). 1, 4, 5, 6-Tetrahydropyrrolo[3, 4-c]pyrazoles: identification of a potent aurora kinase inhibitor with a favorable antitumor kinase inhibition profile. *J. Med. Chem,* Nov 30;49(24), pp. 7247–7251.

Fiedler, W., Mesters, R., Tinnefeld, H., Loges, S., Staib, P., Duhrsen, U., Flasshove, M., Ottmann, O.G., Jung, W., Cavalli, F., Kuse, R., Thomalla, J., Serve, H., O'Farrell, A.M., Jacobs, M., Brega, N.M., Scigalla, P., Hossfeld, D.K., & Berdel, W.E. (2003). A phase 2 clinical study of SU5416 in patients with refractory acute myeloid leukemia. *Blood,* Oct 15;102(8), pp. 2763–2767.

Fiedler, W., Serve, H., Dohner, H., Schwittay, M., Ottmann, O.G., O'Farrell, A.M., Bello, C.L., Allred, R., Manning, W.C., Cherrington, J.M., Louie, S.G., Hong, W., Brega, N.M., Massimini, G., Scigalla, P., Berdel, W.E., & Hossfeld, D.K. (2005). A Phase I study of SU11248 in the treatment of patients with refractory or resistant acute myeloid leukemia (AML) or not amenable to conventional therapy for the disease. *Blood,* Feb 1;105(3), pp. 968–993.

Furukawa, Y., Vu, H.A., Akutsu, M., Odgerel, T., Izumi, T., Tsunoda, S., Matsuo, Y., Kirito, K., Sato, Y., Mano, H., & Kano, Y. (2007). Divergent cytotoxic effects of PKC412 in combination with conventional antileukemic agents in FLT3 mutation-positive versus –negative leukemia cell lines. *Leukemia,* May;21(5), pp. 1005-1014.

Galban, S., Hwang, C., Rumble, J.M., Oetien, K.A., Wright, C.W., Boudreault, A., Durkin, J., Gillard, J.W., Jaquith, J.B., Morris, S.J., & Duckett, C.S. (2009). Cytoprotective effects of IAPs revealed by a small molecule antagonist. *Biochem J,* Feb 1;417(3), pp. 765–771.

Gambacorti-Passerini, C., Barni, R., le Coutre, P., Zucchetti, M., Cabrita, G., Cleris, L., Rossi, F., Gianazza, E., Brueggen, J., Cozens, R., Pioltelli, P., Pogliani, E., Corneo, G., Formelli, F., & D'Incalci, M. (2000). Role of alpha1 acid glycoprotein in the in vivo resistance of human BCR-ABL (+) leukemic cells to the abl inhibitor STI571. *J Natl Cancer Inst,* Oct 18;92(20), pp. 1641-50.

Giles, F.J., Cortes, J., Jones, D., Bergstrom, D., Kantarjian, H., & Freedman, S.J. (2007). MK-0457, a novel kinase inhibitor, is active in patients with chronic myeloid leukemia or acute lymphocytic leukemia with the T315I BCR-ABL mutation. *Blood,* Jan 15;109(2), pp. 500-2.

Giles, F.J., Stopeck, A.T., Silverman, L.R., Lancet, J.E., Cooper, M.A., Hannah, A.L., Cherrington, J.M., O'Farrell, A.M., Yuen, H.A., Louie, S.G., Hong, W., Cortes, J.E., Verstovsek, S., Albitar, M., O'Brien, S.M., Kantarjian, H.M., & Karp, J.E. (2003). SU5416, a small molecule tyrosine kinase receptor inhibitor, has biologic activity in patients with refractory acute myeloid leukemia or myelodysplastic syndromes. *Blood,* Aug 1;102(3), pp. 795–801.

Golas, J. M., Arndt, K., Etienne, C., Lucas, J., Nardin, D., Gibbons, J., Frost, P., Ye, F., Boschelli, D.H., & Boschelli, F. (2003). SKI-606, a 4-anilino-3-quinolinecarbonitrile dual inhibitor of SRC and ABL kinases, is a potent antiproliferative agent against chronic myelogenous leukemia cells in culture and causes regression of K562 xenografts in nude mice. *Cancer Res,* Jan 15;63(2), pp. 375–381.

Goldman, J.M. & Melo, J.V. (2003). Chronic myeloid leukemia-advances in biology and new approaches to treatment. *N Engl J Med* Oct 9;349(15):1451-64.

Gorre, M. E., Mohammed, M., Ellwood, K., Hsu, N., Paquette, R., Rao, P.N., & Sawyers, C.L. (2001). Clinical resistance to STI-571 cancer therapy caused by BCR-ABL gene mutation or amplification. *Science,* Aug 3;293(5531), pp. 876–880.

Gozgit, J.M., Wong, M.J., Wardwell, S., Tyner, J.W., Loriaux, M.M., Mohemmad, Q.K., Narasimhan, N.I., Shakespeare, W.C., Wang, F., Druker, B.J., Clackson, T., Rivera, V.M. (2011). Potent activity of Ponatinib (AP24534) in models of FLT3-driven acute myeloid leukemia and other hematologic malignancies. *Mol Cancer Ther,* Jun;10(6), pp. 1028-1035.

Guerrouahen, B.S., Futami, M., Vaklavas, C., Kanerva, J., Whichard, Z.L., Nwawka, K., Blanchard, E.G., Lee, F.Y., Robinson, L.J., Arceci, R., Kornblau, S.M., Wieder, E., Cayre, Y.E., & Corey, S.J. (2010). Dasatinib inhibits the growth of molecularly heterogeneous myeloid leukemias. *Clin Cancer Res,* Feb 15;16(4), pp. 1149–1158.

Harrison, P.R., Nibbs, R.J., Bartholomew, C., O'Prey, J., Qiu, J., Walker, M., Clark, A.M., Leslie, N., & Ostertag, W. (1997). Molecular mechanisms involved in long-term maintenance of erythroleukaemia cells by stromal cells. *Leukemia,* Apr;11:(suppl 3), pp. 474-477.

Heidel, F., Solem, F.K., Breitenbuecher, F., Lipka, D.B., Kasper, S., Thiede, M.H., Brandts, C., Serve, H., Roesel, J., Giles, F., Feldman, E., Ehninger, G., Schiller, G.J., Nimer, S., Stone, R.M., Wang, Y., Kindler, T., Cohen, P.S., Huber, C., & Fischer, T. (2006). Clinical resistance to the kinase inhibitor PKC412 in acute myeloid leukemia by mutation of Asn-676 in the FLT3 tyrosine kinase domain. *Blood,* Jan 1;107(1), pp. 293-300.

Hennequin, L. F., Allen, J., Breed, J., Curwen, J., Fennell, M., Green, T.P., Lambert-van der Brempt, C., Morgentin, R., Norman, R.A., Olivier, A., Otterbein, L., Ple, P.A., Warin, N., & Costello, G. (2006). N-(5-Chloro-1, 3-benzodioxol-4-yl)-7-[2-(4-methylpiperazin-1-yl)ethoxy]-5- (tetrahydro-2H-pyran-4-yloxy)quinazolin-4-amine, a novel, highly selective, orally available, dual-specific c-Src/Abl kinase inhibitor. *J. Med. Chem,* Nov 2;49(22), pp. 6465–6488.

Hochhaus, A., Kreil, S., Corbin, A.S., La Rosee, P., Muller, M.C., Lahaye, T., Hanfstein, B., Schoch, C., Cross, N.C., Berger, U., Gschaidmeier, H., Druker, B.J., & Hehlmann, R. (2002). Molecular and chromosomal mechanisms of resistance to imatinib (STI571) therapy. *Leukemia,* Nov;16(11), pp. 2190–2196.

Hofmann, W. K., Komor, M., Wassmann, B., Jones, L.C., Gschaidmeier, H., Hoelzer, D., Koeffler, H.P., & Ottmann, O.G. (2003). Presence of the BCR-ABL mutation Glu255Lys prior to STI571 (imatinib) treatment in patients with Ph+ acute lymphoblastic leukemia. *Blood,* July 15;102(2), pp. 659–661.

Horiike, S., Yokota, S., Nakao, M., Iwai, T., Sasai, Y., Kaneko, H., Taniwaki, M., Kashima, K., Fujii, H., Abe, T., & Misawa, S. (1997). Tandem duplications of the FLT3 receptor gene are associated with leukemic transformation of myelodysplasia. *Leukemia,* Sep;11(9), pp. 1442-1446.

Ikezoe, T., Nishioka, C., Tasaka, T., Yang, Y., Komatsu, N., Togitani, K., Koeffler, H.P., & Taguchi, H. (2006). The antitumor effects of sunitinib (formerly SU11248) against a variety of human hematologic malignancies: enchancement of growth inhibition via inhibition of mammalian target of rapamycin signaling. *Mol. Cancer Ther,* Oct;5(10), pp. 2522-2530.

Jiang, J., Paez, J.G., Lee, J.C., Bo, R., Stone, R.M., DeAngelo, D.J., Galinsky, I., Wolpin, B.M., Jonasova, A., Herman, P., Fox, E.A., Boggon, T.J., Ecki, M.J., Weisberg, E., Griffin, J.D., Gilliland, D.G., Meyerson, M., & Sellers, W.R. (2004). Identifying and characterizing a novel activating mutation of the FLT3 tyrosine kinase in AML. *Blood,* Sep 15;104(6), pp. 1855–1858.

Kancha, R.K., Grundler, R., Peschel, C., & Duyster, J. (2007). Sensitivity toward sorafenib and sunitinib varies between different activating and drug-resistant FLT3-ITD mutations. *Exp Hematol,* Oct;35(10), pp. 1522–1526.

Kantarjian, H., Shah, N.P., Hochhaus, A., Cortes, J., Shah, S., Ayala, M., Moiraghi, B., Shen, Z., Mayer, J., Pasquini, R., Nakamae, H., Huguet, F., Boque, C., Chuah, C., Bleickardt, E., Bradley-Garelik, M.B., Zhu, C., Szatrowski, T., Shapiro, D., & Baccarani, M. (2010) Dasatinib versus imatinib in newly diagnosed chronic-phase chronic myeloid leukemia. *N Engl J Med,* June 17;362(24), pp. 2260-2270.

Kasper, S., Breitenbuecher, F., Hoehn, Y., Heidel, F., Lipka, D.B., Markova, B., Huber, C., Kindler, T., & Fischer, T. (2008). The kinase inhibitor LS104 induces apoptosis, enhances cytotoxic effects of chemotherapeutic drugs and is targeting the receptor tyrosine kinase FLT3 in acute myeloid leukemia. *Leuk Res,* Nov;32(11), pp. 1698–1708.

Kelly, L.M., Liu, Q., Kutok, J.L., Williams, I.R., Boulton, C.L., & Gilliland, D.G. (2002a). FLT3 internal tandem duplication mutations associated with human acute myeloid leukemias induce myeloproliferative disease in a murine bone marrow transplant model. *Blood,* Jan 1;99(1), pp. 310–318.

Kelly, L.M., Yu, J.C., Boulton, C.L., Apatira, M.M., Li, J., Sullivan, C.M., Williams, I., Amaral, S.M., Curley, D.P., Duclos, N., Neuberg, D., Scarborough, R.M., Pandey, A., Hollenbach, S., Abe, K., Lokker, N.A., Gilliland, D.G., & Giese, N.A. (2002b). CT53518, a novel selective FLT3 antagonist for the treatment of acute myelogenous leukemia. *Cancer Cell,* Jun;1(5), pp. 421–432.

Kim, K.T., Baird, K., Ahn, J.Y., Meltzer, P., Lilly, M., Levis, M.,& Small, D. (2005). Pim-1 is up-regulated by constitutively activated FLT3 and plays a role in FLT3-mediated cell survival. *Blood,* Feb 15;105(4), pp. 1759–1767.

Kim, K.T., Levis, M., & Small, D. (2006). Constitutively activated FLT3 phosphorylates BAD partially through pim-1. *Br J Haematol,* Sept;134(5), pp. 500–509.

Kindler, T., Breitenbuecher, F., Kasper, S., Estey, E., Giles, F., Feldman, E., Ehninger, G., Schiller, G., Klimek, V., Nimer, S.D., Gratwohl, A., Choudhary, C.R., Mueller-Tidow, C., Serve, H., Gschaidmeier, H., Cohen, P.S., Huber, C., & Fischer, T. (2005). Identification of a novel activating mutation (Y842C) within the activation loop of FLT3 in patients with acute myeloid leukemia (AML). *Blood,* Jan 1;105(1), pp. 335–340.

Kiyoi, H., Towatari, M., Yokota, S., Hamaguchi, M., Ohno, R., Saito, H., & Naoe, T. (1998). Internal tandem duplication of the FLT3 gene is a novel modality of elongation mutation which causes constitutive activation of the product. *Leukemia,* Sep;12(9), pp. 1333-1337.

Knapper, S., Burnett, A.K., Littlewood, T., Kell, W.J., Agrawal, S., Chopra, R., Clark, R., Levis, M.J., & Small, D. (2006). A phase 2 trial of the FLT3 inhibitor lestaurtinib

(CEP701) as first line treatment for older patients with acute myeloid leukemia not considered fit for intensive chemotherapy. *Blood,* Nov 15;108(10), pp. 3262–3270.

Kohl, T.M., Hellinger, C., Ahmed, F., Buske, C., Hiddermann, W., Bohlander, S.K., & Spiekermann, K. (2007). BH3 mimetic ABT-737 neutralizes resistance to FLT3 inhibitor treatment mediated by FLT3independent expression of BCL2 in primary AML blasts. *Leukemia,* Aug;21(8), pp. 1763–1772.

Kondo, M., Horibe, K., Takahashi, Y., Matsumoto, K., Fukuda, M., Inaba, J., Kato, K., Kojima, S., & Matsuyama, T. (1999). Prognostic value of internal tandem duplication of the FLT3 gene in childhood acute myelogenous leukemia. *Med Pediatr Oncol,* Dec;33(6), pp. 525-529.

Konopleva, M., Konoplev, S., Hu, W., Zaritskey, A.Y., Afanasiev, B.V., & Andreeff, M. (2002). Stromal cells prevent apoptosis of AML cells by up-regulation of anti-apoptotic proteins. *Leukemia,* Sept;1(9)6, pp. 1713–1724.

Kornblau, S.M., Womble, M., Qiu, Y.H., Jackson, C.E., Chen, W., Konopleva, M., Estey, E.H., & Andreeff, M. (2006). Simultaneous activation of multiple signal transduction pathways confers poor prognosis in acute myelogenous leukemia. *Blood,* Oct 1;108(7), pp. 2358–2365.

Kornblau, S.M., Singh, N., Qiu, Y., Chen, W., Zhang, N., & Coombes, K.R. (2010). Highly phosphorylated FOXO3A is an adverse prognostic factor in acute myeloid leukemia. *Clin Cancer Res,* Mar 15;16(6), pp. 1865–1874.

Kumagai, M., Manabe, A., Pui, C.H., Behm, F.G., Raimondi, S.C., Hancock, M.L., Mahmoud, H., Crist, W.M., & Campana, D. (1996). Stroma-supported culture in childhood B-lineage acute lymphoblastic leukemia cells predicts treatment outcome. *J Clin Invest,* Feb 1;97(3), pp. 755–760.

Kuroda, J., Puthalakath, H., Cragg, M.S., Kelly, P.N., Bouillet, P., Huang, D.C., Kimura, S., Ottmann, O.G., Druker, B.J., Villunger, A., Roberts, A.W.,& Strasser, A. (2006). Bim and Bad mediate imatinib-induced killing of Bcr/Abl+ leukemic cells, and resistance due to their loss is overcome by a BH3 mimetic. *Proc Natl Acad Sci USA,* Oct 3;103(40), pp. 14907-14912.

Lagneaux, L., Delforge, A., Bron, D., De Bruyn, C., & Stryckmans, P. (1998). Chronic lymphocytic leukemic B cells but not normal B cells are rescued from apoptosis by contact with normal bone marrow stromal cells. *Blood,* Apr 1;91(7), pp. 2387–2396.

Lagneaux, L., Delforge, A., De Bruyn, C., Bernier, M., & Bron, D. (1999). Adhesion to bone marrow stroma inhibits apoptosis of chronic lymphocytic leukemia cells. *Leukemia Lymphoma,* Nov;35(5-6), pp. 445–453.

le Coutre, P., Tassi, E., Varella-Garcia, M., Barni, R., Mologni, L., Cabrita, G., Marchesi, E., Supino, R., & Gambacorti-Passerini, C. (2000). Induction of resistance to the Abelson inhibitor STI571 in human leukemic cells through gene amplification. *Blood,* Mar 1;95(5), pp. 1758–1766.

Leslie, N.R., O'Prey, J., Bartholomew, C., & Harrison, P.R. (1998). An activating mutation in the kit receptor abolishes the stroma requirement for growth of ELM erythroleukemia cells, but does not prevent their differentiation in response to erythropoietin. *Blood,* Dec 15;92(12), pp. 4798-4807.

Levis, M., Allebach, J., Tse, K.F., Zheng, R., Baldwin, B.R., Smith, B.D., Jones-Bolin S., Ruggeri B., Dionne C.,& Small D. (2002). A FLT3-targeted tyrosine kinase inhibitor is cytotoxic to leukemia cells in vitro and in vivo. *Blood,* Jun 1;99(11), pp. 3885–3891.

Levis, M., Pham, R., Smith, B.D., & Small, D. (2004). In vitro studies of a FLT3 inhibitor combined with chemotherapy: sequence of administration is important to achieve synergistic cytotoxic effects. *Blood,* Aug 15;104(4), pp. 1145-1150.

Lierman, E., Lahortiga, I., Van Miegroet , H., Mentens, N., Marynen, P., & Cools, J. (2007). The ability of sorafenib to inhibit oncogenic PDGFRbeta and FLT3 mutants and overcome resistance to other small molecule inhibitors. *Haematologica,* Jan;92(1), pp. 27–34.

Liesveld, J.L., Harbol, A.W., & Abboud, C.N. (1996). Stem cell factor and stromal cell co-culture prevent apoptosis in a subculture of the megakaryoblastic cell line, UT-7. *Leuk Res,* Jul;20(7), pp. 591-600.

Litwin, C., Leong, K.G., Zapf, R., Sutherland, H., Naiman, S.C., & Karsan, A. (2002). Role of the microenvironment in promoting angiogenesis in acute myeloid leukemia. *Am J Hematol,* May;70(1), pp. 22-30.

Liu, Y. & Gray, N.S. (2006). Rational design of inhibitors that bind to inactive kinase conformations. *Nat Chem Biol.* Jul;2(7), pp. 358-64.

Liu, W.M., Stimson, L.A., & Joel, S.P. (2002). The in vitro activity of the tyrosine kinase inhibitor STI571 in BCR-ABL positive chronic myeloid leukaemia cells: synergistic interactions with anti-leukaemic agents. *Br J Cancer,* May 6;86(9), pp. 1472-8.

Liu, Z., Sun, C., Olejniczak E.T.,Meadows R.P., Betz S.F., Oost T., Herrmann J., Wu J.C., & Fesik S.W. (2000). Structural basis for binding of Smac/DIABLO to the XIAP BIR3 domain. *Nature,* Dec 21-28;408(6815), pp. 1004-8.

Lockton, J.A., Smethurst, D., Macpherson, M., Tootell, R., Marshall, A.L., Clack, G., & Gallagher, N.J. (2005). Phase I ascending single and multiple dose studies to assess the safety, tolerability and pharmacokinetics of AZD0530, a highly selective, dual-specific SRC-ABL inhibitor. *J Clin Oncol ASCO Ann Meet Proc,* 23(16S), Part I of II (June 1 Supplement), 3125a.

Lopes de Menezes, D.E., Peng, J., Garrett, E.N., Louie, S.G., Lee, S.H., Wiesmann, M., Tang, Y., Shephard, L., Goldbeck, C., Oei, Y., Ye H., Aukerman, S.L., & Heise, C. (2005). CHIR-258: A potent inhibitor of FLT3 kinase in experimental tumor xenograft models of human acute myelogenous leukemia. *Clin Cancer Res,* July 15;11(14), pp. 5281–5291.

Lyman, S.D., Seaberg, M., Hanna, R., Zappone, J., Brasel, K., Abkowitz, J.L., Prchal, J.T., Schultz, J.C., & Shahidi, N.T. (1995). Plasma/serum levels of flt3 ligand are low in normal individuals and highly elevated in patients with Fanconi anemia and acquired aplastic anemia. *Blood,* Dec 1;86(11), pp. 4091–4096.

Mahon, F. X., Deininger, M.W., Schultheis, B., Chabrol, J., Reiffers, J., Goldman, J.M., & Melo, J.V. (2000). Selection and characterization of BCR-ABL positive cell lines with differential sensitivity to the tyrosine kinase inhibitor STI571: diverse mechanisms of resistance. *Blood,* Aug 1;96(3), pp. 1070–1079.

Manley, P. W., Cowan-Jacob, S.W., Buchdunger, E., Fabbro, D., Fendrich, G., Furet, P., Meyer, T., & Zimmermann, J. (2002). Imatinib: a selective tyrosine kinase inhibitor. *Eur J Cancer,* Sep;38(Suppl 5), pp. S19–S27.

Mattison, R.J., Ostler, K.R., Locke, F.L., & Godley, L.A. (2007). Implications of FLT3 mutations in the therapy of acute myeloid leukemia. *Rev Recent Clin Trials,* May;2(2), pp. 135-141.

Metzelder, S., Wang, Y, Wollmer, E., Wanzel, M., Teichler, S., Chaturvedi, A., Eilers, M., Enghofer, E., Neubauer, A., & Burchert, A. (2009). Compassionate use of sorafenib in FLT3-ITDpositive acute myeloid leukemia: sustained regression before and after allogeneic stem cell transplantation. *Blood,* Jun 25;113(26), pp. 6567–6571.

Michor, F., Hughes, T.P., Iwasa, Y., Branford, S., Shah, N.P., Sawyers, C.L., & Nowak, M.A. (2005). Dynamics of chronic myeloid leukemia. *Nature,* June 30;435(7046), pp. 1267–1270. PMID: 15988530

Mohi, M.G., Boulton, C., Gu, T.L., Sternberg, D.W., Neuberg, D., Griffin, J.D., Gilliland, D.G., & Neel, B.G. (2004). Combination of rapamycin and protein tyrosine kinase (PTK) inhibitors for the treatment of leukemias caused by oncogenic PTKs. *Proc Natl Acad Sci USA,* Mar 2;101(9), pp. 3130-3135.

Mollgard, L., Deneberg, S., Nahi, H., Bengtzen, S., Jonsson-Videsater, K., Fioretos, T., Andersson, A., Paul C., & Lehmann, S. (2008). The FLT3 inhibitor PKC412 in combination with cytostatic drugs in vitro in acute myeloid leukemia. *Cancer Chemother Pharmacol,* Aug;62(3), pp. 439-448.

Mony, U., Jawad, M., Seedhouse, C., Russell, N., & Pallis, M. (2008). Resistance to FLT3 inhibition in an in vitro model of primary AML cells with a stem cell phenotype in a defined microenvironment. *Leukemia,* Jul;22(7), pp. 1395-1401.

Nagar, B., Bornmann, W.G., Pellicena, P., Schindler, T., Veach, D.R., Miller, W.T., Clarkson, B., & Kuriyan, J. (2002). Crystal structures of the kinase domain of c-Abl in complex with the small molecule inhibitors PD173955 and imatinib (STI-571). *Cancer Res,* Aug 1;62(15), pp. 4236–4243.

Nakao, M., Yokota, S., Iwai, T., Kaneko, H., Horiike, S., Kashima, K., Sonoda, Y., Fujimoto, T., & Misawa, S. (1996). Internal tandem duplication of the FLT3 gene found in acute myeloid leukemia. *Leukemia,* Dec;10(12), pp. 1911-1918.

Nelson, E.A., Walker, S.R., Weisberg, E., Bar-Natan, M., Barrett, R., Gashin, L.B., Terrell, S., Klitgaard, J.L., Santo, L., Addorio, M.R., Ebert, B.L., Griffin, J.D., & Frank, D.A. (2011). The STAT5 inhibitor pimozide decreases survival of chronic myelogenous leukemia cells resistant to kinase inhibitors. *Blood,* Mar 24;117(12), pp. 3421-9.

Nishioka, C., Ikezoe, T., Yang, J., Takeuchi, S., Koeffler, H.P., & Yokoyama, A. (2008a). MS-275, a novel histone deacetylase inhibitor with selectivity against HDAC1, induces degradation of FLT3 via inhibition of chaperone function of heat shock protein 90 in AML cells. *Leuk Res,* Sept;32(9), pp. 1382-1392.

Nishioka, C., Ikezoe, T., Yang, J., Takeshita, A., Taniguchi, A., Komatsu, N., Togitani, K., Koeffler, H.P., & Yokoyama, A. (2008b). Blockade of MEK/ERK signaling enhances sunitinib-induced growth inhibition and apoptosis of leukemia cells possessing activating mutations of the FLT3 gene. *Leuk Res,* Jun;32(6), pp. 865-872.

O'Farrell, A.M., Abrams, T.J., Yuen, H.A., Ngai, T.J., Louie, S.G., Yee, K.W., Wong, L.M., Hong, W., Lee, L.B., Town, A., Smolich, B.D., Manning, W.C., Murray, L.J., Heinrich, M.C., & Cherrington, J.M. (2003a). SU11248 is a novel FLT3 tyrosine kinase inhibitor with potent activity in vitro and in vivo. *Blood,* May 1;101(9), pp. 3597–3605.

O'Farrell, A.M., Foran, J.M., Fiedler, W., Serve, H., Paquette, R.L., Cooper, M.A., Yuen, H.A., Louie, S.G., Kim, H., Nicholas, S., Heinrich, M.C., Berdel, W.E., Bello, C., Jacobs, M., Scigalla, P., Manning, W.C., Kelsey, S., & Cherrington, J.M. (2003b). An innovative Phase I clinical study demonstrates inhibition of FLT3 phosphorylation by SU11248 in acute myeloid leukemia patients. *Clin Cancer Res,* Nov 15;9(15), pp. 5465–5476.

O'Farrell, A.M., Yuen, H.A., Smolich, B., Hannah, A.L., Louie, S.G., Hong, W., Stopeck, A.T., Silverman, L.R., Lancet, J.E., Karp, J.E., Albitar, M., Cherrington, J.M., & Giles, F.J.

(2004). Effects of SU5416, a small molecule tyrosine kinase receptor inhibitor, on FLT3 expression and phosphorylation in patients with refractory acute myeloid leukemia. *Leuk Res,* Jul;28(7), pp. 679–689.

O'Hare, T., Walters, D.K., Stoffregen, E.P., Sherbenou, D.W., Heinrich, M.C., Deininger, M.W., & Druker, B.J. (2005). Combined Abl inhibitor therapy for minimizing drug resistance in chronic myeloid leukemia: Src/Abl inhibitors are compatible with imatinib. *Clin Cancer Res,* Oct 1;11(19 Pt 1), pp. 6987-6993.

O'Prey, J., Leslie, N., Itoh, K., Ostertag, W., Bartholomew, C., & Harrison, P.R. (1998). Both stroma and stem cell factor maintain long-term growth of ELM erythroleukemia cells, but only stroma prevents erythroid differentiation in response to erythropoietin and interleukin-3. *Blood,* Mar 1;91(5), pp. 1548-1555.

Pluk, H., Dorey, K., & Superti-Furga, G. (2002). Autoinhibition of c-ABL. *Cell,* Jan 25;108(2), pp. 247–259.

Pratz, K. & Levis, M. (2008). Incorporating FLT3 inhibitors into acute myeloid leukemia treatment regimens. *Leuk Lymphoma* May;49(5), pp. 852–863.

Pratz, K.W., Cortes, J., Roboz, G.J., Rao, N., Arowojolu, O., Stine, A., Shiotsu, Y., Shudo, A., Akinaga, S., Small, D., Karp, J.E., & Levis, M. (2009). A pharmacodynamic study of the FLT3 inhibitor KW-2449 yields insight into the basis for clinical response. *Blood,* Apr 23;113(17), pp. 3938–3946.

Pratz, K., Sato, T., Murphy, K.M., Stine, A., Rajkhowa, T., & Levis, M. (2010). FLT3-mutant allelic burden and clinical status are predictive of response to FLT3 inhibitors in AML. *Blood,* Feb 18;115(7), pp. 1425-32.

Puttini, M., Coluccia, A.M., Boschelli, F., Cleris, L., Marchesi, E., Donella-Deana, A., Ahmed, S., Redaelli, S., Piazza, R., Magistroni, V., Andreoni, F., Scapozza, L., Formelli, F., & Gambacorti-Passerini, C. (2006). *In vitro* and *in vivo* activity of SKI-606, a novel Src-Abl inhibitor, against imatinib resistant Bcr-Abl+ neoplastic cells. *Cancer Res,* Dec 1;66(23), pp. 11314–11322.

Ray, A., Cowan-Jacob, S.W., Manley, PW, Mestan, J, & Griffin, JD. (2007). Identification of BCR-ABL point mutations conferring resistance to the Abl kinase inhibitor AMN107 (nilotinib) by a random mutagenesis study. *Blood,* Jun 1;109(11), pp. 5011–5015.

Rafii, S., Mohle, R., Shapiro, F., Frey, B.M., & Moore, M.A. (1997). Regulation of hematopoiesis by microvascular endothelium. *Leuk Lymphoma,* Nov;27(5-6), pp. 375-386.

Recher, C., Beyne-Rauzy, O., Demur, C., Chicanne, G., Dos Santos, C., Mas, V.M., Benzaquen, D., Laurent, G., Huguet, F., & Payrastre, B. (2005). Antileukemic activity of rapamycin in acute myeloid leukemia. *Blood,* Mar 15;105(6), pp. 2527–2534.

Reindl, C., Bagrintseva, K., Vempati, S., Schnittger, S., Ellwart, J.W., Wenig, K., Hopfner, K.P., Hiddemann, W., & Spiekermann K. (2006). Point mutations in the juxtamembrane domain of FLT3 define a new class of activating mutations in AML. *Blood,* May 1;107(9), pp. 3700–3707.

Rocnik, J.L., Okabe, R., Yu, J.C., Lee, B.H., Giese, N., Schenkein, D.P., & Gilliland, D.G. (2006). Roles of tyrosine 589 and 591 in STAT5 activation and transformation mediated by FLT3-ITD. *Blood,* Aug 15;108(4), pp. 1339–1345.

Roche-Lestienne, C., Soenen-Cornu, V., Grardel-Duflos, N., Lai, J.L., Philippe, N., Facon, T., Fenaux, P., & Preidhomme, C. (2002). Several types of mutations of the ABL gene can be found in chronic myeloid leukemia patients resistant to STI571, and they can pre-exist to the onset of treatment. *Blood,* Aug 1;100(3), pp. 1014–1018.

Roeder, I., Horn, M., Glauche, I., Hochhaus, A., Mueller, M.C., & Loeffler, M. (2006). Dynamic modeling of imatinib-treated chronic myeloid leukemia: functional insights and clinical implications. *Nature Med,* Oct;12(10), pp. 1181–1184.

Rombouts, W.J., Blokland, I., Lowenberg, B., & Ploemacher, R.E. (2000). Biological characteristics and prognosis of adult acute myeloid leukemia with internal tandem duplications in the FLT3 gene. *Leukemia,* Apr;14(4), pp. 675-683.

Rourmiantsev, S., Shah, N.P., Gorre, M.E., Nicoll, J., Brasher, B.B., Sawyers, C.L., & Van Etten, R.A. (2002). Clinical resistance to the kinase inhibitor STI-571 in chronic myeloid leukemia by mutation of Tyr-253 in the ABL kinase domain P-loop. *Proc. Natl Acad. Sci. USA,* Aug 6;99(16), pp. 10700–10705.

Saglio, G., Kim, D.W., Issaragrisil, S., le Coutre, P., Etienne, G., Lobo, C., Pasquini, R., Clark, R.E., Hochhaus, A., Hughes, T.P., Gallagher, N., Hoenekopp, A., Dong, M., Haque, A., Larson, R.A., & Kantarjian, H.M.; ENESTnd Investigators. (2010) Nilotinib versus imatinib for newly diagnosed chronic myeloid leukemia. *N Engl J Med,* June 17;362(24), pp. 2251-2259.

Schindler, T., Bornmann, W., Pellicena, P., Miller, W.T., Clarkson, B., & Kuriyan, J. (2000). Structural mechanism for STI-571 inhibition of Abelson tyrosine kinase. *Science,* Sep 15;289(5486), pp. 1938–1942.

Shah, N. P., Nicoll, J.M., Nagar, B., Gorre, M.E., Paquette, R.L., Kuriyan, J., & Sawyers C.L. (2002). Multiple BCR-ABL kinase domain mutations confer polyclonal resistance to the tyrosine kinase inhibitor imatinib (STI571) in chronic phase and blast crisis chronic myeloid leukemia. *Cancer Cell,* Aug;2(2), pp. 117–125.

Shah, N.P., Tran, C., Lee, F.Y., Chen, P., Norris, D., & Sawyers, C.L. (2004). Overriding imatinib resistance with a novel ABL kinase inhibitor. *Science,* Jun 16;305(5682), pp. 399-401.

Shaked, Y., Cervi, D., Neuman, M., Chen, L., Klement, G., Michaud, C.R., Haeri, M., Pak, B.J., Kerbel, R.S., & Ben-David, Y. (2005). The splenic microenvironment is a source of proangiogenesis/inflammatory mediators accelerating the expansion of murine erythroleukemic cells. *Blood,* Jun 1;105(11), pp. 4500–4507.

Shankar, D.B., Li, J., Tapang, P., Owen, J., Pease, L.J., Dai, Y., Wei, R.Q., Albert, D.H., Bouska, J.J., Osterling, D.J., Guo, J., Marcotte, P.A., Johnson, E.F., Soni, N., Hartandi, K., Michaelides, M.R., Davidsen, S.K., Priceman, S.J., Chang, J.C., Rhodes, K., Shah, N., Moore, T.B., Sakamoto K.M., & Glaser K.B. (2007). ABT-869, a multitargeted receptor tyrosine kinase inhibitor: inhibition of FLT3 phosphorylation and signaling in acute myeloid leukemia. *Blood,* Apr 15;109(8), pp. 3400–3408.

Shih, C.C., Hu, M.C., Hu, J., Medeiros, J., & Forman, S.J. (1999). Long-term *ex vivo* maintenance and expansion of transplantable human hematopoietic stem cells. *Blood,* Sept 1;94(5), pp. 1623-36.

Shiotsu, Y., Kiyoi, H., Ishikawa, Y., Tanizaki, R., Shimizu, M., Umehara, H., Ishii, K., Mori, Y., Ozeki, K., Minami, Y., Abe, A., Maeda, H., Akiyama, T., Kanda, Y., Sato, Y., Akinaga, S., & Naoe, T. (2009). KW-2449, a novel multikinase inhibitor, suppresses the growth of leukemia cells with FLT3 mutations or T315I-mutated BCR/ABL translocation. *Blood,* Aug 20;114(8), pp. 1607–1617.

Smith, B.D., Levis, M., Beran, M., Giles, F., Kantarjian, H., Berg, K., Murphy, K.M., Dauses, T., Allebach, J., & Small, D. (2004). Single-agent CEP-701, a novel FLT3 inhibitor, shows biologic and clinical activity in patients with relapsed or refractory acute myeloid leukemia. *Blood,* May 15;103(10), pp. 3669–3676.

Soverini, S., Martinelli, G., Rosti, G., Bassi, S., Amabile, M., Poerio, A., Giannini, B., Trabacchi, E., Castagnetti, F., Testoni, N., Luatti, S., de Vivo, A., Cilloni, D., Izzo, B., Fava, M., Abruzzese, E., Alberti, D., Pane, F., Saglio, G., & Baccarani, M. (2005). ABL mutations in late chronic phase chronic myeloid leukemia patients with up-front cytogenetic resistance to imatinib are associated with a greater likelihood of progression to blast crisis and shorter survival: a study by the GIMEMA Working Party on Chronic Myeloid Leukemia. *J. Clin. Oncol,* Jun 20;23(18), pp. 4100–4109.

Stirewalt, D.L. & Radich, J.P. (2003). The role of FLT3 in hematopoietic malignancies. *Nat Rev Cancer* Sep;3(9), pp. 650-65.

Stolzel, F., Steudel, C., Oelschlagel, U., Mohr, B., Koch, S., Ehninger, G., & Thiede, C. (2010). Mechanisms of resistance against FLT3ITD positive human acute myeloid leukemia cells. *Ann Hematol,* Jul;89(7), pp. 653-662.

Stone, R.M., De Angelo, J., Galinsky, I., Estey, E., Klimek, V., Grandin, W., Lebwohl, D., Yap, A., Cohen, P., Fox, E., Neuberg, D., Clark, J., Gilliland, D.G., & Griffin, J.D. (2004). *Ann Hematol,* 83(Suppl 1), pp. S89-90.

Strasser, A. (2005). The role of BH3-only proteins in the immune system. *Nat Rev Immunol,* Mar;5(3), pp. 189-200. PMID: 15719025

Tabe, Y., Jin, L., Tsutsumi-Ishii, Y., Xu, Y., McQueen, T., Priebe, W., Mills, G.B., Ohsaka, A., Nagaoka, I., Andreeff, M., & Konopleva, M. (2007). Activation of integrin-linked kinase is a critical prosurvival pathway induced in leukemic cells by bone marrow-derived stromal cells. *Cancer Research,* Jan 15;67(2), pp. 684-694.

Talpaz, M., Shah, N.P., Kantarjian, H., Donato, N., Nicoll, J., Paquette, R., Cortes, J., O'Brien, S., Nicaise, C., Bleickardt, E., Blackwood-Chirchir, M.A., Lyer, V., Chen, T.T., Huang, F., Decillis, A.P., & Sawyers, C.L. (2006). Dasatinib in imatinib-resistant Philadelphia chromosome-positive leukemias. *N Eng J Med,* Jun 15;354(24), pp. 2531-2541.

Verfaillie, CM. (1993). Soluble factor(s) produced by human bone marrow stroma increase cytokine-induced proliferation and maturation of primitive hematopoietic progenitors while preventing their terminal differentiation. *Blood,* Oct 1;82(7), pp. 2045-53.

Von Bubnoff, N., Schneller, F., Peschel, C. & Duyster, J. (2002). *BCR-ABL* gene mutations in relation to clinical resistance of Philadelphia-chromosome-positive leukaemia to STI571: a prospective study. *Lancet,* Feb 9;359(9305), pp. 487–491.

Von Bubnoff, N., Manley, P.W., Mestan, J., Sanger, J., Peschel, C., & Duyster, J. (2006). BCR-ABL resistance screening predicts a limited spectrum of point mutations to be associated with clinical resistance to the Abl kinase inhibitor nilotinib (AMN107). *Blood,* Aug 15;108(4), pp. 1328-1333.

Von Bubnoff, N., Engh, R.A., Aberg, E., Sanger, J., Peschel, C., & Duyster, J. (2009). FMS-like tyrosine kinase 3-internal tandem duplication tyrosine kinase inhibitors display a nonoverlapping profile of resistance mutations in vitro. *Cancer Res,* Apr 1;69(7), pp. 3032–3041.

Weisberg, E. & Griffin, J.D. (2000). Mechanism of resistance to the ABL tyrosine kinase inhibitor STI571 in BCR/ABL-transformed hematopoietic cell lines. *Blood,* Jun 1;95(11), pp. 3498-505.

Weisberg, E., Manley, P.W., Breitenstein, W., Brüggen, J., Cowan-Jacob, S.W., Ray, A., Huntly, B., Fabbro, D., Fendrich, G., Hall-Meyers, E., Kung, A.L., Mestan, J., Daley, G.Q., Callahan, L., Catley, L., Cavazza, C., Azam, M., Neuberg, D., Wright, R.D., Gilliland, D.G., & Griffin, J.D. (2005). Characterization of AMN107, a selective inhibitor of native and mutant Bcr-Abl. *Cancer Cell,* Feb;7(2):129-41. Erratum in: Cancer Cell. 2005 Apr;7(4), pp. 399. Mohammed, Azam [corrected to Azam, Mohammad].

Weisberg, E., Catley, L., Wright, R.D., Moreno, D., Banerji, L., Ray, A., Manley, P.W., Mestan, J.,

Fabbro, D., Jiang, J., Hall-Meyers, E., Callahan, L., DellaGatta, J.L., Kung, A.L., & Griffin, J.D. (2007a). Beneficial effects of combining nilotinib and imatinib in preclinical models of BCR-ABL+ leukemias. *Blood,* Mar 1;109(5), pp. 2112-20.

Weisberg E., Wright R.D., Jiang J., Ray A., Moreno D., Manley P.W., Fabbro D., Hall-Meyers E., Catley L., Podar K., Kung A.L., & Griffin J.D. (2006). Effects of midostaurin, nilotinib, and imatinib against GIST-associated PDGFRA mutants with differential imatinib sensitivity. *Gastroenterology,* Dec;131(6), pp. 1734-42.

Weisberg, E., Boulton, C., Kelly, L.M., Manley, P., Fabbro, D., Meyer, T., Gilliland, D.G., & Griffin, J.D. (2002). Inhibition of mutant FLT3 receptors in leukemia cells by the small molecule tyrosine kinase inhibitor midostaurin. *Cancer Cell,* Jun;1(5), pp. 433-43.

Weisberg, E., Banerji, L., Wright, R.D., Barrett, R., Ray, A., Moreno, D., Catley, L., Jiang, J., Hall-Meyers, E., Sauveur-Michel, M., Stone, R., Galinsky, I., Fox, E., Kung, A.L., & Griffin, J.D. (2008a). Potentiation of antileukemic therapies by the dual PI3K/PDK-1 inhibitor, BAG956: effects on BCR-ABL- and mutant FLT3-expressing cells. *Blood,* Apr 1;111(7), pp. 3723-34.

Weisberg, E., Roesel, J., Bold, G., Furet, P., Jiang, J., Cools, J., Wright, R.D., Nelson, E., Barrett, R., Ray, A., Moreno, D., Hall-Meyers, E., Stone, R., Galinsky, I., Fox, E., Gilliland, G., Daley, J.F., Lazo-Kallanian, S., Kung, A.L., & Griffin, J.D. (2008b). Antileukemic effects of the novel, mutant FLT3 inhibitor NVP-AST487: effects on PKC412-sensitive and –resistant FLT3-expressing cells. *Blood,* Dec 15;112(13), pp. 5161-70.

Weisberg, E., Kung, A.L., Wright, R.D., Moreno, D., Catley, L., Ray, A., Zawel, L., Tran, M., Cools, J., Gilliland, G., Mitsiades, C., McMillin, D.W., Jiang, J., Hall-Meyers, E.,& Griffin, J.D. (2007b). Potentiation of antileukemic therapies by Smac mimetic, LBW242: effects on mutant FLT3-expressing cells. *Mol Cancer Ther,* Jul;6(7), pp. 1951-61.

Weisberg, E., Wright, R.D., McMillin, D.W., Mitsiades, C., Ray, A., Barrett, R., Adamia, S., Stone, R., Galinsky, I., Kung, A.L., & Griffin, J.D. (2008c). Stromal-mediated protection of tyrosine kinase inhibitor-treated BCR-ABL-expressing leukemia cells. *Mol Cancer Ther,* May;7(5), pp. 1121-9.

Weisberg, E., Barrett, R., Liu, Q., Stone, R., Gray, N., & Griffin, J.D. (2009). FLT3 inhibition and mechanisms of drug resistance in mutant FLT3-positive AML. *Drug Resist Updat,* Jun;12(3), pp. 81-9.

Weisberg, E., Choi, H.G., Ray, A., Barrett, R., Zhang, J., Sim, T., Zhou, W., Seeliger, M., Cameron, M., Azam, M., Fletcher, J.A., Debiec-Rychter, M., Mayeda, M., Moreno, D., Kung, A.L., Janne, P.A., Khosravi-Far, R., Melo, J.V., Manley, P.W., Adamia, S., Wu, C., Gray, N., & Griffin, J.D. (2010a). Discovery of a small-molecule type II inhibitor of wild-type and gatekeeper mutants of BCR-ABL, PDGFRalpha, Kit, and Src kinases: novel type II inhibitor of gatekeeper mutants. *Blood,* May 27;115(21), pp. 4206-16.

Weisberg, E., Choi , H.G., Barrett, R., Zhou, W., Zhang, J., Ray, A., Nelson, E.A., Jiang, J., Moreno, D., Stone, R., Galinsky, I., Fox, E., Adamia, S., Kung, A.L., Gray, N.S., & Griffin, J.D. (2010b). Discovery and characterization of novel mutant FLT3 kinase inhibitors. *Mol Cancer Ther,* Sep;9(9), pp. 2468-77.

Weisberg, E., Deng, X., Choi, H.G., Barrett, R., Adamia, S., Ray, A., Moreno, D., Kung, A.L., Gray, N., & Griffin, J.D. (2010c). Beneficial effects of combining a type II ATP competitive inhibitor with an allosteric competitive inhibitor of BCR-ABL for the treatment of imatinib-sensitive and imatinib-resistant CML. *Leukemia,* Jul;24(7), pp. 1375-8.

Weisberg, E., Ray, A., Barrett, R., Nelson, E., Christie, A.L., Porter, D., Straub, C., Zawel, L., Daley, J.F., Lazo-Kallanian, S., Stone, R., Galinsky, I., Frank, D., Kung, A.L., & Griffin, J.D. (2010d). Smac mimetics: implications for enhancement of targeted therapies in leukemia. *Leukemia,* Dec;24(12), pp. 2100-9.

White, D.L., Saunders, V.A., Dang, P., Engler, J., Zannettino, A.C., Cambareri, A.C., Quinn, S.R., Manley, P.W., & Hughes, T.P. (2006). Oct-1 mediated influx is a key determinant of the intracellular uptake of imatinib but not nilotinib (AMN107): reduced OCT-1 activity is the cause of low in vitro sensitivity to imatinib. *Blood,* July 15;108(2), pp. 697-704.

White, D.L., Saunders, V.A., Quinn, S.R., Manley, P.W.,& Hughes, T.P. (2007). Imatinib increases the intracellular concentration of nilotinib, which may explain the observed synergy between these drugs. *Blood,* Apr 15;109(8), pp. 3609-10.

Wu, G., Chai, J., Suber, T.L., Wu, J.W., Du, C., Wang, X., & Shi, Y. (2000). Structural basis of IAP recognition by Smac/DIABLO. *Nature*, Dec 21-28;408(6815), pp. 1008-12.

Wodnar-Filipowicz, A., Lyman, S.D., Gratwohl, A., Tichelli, A., Speck, B., & Nissen, C. (1996). Flt3 ligand level reflects hematopoietic progenitor cell function in aplastic anemia and chemotherapy-induced bone marrow aplasia. *Blood,* Dec 15;88(12), pp. 4493–4499.

Wu, J., Meng, F., Kong, L.Y., Peng, Z., Ying, Y., Bornmann, W.G., Darnay, B.G., Lamothe, B., Sun, H., Talpaz, M., & Donato, N.J. (2008). Association between imatinib-resistant BCR-ABL mutation-negative leukemia and persistent activation of LYN kinase. *J Natl Cancer Inst,* Jul 2;100(13), pp. 926-39.

Yamamoto, Y., Kiyoi, H., Nakano, Y., Suzuki, R., Kodera, Y., Miyawaki, S., Asou, N., Kuriyama, K., Yagasaki, F., Shimazaki, C., Akiyama, H., Saito, K., Nishimura, M., Motoji, T., Shinagawa, K., Takeshita, A., Saito, H., Ueda, R., Ohno, R., & Naoe, T. (2001). Activating mutation of D835 within the activation loop of FLT3 in human hematologic malignancies. *Blood,* Apr 15;97(8), pp. 2434–2439.

Yee, K.W., O'Farrell, A.M., Smolich, B.D., Cherrington, J.M., McMahon, G., Wait, C.L., McGreevey, L.S., Griffith, D.J., & Heinrich, M.C. (2002). SU5416 and SU5614 inhibit kinase activity of wild-type and mutant FLT3 receptor tyrosine kinase. *Blood,* Oct 15;100(8), pp. 2941–2949.

Yee, K.W., Schittenheim, M., O'Farrell, A.M., Town, A.R., McGreevey, L., Bainbridge, T., Cherrington, J.M., & Heinrich, M.C. (2004). Synergistic effect of SU11248 with cytarabine or daunorubicin on FLT3-ITD-positive leukemic cells. *Blood,* Dec 15;104(13), pp. 4202-4209.

Zarrinkar, P.P., Gunawardane, R.N., Cramer, M.D., Gardner, M.F., Brigham, D., Belli, B., Karaman, M.W., Pratz, K.W., Pallares, G., Chao, Q., Sprankle, K.G., Patel, H.K., Levis, M., Armstrong, R.C., James, J.,& Bhagwat, S.S. (2009). AC220 is a uniquely potent and selective inhibitor of FLT3 for the treatment of acute myeloid leukemia (AML). *Blood,* Oct 1;114(14), pp. 2984–2992.

Zeng, Z., Samudio, I.J., Munsell, M., An, J., Huang, Z., Estey, E., Andreeff, M., & Konopleva, M. (2006). Inhibition of CXCR4 with the novel RCP168 peptide overcomes stroma-mediated chemoresistance in chronic and acute leukemias. *Mol Cancer Ther,* Dec;5(12), pp. 3113-21.

Zhang, W., Konopleva, M., Shi, Y.X., McQueen, T., Harris, D., Ling, X., Estrov, Z., Quintas-Cardama, A., Small, D., Cortes, J., Andreeff, M. (2008). Mutant FLT3: a direct target of sorafenib in acute myelogenous leukemia. *J Natl Cancer Inst*, Feb 6;100(3), pp. 184–198.

Zhang, J., Adrian, F.J., Jahnke, W., Cowan-Jacob, S.W., Li, A.G., Iacob, R.E., Sim, T., Powers, J., Dierks, C., Sun, F., Guo, G.R., Ding, Q., Okram, B., Choi, Y., Woiciechowski, A., Deng, X., Liu, G., Fendrich, G., Strauss, A., Vaipai, N., Grzesiek, S., Tuntland, T., Liu, Y., Bursulava, B., Azam, M., Manley, P.W., Engen, J.R., Daley, G.Q., Warmuth, M., & Gray, N.S. (2010). Targeting Bcr–Abl by combining allosteric with ATP-binding-site inhibitors. *Nature,* Jan 28;463(7280), pp. 501-506.

Zhou, J., Bi C., Janakakumara, J.V., Liu, S.C., Chng, W.J., Tay, K.G., Poon, L.F., Xie, Z., Palaniyandi, S., Yu, H., Glaser, K.B., Albert, D.H., Davidsen, S.K., & Chen, C.S. (2009). Enhanced activation of STAT pathways and overexpression of survivin confer resistance to FLT3 inhibitors and could be therapeutic targets in AML. *Blood,* Apr 23;113(17), pp. 4052–4062.

Zwierzina, H., Anderson, J.E., Rollinger-Holzinger, I., Torok-Storb, B., Nuessler, V., & Lyman, S.D. (1999). Endogenous FLT-3 ligand serum levels are associated with disease stage in patients with myelodysplastic syndromes. *Leukemia,* Apr;13(4), pp. 553–557.

4

De Novo Acquisition of BCR-ABL Mutations for CML Acquired Resistance

WenYong Chen, Hongfeng Yuan and Zhiqiang Wang
Department of Cancer Biology, Beckman Research Institute, City of Hope
USA

1. Introduction

Chronic myelogenous leukemia (CML) is a rare and fatal neoplastic disease clinically presented as aberrant accumulation of myeloid cells in bone marrow, blood and spleen. CML occurs in 1 to 2 cases per 100,000 people, and is most common in older people with a median age at diagnosis of around 65. In the United States of America, there are 3500 to 5000 new cases per year (Jemal et al., 2010). If untreated, CML naturally progresses from initial chronic phase to accelerated phase and blast crisis that resembles acute myeloid leukemia. CML is one of the most extensively studied human cancers, and exemplifies that good scientific research can lead to successful treatment of a devastating disease.

In early 1960s, a characteristic small chromosome of CML was identified by Peter Nowell and David Hungerford who worked in University of Pennsylvania and Fox Chase Cancer Center in Philadelphia, respectively, and was subsequently called the Philadelphia (Ph) chromosome (Nowell and Hungerford, 1960; Nowell and Hungerford, 1961). Ph chromosome is found in 95% CML patients. In 1973, Janet Rowley identified that Ph chromosome was a product of reciprocal translocation of chromosome 9 and 22, the t(9;22)(q34;q11) (Rowley, 1973). In early 1980s, the genes involved in translocation were identified as proto-oncogene ABL (human homolog of Abelson leukemia virus gene) on chromosome 9 that was fused to BCR (break cluster region) on chromosome 22 (Groffen et al., 1984), revealing molecular insight of CML. In early 1990s, aberrant tyrosine kinase activity of BCR-ABL and its essential roles in transformation of cells were established by several groups (Daley et al., 1990; Heisterkamp et al., 1990; Lugo et al., 1990). These molecular discoveries provide crucial foundation for drug development for CML treatment.

In 1996, Brian Druker and colleagues reported the first specific ABL kinase inhibitor imatinib mesylate (STI571, CGP 57148, or Gleevec) that effectively inhibited growth of BCR-ABL positive cells (Druker et al., 1996). In 1998, a phase I clinical trial of imatinib was initiated in three centers in the United States (Druker et al., 2001). Imatinib shows magnificent effect on bringing CML patients, especially those in chronic phase, into remission and improving long-term survival and disease management (Druker et al., 2006), and the drug is now the first line treatment for CML.

However, in contrast to chronic CML, patients at advanced phases (accelerated phase and blast crisis) generally have only transient response to imatinib, and relapse quickly (Deininger and Druker, 2003). Even for chronic phase patients, imatinib does not eradicate the disease and it relapses rapidly if imatinib is discontinued (Michor et al., 2005). Multiple mechanisms, both BCR-ABL dependent and independent, have been described or proposed for CML drug resistance, including amplification of BCR-ABL, mutations of BCR-ABL, drug pump, leukemia stem cell quiescence, as extensively reviewed before (Apperley, 2007). For the scope of this chapter, we will focus on CML acquired resistance, the resistance developed after initial remission of the disease, through BCR-ABL genetic mutations.

2. Acquisition of genetic mutations of CML through drug selection of pre-existing mutants

Charles Sawyers and colleagues first described that acquired resistance to imatinib is mediated primarily by BCR-ABL mutations, and to a less extent, by amplification of BCR-ABL gene and other mechanisms (Gorre et al., 2001; Shah et al., 2002). These mutations confer various degree of resistance of CML cells to imatinib. Compiled from published data from 2001 to 2007, over 50 unique mutations have been identified in all CML patients, and they are mainly located at the BCR-ABL kinase domain (Apperley, 2007). We have updated this mutation profile by adding data published from 2008 to 2010 (Chien et al., 2008; Jones et al., 2008; Kim et al., 2009; Lewandowski et al., 2009; Markose et al., 2009; Press, 2010). The ten most common mutations representing 74% of total mutations (Fig. 1) exhibit similar patterns as shown before (Apperley, 2007). T315I remains as the most frequent mutation followed by Y253 and E255 mutations. Some minor changes are noticed: G250A/E moves to the 4th place ahead of M351T whereas M244V moves to the 10th place.

The four critical regions of BCR-ABL kinase domain are the prime targets for these mutations: T315I mutation for imatinib binding site, mutations on Y253, E255 and G250 for ATP binding site or P-loop, mutations on M351, E355 and F359 for catalytic domain and mutations on H396 for activation loop (Nagar et al., 2002; Schindler et al., 2000). M244V mutation occurs in close proximity to the P-loop and F317 mutations close to imatinib binding site. Although it is not functionally clear about the significance of every mutation detected, the profile highlights the importance of those high frequency mutations. T315I mutant BCR-ABL is resistant to inhibition by the second generation of tyrosine kinase inhibitors nilotinib (von Bubnoff et al., 2006; Weisberg et al., 2005) and dasatinib (Shah et al., 2004), which inhibit most other BCR-ABL mutations. T315I and P-loop mutations are associated with reduced survival and poor prognosis in patients (Nicolini et al., 2006). Y253F and E255K mutations increase BCR-ABL transformation capability whereas T315I mutation affects oncogenicity by altering P-loop phosphorylation (Griswold et al., 2006; Skaggs et al., 2006).

Progression of chronic phase to advanced phases may require additional alterations of CML genome beyond BCR-ABL (Perrotti et al., 2010). It is perceived that mutation mechanisms may be different in chronic phase from that in blast crisis CML cells. We have plotted ten most frequent mutations in chronic phase CML (Fig. 1) collected from data published from 2001 to 2009 (according to Table S2 in Klemm et al., 2009). The ten most common mutations representing 78% of total mutations in chronic phase are the same amino acids at the BCR-ABL kinase domain as seen in the all CML profile. Noticeably, M351T, instead of T315I, mutation is the most frequent mutation in chronic CML. It is evident that there is substantial increase of T315I mutation and reduction of M244V mutation in all CML profile, suggesting T315I is more favored and M244V is less favored towards the advanced phases. In addition, the most frequent mutations are clustered more tightly according to the functional regions of the kinase domain in all CML profile than in chronic CML profile. Although the above difference may suggest the increased functional selection for drug resistance in advanced CML cells, mechanisms underlying such difference are unknown.

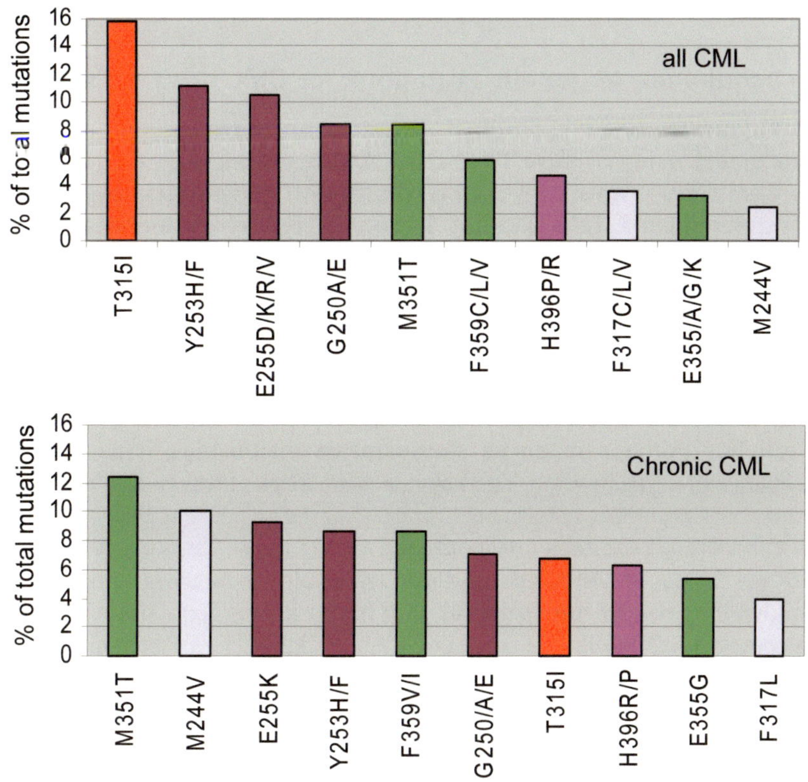

Fig. 1. The top ten mutations of BCR-ABL in all or chronic CML patients
Upper panel: Ten most frequent mutations in all CML. The profile was created by adding 344 mutation cases published between 2008 to 2010 to the previously published profile (Apperley, 2007). Lower panel: Ten most frequent mutations in chronic CML. The profile was created according to the previously compiled data containing 572 total mutation cases published from 2001 to 2009 (Klemm et al., 2009). Mutations in the regions of BCR-ABL kinase domain are color-coded: red for imatinib binding site, maroon for ATP binding site, green for catalytic domain, fuchsia for activation loop, and light blue for amino acids adjacent to those regions.

Charles Sawyers and colleagues were also among the first to identify mutations of BCR-ABL kinase domain in CML patients before imatinib treatment (Roche-Lestienne et al., 2002; Shah et al., 2002), and proposed that BCR-ABL mutations in relapsed CML patients upon imatinib treatment are a result of selection of pre-existing mutant clones (Shah and Sawyers, 2003). This model has been validated by subsequent studies from multiple groups identifying such mutations (Ernst et al., 2008; Roche-Lestienne et al., 2003; Willis et al., 2005). Mathematical modeling further provides support for rapid expansion of pre-existing mutant clones for fast relapse in CML patients (Michor et al., 2005). However, the rate of BCR-ABL mutations found in CML patients prior to imatinib exposure is around 21%, even using high sensitivity methods for detection (Ernst et al., 2008; Roche-Lestienne et al., 2002; Willis et al., 2005), as compared to 40% to 90% in relapsed patients. This difference could be blamed to the insufficient sensitivity of detection methods. Alternatively, additional mechanisms for BCR-ABL mutations may exist and accentuate the mutations.

3. *De novo* acquisition of genetic mutations for CML drug resistance

To address mechanisms of CML acquired resistance, we have recently developed a novel tissue culture model using a naïve blast crisis CML cell line KCL-22 (Yuan et al., 2010). KCL-22 cells were derived from a female blast crisis CML patient, and were characterized as immature undifferentiated cells lacking lymphoid cell characteristics (Kubonishi and Miyoshi, 1983). KCL-22 cells are positive for myeloid cell markers including myeloid progenitor cell marker CD33. KCL-22 cells harbor two Ph chromosomes but do not have detectable BCR-ABL mutations (Yuan et al., 2010). In contrast to resistance of blast crisis CML in vivo, most blast crisis CML cell lines in culture are very sensitive to 1 μM imatinib with exception of KCL-22 (Deininger et al., 1997). Imatinib also kills KCL-22 cells, but it requires higher concentrations and takes longer time (Yuan et al., 2010). This unique feature of KCL-22 cell line perhaps made us successful in establishing it as a new model for acquired resistance of CML in vitro. The key characteristics of this model are summarized as follows:

1. High relevance: KCL-22 cells are incubated with in vivo therapeutic concentrations of imatinib, i.e. 2.5 to 10 μM. Cells undergo gradually increasing apoptosis for about a week followed by re-growing (relapse) with homogenous acquisition of T315I mutation.
2. Easy to use: KCL-22 cell line is commercially available from German Collection of Cell Culture. Cells are easy to grow in standard RPMI 1640 medium supplied with 10% fetal bovine serum, and no additional growth factors are needed. One single dose of imatinib treatment is sufficient.
3. Rapid turnaround: Relapse occurs in about two weeks with initial relapsed cells microscopically visible as small clusters of enlarged and sometimes irregularly shaped cells after around eight days of drug treatment.
4. High reproducibility: Multiple persons in the lab have used this model and it produces highly consistent results among them.

This model provides a novel tool for us to look into the process of acquisition of BCR-ABL mutations on the endogenous BCR-ABL in blast crisis CML cells, and has already provided valuable information in our initial study (Yuan et al., 2010) as summarized below.

1. Acquisition of BCR-ABL mutations does not require pre-existing mutant clones derived from the original patient, as clonal cells without an initial mutation can regenerate mutations and relapse on imatinib. The mutations do not derive from a fixed subpopulation of pre-mutant cells.
2. Acquisition of BCR-ABL mutations does not provoke additional chromosomal rearrangement, is not a result of mutator phenotype of KCL-22 cells, and can not be blocked by standard anti-oxidant treatment.
3. Acquisition of BCR-ABL mutations is a dynamic process influenced by culture and environmental conditions. This is supported by several lines of evidence. First, clonal KCL-22 cells exhibit great difference for BCR-ABL mutations whereas mutations on HPRT gene are relatively stable among clones. Second, clonal KCL-22 cells can acquire different single mutations for each clone, suggesting change of mutation hot spots after

cloning process. We have identified three clones that can acquire T315I, E255K and Y253H mutation, respectively. These three mutations have the highest frequency in human patients shown in Fig. 1. Third, the ability for acquisition of BCR-ABL mutations diminishes in parental KCL-22 cells after they are cultured continuously for more than 30 passages. Finally, we have found that the quality of fetal bovine serum can affect BCR-ABL mutation rate. We routinely use Hyclone characterized fetal bovine serum (Cat# SH30071.03) for mutation study, which typically produces consistent results among batches. However, when Hyclone serum was compared side by side with two other brands of fetal bovine serum, a noticeable reduction of BCR-ABL mutation rate was found in other brands (Fig. 2).

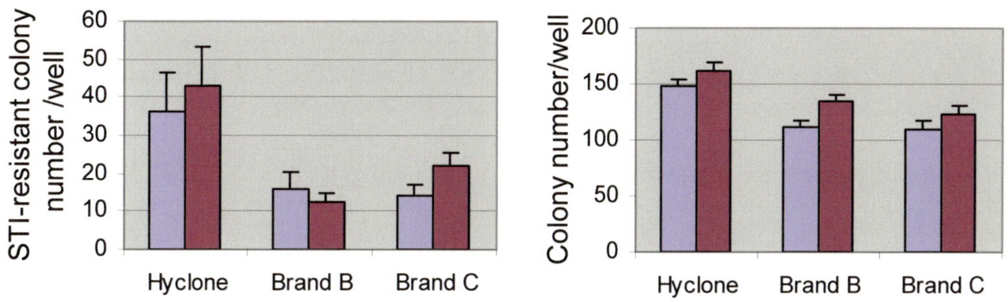

Fig. 2. Tissue culture conditions affect BCR-ABL mutations
Comparison of Hyclone characterized fetal bovine serum with two other brands of fetal bovine serum. KCL-22 cells were incubated with medium supplied with these sera, respectively, for two days, and then seeded onto soft agar for colony formation assay. Left panel, $1x10^6$ cells seeded per well with 2.5 μM imatinib. Right panel: plating efficiency with 500 cells seeded per well. Two independent batches of each serum (colored as blue and maroon) were tested.

4. Acquisition of BCR-ABL mutations depends on expression of BCR-ABL, since knockdown of BCR-ABL blocks KCL-22 cell relapse and mutations. By over-expression of kinase-inactive BCR-ABL, intriguingly, it was found that BCR-ABL kinase activity is not absolutely required for acquisition of mutations.
5. The endogenous BCR-ABL translocation locus significantly influences BCR-ABL mutations, as the mutation rate on the endogenous locus is nearly 10 times higher than that of the randomly integrated BCR-ABL cDNA as illustrated in Fig. 3. This finding reveals a previously unrecognized role of the translocation locus itself in driving BCR-ABL mutagenesis, suggesting possible involvement of the local epigenome for BCR-ABL mutations that will be discussed further below.

Our extensive analyses of BCR-ABL mutations in KCL-22 cells lead to the conclusion that mutations can be acquired *de novo* after imatinib treatment, although precise molecular mechanisms are yet to be uncovered. Such *de novo* acquisition of mutations may provide an alternative mechanism for clinical resistance of CML to tyrosine kinase inhibitors (Fig. 4). This is particularly important given that the majority of CML patients at the time of diagnosis do not harbor detectable BCR-ABL mutations. *De novo* acquisition of BCR-ABL mutations does not necessarily have to operate exclusively from selection of pre-existing mutations. It is anticipated that these two modes of acquisition of BCR-ABL mutations may work in concert in certain patients leading to even faster relapse on the drug treatment. Therefore, we propose that *de novo* mutation acquisition and selection of pre-existing mutations are integrated processes for acquired resistance.

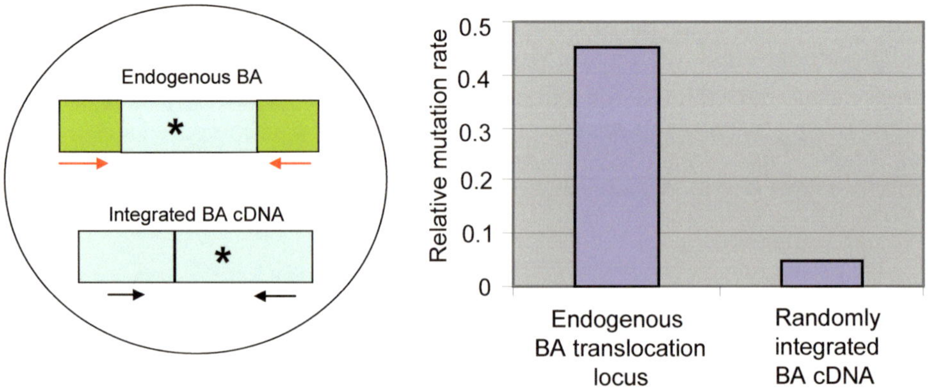

Fig. 3. Mutations on the endogenous BCR-ABL versus integrated BCR-ABL cDNA. Left, endogenous BCR-ABL (BA) was amplified by intron primers and integrated BCR-ABL was amplified by exon primers for mutation detection. Green for introns, blue for exons, asterisk for T315 mutation, and arrows for PCR primers. Right, relative mutation rate was the ratio of the number of clones bearing mutated endogenous BA or integrated BA cDNA divided by total number of clones, according to Yuan et al., 2010.

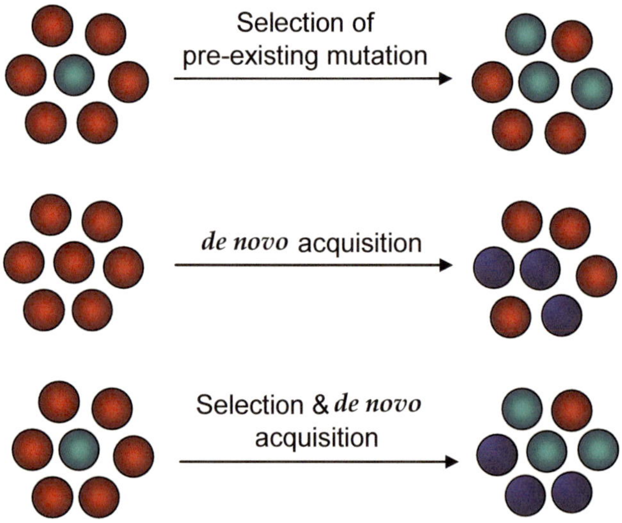

Fig. 4. Two modes of acquisition of BCR-ABL mutations for CML acquired resistance. Clinical relapse of CML on tyrosine kinase may be mediated by selection of pre-existing BCR-ABL mutant cells (green), *de novo* acquisition of BCR-ABL mutations (blue), or the combination of both. Non-mutant leukemia cells are in red. Two types of mutation acquisition could happen on the same amino acids.

Although the clinical readout for *de novo* acquisition and selection of pre-existing mutations are the same, i.e. relapse of the disease due to mutations, the implication for disease management caused by these two modes of mutation acquisition could be different. Whereas strong tyrosine kinase inhibitors may be needed to suppress expansion of pre-existing mutant cells, prevention of *de novo* mutation acquisition by alternative strategies may help block relapse of CML in this category as detailed later.

4. Search for molecular evidence of *de novo* acquisition of mutations in human CML patients

So far, *de novo* acquisition of mutations has not yet been proved in patients. As described above, *de novo* mutation acquisition happens rapidly in the KCL-22 cell model in which early relapsed cells are microscopically visible after eight days of imatinib treatment. We have further found that mutations may likely form as early as two days after imatinib treatment (unpublished data). This rapid generation of mutations may prevent the appropriate use of mathematical models (Michor et al., 2005) to effectively distinguish between *de novo* mutation acquisition versus selection of pre-existing mutations. Separation of these two modes of mutation acquisition is further confounded by pre-existing mutations that may not be detected truly due to insufficient method sensitivity or by non-representative sample collection for analysis. It is currently unclear about the molecular signature of *de novo* mutation acquisition in CML patients or how to track this type of mutagenesis. However, mutations in clonal KCL-22 cells may provide a clue.

The mutation hot spots are different in three KCL-22 clones (clone L1 for E255K, clone L7 for Y253H and clone Ag 11 for T315I) (Yuan et al., 2010). When the codon changes are examined (TAC to CAC for Y253H, GAG to AAG for E255K, and ACT to ATT for T315I), a common molecular feature for these three mutations can be easily identified, namely, they are all transition mutations. It is important to note that both Y253 and E255 codons can acquire either transition or transversion mutation. Since these clonal cells are genetically identical, switching mutation hot spot from one transition mutation spot to another transition spot but not transversion, indicating that transition mutation is easier to be adapted on the BCR-ABL locus for kinase domain mutation. In line with this notion, frequencies for transition mutations for both Y253 and E255 codons are significantly higher than their transversion counterparts, Y253F and E255V in CML patients (Hochhaus et al., 2002; Press, 2010). Importantly, most of high frequency mutations shown in Fig. 1 are transition mutations. Further supporting this, a recent study shows that AID (activation-induced cytidine deaminase) promotes transition mutations in Ph^+ B lymphoid blast crisis CML (Klemm et al., 2009). However, AID is activated in B lymphoid CML, but not in myeloid blast crisis CML including KCL-22 cells (Klemm et al., 2009), there may be additional mechanisms to enhance transitional mutations in myeloid blast crisis CML that makes up about 60% of all blast crisis CML (Calabretta and Perrotti, 2004). On the other hand, genetic mutations tend to have bias towards transition mutations (Wakeley, 1996). Therefore, additional studies including rigorous analysis of clinical samples are needed to explore if transition mutations may indeed play a role in *de novo* acquisition of mutations in CML patients.

5. Mechanistic basis for integration of *de novo* mutation acquisition and selection of pre-existing mutations for drug resistance

A key question about *de novo* acquisition of mutations is how it arises and integrates with selection of pre-existing mutations. The selection model for drug resistance is rooted in

Darwinian genetics, in which mutations can randomly form without providing survival advantage until environmental stress is imposed. It has been well recognized that mammalian genome is under constant genotoxic assault from intrinsic or extrinsic source, and DNA damage contributes significantly to genetic mutations (Friedberg, 2003; Wiseman and Halliwell, 1996). Transformation of BCR-ABL in hematopoietic progenitor cells increases production of reactive oxygen species (ROS) and DNA damage (Koptyra et al., 2006). Expression of BCR-ABL alters functions of cellular DNA damage repair machineries, especially for double-strand break (DSB) repair, which promotes CML genetic instability (Melo and Barnes, 2007). It is reasonable to believe that increased DNA damage and genetic instability would predispose CML cells to form mutations prior to drug treatment.

In the past two decades, significant progresses have been made in the understanding of epigenetics and epigenomics for their roles in shaping gene functions, particularly in cancer development (Jones and Baylin, 2007). Unlike genetic changes, epigenetic/ epigenomic changes are versatile and reversible, which bring dynamics to genetic codes and bridge genetic alterations to environmental changes. Epigenomics plays important roles in DNA damage repair, best studied for DSB repair. Several chromatin remodeling complexes are participated in modifying local chromatin structure to facilitate DNA damage repair (Rossetto et al., 2010). Epigenetic regulation of chemoresistance is a burgeoning field, and little is understood how it is involved in acquisition of genetic mutations for drug resistance.

We propose the following model as illustrated in Fig.5: Acquisition of BCR-ABL mutation is a multi-step process involving at least three core processes: DNA damage initiation, DNA damage repair and survival of newly mutated cells. These core processes are bound together through local epigenome that may serve as a sensor for stress signals and influence either exposure of local DNA to damage, repair process or cell survival. BCR-ABL locus may sustain constant DNA damage and repair, and the status of such DNA damage and repair determines whether the eventual relapse is mediated by selection of pre-existing mutations or *de novo* acquisition of mutations under stress.

Based on this model, we predict that under the steady state, the BCR-ABL locus has ongoing DNA damage and repair, and most of cells do not harbor mutations because most of DNA damage is repaired correctly. Inappropriate repair will lead to low incidence of mutations and allow selection of such pre-existing mutations for cell survival and relapse during chemotherapy. On the other hand, chemotherapy, including but not limited to imatinib, may provide an extrinsic stress signal through epigenome to the locus, which may either increase local DNA damage load or interfere functions of repair machineries, accentuating the mutagenesis process and resulting in *de novo* acquisition of mutations.

The definition of pre-existing mutations or *de novo* acquisition of mutations is based on the readout of DNA sequencing. However, DNA sequencing only detects completed mutations but not DNA damage. Therefore, a damaged base undetectable as a mutation by sequencing may emerge as a mutation, if it is not repaired on time or is repaired improperly. Alternatively, a mutation may emerge as a result of new DNA damage elicited by extrinsic stress. Consequently, *de novo* mutation acquisition would not require a fixed subpopulation as we have shown (Yuan et al., 2010), and it would be a dynamic process if environmental changes, such as cell growth conditions and nutrients, affect local epigenome and subsequently interfere the repair process.

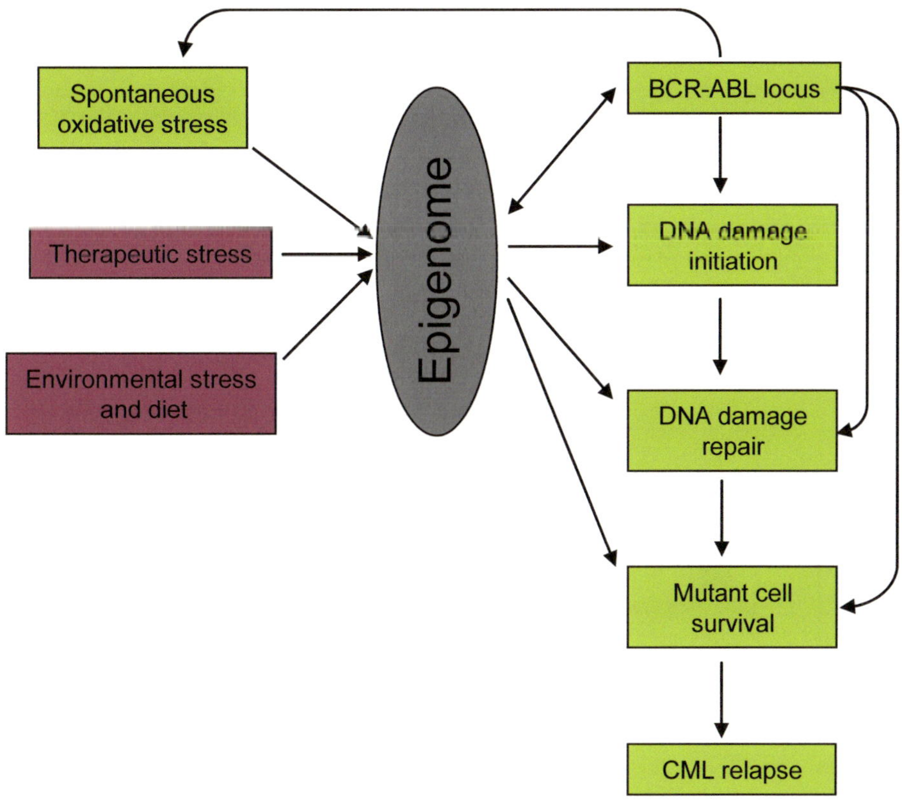

Fig. 5. An epigenome model for acquisition of BCR-ABL mutations
Acquisition of BCR-ABL mutations is a multi-step process that is regulated by BCR-ABL local epigenome. The epigenome is an important sensor of intrinsic oxidative stress signal (green) or extrinsic stress signal (red) including therapeutic or environmental stress, which in turn affects DNA damage, repair and cell survival, leading to maturation of genetic mutations for acquired resistance of CML.

6. New opportunities for studying molecular mechanisms of acquired resistance

In the coming years, it is anticipated that some steps of molecular regulation of mutation acquisition can be answered using the KCL-22 cell model. Here we discuss some steps that need obvious attention. Understanding these mutagenesis steps may help design new strategies to block BCR-ABL mutagenesis.

1. **Regulation of DNA damage initiation.** The very origin of mutations, where DNA damage is from, remains to be clearly defined. Many chemotherapeutic agents deliberately induce DNA damage to kill cancer cells. In contrast, imatinib treatment reduces bulk ROS production and DNA damage response measured by γH2AX (Yuan et al., 2010). It has been shown that anti-oxidants can inhibit BCR-ABL induced ROS production, DNA damage and mutations (Koptyra et al., 2006). However, anti-oxidants vitamin E and N-acetylcysteine, even in excessive amount, are unable to block acquisition of BCR-ABL mutations in KCL-22 cells (Yuan et al., 2010). There are several

possibilities for this observation: these anti-oxidants do not have sufficient potency, the DNA damage is too severe to be blocked, the anti-oxidants are inappropriate for the type of stress and damage in these cells, and the BCR-ABL locus is not accessible for these agents in KCL-22 cells. It is formally possible that there might be other sources of DNA damage.

One interesting but not surprising observation is that after imatinib treatment, ROS level in early apoptotic cells surges by more than 100 folds (Yuan et al., 2010) (Fig. 6). This high level of ROS may initiate cell death pathway. It is provocative to speculate that mutant cells might be derived from rare early apoptotic cells as they somehow abandon apoptosis process but sustain substantial DNA damage, which could not be blocked by treatment with standard anti-oxidants, and would thus lead to genetic mutations.

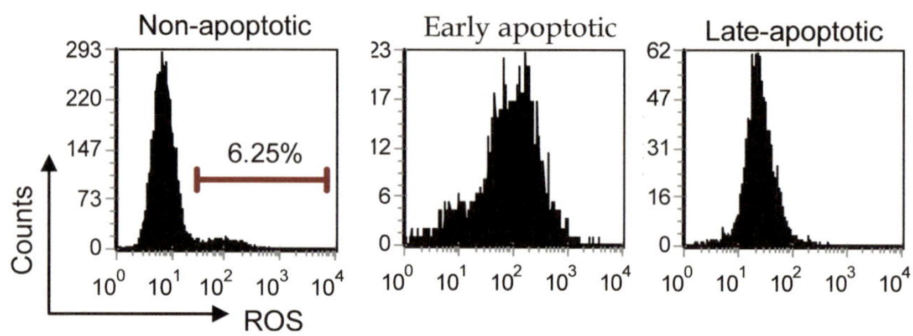

Fig. 6. ROS levels in different apoptotic fractions of KCL-22 cells after imatinib treatment.

2. **Regulation of DNA damage repair**. BCR-ABL alters functions of both homologous recombination (HR) and non-homologous end joining (NHEJ) repair machineries for DSB repair (Melo and Barnes, 2007). NHEJ is the major repair pathway in higher eukaryotes (Khanna and Jackson, 2001). NHEJ repair consists of both classic and alternative pathways. Classic NHEJ has core components KU70/86 and DNA-PKcs. When classic NHEJ is inhibited, alternative NHEJ that is independent of KU70/86 and DNA-PKcs will be activated. BCR-ABL inhibits classic NHEJ by degrading the key NHEJ factor DNA-PKcs (Deutsch et al., 2001). Recently, it has been found that BCR-ABL activates alterative NHEJ through upregulation of Werner Syndrome protein (WRN) and DNA ligase IIIa in CML cells (Sallmyr et al., 2008). For HR repair, BCR-ABL increases expression of RAD51, a central HR factor, which abnormally increases DNA repair and enhances CML drug resistance (Slupianek et al., 2001). In addition, BCR-ABL expression compromises repair fidelity and increases DNA repair errors in CML cells (Nowicki et al., 2004). It will be interesting to determine whether the above mentioned repair mechanisms and factors, and perhaps other repair mechanisms, may be involved in acquisition of BCR-ABL mutations for acquired resistance to imatinib.
3. **Regulation of survival of emerging mutant cells.** The newly relapsed KCL-22 cells exhibit morphological enlargement and irregularity with significant increase of G2/M fraction (Yuan et al., 2010). This indicates that newly relapsed cells may likely suffer mitotic crisis as they slowly progress through cell cycle. This is perhaps the last and critical step for the completion of mutagenesis process to allow full outgrowth of mutant cells. Molecular machineries involved in mitotic regulation might play a role in survival of newly relapsed CML cells. Among them, Aurora serine/threonine kinases are critically involved in regulating mammalian cell division (Keen and Taylor, 2004;

Marumoto et al., 2005). Aurora A over-expression overrides the mitotic spindle assembly checkpoint and promotes cancer cells resistance to chemotherapy (Anand et al., 2003). Interestingly, the pan-Aurora kinase inhibitor VX-680 not only inhibits Aurora kinases but also suppresses T315I BCR-ABL through distinct structural mechanisms (Carter et al., 2005; Young et al., 2006). Another mitotic kinase Polo-like kinase 1 (PLK1) is also known to mediate cancer chemoresistance (Luo et al., 2009). It remains to be determined if these and other mitotic regulators may play a role in CML acquired resistance.

4. **Regulation of epigenome.** Epigenome is a central component in our model. Identifying epigenetic factors involved in acquired resistance will significantly help us understand the dynamic mutation acquisition process. DNA methylation plays an important role in genetic mutations (Jones and Baylin, 2002). Methylation of cytosine at CpG sites significantly increases C to T transition mutation because of the spontaneous hydrolytic deamination of methylated cytosine. Cytosine methylation in gene coding regions is associated with mutation hot spots of certain tumor suppressor genes, such as p53, in cancer.

Histone modifications are essential for DSB repair. Within minutes of DSB, histone H2A variant H2AX is phosphorylated and recruited to damage foci, which is followed by accumulation of DNA repair and chromatin remodeling factors (Rossetto et al., 2010). Several types of chromatin remodeling occur on and surround DSB sites. ATP-dependent chromatin remodeling complex INO80 is rapidly recruited by γH2AX (Downs et al., 2004; Morrison et al., 2004; van Attikum et al., 2004). Recruitment of acetyltransferases and localized acetylation of histone H3 and H4 helps maintain open chromatin for repair (Tamburini and Tyler, 2005). Methylation of histone H4K20 also helps recruitment of repair factors through direct protein interaction (Botuyan et al., 2006; Sanders et al., 2004). When repair is completed, local deacetylation mediated by histone deacetylases restores chromatin structure. Importantly, the ability to modulate histone acetylation and deacetylation is essential for cell viability following HR repair, likely due to its signaling to prevent persistent activation of DNA damage checkpoint (Tamburini and Tyler, 2005). In addition, class III histone deacetylase SIRT1 is also recruited to DSB sites (O'Hagan et al., 2008) and regulates DNA damage response (Oberdoerffer et al., 2008; Yuan et al., 2007). It would be of great interest to define which and how chromatin modifiers response to therapeutic and environmental stress signals to mediate DSB repair and BCR-ABL mutagenesis.

7. Implication of *de novo* acquisition of genetic mutations in leukemia management

Blocking outgrowth of mutant BCR-ABL clones has clear therapeutic significance, regardless how the mutations may be acquired. However, strategies used to overcome resistance may be different for pre-exiting mutations and *de novo* acquired mutations. The former demands more and more potent BCR-ABL inhibitors, which could lead to stronger resistance each time. This has been proved with sequential use of kinase inhibitors, resulting in selection of compound drug-resistant mutations (Shah et al., 2007). More potent third generation of tyrosine kinase inhibitors have been developed (Quintas-Cardama et al., 2010), including AP24534 that inhibits all tested BCR-ABL mutations and blocks outgrowth of mutant clones (O'Hare et al., 2009). Clinical resistance to the third generation of tyrosine kinase inhibitors remains to be determined.

For mutations acquired *de novo*, however, a prevention strategy may be more appropriate and effective to block mutant cells from emergence at the beginning. With better understanding of mechanisms of mutations described above, it is expected that a new agent may be devised to modulate DNA damage initiation, repair, epigenome remodeling, or survival of newly emerged mutant cells, which will prevent CML acquired resistance in future. A combination therapy may be adapted with such a new agent and imatinib or other tyrosine kinase inhibitors. Alternatively, it is also reasonable to speculate that a multi-target agent can be developed to incorporate these features, for example, a drug that both inhibits BCR-ABL tyrosine kinase and modulates epigenome. We anticipate different ways to overcome resistance depending on which steps and factors the drug would target to block mutagenesis. We expect that such a strategy may also have broader implication for management of other types of leukemia to overcome drug resistance.

8. Acknowledgements

This study is supported by the following grants: a career development award from the STOPCANCER Foundation, W81XWH-06-1-0268 from US Department of Defense, a translational research grant from the V-Foundation, and NCI R01 CA143421 to W.Y.C. The core facilities used in this study were supported by NCI P30 CA033572. The contents are solely the responsibility of the authors and do not represent the official views of the National Cancer Institute or NIH.

9. References

Anand, S., Penrhyn-Lowe, S., and Venkitaraman, A.R. (2003). AURORA-A amplification overrides the mitotic spindle assembly checkpoint, inducing resistance to Taxol. Cancer Cell 3, 51-62.

Apperley, J.F. (2007). Part I: mechanisms of resistance to imatinib in chronic myeloid leukaemia. Lancet Oncol 8, 1018-1029.

Botuyan, M.V., Lee, J., Ward, I.M., Kim, J.E., Thompson, J.R., Chen, J., and Mer, G. (2006). Structural basis for the methylation state-specific recognition of histone H4-K20 by 53BP1 and Crb2 in DNA repair. Cell 127, 1361-1373.

Calabretta, B., and Perrotti, D. (2004). The biology of CML blast crisis. Blood 103, 4010-4022.

Carter, T.A., Wodicka, L.M., Shah, N.P., Velasco, A.M., Fabian, M.A., Treiber, D.K., Milanov, Z.V., Atteridge, C.E., Biggs, W.H., 3rd, Edeen, P.T., et al. (2005). Inhibition of drug-resistant mutants of ABL, KIT, and EGF receptor kinases. Proc Natl Acad Sci U S A 102, 11011-11016.

Chien, J.H., Tang, J.L., Chen, R.L., Li, C.C., and Lee, C.P. (2008). Detection of BCR-ABL gene mutations in Philadelphia chromosome positive leukemia patients resistant to STI-571 cancer therapy. Leukemia research 32, 1724-1734.

Daley, G.Q., Van Etten, R.A., and Baltimore, D. (1990). Induction of chronic myelogenous leukemia in mice by the P210bcr/abl gene of the Philadelphia chromosome. Science 247, 824-830.

Deininger, M.W., and Druker, B.J. (2003). Specific targeted therapy of chronic myelogenous leukemia with imatinib. Pharmacol Rev 55, 401-423.

Deininger, M.W., Goldman, J.M., Lydon, N., and Melo, J.V. (1997). The tyrosine kinase inhibitor CGP57148B selectively inhibits the growth of BCR-ABL-positive cells. Blood 90, 3691-3698.

Deutsch, E., Dugray, A., AbdulKarim, B., Marangoni, E., Maggiorella, L., Vaganay, S., M'Kacher, R., Rasy, S.D., Eschwege, F., Vainchenker, W., et al. (2001). BCR-ABL down-regulates the DNA repair protein DNA-PKcs. Blood 97, 2084-2090.

Downs, J.A., Allard, S., Jobin-Robitaille, O., Javaheri, A., Auger, A., Bouchard, N., Kron, S.J., Jackson, S.P., and Cote, J. (2004). Binding of chromatin-modifying activities to phosphorylated histone H2A at DNA damage sites. Mol Cell 16, 979-990.

Druker, B.J., Guilhot, F., O'Brien, S.G., Gathmann, I., Kantarjian, H., Gattermann, N., Deininger, M.W., Silver, R.T., Goldman, J.M., Stone, R.M., et al. (2006). Five year follow-up of patients receiving imatinib for chronic myeloid leukemia. N Engl J Med 355, 2408-2417.

Druker, B.J., Talpaz, M., Resta, D.J., Peng, B., Buchdunger, E., Ford, J.M., Lydon, N.B., Kantarjian, H., Capdeville, R., Ohno-Jones, S., et al. (2001). Efficacy and safety of a specific inhibitor of the BCR-ABL tyrosine kinase in chronic myeloid leukemia. N Engl J Med 344, 1031-1037.

Druker, B.J., Tamura, S., Buchdunger, E., Ohno, S., Segal, G.M., Fanning, S., Zimmermann, J., and Lydon, N.B. (1996). Effects of a selective inhibitor of the Abl tyrosine kinase on the growth of Bcr-Abl positive cells. Nat Med 2, 561-566.

Ernst, T., Erben, P., Muller, M.C., Paschka, P., Schenk, T., Hoffmann, J., Kreil, S., La Rosee, P., Hehlmann, R., and Hochhaus, A. (2008). Dynamics of BCR-ABL mutated clones prior to hematologic or cytogenetic resistance to imatinib. Haematologica 93, 186-192.

Friedberg, E.C. (2003). DNA damage and repair. Nature 421, 436-440.

Gorre, M.E., Mohammed, M., Ellwood, K., Hsu, N., Paquette, R., Rao, P.N., and Sawyers, C.L. (2001). Clinical resistance to STI-571 cancer therapy caused by BCR-ABL gene mutation or amplification. Science 293, 876-880.

Griswold, I.J., MacPartlin, M., Bumm, T., Goss, V.L., O'Hare, T., Lee, K.A., Corbin, A.S., Stoffregen, E.P., Smith, C., Johnson, K., et al. (2006). Kinase domain mutants of Bcr-Abl exhibit altered transformation potency, kinase activity, and substrate utilization, irrespective of sensitivity to imatinib. Mol Cell Biol 26, 6082-6093.

Groffen, J., Stephenson, J.R., Heisterkamp, N., de Klein, A., Bartram, C.R., and Grosveld, G. (1984). Philadelphia chromosomal breakpoints are clustered within a limited region, bcr, on chromosome 22. Cell 36, 93-99.

Heisterkamp, N., Jenster, G., ten Hoeve, J., Zovich, D., Pattengale, P.K., and Groffen, J. (1990). Acute leukaemia in bcr/abl transgenic mice. Nature 344, 251-253.

Hochhaus, A., Kreil, S., Corbin, A.S., La Rosee, P., Muller, M.C., Lahaye, T., Hanfstein, B., Schoch, C., Cross, N.C., Berger, U., et al. (2002). Molecular and chromosomal mechanisms of resistance to imatinib (STI571) therapy. Leukemia 16, 2190-2196.

Jemal, A., Siegel, R., Xu, J., and Ward, E. (2010). Cancer statistics, 2010. CA: a cancer journal for clinicians 60, 277-300.

Jones, D., Thomas, D., Yin, C.C., O'Brien, S., Cortes, J.E., Jabbour, E., Breeden, M., Giles, F.J., Zhao, W., and Kantarjian, H.M. (2008). Kinase domain point mutations in Philadelphia chromosome-positive acute lymphoblastic leukemia emerge after therapy with BCR-ABL kinase inhibitors. Cancer 113, 985-994.

Jones, P.A., and Baylin, S.B. (2002). The fundamental role of epigenetic events in cancer. Nat Rev Genet 3, 415-428.

Jones, P.A., and Baylin, S.B. (2007). The epigenomics of cancer. Cell 128, 683-692.

Keen, N., and Taylor, S. (2004). Aurora-kinase inhibitors as anticancer agents. Nat Rev Cancer 4, 927-936.

Khanna, K.K., and Jackson, S.P. (2001). DNA double-strand breaks: signaling, repair and the cancer connection. Nat Genet 27, 247-254.

Kim, S.H., Kim, D., Kim, D.W., Goh, H.G., Jang, S.E., Lee, J., Kim, W.S., Kweon, I.Y., and Park, S.H. (2009). Analysis of Bcr-Abl kinase domain mutations in Korean chronic myeloid leukaemia patients: poor clinical outcome of P-loop and T315I mutation is disease phase dependent. Hematological oncology 27, 190-197.

Klemm, L., Duy, C., Iacobucci, I., Kuchen, S., von Levetzow, G., Feldhahn, N., Henke, N., Li, Z., Hoffmann, T.K., Kim, Y.M., et al. (2009). The B cell mutator AID promotes B lymphoid blast crisis and drug resistance in chronic myeloid leukemia. Cancer Cell 16, 232-245.

Koptyra, M., Falinski, R., Nowicki, M.O., Stoklosa, T., Majsterek, I., Nieborowska-Skorska, M., Blasiak, J., and Skorski, T. (2006). BCR/ABL kinase induces self-mutagenesis via reactive oxygen species to encode imatinib resistance. Blood 108, 319-327.

Kubonishi, I., and Miyoshi, I. (1983). Establishment of a Ph1 chromosome-positive cell line from chronic myelogenous leukemia in blast crisis. International journal of cell cloning 1, 105-117.

Lewandowski, K., Warzocha, K., Hellmann, A., Skotnicki, A., Prejzner, W., Foryciarz, K., Sacha, T., Gniot, M., Majewski, M., Solarska, I., et al. (2009). Frequency of BCR-ABL gene mutations in Polish patients with chronic myeloid leukemia treated with imatinib: a final report of the MAPTEST study. Polskie Archiwum Medycyny Wewnetrznej 119, 789-794.

Lugo, T.G., Pendergast, A.M., Muller, A.J., and Witte, O.N. (1990). Tyrosine kinase activity and transformation potency of bcr-abl oncogene products. Science 247, 1079-1082.

Luo, J., Emanuele, M.J., Li, D., Creighton, C.J., Schlabach, M.R., Westbrook, T.F., Wong, K.K., and Elledge, S.J. (2009). A genome-wide RNAi screen identifies multiple synthetic lethal interactions with the Ras oncogene. Cell 137, 835-848.

Markose, P., Chendamarai, E., Balasubramanian, P., Velayudhan, S.R., Srivastava, V.M., Mathews, V., George, B., Viswabandya, A., Srivastava, A., and Chandy, M. (2009). Spectrum of BCR-ABL kinase domain mutations in patients with chronic myeloid leukemia from India with suspected resistance to imatinib-mutations are rare and have different distributions. Leukemia & lymphoma 50, 2092-2095.

Marumoto, T., Zhang, D., and Saya, H. (2005). Aurora-A - a guardian of poles. Nat Rev Cancer 5, 42-50.

Melo, J.V., and Barnes, D.J. (2007). Chronic myeloid leukaemia as a model of disease evolution in human cancer. Nat Rev Cancer 7, 441-453.

Michor, F., Hughes, T.P., Iwasa, Y., Branford, S., Shah, N.P., Sawyers, C.L., and Nowak, M.A. (2005). Dynamics of chronic myeloid leukaemia. Nature 435, 1267-1270.

Morrison, A.J., Highland, J., Krogan, N.J., Arbel-Eden, A., Greenblatt, J.F., Haber, J.E., and Shen, X. (2004). INO80 and gamma-H2AX interaction links ATP-dependent chromatin remodeling to DNA damage repair. Cell 119, 767-775.

Nagar, B., Bornmann, W.G., Pellicena, P., Schindler, T., Veach, D.R., Miller, W.T., Clarkson, B., and Kuriyan, J. (2002). Crystal structures of the kinase domain of c-Abl in complex with the small molecule inhibitors PD173955 and imatinib (STI-571). Cancer Res 62, 4236-4243.

Nicolini, F.E., Corm, S., Le, Q.H., Sorel, N., Hayette, S., Bories, D., Leguay, T., Roy, L., Giraudier, S., Tulliez, M., et al. (2006). Mutation status and clinical outcome of 89 imatinib mesylate-resistant chronic myelogenous leukemia patients: a retrospective analysis from the French intergroup of CML (Fi(phi)-LMC GROUP). Leukemia 20, 1061-1066.

Nowell, P., and Hungerford, D. (1960). A minute chromosome in human chronic granulocytic leukemia. Science 132, 1497.

Nowell, P.C., and Hungerford, D.A. (1961). Chromosome studies in human leukemia. II. Chronic granulocytic leukemia. J Natl Cancer Inst 27, 1013-1035.

Nowicki, M.O., Falinski, R., Koptyra, M., Slupianek, A., Stoklosa, T., Gloc, E., Nieborowska-Skorska, M., Blasiak, J., and Skorski, T. (2004). BCR/ABL oncogenic kinase promotes unfaithful repair of the reactive oxygen species-dependent DNA double-strand breaks. Blood 104, 3746-3753.

O'Hagan, H.M., Mohammad, H.P., and Baylin, S.B. (2008). Double strand breaks can initiate gene silencing and SIRT1-dependent onset of DNA methylation in an exogenous promoter CpG island. PLoS genetics 4, e1000155.

O'Hare, T., Shakespeare, W.C., Zhu, X., Eide, C.A., Rivera, V.M., Wang, F., Adrian, L.T., Zhou, T., Huang, W.S., Xu, Q., et al. (2009). AP24534, a pan-BCR-ABL inhibitor for chronic myeloid leukemia, potently inhibits the T315I mutant and overcomes mutation-based resistance. Cancer Cell 16, 401-412.

Oberdoerffer, P., Michan, S., McVay, M., Mostoslavsky, R., Vann, J., Park, S.K., Hartlerode, A., Stegmuller, J., Hafner, A., Loerch, P., et al. (2008). SIRT1 redistribution on chromatin promotes genomic stability but alters gene expression during aging. Cell 135, 907-918.

Perrotti, D., Jamieson, C., Goldman, J., and Skorski, T. (2010). Chronic myeloid leukemia: mechanisms of blastic transformation. J Clin Invest 120, 2254-2264.

Press, R.D. (2010). Major molecular response in CML patients treated with tyrosine kinase inhibitors: the paradigm for monitoring targeted cancer therapy. The oncologist 15, 744-749.

Quintas-Cardama, A., Kantarjian, H., and Cortes, J. (2010). Third-generation tyrosine kinase inhibitors and beyond. Seminars in hematology 47, 371-380.

Roche-Lestienne, C., Lai, J.L., Darre, S., Facon, T., and Preudhomme, C. (2003). A mutation conferring resistance to imatinib at the time of diagnosis of chronic myelogenous leukemia. N Engl J Med 348, 2265-2266.

Roche-Lestienne, C., Soenen-Cornu, V., Grardel-Duflos, N., Lai, J.L., Philippe, N., Facon, T., Fenaux, P., and Preudhomme, C. (2002). Several types of mutations of the Abl gene can be found in chronic myeloid leukemia patients resistant to STI571, and they can pre-exist to the onset of treatment. Blood 100, 1014-1018.

Rossetto, D., Truman, A.W., Kron, S.J., and Cote, J. (2010). Epigenetic modifications in double-strand break DNA damage signaling and repair. Clin Cancer Res 16, 4543-4552.

Rowley, J.D. (1973). Letter: A new consistent chromosomal abnormality in chronic myelogenous leukaemia identified by quinacrine fluorescence and Giemsa staining. Nature 243, 290-293.

Sallmyr, A., Tomkinson, A.E., and Rassool, F.V. (2008). Up-regulation of WRN and DNA ligase IIIalpha in chronic myeloid leukemia: consequences for the repair of DNA double-strand breaks. Blood 112, 1413-1423.

Sanders, S.L., Portoso, M., Mata, J., Bahler, J., Allshire, R.C., and Kouzarides, T. (2004). Methylation of histone H4 lysine 20 controls recruitment of Crb2 to sites of DNA damage. Cell 119, 603-614.

Schindler, T., Bornmann, W., Pellicena, P., Miller, W.T., Clarkson, B., and Kuriyan, J. (2000). Structural mechanism for STI-571 inhibition of abelson tyrosine kinase. Science 289, 1938-1942.

Shah, N.P., Nicoll, J.M., Nagar, B., Gorre, M.E., Paquette, R.L., Kuriyan, J., and Sawyers, C.L. (2002). Multiple BCR-ABL kinase domain mutations confer polyclonal resistance to the tyrosine kinase inhibitor imatinib (STI571) in chronic phase and blast crisis chronic myeloid leukemia. Cancer Cell 2, 117-125.

Shah, N.P., and Sawyers, C.L. (2003). Mechanisms of resistance to STI571 in Philadelphia chromosome-associated leukemias. Oncogene 22, 7389-7395.

Shah, N.P., Skaggs, B.J., Branford, S., Hughes, T.P., Nicoll, J.M., Paquette, R.L., and Sawyers, C.L. (2007). Sequential ABL kinase inhibitor therapy selects for compound drug-resistant BCR-ABL mutations with altered oncogenic potency. J Clin Invest 117, 2562-2569.

Shah, N.P., Tran, C., Lee, F.Y., Chen, P., Norris, D., and Sawyers, C.L. (2004). Overriding imatinib resistance with a novel ABL kinase inhibitor. Science 305, 399-401.

Skaggs, B.J., Gorre, M.E., Ryvkin, A., Burgess, M.R., Xie, Y., Han, Y., Komisopoulou, E., Brown, L.M., Loo, J.A., Landaw, E.M., et al. (2006). Phosphorylation of the ATP-binding loop directs oncogenicity of drug-resistant BCR-ABL mutants. Proc Natl Acad Sci U S A 103, 19466-19471.

Slupianek, A., Schmutte, C., Tombline, G., Nieborowska-Skorska, M., Hoser, G., Nowicki, M.O., Pierce, A.J., Fishel, R., and Skorski, T. (2001). BCR/ABL regulates mammalian RecA homologs, resulting in drug resistance. Mol Cell 8, 795-806.

Tamburini, B.A., and Tyler, J.K. (2005). Localized histone acetylation and deacetylation triggered by the homologous recombination pathway of double-strand DNA repair. Mol Cell Biol 25, 4903-4913.

van Attikum, H., Fritsch, O., Hohn, B., and Gasser, S.M. (2004). Recruitment of the INO80 complex by H2A phosphorylation links ATP-dependent chromatin remodeling with DNA double-strand break repair. Cell 119, 777-788.

von Bubnoff, N., Manley, P.W., Mestan, J., Sanger, J., Peschel, C., and Duyster, J. (2006). Bcr-Abl resistance screening predicts a limited spectrum of point mutations to be associated with clinical resistance to the Abl kinase inhibitor nilotinib (AMN107). Blood 108, 1328-1333.

Wakeley, J. (1996). The excess of transitions among nucleotide substitutions: new methods of estimating transition bias underscore its significance. Trends in ecology & evolution 11, 158-162.

Weisberg, E., Manley, P.W., Breitenstein, W., Bruggen, J., Cowan-Jacob, S.W., Ray, A., Huntly, B., Fabbro, D., Fendrich, G., Hall-Meyers, E., et al. (2005). Characterization of AMN107, a selective inhibitor of native and mutant Bcr-Abl. Cancer Cell 7, 129-141.

Willis, S.G., Lange, T., Demehri, S., Otto, S., Crossman, L., Niederwieser, D., Stoffregen, E.P., McWeeney, S., Kovacs, I., Park, B., et al. (2005). High-sensitivity detection of BCR-ABL kinase domain mutations in imatinib-naive patients: correlation with clonal cytogenetic evolution but not response to therapy. Blood 106, 2128-2137.

Wiseman, H., and Halliwell, B. (1996). Damage to DNA by reactive oxygen and nitrogen species: role in inflammatory disease and progression to cancer. Biochem J 313 (Pt 1), 17-29.

Young, M.A., Shah, N.P., Chao, L.H., Seeliger, M., Milanov, Z.V., Biggs, W.H., 3rd, Treiber, D.K., Patel, H.K., Zarrinkar, P.P., Lockhart, D.J., et al. (2006). Structure of the kinase domain of an imatinib-resistant Abl mutant in complex with the Aurora kinase inhibitor VX-680. Cancer Res 66, 1007-1014.

Yuan, H., Wang, Z., Gao, C., Chen, W., Huang, Q., Yee, J.K., Bhatia, R., and Chen, W.Y. (2010). BCR-ABL gene expression is required for its mutations in a novel KCL-22 cell culture model for acquired resistance of chronic myelogenous leukemia. J Biol Chem 285, 5085-5096.

Yuan, Z., Zhang, X., Sengupta, N., Lane, W.S., and Seto, E. (2007). SIRT1 regulates the function of the Nijmegen breakage syndrome protein. Mol Cell 27, 149-162.

5

Targeting the Chronic Myeloid Leukemia Stem Cell: A Paradigm for the Curative Treatment of Human Malignancies

Adrian Woolfson[1] and Xiaoyan Jiang[2]

[1]*Discovery Medicine and Clinical Pharmacology Oncology, Bristol-Myers Squibb, Princeton,*

[2]*Terry Fox Laboratory, British Columbia Cancer Agency and Departments of Medical Genetics and Medicine, University of British Columbia, Vancouver, BC,*

[1]*US*

[2]*Canada*

1. Introduction

Chronic Myeloid Leukemia (CML) is a clonal myeloproliferative disorder of pluripotent hematopoietic stem/progenitor cells that has been paradigmatic to our understanding of the molecular and cellular basis of human malignancies. It has provided an excellent example of how a specific molecular abnormality can be targeted therapeutically to transform a life-threatening malignancy into a chronic disease. The study of CML has been characterized by a number of 'firsts'. CML was the first malignancy to be: (i) associated with a specific chromosomal abnormality, (ii) associated with a specific molecular alteration (*BCR-ABL*) and (iii) successfully treated with a specifically designed targeted therapeutic agent. As such it seems natural that CML should be the first human malignancy in which a complete medical cure is achieved through the eradication of cancer stem cells. This should be realizable through combining the specific targeting of BCR-ABL and CML stem cells. Once this has been achieved, the challenge will be to successfully transfer the lessons learned from this relatively simple and well-characterized model system to the eradication of cancer stem cells in more complex malignancies.

The treatment of CML has changed dramatically following the introduction into the clinic of the tyrosine kinase inhibitor (TKI) imatinib mesylate and second generation TKIs. These agents directly target the BCR-ABL oncoprotein product of the constitutively active BCR-ABL tyrosine kinase. The specific targeting of BCR-ABL induces durable clinical remission in a high proportion of chronic phase CML (CP-CML) subjects (5 year survival of 89%) (Druker et al, 2006). Although a major molecular response (defined as a 3-log reduction in *BCR-ABL* mutant allele burden) is obtained in many CP-CML patients, only a small number attain PCR negativity as determined by the absence of residual *BCR-ABL* transcripts (Hughes et al, 2003). This is because TKI therapy does not specifically target or eliminate leukemia stem cells (LSCs). Indeed TKI therapy alone is unlikely to ever be curative, as following treatment with TKIs LSCs persist in bone marrow (BM) stem cell niches where they harbor the potential for relapse. The emergence of resistance to TKI monotherapy through the accumulation of somatic kinase domain mutations that interfere with the binding of TKIs to the BCR-ABL ATP-binding site accounts for around 60-90% of relapses (O'Hare et al, 2006). There is consequently a significant unmet medical need for more effective therapeutic strategies that following effective tumor debulking are able to: (i) inhibit the molecular mechanisms responsible for generating the LSC genomic instability phenotype, (ii) target the essential components of the stem cell niche and the BM microenvironment that generate, protect, and nurture LSCs and (iii) efficiently eradicate LSCs. The micro-evolution of TKI resistance in CML is driven by the intrinsic genomic instability of the LSC, which in the presence of the selective pressure of drug, results in the expansion of a relatively predictable and invariant quasispecies of somatic mutants, which have differing degrees of intrinsic and acquired TKI resistance. The frequency of each of these clones oscillates with time, with a unitary or oligoclonal set eventually dominating the structure of the population and the clinical response to TKI therapy. The spectrum of mutants in any individual may be characterized through mutational analysis and subsequently used to select the most appropriate TKI therapy. The persistence of LSCs, however, allows additional drug-resistant mutants to arise, creating a new repertoire of diversity from which the most resistant and fastest growing clones are selected. As a result the therapeutic effects of first- and second-line TKI therapy are eventually circumvented. Clearly the eradication of the LSCs must form both a necessary and essential component of any therapeutic strategies that aim to achieve a deep and sustained molecular and clinical response, and ultimately a cure. In what follows we outline a number of approaches to the characterization of the CML LSC. The profiling and characterization of the LSC phenotype is expected to contribute to the rational design of LSC-targeted therapy, and as such presents an opportunity to establish a general paradigm for the development of cancer stem cell-directed cures for human malignancies.

2. Clinical and therapeutic challenges in the management of CML

CML is a clonal, multi-step and multi-lineage myeloproliferative disease that typically evolves through three phenotypically and clinically distinct stages (Goldman & Melo, 2003; Jiang X. 2007; Savona & Talpaz, 2008; Sloma et al., 2010). The first of these is an indolent chronic phase (CP) characterized at the time of diagnosis by the presence of a deregulated *BCR-ABL*$^+$ clone. This expands inappropriately and comes to dominate the population of BM progenitor cells, while at the same time continuing to produce phenotypically normal mature blood cells. There is, as a result, an excessive output of myeloid precursors and mature granulocytes into the BM and peripheral blood (PB). The second stage is an accelerated phase (AP) characterized by an incremental increase in the disease burden as demonstrated by an increased frequency of leukemic myeloid progenitor/precursor cells. The third stage is a rapidly fatal acute blast crisis phase (BC) characterized by increased genomic instability, deregulated proliferation and loss of differentiation. BC-CML may be categorized as myeloid or lymphoid (pre-B) by the appearance of increased numbers of differentiation-arrested blast cells that reflect the growth of sub-clones of early myeloid or pre-B cells respectively that have acquired additional somatic mutations (Goldman & Melo, 2003; Jiang X. 2007; Savona & Talpaz, 2008; Sloma et al., 2010). The canonical feature of CML is the presence in hematopoietic stem cell (HSC) derived progeny of a Philadelphia chromosome (Ph$^+$) containing a reciprocal t(9;22)(q34;q11) translocation, which generates a clone-specific *BCR-ABL* fusion oncogene. This encodes a chimeric BCR-ABL oncoprotein that has significantly enhanced and constitutive tyrosine kinase activity, which drives the pathogenic features of the disease (Druker et al., 1996; Lugo et al., 1990). It produces a range of biochemical changes that impact the growth-factor dependence, turnover, and genomic stability of primitive CD34+ leukemic cells, whilst at the same time having little impact on their ability to differentiate according to predefined molecular programs (Holyoake et al., 2002; Jiang et al., 2007b; Penserga & Skorski, 2007; Sloma et al., 2010; Valent, 2008).

The identification of an invariant molecular genetic alteration (*BCR-ABL*) in the vast majority of cases of CML has facilitated the development of rational targeted therapy focused on the selective inhibition of the dysregulated tyrosine kinase activity of the encoded BCR-ABL oncoprotein (Druker et al., 1996; Shah et al., 2004; Weisberg et al., 2005). Imatinib mesylate (IM, Novartis, Basel, Swizerland) was the first tyrosine inhibitor to be developed as a molecular targeted drug (Druker et al., 1996). It is a competitive inhibitor of the ATP-binding site of the ABL-kinase domain, and prevents a conformational change of the oncoprotein to its active form, resulting in the elimination of most *BCR-ABL*+ cells (Druker et al., 1996). This relatively selective agent (it also recognizes the ATP-binding site of the c-Kit and platelet-derived growth factor receptors) has been immensely effective in the treatment of subjects with CP-CML (Druker et al., 2006; Druker et al., 2001; Kantarjian et al., 2002; O'Brien et al., 2003). Nevertheless, early relapse and the emergence of IM resistance are observed in 10-20% of subjects in early CP-CML, and up to 40% of those with advanced phase disease including 1-3% of newly diagnosed CML patients that develop sudden blast crisis (Apperley, 2007; Deininger et al., 2005; Forrest et al., 2008; Kantarjian et al., 2003; O'Hare et al., 2006; Valent, 2008). The inability to successfully discontinue IM therapy following at least five years of therapy, the persistence of a reservoir of clonal leukemic stem cells following the attainment of a complete molecular response (CMR), and the uncertain safety profile of long-term TKI treatment, has led to differing views on the most appropriate choice of therapy in CP-CML (Mahon et al., 2010; Ross et al., 2010a; Ross et al., 2010b; Rousselot et al., 2007; Sobrinho-Simoes et al., 2010). Recently, second-line TKIs including Dasatinib (DA,Bristol-Myers Squibb, New York, NY, USA) and Nilotinib (NL, Novatis) have been licensed for use in this indication and represent alternative therapeutic options either first-line or for resistant or intolerant cases. Both drugs have increased potency against the *BCR-ABL* kinase domain mutants most commonly associated with IM resistance. This along with their differing spectrums of inhibitory activity across the human kinome, has translated into increased clinical efficacy in subjects with IM-resistant disease (Carter et al., 2005; Shah et al., 2004; Weisberg et al., 2005). The major cytogenetic response (MCyR) rate following therapy with DA or NL in subjects with IM-resistant CP-CML is approximately 60%, with a complete cytogenetic response (CCyR) rate of 50% (Hochhaus et al., 2008; Kantarjian et al., 2007). Two recent Phase 3 randomized trials in subjects with treatment naïve early stage CP-CML demonstrated that both drugs are more effective than IM at inducing MCyR and major molecular (MMR) responses (Kantarjian et al., 2010; Saglio et al., 2010). DA and NL were subsequently approved by the U.S. Food and Drug Administration (FDA) as first-line therapies in CP-CML. Clinical experience, however, has shown that some subjects experience inadequate responses to all existing TKI therapies, or have an initial response but then progress rapidly (Kantarjian et al., 2006; Talpaz et al., 2006). As is the case in 60% of subjects with IM-resistant disease, the recalcitrant T315I mutation also routinely dominates the observed resistance with DA and NL (Apperley, 2007; Goldman, 2007). As a result these agents have no benefit over IM in subjects whose resistance is thought to be mediated principally by T315I somatic mutants. In spite of this, each TKI has a unique spectrum of activity with respect to most of the other commonly encountered mutations that confer resistance to TKI therapy. Subjects with the V299L, T315A, and F317L/V/I/C mutations, for example, are less sensitive to DA (Muller et al., 2009; Soverini et al., 2011; Soverini et al., 2006), whereas the Y253H, E255K/V and F359V/C/I mutations are less sensitive to treatment with NL (Hughes et al., 2009; Soverini et al., 2011). Several third-generation tyrosine kinase inhibitors have been developed, including ponatinib (AP24534, ARIAD, Cambridge, Massachusetts, US) (O'Hare et al., 2009), which is an orally active multi-targeted kinase inhibitor that targets both the wild type and a broad spectrum of mutant forms of BCR-ABL. It was specifically designed to inhibit the autophosphorylation of wild-type and T315I mutant BCR-ABL and is active against most of the commonly encountered IM-resistant mutations including G250E, Y253F and E255K (O'Hare et al., 2009). In a phase 1 study 38 patients with CP-CML, 66% achieved a MCyR and 53% a CCyR. Most significantly, a total of 89% (nine subjects) of the subjects harboring a T315I mutation attained a CCyR (Santos & Quintas-Cardama, 2011). The effectiveness of long-term therapy with ponatinib in IM-resistant patients, however, has yet to be determined. Allogeneic hematopoietic stem cell transplantation (allo-HSCT) is currently the only therapeutic option for CML that has curative potential. Its use, however, is restricted to subjects of less than 50 years that have a suitable donor, and even this highly selected group has a high risk of procedure-related morbidity and mortality (Forrest et al., 2008). The salvage rate for subjects with advanced phase disease, especially BC-CML, is poor even with allo-HSCT, with the vast majority dying as a result of their disease within a few years. There is consequently a significant unmet medical need for therapeutic options that prevent the emergence of resistant sub-clones and that can be administered with curative intent as a result of the selective targeting of LSCs.

3. Properties of CML stem/progenitor cells that generate TKI resistance

Primitive quiescent CML stem cells are relatively unresponsive to TKIs (Copland et al., 2006; Graham et al., 2002; Jorgensen et al., 2007) and possess unique features that predispose them to intrinsic and acquired resistance to BCR-ABL targeted therapeutics (Chu et al., 2005; Jiang et al., 2007a; Jiang et al., 2007b; Jiang et al., 2007c; Konig et al., 2008; Sorel et al., 2004). Evidence further suggests that LSCs are responsible for relapse following the discontinuation of IM therapy (Mahon et al., 2010; Ross et al., 2010a; Ross et al., 2010b; Rousselot et al., 2007; Sobrinho-Simoes et al., 2010). The elimination of the LSCs responsible for disease perpetuation and for the intrinsic and acquired TKI resistance observed in CML therefore represents the next logical step in the treatment of CML. An essential component of this enterprise, involves the molecular characterization of the CML stem cell phenotype, BM microenvironment and the stem niche that foster the origin, development, growth and survival of LSCs.

The relative insensitivity of primitive CML cells to treatment with IM was first reported in a quiescent subset of $CD34^+$ CML cells using a carboxy-fluorescein diacetate succinimidyl diester (CFSE) staining cell division tracking assay (Graham et al., 2002; Holyoake et al., 1999). This demonstrated that 3 days of exposure of CML cells *in vitro* to concentrations of IM that were several-fold higher than those achieved in the plasma of subjects treated with 400 mg IM daily, failed to eliminate most of the primitive quiescent CML cells (Graham et al., 2002). In contrast, cells with replicative competency during the same interval were eliminated. A similar insensitivity of this subset of cells to DA and NL has also been demonstrated (Copland et al., 2006; Jorgensen et al., 2007). Subsequent studies using assays for long-term culture-initiating cells (LTC-ICs) and colony forming assays (CFCs) have

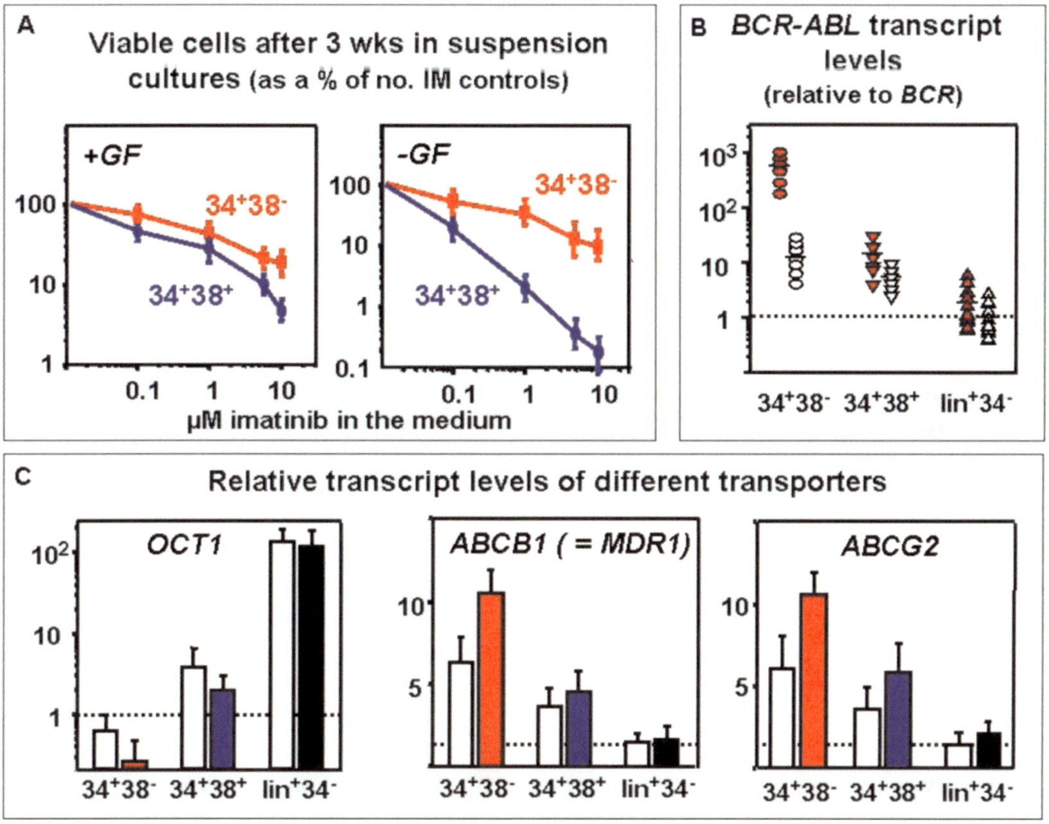

Fig. 1. Unique features of CML stem cells promoting their resistance to BCR-ABL-targeted therapies. (A) Suspension cultures were initiated with FACS-purified lin$^-$CD34$^+$CD38$^-$ and lin$^-$CD34$^+$CD38$^+$ CML cells and maintained for 3 weeks in the presence or absence of growth factors and variable concentrations of imatinib (IM). The differential IM sensitivity of lin$^-$CD34$^+$CD38$^-$ and lin$^-$CD34$^+$CD38$^+$ CML cells to IM *in vitro* is markedly enhanced under growth factor-deprived conditions. (B) *BCR-ABL* transcript levels relative to *BCR* were measured in RNA isolated from different subsets of cells. Expression of *BCR-ABL* is highly deregulated in lin$^-$CD34$^+$CD38$^-$ stem-cell enriched population as compared to their more mature progenitor cells (lin$^-$CD34$^+$CD38$^+$) and differentiated cells (lin$^+$CD34$^-$). (C) *OCT1, ABCB1* and *ABCG2* transcript levels relative to *GAPDH* were measured in different subsets of CP-CML and normal BM cells. A reduced level of *OCT1* and elevated levels of *ABCB1* and *ABCG2* were detected in lin$^-$CD34$^+$CD38$^-$ stem-cell enriched population as compared to their more mature progenitor cells. The combination of very low expression of *OCT1* (low IM uptake), highly elevated expression of *ABCB1* and *ABCG2* (high efflux of IM and other drugs) and elevated expression of *BCR-ABL* in *CML* stem cells indicates that their general insensitivity to IM and other therapeutics is likely to be explained by multiple abnormal mechanisms.

indicated that although IM is able to inhibit the proliferation of primitive CML cells *in vitro*, it does not induce concurrent apoptosis (Holtz et al., 2005; Holtz et al., 2002). We have shown that the ability of IM to inhibit primitive CML cells depends on their differentiation status (Jiang et al., 2007c). In these experiments, stem cell and progenitor cell enriched CML cell fractions ($lin^-CD34^+CD38^-$ and $lin^-CD34^+CD38^+$ cells, respectively) were isolated and cultured in the presence of varying concentrations of IM for a more prolonged period than in the earlier studies with primary quiescent CML cells (3 weeks vs. 3 to 12 days). The inhibitory effect of IM on the yield of viable cells following a 3 week exposure period was found to be much less (~10- to 20-fold) pronounced in cultures initiated with more primitive $lin^-CD34^+CD38^-$ CML cells as compared with the more differentiated $lin^-CD34^+CD38^+$ cells (Figure 1A). Taken together, these findings suggest that the most primitive CML cells are much less sensitive to IM than the differentiated bulk population. The fact that Ph^+CD34^+ CFCs and LTC-ICs remain detectable in subjects with CML that have achieved hematological remission following treatment with IM, suggests that these *in vitro* findings are likely to translate into the clinic (Bhatia et al., 2003; Chu et al., 2005). They are further supported by a recent report revealing the presence of *BCR-ABL*+ cells in LTC-ICs of CML patients that have achieved prolonged clinical remission following treatment with either interferon-alpha, IM or DA (Chomel et al., 2011). However, whereas most CML cells are oncogene addicted and sensitive to TKI treatment, the growth and survival of CML LSCs do not appear to be BCR-ABL tyrosine kinase activity dependent (Corbin et al., 2011). This suggests that alternative pathways may be active in CML LSCs that drive their proliferation and self-renewal in a BCR-ABL independent manner. Combination therapies aimed at targeting critical components of these pathways are likely to be of key importance in the derivation of a logical CML LSC eradication strategy.

Other studies have shown that CML stem/progenitor cells have multiple unique features that would be expected to contribute to the observed intrinsic and acquired resistance to *BCR-ABL* directed therapeutics (Copland, 2009; Engler et al., 2010; Jiang et al., 2007a; Jiang et al., 2007b; Jiang et al., 2007c). These include: (i) elevated levels of *BCR-ABL* expression and kinase activity in CML stem cells as compared with their more mature progeny (Figure 1B) in a manner that is cell cycle status independent (Barnes et al., 2005; Copland et al., 2006; Jamieson et al., 2004; Jiang et al., 2007b; Jiang et al., 2008; Jiang et al., 2007c), (ii) a corresponding reduced (almost undetectable) level of the transporter gene *OCT1* that is the principal regulator of IM uptake (Figure 1C) (Thomas et al., 2004; White et al., 2006) and whose decreased levels would be expected to reduce the ability of cells to take up IM (Engler et al., 2010; Jiang et al., 2007c) and (iii) elevated levels of expression of the ABC transporter genes *ABCB1(MDR)* and *ABCG2* (Figure 1C) which enhance the cellular efflux of IM and other drugs (Jiang et al., 2007c; Jordanides et al., 2006; Lepper et al., 2005). The combination of an exceptionally low level of *OCT1* expression which impedes cellular IM uptake, a highly elevated expression of *ABCB1* and *ABCG2* which produces a high rate of cellular IM efflux, and elevated expression of the *BCR-ABL* oncogene in CML stem cells, indicates that their insensitivity to IM and other therapeutics is in part explained by a unique portfolio of protective mechanisms (Jiang et al., 2007b; Jiang et al., 2007c). Interestingly studies in a cohort of 30 CML patients have shown that IM-non-responders have lower *OCT1* transcript levels than IM-responders (Crossman et al., 2005), and that the functional activity of the encoded OCT1 protein, as measured by the OCT1-mediated influx of IM into primary CML cells, is predictive of the long-term outcome of CP-CML subjects treated with IM (White et al., 2010; White et al., 2006). This suggests that measurement of OCT1 expression might provide a useful predictor of the long-term risk of resistance acquisition in subjects with IM-treated CML.

In order to determine whether the unique properties of CD34$^+$ stem/progenitor cells derived from treatment-naïve CML patients correlate with the subsequent clinical response of the patients to IM therapy, we conducted a retrospective analysis of pre-treatment CD34$^+$ PB cells obtained from 25 IM-treated CP-CML subjects with documented clinical outcomes (Jiang et al., 2010). Following the isolation of CD34$^+$ cells from pre-treatment samples, we measured their *in vitro* CFC sensitivity to IM, expression levels of *BCR-ABL*, *OCT1*, *ABCB1/MDR*, and *ABCG2*, and the frequency of *BCR-ABL* tyrosine kinase domain somatic mutations. The data were segregated and analyzed according to whether they were from the 11 clinically defined IM-responders or the 14 IM non-responders. This confirmed the reported features of CD34$^+$ CML cells, and identified two further features that differed significantly between the two groups. These were the responses of the pre-treatment CFCs to IM exposure *in vitro* ($P<0.0001$) and the frequency of mutant *BCR-ABL* transcripts in CD34$^+$ cells ($P=0.0025$) suggesting that these parameters might form the basis of a prospective test for the optimization of CP-CML management (Jiang et al., 2010).

4. Genomic instability and a mutator phenotype as an invariant feature of CML LSCs

The genomic instability of primitive CML cells induced by the presence of the *BCR-ABL* fusion oncogene has long been thought to be a critical feature of CML. However, it is only in the last decade that data from CML cell lines and transgenic mice have provided definitive evidence that the *BCR-ABL* oncogene is necessary for the induction of genomic instability in hematopoietic cells (Brain et al., 2002; Brain et al., 2003; Canitrot et al., 1999). *BCR-ABL* is able, for example, to induce a mutator phenotype in *BCR-ABL* transfected murine cells. It also produces elevated levels of reactive oxygen species (ROS)-dependent DNA damage as compared with non-transfected controls. This damage to genomic DNA is likely to contribute to the accumulation of the somatic point mutations found in the ATP-binding site of the constitutively expressed BCR-ABL tyrosine kinase, and which are responsible for most cases of TKI resistance (Koptyra et al., 2006; Skorski, 2008). Interestingly, the ROS-dependent mutations in *BCR-ABL* transfected cells were principally detected in a gene encoding the Na^+K^+ATPase *Atp1a1* (Koptyra et al., 2006). Mutant *ATP1A1* transcripts including those containing point mutations, insertions and deletions have been reported at high frequency (15-34%) in CD34$^+$ CML cells rescued from IM nonresponders, a mutational rate similar to that observed in the *BCR-ABL* kinase domain of CML subjects. These mutations are not seen in CD34$^+$ BM cells derived from healthy controls (Jiang et al., 2010). This and other data suggest that *BCR-ABL* induces a mutator phenotype, which results in the genome-wide instability of primitive CML cells.

Investigations into the cellular and molecular causes of IM resistance have shown that the acquisition of somatic mutations in the *BCR-ABL* kinase-encoding domain that reduce the efficiency of IM binding to the ATP binding site represents the most common mechanism of resistance (accounting for 60-80% of relapses) (Deininger et al., 2005; O'Hare et al., 2006; Soverini et al., 2011; Valent, 2008). Copy number amplifications of *BCR-ABL* in contrast are rare (<10% of cases) (Gorre et al., 2001; Hochhaus et al., 2002; Tauchi & Ohyashiki, 2004).

More than 90 different *BCR-ABL* kinase domain point mutations have been reported at varying frequencies in IM-resistant subjects (Apperley, 2007; Hughes et al., 2006; Shah et al., 2002; Soverini et al., 2011). Of these 15 specific amino acid substitutions account for more than 85% of the mutations at the protein sequence level. The mutations responsible for 66% of reported cases, furthermore, have been shown to occur at only six different positions (G250E, Y253F/H, E255K/V, T315I, F359V, H396R/P). The T315I mutation, which confers resistance to IM, DA and NL, is the most frequently detected mutation in IM-resistant patients and is the hardest mutant to treat (Apperley, 2007; Carter et al., 2005; Shah et al., 2004; Soverini et al., 2011; Weisberg et al., 2005). *BCR-ABL* kinase domain mutations are found in IM-naïve patients but not in the germline of healthy controls, indicating that at least some of the mutations are somatically generated prior to the presence of drug selection, and that the increased frequency of mutations observed following TKI therapy occurs as a result of drug-induced selection and associated clonal expansion (Roche-Lestienne et al., 2003; Roche-Lestienne et al., 2002; Willis et al., 2005). The somatic mutations themselves arise as a consequence of underlying genomic instability, which may reflect impaired processes of DNA repair in LSCs. Although some of the mutants are adaptive under the selective pressure of drug exposure, the majority diminish in frequency in the presence of TKI selection. We and others have demonstrated that the *BCR-ABL* fusion gene in $CD34^+$ leukemic progenitor cells (Chu et al., 2005; Jiang et al., 2010) and $CD34^+CD38^-$ stem cell-enriched cells is itself highly unstable (Jiang et al., 2007a) This is reflected in the unusually high frequency of *BCR-ABL* mutations that accumulate in the $CD34^+CD38^-$ compartment in the presence or absence of IM selection. The rapid acquisition of somatic mutations in *BCR-ABL* is also observed in the progeny of CML cells stimulated to proliferate and differentiate *in vitro* (Figure 2) (Jiang et al., 2007a). The rapid and prolific generation of *BCR-ABL* somatic mutants in primary CML cells *in vitro* extends recent findings in *BCR-ABL*-transduced murine BaF3 cells (von Bubnoff et al., 2005), and adult BM cells (Flamant & Turhan, 2005) and indicates that primitive leukemic CML cells have an intrinsically high rate of mutation, and a tendency to fix new somatic point mutations irrespective of the presence or absence of drug. The nature and timing of these apparently stochastic events relative to the size of the primary LSC clone at the time diagnosis and the timing, nature and extent of TKI therapy, may to some extent explain the variable clinical responses observed in different subjects (Jiang et al., 2007a; Roche-Lestienne et al., 2003; Shah et al., 2002; Sorel et al., 2004). A recent study shows that CML subjects defined retrospectively as either IM responders or IM non-responders display significant differences in the frequency of mutant *BCR-ABL* transcripts present in their pre-treatment $CD34^+$ cells (P=0.0025), with some of the highly resistant *BCR-ABL* kinase domain somatic mutants such as T315I being amplified from the $CD34^+$ cells of IM non-responsive subjects (Jiang et al., 2010). Overall this suggests that primary CML stem/progenitor cells have a high degree of focal and possibly genome-wide instability, emphasizing the importance of taking the properties of these cells into account when considering new therapeutic approaches. The unique properties of leukemia stem/progenitor cells may, furthermore, help predict individual responses to TKI therapies and in so doing improve clinical management by facilitating personalized treatment decisions.

One approach to targeting the LSC involves defining and inhibiting the generative mechanism causal to the observed genomic instability in LSCs. The ROS that are induced by *BCR-ABL* are known to cause many types of DNA damage including double-strand breaks (DSBs). It has been shown that the error-prone repair of DSBs by non-homologous end-joining (NHEJ) may be responsible for at least some of the somatic point mutations observed

A

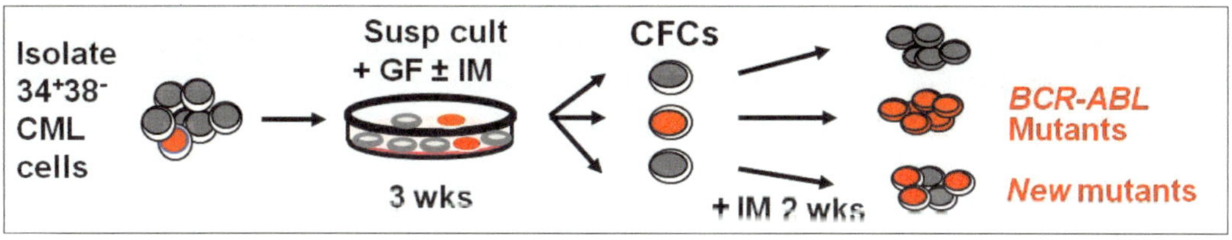

B

No. of colonies of each mutant type	Wt	Mt	Wt + Mt
Start 34+38- cells	20/26	6/26	-
3 wk - IM	5/18	1/18	12/18
3 wk + IM	3/19	2/19	14/19

C

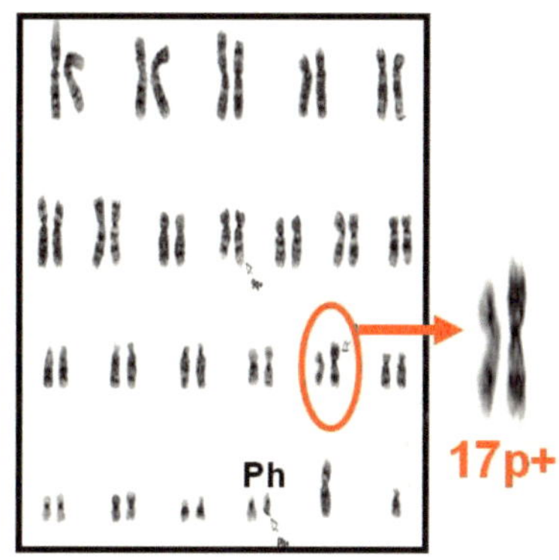

Fig. 2. CML stem cells are highly unstable and generate a high frequency of *BCR-ABL* kinase domain mutations both *in vitro* and *in vivo*. (A) Suspension cultures were initiated with FACS-purified lin-CD34+CD38- stem cell-enriched population and maintained for 3 weeks in the presence or absence of growth factors and IM. The cells harvested from the 3-week cultures were then assayed for CFCs. Mutational analysis was then performed for the detection of *BCR-ABL* kinase domain mutations in freshly isolated lin-CD34+CD38- cells and their CFC progenies. (B) Pre-existing *BCR-ABL* kinase domain mutations could be detected in freshly isolated lin-CD34+CD38- stem cells and new mutations appeared during the growth of primitive CML cells *in vitro*. (C) Chromosomal abnormalities, such as 17 p+, could be observed from single colonies generated from the cells present after 3 weeks in culture with IM.

in early CML and also the large deletions seen in later-stage CML. This is supported by evidence which suggests that key protein components of the major NHEJ pathway, WRN and DNA ligase IIIα that form a molecular complex which is recruited to DSBs, are up-regulated in CML (Sallmyr et al., 2008). There is also evidence that ROS-induced DSBs are repaired, at least to some extent, by single-strand annealing (SSA). This is a rare and very unfaithful repair mechanism whose activity has been shown to be stimulated by *BCR-ABL*. Interestingly the activation of this repair mechanism is attenuated by IM therapy (Cramer et al., 2008). The presence of multiple alternative error-prone mechanisms for repairing DSBs, raises the possibility that the differential recruitment of these alternative repair pathways itself evolves as the disease progresses from CP to BC.

One approach to identifying the generative mechanism that underlies the observed genomic instability in CML, is to generate a compendium of *BCR-ABL* kinase domain somatic mutations to determine if the mutator phenotype observed in LSCs is associated with a distinct mutational signature. In order to establish whether CML is characterized by a distinct mutational imprint, we analyzed *BCR-ABL* tyrosine kinase domain sequence data from 15 IM-naïve and 316 IM-resistant CP-CML subjects (Grant et al., 2010). This revealed a distinct and non-random distribution of *BCR-ABL* kinase domain mutations with apparent hot spot regions located at codon positions 1 and 2, and several other distinct features that are commensurate with the activity of a distinct mutator. These include a propensity for transitions relative to unselected regions of the human genome across all codon positions, a T-to-C mutational hotspot at codon position 2, a near lack of mutations at codon position 3, and an overall under-representation of C-to-T mutations. These results provide evidence for the activity of a distinct mutator that is active in LSCs, and it is interesting that the frequently observed M244V and D276G mutations arise from T-to-C transitions, both of which are predicted consequences of putative CML LSC mutator activity. The clinically most problematic mutation, T315I, is interestingly generated by a C-to-T transition, indicating the imprint of intense drug-mediated selection. This characteristic mutational signature may provide insights into the mechanism that contributes to the observed genomic instability in LSCs, and which may act in concert with the error-prone repair of DSBs. Candidate mutators include the *MYC* oncogene, which is known to result in aberrant DNA synthesis and which has been shown to be over-expressed in CML subjects at the time of diagnosis. Higher expression levels have, furthermore, been shown to correlate with a poor clinical response to IM. Interestingly *MYC* levels do not directly correlate with *BCR-ABL* levels in subjects treated with IM (Albajar et al., 2011).

5. Strategies for the eradication of leukemic stem cells

The existence of both intrinsic and acquired resistance to TKIs in CML stem cells has prompted considerable interest in identifying multi-targeted therapeutic strategies able to combat the emergence of resistant clones by eliminating the LSCs that generate them. It has been hypothesized that combination strategies able to target both proliferating and primitive quiescent leukemic cells will significantly improve clinical outcomes in CML (Jiang X. 2007; Savona & Talpaz, 2008; Sloma et al., 2010). There is no doubt that the development of stem cell-directed therapies will be critical to the attainment of prolonged remission and ultimately TKI cessation and cure. As expected, the use of molecularly targeted agents such as IM results in the elimination of the majority of the more differentiated leukemic cells, but leaves primitive stem cells largely untouched. So although able to effect a significant initial reduction in leukemic cells of a more mature differentiation stage, LSCs eventually repopulate the malignant cell population following or during ongoing TKI therapy, generating new resistant mutants that leads to disease persistence and clinical recurrence. This situation recapitulates the elimination of rapidly cycling cells and sparing of quiescent leukemic stem cells seen in the deployment of conventional chemotherapeutics. Whereas monotherapy using agents that directly target LSCs may result in only a minimal observable initial response, in the absence of LSCs the leukemia is not expected to be maintained or expanded. Most importantly, the micro-evolutionary process that continuously and dynamically generates a spectrum of mutant clones will be disabled. As a result the disease burden would be expected to decline incrementally, providing significantly improved long-term outcomes. Combination with TKIs or other agents that target proliferating cells of a more mature phenotype will though continue to be essential for debulking. In the situation where resistant clones with *BCR-ABL* kinase domain mutations and/or other critical mutations are already present at high frequency, the simultaneous targeting of the mutant clonal population with a second generation TKI will be necessary if molecular cure is to be achieved. This process will be facilitated by the development of new and more effective classes of debulking agents. A switch pocket inhibitor DCC-2036, for example, has been developed which targets the hydrophobic pockets distant from the catalytic region that regulate the transition between the active and inactive state of BCR-ABL. This drug appears to successfully inhibit the majority of TKI-resistant mutants, including the critically important T315I gatekeeper mutation (Chan et al., 2011). DCC-2036 inhibits the BCR-ABL oncoprotein in both its active and inactive conformation by inducing and stabilizing the type II inactive conformation. It is highly effective in suppressing the growth of transduced wild-type *BCR-ABL* murine cells, including cells transduced with the T315I mutant both *in vitro* and *in vivo* (Chan et al., 2011). A phase I trial of DCC-2036 in IM resistant subjects carrying either the T315I mutation or two or more alternative TKI mutations is currently underway. However, although useful in the management of TKI-resistant mutations, DCC-2036 alone is unlikely to target LSCs.

Global gene expression analysis and transcriptome profiling, including the identification of deregulated micro-RNAs (miRs) and the genes they target using next-generation sequencing technologies, have been applied in order to facilitate the identification of new molecular targets and biomarkers able to predict TKI responsivity in primary CML cells, IM resistant cells and *BCR-ABL*-transduced cells. Several studies have compared the transcriptome of $CD34^+$ progenitor cells and $CD34^+CD38^-$ stem cell-enriched leukemic cells with their healthy counterparts. These studies have confirmed the functional relevance of the activation of the JAK/STAT, PI3K/AKT, RAS/MAPK and NFκB pathways in LSCs (Janssen et al., 2005; Jongen-Lavrencic et al., 2005; Kronenwett et al., 2005; Nowicki et al., 2003; Radich et al., 2006; Salesse & Verfaillie, 2003; Yong et al., 2006; Zhao et al., 2008). These studies have also identified differentially expressed genes that are involved in the regulation of DNA repair, cell cycle control, cell adhesion, and homing, as well as genes and transcription factors involved in drug metabolism (Diaz-Blanco et al., 2007; Kronenwett et al., 2005; Salesse & Verfaillie, 2003; Yong et al., 2006; Zhao et al., 2008). Several miRs and their target genes, including *miR-203, miR-328* and *miR-17-92* cluster, have been shown to regulate *BCR-ABL* and the expression of other genes known to be critical to the generation and maintenance of the CML phenotype (Bueno et al., 2008; Eiring et al., 2010; Venturini et al., 2007), indicating the potential utility of Micro-RNA profiling in the identification of novel targets for LSC-directed therapies. Of note, several new potential targets have been identified which regulate the maintenance of self-renewal, quiescence and expansion of CML stem and progenitor cells. These include promyelocytic leukemia protein (PML), β-Catenin, RNA-binding proteins (RBPs) and the *BMI1* and *FOXO* transcription factors, suggesting that the specific targeting of these proteins in conjunction with TKIs, may help eliminate residual CML LSCs (Copland, 2009; Eiring et al., 2008; Hu et al., 2009; Ito et al., 2008; Naka et al., 2010; Park et al., 2003; Rizo et al., 2010; Zhao et al., 2007).

The systematic applications of these and other new technologies have resulted in significant advances in our understanding of the molecular properties of CML stem and progenitor cells. They are also helping to define the nature of the BM microenvironment and stem cell niche that support the growth and differentiation of LSCs. The specific targeting of the BM microenvironment and stem cell niche represent alternative and indirect strategies for the elimination of LSCs (Figure 3). The chemokine receptor CXCR4, for example, which is central to stem cell localization and a known chemo-attractant for hematopoietic cells, is induced by IM and causes CML cell migration to the BM and promotes the survival of quiescent CML progenitors (Jin et al., 2008). This suggests a possible mechanism of IM resistance working through the cross-talk between CML stem/progenitor cells and their BM microenvironment niches, and suggests a rationale for the combination of CXCR4 antagonists with TKIs so as to more effectively eliminate IM-resistant LSCs.

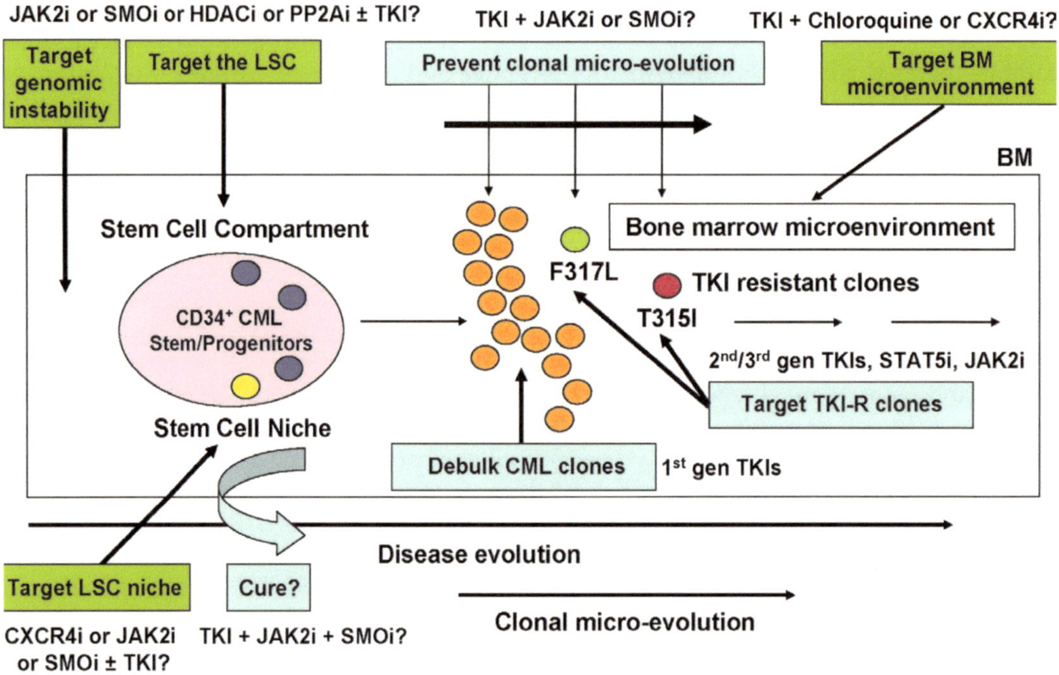

Fig. 3. **Targeting the CML stem cell.** Schematic diagram of the stem cell compartment and stem cell niche, indicating the specific targets of conventional first line TKI drugs, second and third generation TKIs, and the opportunities for targeting the CML stem cells either directly, or through the targeting and manipulation of the stem cell niche or bone marrow microenvironment.

Components of the sonic hedgehog signalling pathway, including the smoothened transmembrane protein (SMO), have similarly been shown to play a critical role in normal and leukemic stem cell development, proliferation and self-renewal, including the regulation of the epithelial-mesenchymal transition (Varjosalo & Taipale, 2008). Knockdown or inhibition of *SMO* impairs HSC self-renewal and abrogates or delays the appearance of CML in several *in vitro* and *in vivo* models (Dierks et al., 2008; Zhao et al., 2009). Conversely, SMO over-activity has been demonstrated in CML cells, with their proliferation being more SMO-dependent than that of healthy HSCs. Clinical trials evaluating the effects of SMO pathway antagonists developed by a number of different pharmaceutical companies and the relevance of this pathway are currently under way in a range of different malignant indications. The combination of NL with the SMO inhibitor LDE225 and DA with PF-04449913 has been reported as having additive effects on the inhibition of primitive CML cells *in vitro* and *in vivo* (Mar et al., 2011). Another study indicates that a combination of histone deacetylase inhibitors (HDACis, e.g. LAQ824) with IM is effective in targeting quiescent CML stem cells (Figure 3). This study also suggests that an IM/HDAC combination inhibits several genes that regulate hematopoietic stem cell maintenance and survival (Zhang et al., 2010). Another study demonstrates that the targeting of autophagy, a process that allows cells to adapt to environmental stresses, enhances the effects of TKIs in *BCR-ABL*+ cell lines and in primary CML stem and progenitor cells (Bellodi et al., 2009). IM induces autophagy in BC-CML cell lines and in primary CML cells, and is associated with endoplasmic reticulum (ER) stress that is mechanistically non-overlapping with IM-induced apoptosis. Combination treatment with TKIs and inhibitors of autophagy such as chloroquine, is more effective in eliminating CML stem and progenitor cells *in vitro* than TKIs or autophagy inhibitors alone (Bellodi et al., 2009). The effectiveness of this combination treatment in eliminating primary CML stem and progenitor cells *in vivo*, however, remains to be seen. Other promising therapeutic strategies include the induction of protein phosphatase-2A activation by FTY720, which inhibits the survival and self-renewal of CML progenitor cells (Neviani et al., 2007; Neviani et al., 2005). A farnesyltransferase inhibitor (BMS-214662) was also found to target primitive quiescent CML cells, indicating a possible role for this class of inhibitors (Copland et al., 2008).

We have been pursuing a strategy based on the targeting of JAK2 with a view to inhibiting the activity of a biologically important multi-molecular complex that we have identified comprising AHI-1 (a novel signalling molecule encoded by the Abelson helper integration site 1 gene), the BCR-ABL fusion oncoprotein and JAK2 kinase (Zhou et al., 2008). *AHI-1* is upregulated in highly enriched populations of CML stem cells in which the levels of *BCR-ABL* transcripts are also elevated (Jiang et al., 2004; Jiang et al., 2007c). Interestingly, overexpression of *AHI-1* confers a growth advantage *in vitro* and results in leukemia *in vivo*, synergizing with *BCR-ABL* to enhance these outcomes (Zhou et al., 2008). Conversely, the stable suppression of *AHI-1* in CD34+ CML cells using small interfering RNA, reduces their growth autonomy *in vitro*. Importantly, this newly defined AHI-1-BCR-ABL-JAK2 molecular interaction complex appears to mediate leukemic stem cell transformation and plays an important role in the TKI response/resistance of primary CML stem and progenitor cells. JAK2 itself is known to interact with the C-terminus of BCR-ABL, and is one of the most prominent targets of BCR-ABL in *BCR-ABL* transformed CML cells (Miyamoto et al., 2001; Samanta et al., 2006; Xie et al., 2001). BCR-ABL has also been found to interact with the IL-3/GM-CSF receptor, which subsequently contributes to the downstream activation of JAK2 (Wilson-Rawls et al., 1997). Furthermore, in primitive CML cells, *BCR-ABL* expression stimulates the production of IL-3, G-CSF and GM-CSF which, following binding to their cognate receptors, further contributes to the CML progenitor cell resistance to TKIs via the activation of the JAK2/STAT5 pathway (Jiang et al., 1999; Wang et al., 2007). High *STAT5* levels have also been shown to mediate acquired IM-resistance in CML cells and the STAT5 inhibitor pimozide was shown to reduce their survival (Nelson et al., 2011; Warsch et al., 2011). Therefore, targeting the activity of JAK2 could provide an excellent strategy to complement the inhibition of BCR-ABL kinase activity in primary CML stem cells (Figure 4). Indeed, recent studies have demonstrated that JAK2 inhibitors (TG101209, WP1193) and a dual kinase inhibitor of JAK2 and ABL kinases (ON044580) induced apoptosis in IM-sensitive and IM-resistant CML cell lines (Samanta et al., 2011; Samanta et al., 2010) and that treatment with TKIs in combination with TG101209 results in greater inhibition of CML stem and progenitor cells as compared to when the same cells are treated with either TKIs or TG101209 alone or a combination of TKIs (DeGeer et al., 2010; DeGeer et al., 2009). Several

JAK2 inhibitors with varying degrees of intra-JAK family and intra-kinome selectivity are currently in various stages of clinical development. However, the myelosuppressive effects of these inhibitors on normal hematopoietic stem/progenitor cells remain a concern. The development of highly selective and less toxic (fewer hits across the kinome) JAK2 inhibitors in combination with first or second generation TKIs provides an attractive option for the specific targeting of LSCs (Figure 3 and 4). The permanent eradication of the leukemia stem cell in conjunction with tumor debulking, is expected to result in a functional cure, and in so doing to provide the study of CML with its ultimate crowning achievement. Importantly it should also provide molecular medicine with a general paradigm for the medical cure of cancer through stem cell eradication that with appropriate modifications should be applicable to multiple tumor types.

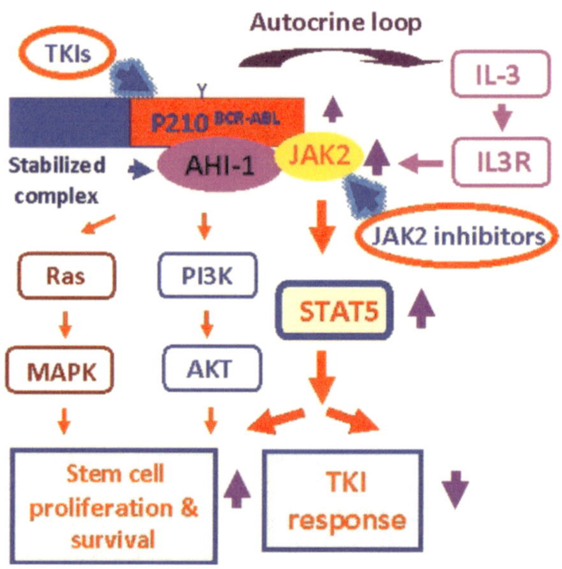

Fig. 4. Model of the targeting of the AHI-1-BCR-ABL-JAK2 complex in CML stem cells by combination treatment of TKI and JAK2 inhibitors. Schematic diagram of the AHI-1-BCR-ABL-JAK2 interaction complex that regulates constitutive activation of BCR-ABL and JAK2/STAT5 and results in increased proliferation and a reduced TKI response in CML stem and progenitor cells. Targeting both BCR-ABL and JAK2 activities to destabilize this protein interaction complex may represent a potential therapeutic option for CML.

6. Conclusion

The discovery of tyrosine kinase inhibitors marked a major advance in CML therapy and other cancers. Although highly successful, selective tyrosine kinase inhibition has not resulted in a functional cure. As CML is driven by genetically unstable pluripotent leukemic stem cells, therapeutic approaches that target these cells will be required for definitive curative therapies. The systematic characterization of the unique biological properties of CML LSCs promises to deliver new insights into the process of malignant transformation and disease progression. As it comprises a relatively simple and well-understood model system, it is envisaged that the elimination of LSCs in CML will provide a general paradigm for cancer stem cell eradication and the consequent provision for the basis of medical cures across a broad range of different malignancies.

7. Acknowledgment

The preparation of this book chapter was enabled by support from research grants from the Canadian Cancer Society (Grant# 700289), the leukemia & Lymphoma Society of Canada and the Cancer Research Society (X. J). X. Jiang is Michael Smith Foundation for Health Research Scholar.

8. Conflict-of-interest disclosure

A. Woolfson is an employee of Bristol-Myers Squibb, some of whose products are discussed in this chapter.

9. References

Albajar, M., Gomez-Casares, M.T., Llorca, J., Mauleon, I., Vaque, J.P., Acosta, J.C., Bermúdez, A., Donato, N., Delgado, M.D. & Leon, J. (2011). MYC in chronic myeloid leukemia: Induction of aberrant DNA synthesis and association with poor response to Imatinib. *Mol. Cancer Res.*, Vol.9, 564-576

Apperley, J.F. (2007). Part I: mechanisms of resistance to imatinib in chronic myeloid leukaemia. *Lancet Oncol.*, Vol.8, 1018-1029

Barnes, D.J., Palaiologou, D., Panousopoulou, E., Schultheis, B., Yong, A.S., Wong, A., Pattacini, L., Goldman, J.M. & Melo, J.V. (2005). Bcr-Abl expression levels determine the rate of development of resistance to imatinib mesylate in chronic myeloid leukemia. *Cancer Res.*, Vol.65, 8912-8919

Bellodi, C., Lidonnici, M.R., Hamilton, A., Helgason, G.V., Soliera, A.R., Ronchetti, M., Galavotti, S., Young, K.W., Selmi, T., Yacobi, R., Van Etten, R.A., Donato, N., Hunter, A., Dinsdale, D., Tirro, E., Vigneri, P., Nicotera, P., Dyer, M.J., Holyoake, T., Salomoni, P. & Calabretta, B. (2009). Targeting autophagy potentiates tyrosine kinase inhibitor-induced cell death in Philadelphia chromosome-positive cells, including primary CML stem cells. *J. Clin. Invest.*, Vol.119, 1109-1123

Bhatia, R., Holtz, M., Niu, N., Gray, R., Snyder, D.S., Sawyers, C.L., Arber, D.A., Slovak, M.L. & Forman, S.J. (2003). Persistence of malignant hematopoietic progenitors in chronic myelogenous leukemia patients in complete cytogenetic remission following imatinib mesylate treatment. *Blood*, Vol.101, 4701-4707

Brain, J., Saksena, A. & Laneuville, P. (2002). The kinase inhibitor STI571 reverses the Bcr-Abl induced point mutation frequencies observed in pre-leukemic $P190^{Bcr\text{-}Abl}$ transgenic mice. *Leuk. Res.*, Vol.26, 1011-1016

Brain, J.M., Goodyer, N. & Laneuville, P. (2003). Measurement of genomic instability in preleukemic $P190^{BCR/ABL}$ transgenic mice using inter-simple sequence repeat polymerase chain reaction. *Cancer Res.*, Vol.63, 4895-4898

Bueno, M.J., Perez De Castro, I., Gomez de Cedron, M., Santos, J., Calin, G.A., Ciqudosa, J.C., Croce, C.M., Fernandez-Piqueras, J. & Malumbres, M. (2008). Genetic and epigenetic silencing of microRNA-203 enhances ABL1 and BCR-ABL1 oncogene expression. *Cancer Cell*, Vol.13, 496-506

Canitrot, Y., Lautier, D., Laurent, G., Frechet, M., Ahmed, A., Turhan, A.G., Salles, B., Cazaux, C. & Hoffmann, J.S. (1999). Mutator phenotype of BCR-ABL transfected Ba/F3 cell lines and its association with enhanced expression of DNA polymerase b. *Oncogene,* Vol.18, 2676-2680

Carter, T.A., Wodicka, L.M., Shah, N.P., Velasco, A.M., Fabian, M.A., Treiber, D.K., Milanov, Z.V., Atteridge, C.E., Biggs, W.H.I., Edeen, P.T., Floyd, M., Ford, J.M., Grotzfeld, R.M., Herrgard, S., Insko, D.E., Mehta, S.A., Patel, H.K., Pao, W., Sawyers, C.L., Varmus, H., Zarrinkar, P.P. & Lockhart, D.J. (2005). Inhibition of drug-resistant mutants of ABL, KIT, and EGF receptor kinases. *Proceedings of the National Academy of Sciences USA,* Vol.102, 11011-11016

Chan, W.W., Wise, S.C., Kaufman, M.D., Ahn, Y.M., Ensinger, C.L., Haack, T., Hood, M.M., Jones, J., Lord, J.W., Lu, W.P., Miller, D., Patt, W.C., Smith, B.D., Petillo, P.A., Rutkoski, T.J., Telikepalli, H., Vogeti, L., Yao, T., Clark, R., Evangelista, P., Gavrilescu, L.C., Lazarides, K., Zaleskas, V.M., Stewart, L.J., Van Etten, R.A. & Flynn, D.l. (2011). Conformational control inhibition of the BCR-ABL1 tyrosine kinase, including the gatekeeper T315I mutant, by the switch-control inhibitor DCC-2036. *Cancer Cell,* Vol.12, 556-568

Chomel, J.C., Bonnet, M.L., Sorel, N., Bertrand, A., Meunier, M.C., Fichelson, S., Melkus, M., Bennaceur-Griscelli, A., Guilhot, F. & Turhan, A.G. (2011). Leukemic stem cell persistency in chronic myeloid leukemia patients with sustained undetectable molecular residual disease. *Blood,* Vol. 51, 2103-11

Chu, S., Xu, H., Shah, N.P., Snyder, D.S., Forman, S.J., Sawyers, C.L. & Bhatia, R. (2005). Detection of BCR-ABL kinase mutations in $CD34^+$ cells from chronic myelogenous leukemia patients in complete cytogenetic remission on imatinib mesylate treatment. *Blood,* Vol.105, 2093-2098

Copland, M. (2009). Chronic myelogenous leukemia stem cells: What's new? *Curr. Hematol. Malig. Rep.,* Vol.4, 66-73

Copland, M., Hamilton, A., Elrick, L.J., Baird, J.W., Allan, E.K., Jordanides, N., Barow, M., Mountford, J.C. & Holyoake, T.L. (2006). Dasatinib (BMS-354825) targets an earlier progenitor population than imatinib in primary CML, but does not eliminate the quiescent fraction. *Blood,* Vol.107, 4532-4539

Copland, M., Pellicano, F., Richmond, L., Allan, E.K., Hamilton, A., Lee, F.Y., Weinmann, R. & Holyoake, T.L. (2008). BMS-214662 potently induces apoptosis of chronic myeloid leukemia stem and progenitor cells and synergizes with tyrosine kinase inhibitors. *Blood,* Vol.111, 2843-2853

Corbin, A.S., Agarwal, A., Loriaux, M., Cortes, J., Deininger, M.W. & Druker, B.J. (2011). Human chronic myeloid leukemia stem cells are insensitive to imatinib despite inhibition of BCR-ABL activity. *J. Clin. Invest.,* Vol.121, 396-409

Cramer, K., Nieborowska-Skorska, M., Koptyra, M., Slupianek, A., Penserga, E.T.P., Eaves, C.J., Aulitzky, W. & Skorski, T. (2008). BCR/ABL and other kinases from chronic myeloproliferative disorders stimulate single-strand annealing, an unfaithful DNA double-strand break repair. *Cancer Res.,* Vol.68, 6884-6888

Crossman, L.C., Druker, B.J., Deininger, M.W., Pirmohamed, M., Wang, L. & Clark, R.E. (2005). hOCT 1 and resistance to imatinib. *Blood,* Vol.106, 1133-1134

DeGeer, D., Gallipoli, P., Chen, M., Sloma, I., Jorgensen, H., Forrest, D., Lambie, K., Nakamoto, H., Saw, K.M., Chan, M., Newmarch, K., Zhou, L., Turhan, A.,

Arlinghaus, R., Eaves, A., Eaves, C., Holyoake, T. & Jiang, X. (2010). Combined targeting of BCR-ABL and JAK2 with ABL and JAK2 inhibitors is effective against CML patients' leukemic stem/progenitor cells. *Blood,* Vol.116.1393.

DeGeer, D., Newmarch, K., Zhou, L., Chen, M., Saw, K.M., Turhan, A. & Jiang, X. (2009). A novel AHI-1-BCR-ABL-JAK2 interaction complex mediates cellular resistance to tyrosine kinase inhibitors in CML. *Blood,* Vol.114, 21.

Deininger, M., Buchdunger, E. & Druker, B.J. (2005). The development of imatinib as a therapeutic agent for chronic myeloid leukemia. *Blood,* Vol.105, 2640-2653

Diaz-Blanco, E., Bruns, I., Neumann, F., Fischer, J.C., Graef, T., Rosskopf, M., Brors, B., Pechtel, S., Bork, S., Koch, A., Baer, A., Rohr, U.P., Kobbe, G., Haeseler, A., Gattermann, N., Haas, R. & Kronenwett, R. (2007). Molecular signature of $CD34^+$ hematopoietic stem and progenitor cells of patients with CML in chronic phase. *Leukemia,* Vol.21, 494-504

Dierks, C., Beigi, R., Guo, G.R., Zirlik, K., Stegert, M.R., Manley, P., Trussell, C., Schmitt-Graeff, A., Landwerlin, K., Veelken, H. & Warmuth, M. (2008). Expansion of Bcr-Abl-positive leukemic stem cells is dependent on Hedgehog pathway activation. *Cancer Cell,* Vol.14, 238-249

Druker, B.J., Guilhot, F., O'Brien, S.G., Gathmann, I., Kantarjian, H., Gattermann, N., Deininger, M.W., Silver, R.T., Goldman, J.M., Stone, R.M., Cervantes, F., Hochhaus, A., Powell, B.L., Gabrilove, J.L., Rousselot, P., Reiffers, J., Cornelissen, J.J., Hughes, T., Agis, H., Fischer, T., Verhoef, G., Shepherd, J., Saglio, G., Gratwohl, A., Nielsen, J.L., Radich, J.P., Simonsson, B., Taylor, K., Baccarani, M., So, C., Letvak, L. & Larson, R.A. (2006). Five-year follow-up of patients receiving imatinib for chronic myeloid leukemia. *N. Engl. J. Med.,* Vol.355, 2408-2417

Druker, B.J., Talpaz, M., Resta, D.J., Peng, B., Buchdunger, E., Ford, J.M., Lydon, N.B., Kantarjian, H., Capdeville, R., Ohno-Jones, S. & Sawyers, C.L. (2001). Efficacy and safety of a specific inhibitor of the BCR-ABL tyrosine kinase in chronic myeloid leukemia. *N. Engl. J. Med.,* Vol.344, 1031-1037

Druker, B.J., Tamura, S., Buchdunger, E., Ohno, S., Segal, G.M., Fanning, S., Zimmermann, J. & Lydon, N.B. (1996). Effects of a selective inhibitor of the Abl tyrosine kinase on the growth of Bcr-Abl positive cells. *Nat. Med.,* Vol.2, 561-566

Eiring, A.M., Harb, J.G., Neviani, P., Garton, C., Oaks, J.J., Spizzo, R., Liu, S., Schwind, S., Santhanam, R., Hickey, C.J., Becker, H., Chandler, J.C., Andino, R., Cortes, J., Hokland, P., Huettner, C.S., Bhatia, R., Roy, D.C., Liebhaber, S.A., Caliqiuri, M.A., Marcucci, G., Garzon, R., Croce, C.M., Calin, G.A. & Perrotti, D. (2010). miR-328 functions as an RNA decoy to modulate hnRNP E2 regulation of mRNA translation in leukemic blasts. *Cell,* Vol.140, 652-665

Eiring, A.M., Neviani, P., Santhanam, R., Oaks, J.J., Chang, J.S., Notari, M., Willis, W., Gambacorti-Passerini, C., Volinia, S., Marcucci, G., Caligiuri, M.A., Leone, G.W. & Perrotti, D. (2008). Identification of novel posttranscriptional targets of the BCR/ABL oncoprotein by ribonomics: requirement of E2F3 for BCR/ABL leukemogenesis. *Blood,* Vol.111, 816-828

Engler, J.R., Frede, A., Saunders, V.A., Zannettino, A.C., Hughes, T.P. & White, D.L. (2010). Chronic myeloid leukemia CD34+ cells have reduced uptake of imatinib due to low OCT-1 activity. *Leukemia,* Vol.24, 765-770

Flamant, S. & Turhan, A.G. (2005). Occurrence of de novo ABL kinase domain mutations in primary bone marrow cells after BCR-ABL gene transfer and Imatinib mesylate selection. *Leukemia,* Vol.19, 1265-1267

Forrest, D.L., Jiang, X., Eaves, C.J. & Smith, C.L. (2008). An approach to the management of chronic myeloid leukemia in British Columbia. *Curr. Oncol.,* Vol.15, 48-55

Goldman, J.M. (2007). How I treat chronic myeloid leukemia in the imatinib era. *Blood,* Vol.110, 2828-2837

Goldman, J.M. & Melo, J.V. (2003). Chronic myeloid leukemia--advances in biology and new approaches to treatment. *N. Engl. J. Med.,* Vol.349, 1451-1464

Gorre, M.E., Mohammed, M., Ellwood, K., Hsu, N., Paquette, R., Rao, P.N. & Sawyers, C.L. (2001). Clinical resistance to STI-571 cancer therapy caused by BCR-ABL gene mutation or amplification. *Science,* Vol.293, 876-880

Graham, S.M., Jorgensen, H.G., Allan, E., Pearson, C., Alcorn, M.J., Richmond, L. & Holyoake, T.L. (2002). Primitive, quiescent, Philadelphia-positive stem cells from patients with chronic myeloid leukemia are insensitive to STI571 in vitro. *Blood,* Vol.99, 319-325

Grant, H., Jiang, X., Stebbing, J., Foroni, L., Craddock, C., Griffiths, M., Clark, R.E., O'Brien, S., Khorashad, J.S., Gerrard, G., Wang, L., Irving, J.A.E., Wang, M., Karran, L., Dyer, M.J.S., Forrest, D., Page, K., Eaves, C.J. & Woolfson, A. (2010). Analysis of BCR-ABL1 tyrosine kinase domain mutational spectra in primitive chronic myeloid leukemia cells suggests a unique mutator phenotype. *Leukemia,* Vol.24, 1817-1821

Hochhaus, A., Baccarani, M., Deininger, M., Apperley, J.F., Lipton, J.H., Goldberg, S.L., Corm, S., Shah, N.P., Cervantes, F., Silver, R.T., Niederwieser, D., Stone, R.M., Dombret, H., Larson, R.A., Roy, L., Hughes, T., Muller, M.C., Ezzeddine, R., Countouriotis, A.M. & Kantarjian, H.M. (2008). Dasatinib induces durable cytogenetic responses in patients with chronic myelogenous leukemia in chronic phase with resistance or intolerance to imatinib. *Leukemia,* Vol.22, 1200-1206

Hochhaus, A., Kreil, S., Corbin, A.S., La Rosee, P., Muller, M.C., Lahaye, T., Hanfstein, B., Schoch, C., Cross, N.C., Berger, U., Gschaidmeier, H., Druker, B.J. & Hehlmann, R. (2002). Molecular and chromosomal mechanisms of resistance to imatinib (STI571) therapy. *Leukemia,* Vol.16, 2190-2196

Holtz, M.S., Forman, S.J. & Bhatia, R. (2005). Nonproliferating CML $CD34^+$ progenitors are resistant to apoptosis induced by a wide range of proapoptotic stimuli. *Leukemia,* Vol.19, 1034-1041

Holtz, M.S., Slovak, M.L., Zhang, F., Sawyers, C.L., Forman, S.J. & Bhatia, R. (2002). Imatinib mesylate (STI571) inhibits growth of primitive malignant progenitors in chronic myelogenous leukemia through reversal of abnormally increased proliferation. *Blood,* Vol.99, 3792-3800

Holyoake, T., Jiang, X., Eaves, C. & Eaves, A. (1999). Isolation of a highly quiescent subpopulation of primitive leukemic cells in chronic myeloid leukemia. *Blood,* Vol.94, 2056-2064

Holyoake, T.L., Jiang, X., Drummond, M.W., Eaves, A.C. & Eaves, C.J. (2002). Elucidating critical mechanisms of deregulated stem cell turnover in the chronic phase of chronic myeloid leukemia. *Leukemia,* Vol.16, 549-558

Hu, Y., Chen, Y., Douglas, L. & Li, S. (2009). beta-Catenin is essential for survival of leukemic stem cells insensitive to kinase inhibition in mice with BCR-ABL-induced chronic myeloid leukemia. *Leukemia,* Vol.23, 109-116

Hughes, T.P., Kaeda, J., Branford, S., Rudzki, Z., Hochhaus, A., Hensley, M.L., Gathmann, I., Bolton, A.E., van Hoomissen, I.C, Goldman, J.M., Radich, J.P. (2003). Frequency of major molecular responses to imatinib or interferon alfa plus cytarabine in newly diagnosed chronic myeloid leukemia. N. Engl. J. Med., Vol.349, 1423- 1432

Hughes, T., Deininger, M., Hochhaus, A., Branford, S., Radich, J., Kaeda, J., Baccarani, M., Cortes, J., Cross, N.C., Druker, B.J., Gabert, J., Grimwade, D., Hehlmann, R., Kamel-Reid, S., Lipton, J.H., Longtine, J., Martinelli, G., Saglio, G., Soverini, S., Stock, W. & Goldman, J.M. (2006). Monitoring CML patients responding to treatment with tyrosine kinase inhibitors: review and recommendations for harmonizing current methodology for detecting BCR-ABL transcripts and kinase domain mutations and for expressing results. *Blood,* Vol.108, 28-37

Hughes, T., Sagilo, G., Branford, S., Soverini, S., Kim, D.W., Muller, M.C., Martinelli, G., Cortes, J., Beppu, L., Gottardi, E., Kim, D., Erben, P., Shou, Y., Hague, A., Gallagher, N., Radich, J. & Hochhaus, A. (2009). Impact of baseline BCR-ABL mutations on response to nilotinib in patients with chronic myeloid leukemia in chronic phase. *J. Clin. Oncol.,* Vol.27, 4204-4210

Ito, K., Bernardi, R., Morotti, A., Matsuoka, S., Saglio, G., Ikeda, Y., Rosenblatt, J., Avigan, D.E., Teruya-Feldstein, J. & Pandolfi, P.P. (2008). PML targeting eradicates quiescent leukaemia-initiating cells. *Nature,* Vol.453, 1072-1078

Jamieson, C.H., Ailles, L.E., Dylla, S.J., Muijtjens, M., Jones, C., Zehnder, J.L., Gotlib, J., Li, K., Manz, M.G., Keating, A., Sawyers, C.L. & Weissman, I.L. (2004). Granulocyte-macrophage progenitors as candidate leukemic stem cells in blast-crisis CML. *N. Engl. J. Med.,* Vol.351, 657-667

Janssen, J.J., Klaver, S.M., Waisfisz, Q., Pasterkamp, G., de Kleijn, D.P., Schuurhuis, G.J. & Ossenkoppele, G.J. (2005). Identification of genes potentially involved in disease transformation of CML. *Leukemia,* Vol.19, 998-1004

Jiang X. (2007). Molecular and cellular mechanisms of deregulated hematopoietic stem cell functions in chronic myeloid leukemia. In: *Cancer Nanotechnology,* pp. 135-157, American Scientific Publishers.

Jiang, X., Forrest, D., Nicolini, F., Turhan, A., Guilhot, J., Yip, C., Holyoake, T., Jorgensen, H., Lambie, K., Saw, K.M., Pang, E., Vukovic, R., Lehn, P., Ringrose, A., Yu, M., Brinkman, R.R., Smith, C., Eaves, A. & Eaves, C. (2010). Properties of $CD34^+$ CML stem/progenitor cells that correlate with different clinical responses to imatinib mesylate. *Blood,* Vol.116, 2112-2121

Jiang, X., Lopez, A., Holyoake, T., Eaves, A. & Eaves, C. (1999). Autocrine production and action of IL-3 and granulocyte colony-stimulating factor in chronic myeloid leukemia. *Proceedings of the National Academy of Sciences USA,* Vol.96, 12804-12809

Jiang, X., Saw, K.M., Eaves, A. & Eaves, C. (2007a). Instability of BCR-ABL gene in primary and cultured chronic myeloid leukemia stem cells. *J. Natl. Cancer Inst.,* Vol.99, 680-693

Jiang, X., Smith, C., Eaves, A. & Eaves, C. (2007b). The challenges of targeting chronic myeloid leukemia stem cells. *Clin. Lymphoma Myeloma,* Vol.7, S71-80

Jiang, X., Zhao, Y., Chan, W.Y., Vercauteren, S., Pang, E., Kennedy, S., Nicolini, F., Eaves, A. & Eaves, C. (2004). Deregulated expression in Ph[+] human leukemias of AHI-1, a gene activated by insertional mutagenesis in mouse models of leukemia. *Blood,* Vol.103, 3897-3904

Jiang, X., Zhao, Y., Forrest, D., Smith, C., Eaves, A. & Eaves, C. (2008). Stem cell biomarkers in chronic myeloid leukemia. *Dis. Markers,* Vol.24, 201-216

Jiang, X., Zhao, Y., Smith, C., Gasparetto, M., Turhan, A., Eaves, A. & Eaves, C. (2007c). Chronic myeloid leukemia stem cells possess multiple unique features of resistance to BCR-ABL targeted therapies. *Leukemia,* Vol.21, 926-935

Jin, L., Tabe, Y., Konoplev, S., Xu, Y., Leysath, C.E., Lu, H., Kimura, S., Ohsaka, A., Rios, M.B., Calvert, L., Kantarjian, H., Andreeff, M. & Konopleva, M. (2008). CXCR4 up-regulation by imatinib induces chronic myelogenous leukemia (CML) cell migration to bone marrow stroma and promotes survival of quiescent CML cells. *Mol. Cancer Ther.,* Vol.7, 48-58

Jongen-Lavrencic, M., Salesse, S., Delwel, R. & Verfaillie, C.M. (2005). BCR/ABL-mediated downregulation of genes implicated in cell adhesion and motility leads to impaired migration toward CCR7 ligands CCL19 and CCL21 in primary BCR/ABL-positive cells. *Leukemia,* Vol.19, 373-380

Jordanides, N.E., Jorgensen, H.G., Holyoake, T.L. & Mountford, J.C. (2006). Functional ABCG2 is over-expressed on primary CML CD34+ cells and is inhibited by imatinib mesylate. *Blood,* Vol.108, 1370-1373

Jorgensen, H.G., Allan, E.K., Jordanides, N.E., Mountford, J.C. & Holyoake, T.L. (2007). Nilotinib exerts equipotent antiproliferative effects to imatinib and does not induce apoptosis in CD34+ CML cells. *Blood,* Vol.109, 4016-4019

Kantarjian, H., Giles, F., Wunderle, L., Bhalla, K., O'Brien, S., Wassmann, B., Tanaka, C., Manley, P., Rae, P., Mietlowski, W., Bochinski, K., Hochhaus, A., Griffin, J.D., Hoelzer, D., Albitar, M., Dugan, M., Cortes, J., Alland, L. & Ottmann, O.G. (2006). Nilotinib in imatinib-resistant CML and Philadelphia chromosome-positive ALL. *N. Engl. J. Med.,* Vol.354, 2542-2551

Kantarjian, H., O'Brien, S., Cortes, J., Giles, F., Thomas, D., Kornblau, S., Shan, J., Beth Rios, M., Keating, M., Freireich, E. & Talpaz, M. (2003). Sudden onset of the blastic phase of chronic myelogenous leukemia: patterns and implications. *Cancer,* Vol.98, 81-85

Kantarjian, H., Sawyers, C., Hochhaus, A., Guilhot, F., Schiffer, C., Gambacorti-Passerini, C., Niederwieser, D., Resta, D., Capdeville, R., Zoellner, U., Talpaz, M., Druker, B., Goldman, J., O'Brien, S.G., Russell, N., Fischer, T., Ottmann, O., Cony-Makhoul, P., Facon, T., Stone, R., Miller, C., Tallman, M., Brown, R., Schuster, M., Loughran, T., Gratwohl, A., Mandelli, F., Saglio, G., Lazzarino, M., Russo, D., Baccarani, M. & Morra, E. (2002). Hematologic and cytogenetic responses to imatinib mesylate in chronic myelogenous leukemia. *N. Engl. J. Med.,* Vol.346, 645-652

Kantarjian, H., Shah, N.P., Hochhaus, A., Cortes, J., Shah, S., Ayala, M., Moiraghi, B., Shen, Z., Mayer, J., Pasquini, R., Nakamae, H., Huguet, F., Bogue, C., Chuah, C., Bleickardt, E., Bradley-Garelik, M.B., Zhu, C., Szatrowski, T., Shapiro, D. & Baccarani, M. (2010). Dasatinib versus imatinib in newly diagnosed chronic-phase chronic myeloid leukemia. *N. Engl. J. Med.,* Vol.362, 2260-2270

Kantarjian, H.M., Giles, F., Gattermann, N., Bhalla, K., Alimena, G., Palandri, F., Ossenkoppele, G.J., Nicolini, F.E., O'Brien, S.G., Litzow, M., Bhatia, R., Cervantes,

F., Hague, A., Shou, Y., Resta, D.J., Weitzman, A., Hochhaus, A. & le Coutre, P. (2007). Nilotinib (formerly AMN107), a highly selective BCR-ABL tyrosine kinase inhibitor, is effective in patients with Philadelphia chromosome-positive chronic myelogenous leukemia in chronic phase following imatinib resistance and intolerance. *Blood,* Vol.110, 3540-3546

Konig, H., Copland, M., Chu, S., Jove, R., Holyoake, T.L. & Bhatia, R. (2008). Effects of dasatinib on SRC kinase activity and downstream intracellular signaling in primitive chronic myelogenous leukemia hematopoietic cells. *Cancer Res.,* Vol.68, 9624-9633

Koptyra, M., Falinski, R., Nowicki, M.O., Stoklosa, T., Majsterek, I., Nieborowska-Skorska, M., Blasiak, J. & Skorski, T. (2006). BCR/ABL kinase induces self-mutagenesis via reactive oxygen species to encode imatinib resistance. *Blood,* Vol.108, 319-327

Kronenwett, R., Butterweck, U., Steidl, U., Kliszewski, S., Neumann, F., Bork, S., Blanco, E.D., Roes, N., Graf, T., Brors, B., Eils, R., Maercker, C., Kobbe, G., Gattermann, N. & Haas, R. (2005). Distinct molecular phenotype of malignant $CD34^+$ hematopoietic stem and progenitor cells in chronic myelogenous leukemia. *Oncogene,* Vol.24, 5313-5324

Lepper, E.R., Nooter, K., Verweij, J., Acharya, M.R., Figg, W.D. & Sparreboom, A. (2005). Mechanisms of resistance to anticancer drugs: the role of the polymorphic ABC transporters ABCB1 and ABCG2. *Pharmacogenomics,* Vol.6, 115-138

Lugo, T.G., Pendergast, A.M., Muller, A.J. & Witte, O.N. (1990). Tyrosine kinase activity and transformation potency of *bcr-abl* oncogene products. *Science,* Vol.247, 1079-1082

Mahon, F.X., Rea, D., Guilhot, J., Guilhot, F., Huguet, F., Nicolini, F., Legros, L., Charbonnier, A., Guerci, A., Varet, B., Etienne, G., Reiffers, J. & Rousselot, P. (2010). Discontinuation of imatinib in patients with chronic myeloid leukaemia who have maintained complete molecular remission for at least 2 years: the prospective, multicentre Stop Imatinib (STIM) trial. *Lancet Oncol.,* Vol.11, 1029-1035

Mar, B.G., Amakye, D., Aifantis, I. & Buonamici, S. (2011). The controversial role of the Hedgehog pathway in normal and malignant hematopoiesis. *Leukemia,* online publication 10 June 2011

Miyamoto, N., Sugita, K., Goi, K., Inukai, T., Lijima, K., Tezuka, T., Kojika, S., Nakamura, M., Kagami, K. & Nakazawa, S. (2001). The JAK2 inhibitor AG490 predominantly abrogates the growth of human B-precursor leukemic cells with 11q23 translocation or Philadelphia chromosome. *Leukemia,* Vol.15, 1758-1768

Muller, M.C., Cortes, J.E., Kim, D.W., Druker, B.J., Erben, P., Pasquini, R., Branford, S., Hughes, T.P., Radich, J.P., Ploughman, L., Mukhopadhyay, J. & Hochhaus, A. (2009). Dasatinib treatment of chronic-phase chronic myeloid leukemia: analysis of responses according to preexisting BCR-ABL mutations. *Blood,* Vol.114, 4944-4953

Naka, K., Hoshii, T., Muraguchi, T., Tadokoro, Y., Ooshio, T., Kondo, Y., Nakao, S., Motoyama, N. & Hirao, A. (2010). TGF-beta-FOXO signalling maintains leukaemia-initiating cells in chronic myeloid leukaemia. *Nature,* Vol.463, 676-680

Nelson, E.A., Walker, S.R., Weisberg, E., Bar-Natan, M., Barrett, R., Gashin, L.B., Terrell, S., Klitgaard, J.L., Santo, L., Addorio, M.R., Ebert, B.L., Griffin, J.D. & Frank, D.A. (2011). The STAT5 inhibitor pimozide decreases survival of chronic myelogenous leukemia cells resistant to kinase inhibitors. *Blood,* Vol.117, 3421-3429

Neviani, P., Santhanam, R., Oaks, J.J., Eiring, A.M., Notari, M., Blaser, B.W., Liu, S., Trotta, R., Muthusamy, N., Gambacorti-Passerini, C., Druker, B.J., Cortes, J., Marcucci, G., Chen, C.S., Verrills, N.M., Roy, D.C., Caligiuri, M.A., Bloomfield, C.D., Byrd, J.C. & Perrotti, D. (2007). FTY720, a new alternative for treating blast crisis chronic myelogenous leukemia and Philadelphia chromosome-positive acute lymphocytic leukemia. *J. Clin. Invest.*, Vol.117, 2408-2421

Neviani, P., Santhanam, R., Trotta, R., Notari, M., Blaser, B.W., Liu, S., Mao, H., Chang, J.S., Galietta, A., Uttam, A., Roy, D.C., Valtieri, M., Bruner-Klisovic, R., Caligiuri, M.A., Bloomfield, C.D., Marcucci, G. & Perrotti, D. (2005). The tumor suppressor PP2A is functionally inactivated in blast crisis CML through the inhibitory activity of the BCR/ABL-regulated SET protein. *Cancer Cell*, Vol.8, 355-368

Nowicki, M.O., Pawlowski, P., Fischer, T., Hess, G., Pawlowski, T. & Skorski, T. (2003). Chronic myelogenous leukemia molecular signature. *Oncogene*, Vol.22, 3952-3963

O'Brien, S.G., Guilhot, F., Larson, R.A., Gathmann, I., Baccarani, M., Cervantes, F., Cornelissen, J.J., Fischer, T., Hochhaus, A., Hughes, T., Lechner, K., Nielsen, J.L., Rousselot, P., Reiffers, J., Saglio, G., Shepherd, J.D., Simonsson, B., Gratwohl, A., Goldman, J.M., Kantarjian, H., Taylor, K., Verhoef, G., Bolton, A.E., Capdeville, R. & Druker, B.J. (2003). Imatinib compared with interferon and low-dose cytarabine for newly diagnosed chronic-phase chronic myeloid leukemia. *J. New. Eng. Med.*, Vol.348, 994-1004

O'Hare, T., Corbin, A.S. & Druker, B.J. (2006). Targeted CML therapy: controlling drug resistance, seeking cure. *Curr. Opin. Genet. Dev.*, Vol.16, 92-99

O'Hare, T., Shakespeare, W.C., Zhu, X., Eide, C.A., Rivera, V.M., Wang, F., Adrian, L.T., Zhou, T., Huang, W.S., Xu, Q., Metcalf, C.A., Tyner, J.W., Loriaux, M.M., Corbin, A.S., Wardwell, S., Ning, Y., Keates, J.A., Wang, Y., Sundaramoorthi, R., Thomas, M., Zhou, D., Snodgrass, J., Commodore, L., Sawyer, T.K., Dalgarno, D.C., Deininger, M.W., Druker, B.J. & Clackson, T. (2009). AP24534, a pan-BCR-ABL inhibitor for chronic myeloid leukemia, potently inhibits the T315I mutant and overcomes mutation-based resistance. *Cancer Cell*, Vol.6, 401-412

Park, I.K., Qian, D., Kiel, M., Becker, M.W., Pihalja, M., Weissman, I.L., Morrison, S.J. & Clarke, M.F. (2003). Bmi-1 is required for maintenance of adult self-renewing haematopoietic stem cells. *Nature*, Vol.423, 302-305

Penserga, E.T. & Skorski, T. (2007). Fusion tyrosine kinases: a result and cause of genomic instability. *Oncogene*, Vol.26, 11-20

Radich, J.P., Dai, H., Mao, M., Oehler, V., Schelter, J., Druker, B., Sawyers, C., Shah, N., Stock, W., Willman, C.L., Friend, S. & Linsley, P.S. (2006). Gene expression changes associated with progression and response in chronic myeloid leukemia. *Proceedings of the National Academy of Sciences USA*, Vol.103, 2794-2799

Rizo, A., Horton, S.J., Olthof, S., Dontje, B., Ausema, A., van Os, R., van den Boom, V., Vellenga, E., de Haan, G. & Schuringa, J.J. (2010). BMI1 collaborates with BCR-ABL in leukemic transformation of human CD34+ cells. *Blood*, Vol.116, 4621-4630

Roche-Lestienne, C., Lai, J.L., Darre, S., Facon, T. & Preudhomme, C. (2003). A mutation conferring resistance to imatinib at the time of diagnosis of chronic myelogenous leukemia. *N. Engl. J. Med.*, Vol.348, 2265-2266

Roche-Lestienne, C., Soenen-Cornu, V., Grardel-Duflos, N., Lai, J.L., Philippe, N., Facon, T., Fenaux, P. & Preudhomme, C. (2002). Several types of mutations of the Abl gene can be found in chronic myeloid leukemia patients resistant to STI571, and they can pre-exist to the onset of treatment. *Blood,* Vol.100, 1014-1018

Ross, D.M., Branford, S., Seymour, J.F., Schwarer, A.P., Arthur, C., Bartley, P.A., Slader, C., Field, C., Dang, P., Filshie, R.J., Mills, A.K., Grigg, A.P., Melo, J.V. & Hughes, T.P. (2010a). Patients with chronic myeloid leukemia who maintain a complete molecular response after stopping imatinib treatment have evidence of persistent leukemia by DNA PCR. *Leukemia,* Vol.24, 1719-1724

Ross, D.M., Hughes, T.P. & Melo, J.V. (2010b). Do we have to kill the last CML cell? *Leukemia,* Vol.25, 193-200

Rousselot, P., Huguet, F., Rea, D., Legros, L., Cayuela, J.M., Maarek, O., Blanchet, O., Marit, G., Gluckman, E., Reiffers, J., Gardembas, M. & Mahon, F.X. (2007). Imatinib mesylate discontinuation in patients with chronic myelogenous leukemia in complete molecular remission for more than 2 years. *Blood,* Vol.109, 58-60

Saglio, G., Kim, D.W., Issaragrisil, S., le Coutre, P., Etienne, G., Lobo, C., Pasquini, R., Clark, R.E., Hochhaus, A., Hughes, T.P., Gallagher, N., Hoenekopp, A., Dong, M., Hague, A., Larson, R.A. & Kantarjian, H.M. (2010). Nilotinib versus imatinib for newly diagnosed chronic myeloid leukemia. *N. Engl. J. Med.,* Vol.362, 2251-2259

Salesse, S. & Verfaillie, C.M. (2003). BCR/ABL-mediated increased expression of multiple known and novel genes that may contribute to the pathogenesis of chronic myelogenous leukemia. *Mol. Cancer Ther.,* Vol.2, 173-182

Sallmyr, A., Tomkinson, A.E. & Rassol, F.V. (2008). Up-regulation of WRN and DNA ligase IIIá in chronic myeloid leukemia: consequences for the repair of double-strand breaks. *Blood,* Vol.112, 1413-1423

Samanta, A., Perazzona, B., Chakraborty, S., Sun, X., Modi, H., Bhatia, R., Priebe, W. & Arlinghaus, R. (2011). Janus kinase 2 regulates Bcr-Abl signaling in chronic myeloid leukemia. *Leukemia,* Vol.25, 463-472

Samanta, A.K., Chakraborty, S.N., Wang, Y., Schlette, E., Reddy, E.P. & Arlighhaus, R.B. (2010). Destabilization of Bcr-Abl/Jak2 network by a Jak2/Abl kinase inhibitor ON044580 overcomes drug resistance in blast crisis chronic myelogenous leukemia (CML). *Genes Cancer,* Vol.1, 346-359

Samanta, A.K., Lin, H., Sun, T., Kantarjian, H. & Arlinghaus, R.B. (2006). Janus kinase 2: a critical target in chronic myelogenous leukemia. *Cancer Res.,* Vol.66, 6468-6472

Santos, F.P. & Quintas-Cardama, A. (2011). New drugs for chronic myelogenous leukemia. *Curr. Hematol. Malig. Rep.,* Vol.6, 96-103

Savona, M. & Talpaz, M. (2008). Getting to the stem of chronic myeloid leukaemia. *Nat. Rev. Cancer,* Vol.8, 341-350

Shah, N.P., Nicoll, J.M., Nagar, B., Gorre, M.E., Paquette, R.L., Kuriyan, J. & Sawyers, C.L. (2002). Multiple BCR-ABL kinase domain mutations confer polyclonal resistance to the tyrosine kinase inhibitor imatinib (STI571) in chronic phase and blast crisis chronic myeloid leukemia. *Cancer Cell,* Vol.2, 117-125

Shah, N.P., Tran, C., Lee, F.Y., Chen, P., Norris, D. & Sawyers, C.L. (2004). Overriding imatinib resistance with a novel ABL kinase inhibitor. *Science,* Vol.305, 399-401

Skorski, T. (2008). BCR/ABL, DNA damage and DNA repair: implications for new treatment concepts. *Leuk. Lymphoma,* Vol.49, 610-614

Sloma, I., Jiang, X., Eaves, A.C. & Eaves, C.J. (2010). Insights into the stem cells of chronic myeloid leukemia. *Leukemia,* Vol.24, 1823-1833

Sobrinho-Simoes, M., Wilczek, V., Score, J., Cross, N.C., Apperley, J.F. & Melo, J.V. (2010). In search of the original leukemic clone in chronic myeloid leukemia patients in complete molecular remission after stem cell transplantation or imatinib. *Blood,* Vol.116, 1329-1335

Sorel, N., Bonnet, M.L., Guillier, M., Guilhot, F., Brizard, A. & Turhan, A.G. (2004). Evidence of ABL-kinase domain mutations in highly purified primitive stem cell populations of patients with chronic myelogenous leukemia. *Biochem. Biophys. Res. Commun.,* Vol.323, 728-730

Soverini, S., Hochhaus, A., Nicolini, F.E., Gruber, F., Lange, T., Saglio, G., Pane, F., Muller, M.C., Ernst, T., Rosti, G., Porkka, K., Baccarani, M., Cross, N.C. & Martinelli, G. (2011). BCR-ABL kinase domain mutation analysis in chronic myeloid leukemia patients treated with tyrosine kinase inhibitors: recommendations from an expert panel on behalf of European LeukemiaNet. *Blood,* Vol.118, 1208-1215

Soverini, S., Martinelli, G., Colarossi, S., Gnani, A., Castagnetti, F., Rosti, G., Bosi, C., Paolini, S., Rondoni, M., Piccaluga, P.P., Palandri, F., Giannoulia, P., Marzocchi, G., Luatti, S., Testoni, N., Iacobucci, I., Cilloni, D., Saglio, G. & Baccarani, M. (2006). Presence or the emergence of a F317L BCR-ABL mutation may be associated with resistance to dasatinib in Philadelphia chromosome-positive leukemia. *J. Clin. Oncol.,* Vol.24, e51-e52

Talpaz, M., Shah, N.P., Kantarjian, H., Donato, N., Nicoll, J., Paquette, R., Cortes, J., O'Brien, S., Nicaise, C., Bleickardt, E., Blackwood-Chirchir, M.A., Iyer, V., Chen, T.T., Huang, F., Decillis, A.P. & Sawyers, C.L. (2006). Dasatinib in imatinib-resistant Philadelphia chromosome-positive leukemias. *N. Engl. J. Med.,* Vol.354, 2531-2541

Tauchi, T. & Ohyashiki, K. (2004). Molecular mechanisms of resistance of leukemia to imatinib mesylate. *Leuk. Res.,* Vol.28, S39-S45

Thomas, J., Wang, L., Clark, R.E. & Pirmohamed, M. (2004). Active transport of imatinib into and out of cells: implications for drug resistance. *Blood,* Vol.104, 3739-3745

Valent, P. (2008). Emerging stem cell concepts for imatinib-resistant chronic myeloid leukaemia: implications for the biology, management, and therapy of the disease. *Br. J. Haematol.,* Vol.142, 361-378

Varjosalo, M. & Taipale, J. (2008). Hedgehog: functions and mechanisms. *Genes Dev.,* Vol.22, 2454-2472

Venturini, L., Battmer, K., Castoldi, M., Schultheis, B., Hochhaus, A., Muckenthaler, M.U., Ganser, A., Eder, M. & Scherr, M. (2007). Expression of the miR-17-92 polycistron in chronic myeloid leukemia (CML) CD34+ cells. *Blood,* Vol.109, 4399-4405

von Bubnoff, N., Veach, D.R., van der Kuip, H., Aulitzky, W.E., Sanger, J., Seipel, P., Bornmann, W.G., Peschel, C., Clarkson, B. & Duyster, J. (2005). A cell-based screen for resistance of Bcr-Abl-positive leukemia identifies the mutation pattern for PD166326, an alternative Abl kinase inhibitor. *Blood,* Vol.105, 1652-1659

Wang, Y., Cai, D., Brendel, C., Barett, C., Erben, P., Manley, P.W., Hochhaus, A., Neubauer, A. & Burchert, A. (2007). Adaptive secretion of granulocyte-macrophage colony-stimulating factor (GM-CSF) mediates imatinib and nilotinib resistance in BCR/ABL^{+} progenitors via JAK-2/STAT-5 pathway activation. *Blood,* Vol.109, 2147-2155

Warsch, W., Kollmann, K., Eckelhart, E., Fajmann, S., Cerny-Reiterer, S., Holbl, A., Gleixner, K.V., Dworzak, M., Mayerhofer, M., Hoermann, G., Herrmann, H., Sillaber, C.,

Egger, G., Valent, P., Moriggl, R. & Sexl, V. (2011). High STAT5 levels mediate imatinib resistance and indicate disease progression in chronic myeloid leukemia. *Blood*, Vol.117, 3409-3420

Weisberg, E., Manley, P.W., Breitenstein, W., Bruggen, J., Cowan-Jacob, S.W., Ray, A., Huntly, B., Fabbro, D., Fendrich, G., Hall-Meyers, E., Kung, A.L., Mestan, J., Daley, G.Q., Callahan, L., Catley, L., Cavazza, C., Azam, M., Neuberg, D., Wright, R.D., Gilliland, D.G. & Griffin, J.D. (2005). Characterization of AMN107, a selective inhibitor of native and mutant Bcr-Abl. *Cancer Cell*, Vol.7, 129-141

White, D.L., Dang, P., Engler, J., Frede, A., Zrim, S., Osborn, M., Saunders, V.A., Manley, P.W. & Hughes, T.P. (2010). Functional activity of the OCT-1 protein is predictive of long-term outcome in patients with chronic-phase chronic myeloid leukemia treated with Imatinib. *J. Clin. Oncol.*, Vol.28, 2761-2767

White, D.L., Saunders, V.A., Dang, P., Engler, J., Zannettino, A.C., Cambareri, A.C., Quinn, S.R., Manley, P.W. & Hughes, T.P. (2006). OCT-1 mediated influx is a key determinant of the intracellular uptake of imatinib but not nilotinib (AMN107); reduced OCT-1 activity is the cause of low in vitro sensitivity to imatinib. *Blood*, Vol.108, 697-704

Willis, S.G., Lange, T., Demehri, S., Otto, S., Crossman, L., Niederwieser, D., Stoffregen, E.P., McWeeney, S., Kovacs, I., Park, B., Druker, B.J. & Deininger, M.W. (2005). High-sensitivity detection of BCR-ABL kinase domain mutations in imatinib-naive patients: correlation with clonal cytogenetic evolution but not response to therapy. *Blood*, Vol.106, 2128-2137

Wilson-Rawls, J., Liu, J., Laneuville, P. & Arlinghaus, R.B. (1997). P210 Bcr-Abl interacts with the interleukin-3 beta c subunit and constitutively activates Jak2. *Leukemia*, Vol.11 , 428-431

Xie, S., Wang, Y., Liu, J., Sun, T., Wilson, M.B., Smithgall, T.E. & Arlinghaus, R.B. (2001). Involvement of Jak2 tyrosine phosphorylation in Bcr-Abl transformation. *Oncogene*, Vol.20, 6188-6195

Yong, A.S., Szydlo, R.M., Goldman, J.M., Apperley, J.F. & Melo, J.V. (2006). Molecular profiling of $CD34^+$ cells identifies low expression of CD7, along with high expression of proteinase 3 or elastase, as predictors of longer survival in patients with CML. *Blood*, Vol.107, 205-212

Zhang, B., Strauss, A.C., Chu, S., Li, M., Ho, Y., Shiang, K.D., Snyder, D.S., Huettner, C.S., Shultz, L., Holyoake, T. & Bhatia, R. (2010). Effective targeting of quiescent chronic myelogenous leukemia stem cells by histone deacetylase inhibitors in combination with imatinib mesylate. *Cancer Cell*, Vol.17, 427-442

Zhao, C., Blum, J., Chen, A., Kwon, H.Y., Jung, S.H., Cook, J.M., Lagoo, A. & Reya, T. (2007). Loss of beta-catenin impairs the renewal of normal and CML stem cells in vivo. *Cancer Cell*, Vol.12, 528-541

Zhao, C., Chen, A., Jamieson, C.H., Fereshteh, M., Abrahamsson, A., Blum, J., Kwon, H.Y., Kim, J., Chute, J.P., Rizzieri, D., Munchhof, M., VanArsdale, T., Beachy, P.A. & Reya, T. (2009). Hedgehog signalling is essential for maintenance of cancer stem cells in myeloid leukaemia. *Nature*, Vol.458, 776-779

Zhao, Y., Delaney, A., Raouf, A., Raghuram, K., Li, I., Schnerch, A., Jiang, X., Eaves, A.C., Marra, M.A. & Eaves, C.J. (2008). Differentially expressed and novel transcripts in highly purified chronic phase CML stem cells. *Blood*, Vol.112, 193

Zhou, L.L., Zhao, Y., Ringrose, A., DeGeer, D., Kennah, E., Lin, A.E., Sheng, G., Li, X.J., Turhan, A. & Jiang, X. (2008). AHI-1 interacts with BCR-ABL and modulates BCR-ABL transforming activity and imatinib response of CML stem/progenitor cells. *J. Exp. Med.*, Vol.205, 2657-2671

6

The Proteasome as a Therapeutic Target in Chronic Myeloid Leukemia

Ignacio Pérez-Roger and María Pilar Albero
Universidad CEU Cardenal Herrera
Spain

1. Introduction

Chronic Myeloid Leukemia (CML) appears as a consequence of the reciprocal translocation between chromosomes 9 and 22 which results in the expression of the Bcr-Abl oncoprotein in a hematopoietic stem cell. The tyrosine kinase activity of Bcr-Abl is the direct cause of the disease. Therefore, inhibitors of this kinase activity are being used in the treatment of CML. Imatinib was the first of such inhibitors and is the first line treatment in CML. However, the appearance of Bcr-Abl mutants that are resistant to these inhibitors has emerged as a problem in the treatment of CML. Consequently, the search for new drugs or therapeutic targets is underway.

The proteasome is a multiprotein complex where proteins are degraded in a much regulated manner. Protein degradation at the proteasome is dependent upon ubiquitylation, which, in turn, is mediated by ubiquitin-ligase complexes. By degrading specific proteins, the proteasome is involved in cellular processes as important as cell cycle regulation, proliferation, differentiation and survival. As such, its activity is also related to the transformation of tumor cells. In fact, it has been shown that tumor cells show an increase in proteasome activity. Specifically, Bcr-Abl tyrosine kinase activity results in an increase of proteasome activity and degradation of some negative regulators of cell cycle progression as $p27^{kip1}$. Therefore, proteasome inhibitors could be an alternative in CML treatment.

In this chapter, we will discuss the available data suggesting that proteasome inhibition could be used in the treatment of CML, including those cases in which Bcr-Abl inhibition is not a possibility.

2. Bcr-Abl and its control of the cell cycle and apoptosis

In the t(9;22)(q34;q11) translocation found in CML, the *bcr* (Breakpoint Cluster Region) and *abl* (Abelson Leukemia) genes get fused. As a result, the chimeric tyrosine kinase oncoprotein Bcr-Abl is expressed (Ben-Neriah et al., 1986). Unlike c-Abl that shuttles between the nucleus and the cytoplasm and whose kinase activity is finely tuned, Bcr-Abl is cytoplasmic and its kinase activity is increased and deregulated (Salesse & Verfaillie, 2002). Through phosphorylation of different substrates, Bcr-Abl activates different signal transduction pathways that participate in the control of cellular proliferation, differentiation, migration, adhesion and survival (Afar et al., 1994; Andreu et al., 2005; Bedi et al., 1994;

Gordon et al., 1987; Horita et al., 2000; Jiang et al., 2000; Puil et al., 1994; Salesse & Verfaillie, 2003; Sawyers, 1993).

Several different substrates and partners of Bcr-Abl have been identified so far. Current efforts are directed at linking these pathways to the specific pathologic defects that characterize CML. These defects include increased proliferation and/or decreased apoptosis of a hematopoietic stem cell or progenitor cell (which leads to a massive increase in myeloid cell numbers), premature release of immature myeloid cells into the circulation (probably due to a defect in adherence of myeloid progenitors to marrow stroma) and genetic instability which results in disease progression (Druker, 2008).

Pathways activated by Bcr-Abl include the Ras-Raf-MAPK, the PI3K/Akt and the JAK/STAT pathways. The Ras-Raf-MAPK pathway links Bcr-Abl to the increased proliferative rate. The PI3K/Akt pathway induces survival signals through different mechanisms such as the Ras-Raf pathway, the phosphorylation of Bad, the induction of Bcl-x_L expression and the inhibition of caspase activity. Besides, it controls the activity of several transcription factors involved in the expression of cell cycle regulatory proteins, such as FoxO, belonging to the Forkhead family of transcription factors, and NF-κB (Manning & Cantley, 2007; Medema et al., 2000). Akt also regulates cell growth through mTOR and the control of protein translation and synthesis (Manning & Cantley, 2007). The JAK/STAT pathway is also a target of Bcr-Abl kinase activity. Bcr-Abl induces the expression of the antiapoptotic protein Bcl-x_L through the activation of STAT5, which binds to the promoter of the *bcl-x_L* gene, thus increasing survival of Bcr-Abl expressing cells (Horita et al., 2000).

Bcr-Abl regulates the expression and activity of the cell cycle inhibitor $p27^{kip1}$ through the PI3K/Akt pathway. The inhibition of Bcr-Abl and the inhibition of the PI3K/Akt pathway both result in an increase of $p27^{kip1}$ levels. Bcr-Abl also induces the expression of cyclins D and E and the activity of the cyclin E associated kinase Cdk2, resulting in the phosphorylation and inactivation of the tumor suppressor Retinoblastoma protein (Rb). Consequently, Bcr-Abl expressing cells show a deregulation of one of the main mechanisms controlling cell cycle progression along G1 and into S phase (Andreu et al., 2005).

Therefore, by activating several different signal transduction pathways, Bcr-Abl induces cell proliferation and suppresses apoptosis in CML cells.

3. The proteasome as a therapeutic target

Protein synthesis and degradation are key mechanisms by which protein levels are regulated inside cells. In fact, specific protein degradation has emerged as a very active field of research. Two different machineries are involved in this process: the autophagosome (which will not be considered in this chapter) and the proteasome.

3.1 Protein degradation at the proteasome

The 26S proteasome is a multiprotein complex that can be found in the cytoplasm and in the nucleus of eukaryotic cells. It is composed of a catalytic 20S core and two 19S regulatory subunits. Proteasome assembly and protein degradation are both ATP dependent (Almond & Cohen, 2002; Baumeister et al., 1997; Baumeister et al., 1998). The catalytic core has three activities: chymotryptic, tryptic, and post-glutamyl peptide hydrolytic-like activities.The regulatory subunits are responsible for substrate recognition and unfolding. The proteasome is involved in a wide variety of cellular processes including apoptosis, cell cycle and division, differentiation and development, all of them related directly or indirectly to tumoral transformation (DeSalle & Pagano, 2001).

For a protein to be degraded at the proteasome, it must be labelled with ubiquitin. Ubiquitin is a small polypeptide of 76 aminoacids which is highly conserved in all eukaryotes. Protein ubiquitylation not only can lead to degradation but is also a mechanism involved in intracellular transport. Ubiquitin can be added to proteins as single molecules to one (monoubiquitylation) or several (multiubiquitylation) Lysine residues or as polyubiquitin chains (polyubiquitylation) using one of several Lysine residues of the ubiquitin molecule to form the chain.

Ubiquitylation requires the sequential activity of three enzymes. The C-terminal Glycine of ubiquitin is activated in an ATP dependent process by an E1 ubiquitin-activating enzyme. This reaction results in the formation of a thioester covalent linkage between ubiquitin and a Cysteine residue in E1. Activated ubiquitin is then transferred to the ubiquitin-conjugating enzyme E2 by a trans-esterification reaction. Finally, a ubiquitin-ligase E3 enzyme transfers the ubiquitin molecule to the specific target protein to be degraded, thus acting as the substrate recognizing enzyme. This conserved ubiquitylation cascade allows for different combinations of E1-E2-E3 molecules leading to the recognition, labeling and degradation of multiple target proteins (Hershko & Ciechanover, 1998).

3.2 The proteasome and the cell cycle control

Along the cell cycle, two different E3 complexes are involved in the degradation of regulatory proteins. The SCF complex contains four different subunits: Skp1, Cul1, Roc1/Rbx1 and one of several different F-box proteins. This E3 complex is necessary, for instance, for the degradation of G1 cyclins, leading to the G1/S transition. G2 cyclins, on the other hand, are ubiquitylated by the E3 APC/C (Anaphase Promoting Complex/Cyclosome). The APC/C complex is activated by phosphorylation and its activity is required for mitosis (Murray, 2004).

The F-box protein in the SCF complexes interacts with specific substrates targeting them for degradation. Interaction with Skp1 requires the conserved F-box region. The substrate that is to be degraded needs to be previously phosphorylated. SCF complexes containing the F-box protein β-Trcp ($SCF^{\beta\text{-}Trcp}$) are involved in the degradation of proteins of the NF-κB pathway and of β-catenin. Another important F-box protein is Skp2 (S-phase kinase-interacting protein 2), identified as a protein interacting with cyclin A/Cdk2 complexes (Zhang et al., 1995). Many key regulators of the cell cycle, including the cell cycle inhibitor $p27^{kip1}$, are ubiquitylated by SCF^{Skp2} complexes (Carrano et al., 1999; Sutterluty et al., 1999; Tsvetkov et al., 1999).

The cell cycle inhibitor $p27^{kip1}$ binds to Cdk2-containing complexes, inhibiting its kinase activity and therefore blocking cell cycle progression along G1 and into the S phase. It can also bind to cyclin D-containing complexes, where $p27^{kip1}$ is "sequestered" and maintained away from active cyclin E/Cdk2 complexes (Bouchard et al., 1999; Perez-Roger et al., 1999). $p27^{kip1}$ levels in tumors are useful as a prognostic marker. Degradation of $p27^{kip1}$ at the proteasome requires its previous phosphorylation (at Threonine 187) by the same cyclin E/Cdk2 complexes it inhibits. Next, the SCF^{Skp2} complex recognizes the phosphorylated protein and labels it with a polyubiquitin chain leading to its degradation (Carrano et al., 1999; Montagnoli et al., 1999; Nguyen et al., 1999; Perez-Roger et al., 1999; Perez-Roger et al., 1997; Sheaff et al., 1997; Sutterluty et al., 1999; Tsvetkov et al., 1999; Vlach et al., 1997).

Skp2 expression changes along the cell cycle, being higher in S and G2 and lower in M and G1. Induction of Skp2 in the G1-S transition promotes the degradation of $p27^{kip1}$, allowing cell cycle progression (Andreu et al., 2005; Carrano et al., 1999; Marti et al., 1999; Schneider et al., 2006; Wirbelauer et al., 2000; Zhang et al., 1995). Skp2 is degraded at the proteasome in mitosis, when the APC/C complex becomes active (Wirbelauer et al., 2000). Ectopic expression of Skp2 in quiescent cells is sufficient to induce cell cycle entry, making Skp2 a potent oncoprotein. In many tumors, the levels of Skp2 and of $p27^{kip1}$ are inversely proportional: low Skp2 correlates with high $p27^{kip1}$ and slow growing tumors, whereas high Skp2 correlates with low $p27^{kip1}$ and fast growing tumors.

3.3 Proteasome inhibition: Bortezomib

The relationship between the ubiquitin-proteasome system (UPS) and the regulation of cellular proliferation, differentiation, survival and transformation led to considering the proteasome as a suitable target in cancer therapy (Adams, 2004). Proteasome inhibitors block protein degradation, causing the accumulation of damaged proteins and inducing the heat shock response and cell death (Concannon et al., 2007; Friedman & Xue, 2004).

Among the several proteasome inhibitors described, Bortezomib has been approved by the FDA for treatment of Multiple Myeloma and Mantle Cell Lymphoma (Ocio et al., 2008; Perez-Galan et al., 2006). Bortezomib is a dipeptdyl boronic acid that inhibits specifically and reversibly the chymotrypsine like activity of the proteasome, thought to be the rate limiting step of proteasome degradation (Eldridge & O'Brien, 2010; Jung et al., 2004; Richardson et al., 2006).

Surprisingly, Bortezomib appears to be quite selective against tumor cells. For some reason, normal cells seem to be more resistant to proteasome inhibition. One of the molecular effects of Bortezomib in several (but not all) cell types is the inhibition of the NF-κB pathway involved in suppressing apoptosis and increasing cell survival and resistance to cytotoxic agents (Baud & Karin, 2009). Some cases of Multiple Myeloma show an increase in NF-κB signaling making them especially sensitive to Bortezomib. Other probably important targets of Bortezomib are p53, p21, p27, Bax, Smac/Diablo and p44/42MAPK, all of them involved in the regulation of cell proliferation and/or survival (Voorhees et al., 2003).

4. Inhibition of the proteasome in CML

Proteasome activity is necessary for all cells to maintain the appropriate balance between protein synthesis and degradation. Therefore, proteasome inhibitors have a highly cytotoxic effect. However, cancer cells seem to be more sensitive to proteasome inhibition than control or normal cells.

4.1 Bcr-Abl and the proteasome

Bcr-Abl activity down-regulates the level of the cell cycle inhibitor $p27^{kip1}$ in different cell models expressing Bcr-Abl endogenously (like K562) or exogenously (like Mo7e and BaF/3) and in primary CML CD34+ cells. Moreover, exogenous $p27^{kip1}$ expression partially antagonizes the effect of Bcr-Abl on proliferation (Albero et al., 2010; Andreu et al., 2005; Bretones et al., 2011; Jonuleit et al., 2000). By inhibiting the tyrosine kinase activity of Bcr-Abl with Imatinib, the half-life of $p27^{kip1}$ is increased, meaning that Bcr-Abl induces the degradation of $p27^{kip1}$. At the same time, the expression of Skp2 decreases and when the expression of Skp2 is silenced in Bcr-Abl expressing cells, the levels of p27^{kip1} increase, showing again the inverse relationship between these two proteins. The regulation of p27^{kip1} expression by Bcr-Abl depends mainly on the PI3K/Akt pathway. This can be demonstrated because when cells are treated with either the Bcr-Abl inhibitor Imatinib or the PI3K inhibitor LY294002 the effects are quite similar. These effects are threefold (Fig. 1): first, Akt phosphorylates and inactivates FoxO transcription factors, involved in the regulation of p27^{kip1} gene transcription; second, Bcr-Abl induces the expression of Skp2 through the Akt pathway, which results in the proteasomal degradation of p27^{kip1} (Andreu et al., 2005); third, Akt also phosphorylates p27^{kip1} directly, preventing its translocation to the nucleus where it inhibits the cyclin/Cdk complexes controlling the cell cycle (Liang et al., 2002).

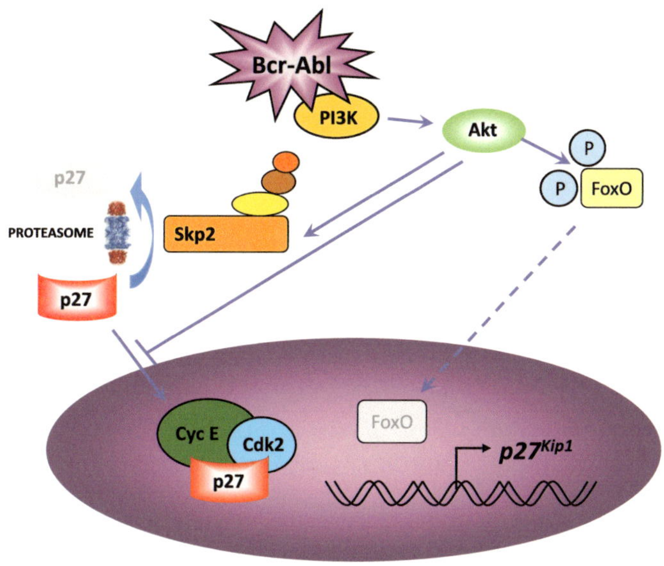

Fig. 1. Bcr-Abl regulation of the level and activity of p27^{kip1} includes transcriptional inhibition, misslocalization and proteasomal degradation.

Apart from the regulation of key proteins controlling cell cycle progression, there is a direct relationship between Bcr-Abl and the proteasome. Exogenous expression of Bcr-Abl in cells directly increases the activity of the proteasome and siRNA knock down of Bcr-Abl expression in K562 cells is associated with a decrease of all three proteasome activities (Crawford et al., 2009).

As Bcr-Abl regulates the activity of the proteasome and induces the proteasomal degradation of several proteins, Bortezomib was proposed as a therapeutic alternative to Imatinib, especially in CML cases of Imatinib resistance.

4.2 Molecular changes in CML cells treated with Bortezomib

Proteasome inhibition with Bortezomib in Bcr-Abl expressing cell models or primary CD34+ cells from CML patients results in a cell cycle inhibition and induction of apoptosis (Albero et al., 2010; Gatto et al., 2003; Jagani et al., 2009). Different key regulators are affected by Bortezomib leading to the detection of apoptosis markers, such as the activation (cleavage) of caspases (3, 8 and 9), or the down-regulation of Bcl-x_L and induction of Bim. Among these key events, Bortezomib treatment reverses the Bcr-Abl suppression of FoxO proteins and blocks the activation of NF-κB.

Although apoptosis induction is a commonplace of Bortezomib treatment, the inhibition of the cell cycle can be at the G1/S transition or at the G2/M boundary, depending on the cell models used (Albero et al., 2010; Gatto et al., 2003). The cell cycle inhibition at the G1/S transition can be explained by the accumulation of $p27^{kip1}$ in Bortezomib treated cells (Fig. 2). This accumulation inhibits the kinase activity of cyclin/Cdk complexes, which results in the dephosphorylation (activation) of Rb, blocking the cell cycle at the restriction point by the sequestration and inactivation of E2F transcription factors. The dephosphorylation of Rb is followed by its caspase-dependent processing and degradation, something associated with the induction of apoptosis. As a consequence of the impact on Rb phosphorylation, Bortezomib treatment also results in the down-regulation of cyclin A expression (Albero et al., 2010).

In cell lines derived from CML patients in blast crisis, Bortezomib induces the accumulation of IκBα, correlating with a decrease in the NF-κB DNA binding activity in the nucleus at the same time (Gatto et al., 2003). However, this effect was only transient and perhaps does not explain the cellular effects of Bortezomib. In contrast, in Baf/3-derived cell lines exogenously expressing Bcr-Abl, there was no effect of Bortezomib on NF-κB activity (Albero et al., 2010). However, in this same study, the non-canonical NF-κB pathway was analyzed and the results show that Bortezomib prevents the activation of NF-κB2. This protein is activated by proteolysis from a 100 kDa precursor to yield the 52 kDa active form in a proteasome dependent manner (Barre & Perkins, 2007). As NF-κB2 is not activated, the expression of two of its regulated targets, Skp2 and Myc, is also inhibited (Albero et al., 2010; Barre & Perkins, 2007; Schneider et al., 2006). This effect, in turn, would reinforce the effect of Bortezomib on the accumulation of $p27^{kip1}$ (Fig. 2) leading to the dephosphorylation of Rb and the cell cycle inhibition at the G1/S transition (Albero et al., 2010).

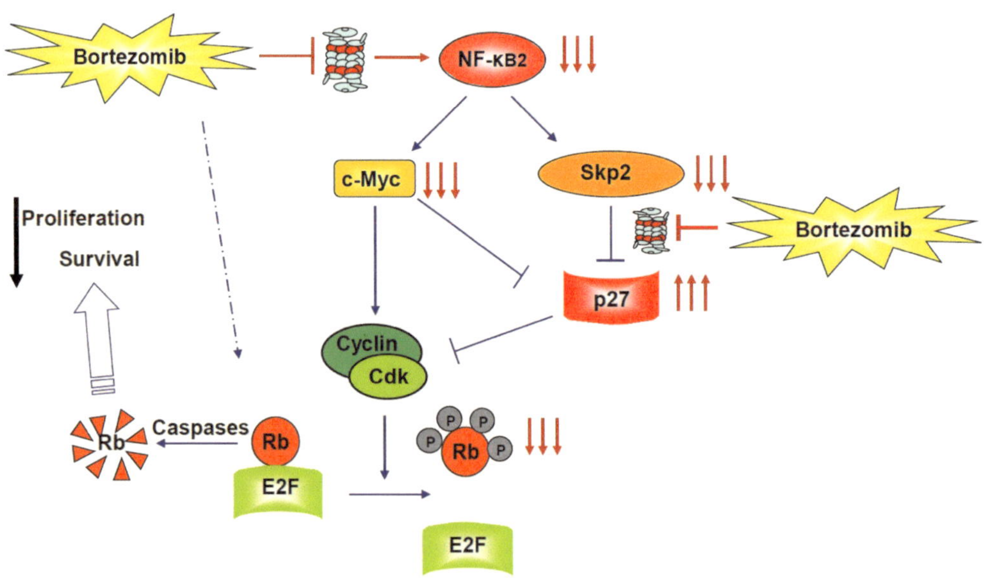

Fig. 2. Possible molecular mechanism leading to cell cycle arrest in G1 and apoptosis in CML cells treated with Bortezomib, as proposed (Albero et al., 2010).

4.3 Effect of Bortezomib on Imatinib resistant CML cells

As Bortezomib inhibition of the cell cycle and induction of apoptosis is independent of Bcr-Abl kinase activity it should be effective even in Imatinib resistant cases. Several different reports show the effect of Bortezomib on cells resistant to Imatinib, using cell lines exogenously expressing wild type and mutant forms of Bcr-Abl, primary CD34+ cells and cell lines derived from patients in blast crisis resistant to Imatinib, or CML cell lines selected for Imatinib resistance by chronic exposure to the inhibitor. In all these cases, Bortezomib induces apoptosis of Bcr-Abl expressing cells regardless of the mutational status of the protein, and at concentrations at which control cells are not sensitive (Albero et al., 2010; Colado et al., 2008; Crawford et al., 2009; Gatto et al., 2003; Heaney et al., 2010; Jagani et al., 2009). As these studies include the highly resistant gate keeper mutant T315I, it is clear that Bortezomib could be an alternative to Imatinib when this treatment is ineffective.
Another source of Imatinib resistant cells is the population of primitive, quiescent hematopoietic CML stem cells (Graham et al., 2002). During Imatinib treatment, there is an initial phase in which Bcr-Abl transcripts decrease rapidly, followed by a second phase in which this decrease is slower. This is probably due to the different sensitivity of CML cell subpopulations to Imatinib. Differentiated cells are more sensitive to Imatinib, whereas primitive CML stem cells are less sensitive to Imatinib. This difference could be due to the almost quiescent state of CML stem cells. This subpopulation of cells (Lin-CD34+) represents approximately 0.5% of the CD34+ cells but are likely to be responsible for the minimal residual disease found in Imatinib treated patients and to relapse if the treatment is interrupted. It is estimated that up to 10^6 lekemia cells may remain in patients with no detectable Bcr-Abl transcripts and therefore it is recommended that Imatinib treatment is not interrupted (Bhatia et al., 2003; Graham et al., 2002; Holyoake et al., 1999; Holyoake et al., 2001; Quintas-Cardama et al., 2009).
Bortezomib is also effective against the quiescent CML stem cells in different assays (Heaney et al., 2010). Bortezomib treatment induces apoptosis of CD34+ cells from chronic phase CML patients at diagnosis, with the accumulation of ubiquitylated proteins but with no effect on the kinase activity of Bcr-Abl. The primitive CD34+CD38- population that includes the quiescent CML stem cells is also sensitive to Bortezomib, which reduces the long-term colony formation capability of the cells. Finally, Bortezomib treatment also leads to a significant reduction in the engraftment potential of human CD34+ CML cells, although in this experiment there were still detectable Bcr-Abl positive cells. However, the effect of Bortezomib is not specific for CML cells, as it induces apoptosis also in normal CD34+CD38- hematopoietic stem cells (Heaney et al., 2010).

5. Conclusion

Imatinib is the first and so far the best example of rational design of anticancer therapeutic drugs. However, it is not able to cure and in some cases its efficacy is reduced due to Bcr-Abl dependent and independent mechanisms of resistance. In this context, the relationship between Bcr-Abl and the proteasome is worth exploiting. In fact, the proteasome inhibitor Bortezomib has shown its potential *in vitro* and in animal models. Nevertheless, proteasome inhibition is cytotoxic to all cell types. Therefore, the future of Bortezomib and other "non-specific" inhibitors or drugs may lie in the search for synergies with other "specific" drugs aimed to the molecular events characteristic of the tumor. In Chronic Myeloid Leukemia, inhibiting the proteasome with Bortezomib and inhibiting the kinase activity of Bcr-Abl with Imatinib or one of the new compounds may prove the right combination to tackle the problems of Bcr-Abl mutations and the Imatinib resistant leukemia stem cell. This could be a good starting point for this kind of combined therapies in other tumors where the search for a "specific" therapy is still ongoing.

6. Acknowledgement

Financial support: IPR receives grants from the Instituto de Salud Carlos III (PI10/00109) and from the Universidad CEU Cardenal Herrera (Programa Banco Santander Copernicus and PRUCH).

7. References

Adams, J. (2004). The proteasome: a suitable antineoplastic target. Nat Rev Cancer, Vol.4, No.5, (May), pp. 349-360

Afar, D.E., Goga, A., McLaughlin, J., Witte, O.N. & Sawyers, C.L. (1994). Differential complementation of Bcr-Abl point mutants with c-Myc. Science, Vol.264, No.5157, (Apr 15), pp. 424-426

Albero, M.P., Vaquer, J.M., Andreu, E.J., Villanueva, J.J., Franch, L., Ivorra, C., Poch, E., Agirre, X., Prosper, F. & Perez-Roger, I. (2010). Bortezomib decreases Rb phosphorylation and induces caspase-dependent apoptosis in Imatinib-sensitive and -resistant Bcr-Abl1-expressing cells. Oncogene, Vol.29, No.22, (Jun 3), pp. 3276-3286

Almond, J.B. & Cohen, G.M. (2002). The proteasome: a novel target for cancer chemotherapy. Leukemia, Vol.16, No.4, (Apr), pp. 433-443

Andreu, E.J., Lledo, E., Poch, E., Ivorra, C., Albero, M.P., Martinez-Climent, J.A., Montiel-Duarte, C., Rifon, J., Perez-Calvo, J., Arbona, C., Prosper, F. & Perez-Roger, I. (2005). BCR-ABL induces the expression of Skp2 through the PI3K pathway to promote p27Kip1 degradation and proliferation of chronic myelogenous leukemia cells. Cancer Res, Vol.65, No.8, (Apr 15), pp. 3264-3272

Barre, B. & Perkins, N.D. (2007). A cell cycle regulatory network controlling NF-kappaB subunit activity and function. Embo J, Vol.26, No.23, (Nov 28), pp. 4841-4855

Baud, V. & Karin, M. (2009). Is NF-kappaB a good target for cancer therapy? Hopes and pitfalls. Nat Rev Drug Discov, Vol.8, No.1, (Jan), pp. 33-40

Baumeister, W., Cejka, Z., Kania, M. & Seemuller, E. (1997). The proteasome: a macromolecular assembly designed to confine proteolysis to a nanocompartment. Biol Chem, Vol.378, No.3-4, (Mar-Apr), pp. 121-130

Baumeister, W., Walz, J., Zuhl, F. & Seemuller, E. (1998). The proteasome: paradigm of a self-compartmentalizing protease. Cell, Vol.92, No.3, (Feb 6), pp. 367-380

Bedi, A., Zehnbauer, B.A., Barber, J.P., Sharkis, S.J. & Jones, R.J. (1994). Inhibition of apoptosis by BCR-ABL in chronic myeloid leukemia. Blood, Vol.83, No.8, (Apr 15), pp. 2038-2044

Ben-Neriah, Y., Daley, G.Q., Mes-Masson, A.M., Witte, O.N. & Baltimore, D. (1986). The chronic myelogenous leukemia-specific P210 protein is the product of the bcr/abl hybrid gene. Science, Vol.233, No.4760, (Jul 11), pp. 212-214

Bhatia, R., Holtz, M., Niu, N., Gray, R., Snyder, D.S., Sawyers, C.L., Arber, D.A., Slovak, M.L. & Forman, S.J. (2003). Persistence of malignant hematopoietic progenitors in chronic myelogenous leukemia patients in complete cytogenetic remission following imatinib mesylate treatment. Blood, Vol.101, No.12, (Jun 15), pp. 4701-4707

Bouchard, C., Thieke, K., Maier, A., Saffrich, R., Hanley-Hyde, J., Ansorge, W., Reed, S., Sicinski, P., Bartek, J. & Eilers, M. (1999). Direct induction of cyclin D2 by Myc contributes to cell cycle progression and sequestration of p27. Embo J, Vol.18, No.19, pp. 5321-5333.

Bretones, G., Acosta, J.C., Caraballo, J.M., Ferrandiz, N., Gomez-Casares, M.T., Albajar, M., Blanco, R., Ruiz, P., Hung, W.C., Albero, M.P., Perez-Roger, I. & Leon, J. (2011). SKP2 oncogene is a direct MYC target gene and MYC down-regulates p27(KIP1) through SKP2 in human leukemia cells. J Biol Chem, Vol.286, No.11, (Mar 18), pp. 9815-9825

Carrano, A.C., Eytan, E., Hershko, A. & Pagano, M. (1999). SKP2 is required for ubiquitin-mediated degradation of the CDK inhibitor p27. Nat Cell Biol, Vol.1, No.4, (Aug), pp. 193-199

Colado, E., Alvarez-Fernandez, S., Maiso, P., Martin-Sanchez, J., Vidriales, M.B., Garayoa, M., Ocio, E.M., Montero, J.C., Pandiella, A. & San Miguel, J.F. (2008). The effect of the proteasome inhibitor bortezomib on acute myeloid leukemia cells and drug resistance associated with the CD34+ immature phenotype. Haematologica, Vol.93, No.1, (Jan), pp. 57-66

Concannon, C.G., Koehler, B.F., Reimertz, C., Murphy, B.M., Bonner, C., Thurow, N., Ward, M.W., Villunger, A., Strasser, A., Kogel, D. & Prehn, J.H. (2007). Apoptosis induced by proteasome inhibition in cancer cells: predominant role of the p53/PUMA pathway. Oncogene, Vol.26, No.12, (Mar 15), pp. 1681-1692

Crawford, L.J., Windrum, P., Magill, L., Melo, J.V., McCallum, L., McMullin, M.F., Ovaa, H., Walker, B. & Irvine, A.E. (2009). Proteasome proteolytic profile is linked to Bcr-Abl expression. Exp Hematol, Vol.37, No.3, (Mar), pp. 357-366

DeSalle, L.M. & Pagano, M. (2001). Regulation of the G1 to S transition by the ubiquitin pathway. FEBS Lett, Vol.490, No.3, (Feb 16), pp. 179-189

Druker, B.J. (2008). Translation of the Philadelphia chromosome into therapy for CML. Blood, Vol.112, No.13, (Dec 15), pp. 4808-4817

Eldridge, A.G. & O'Brien, T. (2010). Therapeutic strategies within the ubiquitin proteasome system. Cell Death Differ, Vol.17, No.1, (Jan), pp. 4-13

Friedman, J. & Xue, D. (2004). To live or die by the sword: the regulation of apoptosis by the proteasome. Dev Cell, Vol.6, No.4, (Apr), pp. 460-461

Gatto, S., Scappini, B., Pham, L., Onida, F., Milella, M., Ball, G., Ricci, C., Divoky, V., Verstovsek, S., Kantarjian, H.M., Keating, M.J., Cortes-Franco, J.E. & Beran, M. (2003). The proteasome inhibitor PS-341 inhibits growth and induces apoptosis in

Bcr/Abl-positive cell lines sensitive and resistant to imatinib mesylate. Haematologica, Vol.88, No.8, (Aug), pp. 853-863

Gordon, M.Y., Dowding, C.R., Riley, G.P., Goldman, J.M. & Greaves, M.F. (1987). Altered adhesive interactions with marrow stroma of haematopoietic progenitor cells in chronic myeloid leukaemia. Nature, Vol.328, No.6128, (Jul 23-29), pp. 342-344

Graham, S.M., Jorgensen, H.G., Allan, E., Pearson, C., Alcorn, M.J., Richmond, L. & Holyoake, T.L. (2002). Primitive, quiescent, Philadelphia-positive stem cells from patients with chronic myeloid leukemia are insensitive to STI571 in vitro. Blood, Vol.99, No.1, (Jan 1), pp. 319-325

Heaney, N.B., Pellicano, F., Zhang, B., Crawford, L., Chu, S., Kazmi, S.M., Allan, E.K., Jorgensen, H.G., Irvine, A.E., Bhatia, R. & Holyoake, T.L. (2010). Bortezomib induces apoptosis in primitive chronic myeloid leukemia cells including LTC-IC and NOD/SCID repopulating cells. Blood, Vol.115, No.11, (Mar 18), pp. 2241-2250

Hershko, A. & Ciechanover, A. (1998). The ubiquitin system. Annu Rev Biochem, Vol.67, pp. 425-479

Holyoake, T., Jiang, X., Eaves, C. & Eaves, A. (1999). Isolation of a highly quiescent subpopulation of primitive leukemic cells in chronic myeloid leukemia. Blood, Vol.94, No.6, (Sep 15), pp. 2056-2064

Holyoake, T.L., Jiang, X., Jorgensen, H.G., Graham, S., Alcorn, M.J., Laird, C., Eaves, A.C. & Eaves, C.J. (2001). Primitive quiescent leukemic cells from patients with chronic myeloid leukemia spontaneously initiate factor-independent growth in vitro in association with up-regulation of expression of interleukin-3. Blood, Vol.97, No.3, (Feb 1), pp. 720-728

Horita, M., Andreu, E.J., Benito, A., Arbona, C., Sanz, C., Benet, I., Prosper, F. & Fernandez-Luna, J.L. (2000). Blockade of the Bcr-Abl kinase activity induces apoptosis of chronic myelogenous leukemia cells by suppressing signal transducer and activator of transcription 5-dependent expression of Bcl-xL. J Exp Med, Vol.191, No.6, (Mar 20), pp. 977-984

Jagani, Z., Song, K., Kutok, J.L., Dewar, M.R., Melet, A., Santos, T., Grassian, A., Ghaffari, S., Wu, C., Yeckes-Rodin, H., Ren, R., Miller, K. & Khosravi-Far, R. (2009). Proteasome inhibition causes regression of leukemia and abrogates BCR-ABL-induced evasion of apoptosis in part through regulation of forkhead tumor suppressors. Cancer Res, Vol.69, No.16, (Aug 15), pp. 6546-6555

Jiang, Y., Zhao, R.C. & Verfaillie, C.M. (2000). Abnormal integrin-mediated regulation of chronic myelogenous leukemia CD34+ cell proliferation: BCR/ABL up-regulates the cyclin-dependent kinase inhibitor, p27Kip, which is relocated to the cell cytoplasm and incapable of regulating cdk2 activity. Proc Natl Acad Sci U S A, Vol.97, No.19, (Sep 12), pp. 10538-10543

Jonuleit, T., van der Kuip, H., Miething, C., Michels, H., Hallek, M., Duyster, J. & Aulitzky, W.E. (2000). Bcr-Abl kinase down-regulates cyclin-dependent kinase inhibitor p27 in human and murine cell lines. Blood, Vol.96, No.5, pp. 1933-1939.

Jung, L., Holle, L. & Dalton, W.S. (2004). Discovery, Development, and clinical applications of bortezomib. Oncology (Williston Park), Vol.18, No.14 Suppl 11, (Dec), pp. 4-13

Liang, J., Zubovitz, J., Petrocelli, T., Kotchetkov, R., Connor, M.K., Han, K., Lee, J.H., Ciarallo, S., Catzavelos, C., Beniston, R., Franssen, E. & Slingerland, J.M. (2002). PKB/Akt phosphorylates p27, impairs nuclear import of p27 and opposes p27-mediated G1 arrest. Nat Med, Vol.8, No.10, pp. 1153-1160.

Manning, B.D. & Cantley, L.C. (2007). AKT/PKB signaling: navigating downstream. Cell, Vol.129, No.7, (Jun 29), pp. 1261-1274

Marti, A., Wirbelauer, C., Scheffner, M. & Krek, W. (1999). Interaction between ubiquitin-protein ligase SCFSKP2 and E2F-1 underlies the regulation of E2F-1 degradation. Nat Cell Biol, Vol.1, No.1, (May), pp. 14-19

Medema, R.H., Kops, G.J., Bos, J.L. & Burgering, B.M. (2000). AFX-like Forkhead transcription factors mediate cell-cycle regulation by Ras and PKB through p27kip1. Nature, Vol.404, No.6779, (Apr 13), pp. 782-787

Montagnoli, A., Fiore, F., Eytan, E., Carrano, A.C., Draetta, G.F., Hershko, A. & Pagano, M. (1999). Ubiquitination of p27 is regulated by Cdk-dependent phosphorylation and trimeric complex formation. Genes Dev, Vol.13, No.9, (May 1), pp. 1181-1189

Murray, A.W. (2004). Recycling the cell cycle: cyclins revisited. Cell, Vol.116, No.2, (Jan 23), pp. 221-234

Nguyen, H., Gitig, D.M. & Koff, A. (1999). Cell-free degradation of p27(kip1), a G1 cyclin-dependent kinase inhibitor, is dependent on CDK2 activity and the proteasome. Mol Cell Biol, Vol.19, No.2, (Feb), pp. 1190-1201

Ocio, E.M., Mateos, M.V., Maiso, P., Pandiella, A. & San-Miguel, J.F. (2008). New drugs in multiple myeloma: mechanisms of action and phase I/II clinical findings. Lancet Oncol, Vol.9, No.12, (Dec), pp. 1157-1165

Perez-Galan, P., Roue, G., Villamor, N., Montserrat, E., Campo, E. & Colomer, D. (2006). The proteasome inhibitor bortezomib induces apoptosis in mantle-cell lymphoma through generation of ROS and Noxa activation independent of p53 status. Blood, Vol.107, No.1, (Jan 1), pp. 257-264

Perez-Roger, I., Kim, S.H., Griffiths, B., Sewing, A. & Land, H. (1999). Cyclins D1 and D2 mediate myc-induced proliferation via sequestration of p27(Kip1) and p21(Cip1). Embo J, Vol.18, No.19, pp. 5310-5320.

Perez-Roger, I., Solomon, D.L., Sewing, A. & Land, H. (1997). Myc activation of cyclin E/Cdk2 kinase involves induction of cyclin E gene transcription and inhibition of p27(Kip1) binding to newly formed complexes. Oncogene, Vol.14, No.20, pp. 2373-2381.

Puil, L., Liu, J., Gish, G., Mbamalu, G., Bowtell, D., Pelicci, P.G., Arlinghaus, R. & Pawson, T. (1994). Bcr-Abl oncoproteins bind directly to activators of the Ras signalling pathway. Embo J, Vol.13, No.4, (Feb 15), pp. 764-773

Quintas-Cardama, A., Kantarjian, H.M. & Cortes, J.E. (2009). Mechanisms of primary and secondary resistance to imatinib in chronic myeloid leukemia. Cancer Control, Vol.16, No.2, (Apr), pp. 122-131

Richardson, P.G., Mitsiades, C., Hideshima, T. & Anderson, K.C. (2006). Bortezomib: proteasome inhibition as an effective anticancer therapy. Annu Rev Med, Vol.57, pp. 33-47

Salesse, S. & Verfaillie, C.M. (2002). BCR/ABL: from molecular mechanisms of leukemia induction to treatment of chronic myelogenous leukemia. Oncogene, Vol.21, No.56, (Dec 9), pp. 8547-8559

Salesse, S. & Verfaillie, C.M. (2003). BCR/ABL-mediated Increased Expression of Multiple Known and Novel Genes That May Contribute to the Pathogenesis of Chronic Myelogenous Leukemia. Mol Cancer Ther, Vol.2, No.2, (February 1, 2003), pp. 173-182

Sawyers, C.L. (1993). Molecular consequences of the BCR-ABL translocation in chronic myelogenous leukemia. Leuk Lymphoma, Vol.11 Suppl 2, pp. 101-103

Schneider, G., Saur, D., Siveke, J.T., Fritsch, R., Greten, F.R. & Schmid, R.M. (2006). IKKalpha controls p52/RelB at the skp2 gene promoter to regulate G1- to S-phase progression. Embo J, Vol.25, No.16, (Aug 23), pp. 3801-3812

Sheaff, R.J., Groudine, M., Gordon, M., Roberts, J.M. & Clurman, B.E. (1997). Cyclin E-CDK2 is a regulator of p27Kip1. Genes Dev, Vol.11, No.11, (Jun 1), pp. 1464-1478

Sutterluty, H., Chatelain, E., Marti, A., Wirbelauer, C., Senften, M., Muller, U. & Krek, W. (1999). p45SKP2 promotes p27Kip1 degradation and induces S phase in quiescent cells. Nat Cell Biol, Vol.1, No.4, (Aug), pp. 207-214

Tsvetkov, L.M., Yeh, K.H., Lee, S.J., Sun, H. & Zhang, H. (1999). p27(Kip1) ubiquitination and degradation is regulated by the SCF(Skp2) complex through phosphorylated Thr187 in p27. Curr Biol, Vol.9, No.12, (Jun 17), pp. 661-664

Vlach, J., Hennecke, S. & Amati, B. (1997). Phosphorylation-dependent degradation of the cyclin-dependent kinase inhibitor p27. Embo J, Vol.16, No.17, (Sep 1), pp. 5334-5344

Voorhees, P.M., Dees, E.C., O'Neil, B. & Orlowski, R.Z. (2003). The proteasome as a target for cancer therapy. Clin Cancer Res, Vol.9, No.17, (Dec 15), pp. 6316-6325

Wirbelauer, C., Sutterluty, H., Blondel, M., Gstaiger, M., Peter, M., Reymond, F. & Krek, W. (2000). The F-box protein Skp2 is a ubiquitylation target of a Cul1-based core ubiquitin ligase complex: evidence for a role of Cul1 in the suppression of Skp2 expression in quiescent fibroblasts. Embo J, Vol.19, No.20, (Oct 16), pp. 5362-5375

Zhang, H., Kobayashi, R., Galaktionov, K. & Beach, D. (1995). p19Skp1 and p45Skp2 are essential elements of the cyclin A-CDK2 S phase kinase. Cell, Vol.82, No.6, (Sep 22), pp. 915-925

7

Ser/Thr Phosphatases: The New Frontier for Myeloid Leukemia Therapy?

Amanda M. Smith, Kathryn G. Roberts and Nicole M. Verrills
School of Biomedical Sciences, University of Newcastle and Hunter Medical Research Institute, Newcastle, NSW, Australia

1. Introduction

Myeloid leukemias are characterised by mutation and altered expression of a range of tyrosine kinases. Over 90% of chronic myeloid leukemias (CML) harbour the Philadelphia chromosome, resulting in expression of the BCR/ABL fusion protein, a constitutively active tyrosine kinase that is essential for survival of the CML cells. Acute myeloid leukemia (AML) is a heterogeneous disease characterised by mutations and dysregulation of a range of tyrosine kinases including the receptors Fms-like tyrosine kinase (Flt-3), c-KIT and platelet derived growth factor receptor (PDGFR). Tyrosine kinases represent powerful therapeutic targets, as the archetypical example of imatinib has shown for CML. However, many patients develop resistance to imatinib and other second generation inhibitors. Furthermore, trials of tyrosine kinase inhibitors for AML have thus far proven disappointing. Thus novel therapeutic targets are needed in order to improve the survival of myeloid leukemia patients.

Oncogenic tyrosine kinases induce activation of a variety of signaling pathways required for the growth and survival of leukemia cells, such as the Ras/MAPK, PI3K/Akt, and JAK/STAT pathways. In addition to protein kinases, the rate and duration of protein phosphorylation is tightly regulated by the activity of protein phosphatases, and in normal cells the reversal of protein phosphorylation by phosphatases is essential for providing the fine-tuning of signaling pathways and maintaining a balance in cellular physiology. While much of the focus for targeted therapies in leukemia therapy has concentrated on the kinases responsible for phosphorylation events, relatively little attention has been given to the role that protein phosphatases play. However, research over the past decade has now begun to highlight the importance of protein phosphatases in leukemia and their potential as targets for novel therapies. In particular, the ser/thr phosphatase PP2A has emerged as an important tumor suppressor in myeloid leukemias and strategies aimed at reactivating this complex enzyme show great promise for a new generation of leukemia therapies.

2. Protein phosphorylation in cellular signaling

Signal transduction via a network of cellular communication pathways enables modulation of essential cellular functions such as proliferation, differentiation, survival, adhesion, motility and death. Phosphorylation is the most common mechanism for the propagation of

intracellular signals. The net phosphorylation state relies on a delicate balance between protein kinases, which catalyse phosphate addition, and protein phosphatases, catalysing phosphate removal. The role of protein kinases in the cellular signaling pathways controlling biological functions has been extensively studied and protein kinases are currently the pharmaceutical industry's second largest drug target (Cohen 2002). In contrast, the role of phosphatases in disease has only recently come to the forefront of research.
Proteins are primarily phosphorylated on Serine (Ser), Threonine (Thr) and Tyrosine (Tyr) residues, each accounting for approximately 86, 12 and 2% of the human phosphoproteome respectively (Olsen *et al.* 2006). Around 2% of the human genome encodes a protein kinase gene, totalling 518 genes, of which 428 are known or predicted to phosphorylate Ser or Thr residues, and 90 encode protein tyrosine kinases (Alonso *et al.* 2004; Manning *et al.* 2002). In contrast, the human genome only encodes 147 phosphatase catalytic subunit genes. Of these, 107 encode a protein tyrosine phosphatase (PTP), a number that is comparable with the opposing tyrosine kinase genes (Alonso *et al.* 2004). Interestingly, while 98% of phosphoprotein sites are Ser and Thr residues, only a handful of the total protein phosphatases are specific for these amino acids (Moorhead *et al.* 2007). The unique way in which Ser/Thr phosphatases are regulated explains the difference in the number of Ser/Thr phosphatase catalytic subunits compared to PTPs. The evolution of PTPs has developed through the addition of discrete modular domains onto a core catalytic domain that define the function of the enzyme. In contrast, Ser/Thr phosphatases consist of a relatively simple catalytic subunit that reversibly binds to additional regulatory or interacting partner proteins which target the complex to specific subcellular locations and substrates, and ultimately control their activity.

3. Classification of protein phosphatases

Protein phosphatases can be classified into three main classes based on characteristics such as sequence, structure and phosphoamino-acid specificity. According to substrate specificity the largest phosphatase class is the ser/thr specific phosphoprotein phosphatase (PPP) family including PP1, PP2A, PP2B and PP4-PP7. The metallo-protein phosphatase dependant (PPM) family, made up mainly of PP2C, also functions against serine and threonine residues. Protein tyrosine phosphatases (PTP) form the second group and the aspartate-based or dual specificity protein phosphatases (DUSPs) the third. Genetic sequencing and analysis maintained these rules of partition, however it has recently been shown that particular Ser/Thr phosphatases can also dephosphorylate Tyr residues and various enzymes that fall into the dual specificity category based on their genetic sequence can selectively function on Ser, Thr, Tyr, phosphoinositides or RNA (Alonso *et al.* 2004; Begley and Dixon 2005).

4. PTPs in myeloid leukemias

The role of PTPs in cancer has been recently reviewed (Jiang and Zhang 2008; Julien *et al.* 2011; Lopez-Ruiz *et al.* 2011; Ruela-de-Sousa *et al.* 2011) and will not be discussed in detail here. However it should be noted that PTPs can act as either tumor suppressors or oncogenes in both solid tumors and leukaemais. For example, SHP1, a non-receptor PTP, displays tumor suppressive properties. SHP1 associates with a number of signaling molecules including CD5, the IL-3 receptor, CD22, the B-cell receptor, c-KIT and BCR/ABL

(Bruecher-Encke *et al.* 2001; Lorenz *et al.* 1996; Zhang *et al.* 2000), and these interactions exert primarily inhibitory effects on the signaling pathways. Silencing of the SHP1 gene via promotor methylation has been identified as a common event in a range of leukemias and lymphomas, and has been suggested as a potential marker for disease progression (Chim *et al.* 2004; Johan *et al.* 2005; Oka *et al.* 2002; Zhang *et al.* 2000). Other PTPs implicated as tumor suppressors in myeloid leukemias include PTEN, PTPN2, DEP-1, and DUSP-16. In contrast, SHP2 displays oncogenic properties as it promotes growth and survival pathways due to its dephosphorylating activity toward negative regulators of the Ras/Erk and PI3K/Akt signaling pathways (Neel *et al.* 2003). Somatic mutations in the SHP2 gene occur in around 30% of sporadic juvenile myelomonocytic leukemia (JMML) cases (Tartaglia *et al.* 2003), 6% of childhood acute lymphoblastic leukemia (ALL) (Tartaglia *et al.* 2004) and 5% of AML (Bentires-Alj *et al.* 2004; Tartaglia and Gelb 2005; Tartaglia *et al.* 2004; Tartaglia *et al.* 2005). Other PTPs with potential oncogenic roles in leukemia include CD45, Cdc25, and DUSP-7.

5. Ser/Thr phosphatases

In the early 1980s Ingebritsen and Cohen utilised a number of characteristics of phosphatases to pioneer nomenclature classes for the various enzymes (Ingebritsen and Cohen 1983a). Biochemical assays, sensitivity to endogenous inhibitors and the limited knowledge of substrate specificity at the time were originally used to classify the Ser/Thr phosphatases as either type 1 (PP1) or type 2 (PP2). PP1 specifically dephosphorylates the β subunit of phosphorylase kinase and is inhibited by nanomolar concentrations of the two small heat- and acid-stable proteins, termed inhibitor-1 (I-1) (Nimmo and Cohen 1978) and inhibitor-2 (I-2) (Foulkes and Cohen 1980). PP2 phosphatases preferentially dephosphorylate the α-subunit of phosphorylase kinase and are insensitive to I-1 and I-2 (Cohen 1989; Ingebritsen and Cohen 1983a; Ingebritsen and Cohen 1983b). PP2 phosphatases could in turn be subclassified into three distinct enzymes, PP2A, PP2B, and PP2C in a number of ways, but most simply by their metal-ion requirement. PP2A does not require a metal ion, however, PP2B and PP2C are Ca^{2+} and Mg^{2+} dependent respectively (Ingebritsen and Cohen 1983a; Ingebritsen and Cohen 1983b; Moorhead *et al.* 2007). More recently the Ser/Thr phosphatases were re-defined according to their structurally distinct gene family as part of the phosphoprotein phosphatase (PPP) family comprising PP1, PP2A, PP2B, PP4, PP5, PP6 and PP7 catalytic subunits, or protein phosphatase Mg^{2+}- or Mn^{2+}-dependent (PPM) family primarily composed of the PP2C catalytic subunit. The majority of Ser/Thr phosphatase activity in vivo is accounted for by the PPP family members PP1, PP2A and PP2B, together with PP2C of the PPM family (Barford *et al.* 1998). In the majority of cases they operate in hetero-oligomeric complexes interacting with an increasing diversity of targeting and regulatory subunits (Gallego and Virshup 2005).

6. Protein phosphatase 2A (PP2A)

The past decade has seen a surge in research into the PPP family member, PP2A, most notably due to the discoveries indicating its important role as a tumor suppressor. In particular PP2A has been implicated as a major player in myeloid leukemias and as a potential target for novel therapeutic strategies. In order to study the role of PP2A in leukemogenesis, understanding the structure and function of this complex enzyme is imperative, and as such is summarised below.

6.1 Structure and regulation of PP2A

PP2A is not a single phosphatase, but essentially encompasses a group of oligomeric enzymes consisting of a well conserved catalytic and structural subunit, together with the addition of one of a variety of regulatory subunits (Fig. 1). It makes up 1% of total cellular proteins and along with PP1, accounts for over 90% of serine/threonine phosphatase activity in the cell (Eichhorn *et al.* 2009). The PP2A core enzyme consists of a structural subunit (PP2A-A/PR65) and a catalytic subunit (PP2Ac). In mammals, two distinct genes (α and β) encode closely related versions of both the A (Hemmings *et al.* 1990) and C subunits (Arino *et al.* 1988). A third regulatory subunit (PP2A B) binds to the AC heterodimer, and determines both the substrate specificity and cellular localisation of PP2A holoenzyme complexes. Three B subunit families have been identified to date: B/B55/PR55 (Mayer *et al.* 1991; Strack *et al.* 1999; Zolnierowicz *et al.* 1994), B'/B56/PR61 (McCright *et al.* 1996; McCright and Virshup 1995), B"/PR72/130/PR70/48 (Hendrix *et al.* 1993; Stevens *et al.* 2003; Yan *et al.* 2000). Regulation of PP2A activity is accomplished primarily by members of its regulatory subunits. An additional level of regulation is introduced by post-translational modification of the catalytic subunit, which can undergo methylation and phosphorylation (Janssens *et al.* 2008), as well as the interaction with a vast array of other cellular and viral proteins such as SET, CIP2A and the SV40 small T antigen (Janssens and Goris 2001; Sablina and Hahn 2008). The use of specific PP2A inhibitors, PP2A activators and molecular genetics tools both *in vitro* and *in vivo* have exposed a role for PP2A in cell morphology, cell cycle regulation, development and apoptosis.

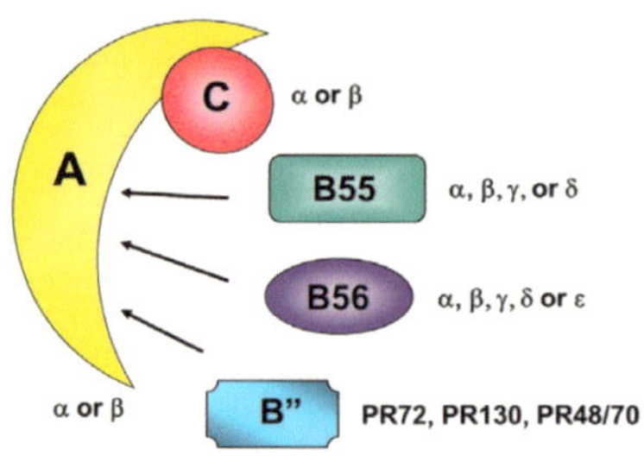

Fig. 1. Schematic of PP2A holoenzymes

6.2 PP2A in cellular signaling

PP2A has been implicated in a wide range of cellular signaling pathways, many of which are involved in cellular proliferation, apoptosis and differentiation, and as such are important in tumorigenesis. Since PP2A is one of the most abundant cellular phosphatases, it is not surprising that PP2A can exert opposing roles on similar pathways by acting at different levels. Recent work indicates that this substrate specificity is mediated by distinct PP2A complexes.

6.2.1 PP2A and MAPK signaling

A major function of PP2A is regulation of the MAPK signaling pathway. Interestingly, PP2A can exert both inhibitory and activating effects in a context-dependent manner (Fig. 2). PP2A acts negatively via the dephosphorylation of MEK (Heriche *et al.* 1997; Sontag *et al.* 1993) and ERK both *in vitro* and in mammalian cells (Alessi *et al.* 1995; Wang *et al.* 2003; Zhou *et al.* 2002). Specific knockdown of B56β and B56γ, but not B55 family subunits in NIH3T3 mouse fibroblasts increases basal ERK activation and prolongs ERK signal during stimulation in the absence of pMEK (Fig. 3A) (Letourneux *et al.* 2006). More recent evidence indicates that PP2A activates Ras-dependent MAPK signaling at the level of Raf-1 and its scaffolding protein Kinase Suppressor of Ras-1 (KSR1) (Abraham *et al.* 2000; Jaumot and Hancock 2001; Kubicek *et al.* 2002; Ory *et al.* 2003). Dephosphorylation of KSR1 (Ser329) and Raf-1 (Ser259) by B55α-containing PP2A complexes induces membrane translocation and increases the kinase activity of both proteins in several mammalian cell models, including NIH3T3, COS and HEK293 cells (Fig. 3B) (Abraham *et al.* 2000; Adams *et al.* 2005; Dougherty *et al.* 2005; Ory *et al.* 2003). Taken together, these studies provide biochemical mechanisms for how PP2A functions as a negative and positive regulator of MAPK signaling, depending on the specific regulatory subunit and substrate involved.

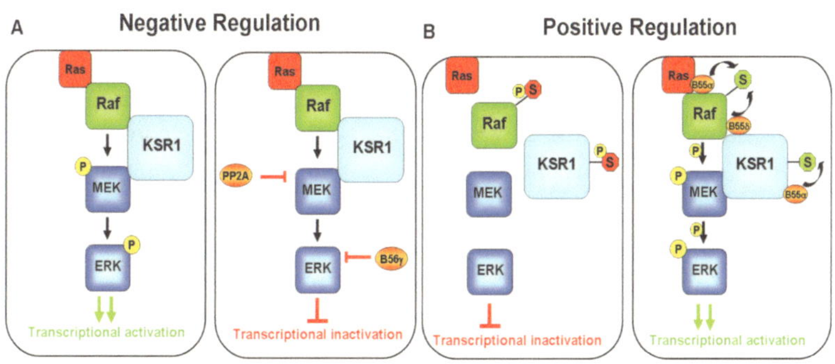

Fig. 2. Schematic overview of MAPK signaling regulation by PP2A
A) PP2A holoenzymes containing B56 family members negatively regulate MAPK signaling by inactivating MEK and ERK. **B)** In the inactive state, Raf and KSR1 are phosphorylated on Ser259 and Ser329, respectively, and are located within the cytoplasm. Upon stimulation, B55α-containing PP2A complexes dephosphorylate these residues, which results in protein activation and translocation to the plasma membrane. This facilitates the Ras/Raf interaction and induces transcriptional activation.

6.2.2 PP2A and PI3K/Akt signaling

The normal function of Akt is tightly modulated by phosphorylation events on Thr308 or Ser473 (Sarbassov *et al.* 2005; Vanhaesebroeck and Alessi 2000), and PP2A is the major phosphatase targeting these residues *in vitro* (Borgatti *et al.* 2003; Ivaska *et al.* 2002; Resjo *et al.* 2002). Over-expression of B55α-containing PP2A holoenzymes in the pro-lymphoid FL5.12 cell line substantially dephosphorylates Akt at Thr308 and results in subsequent growth suppression (Kuo *et al.* 2008). Conversely, Aα downregulation impairs Akt phosphorylation in neuronal cells, implicating PP2A as a positive regulator of the PI3K/Akt survival signaling cascade (Strack *et al.* 2004). An intriguing study by Andrabi *et al.* , demonstrated that Akt can act as a pro- or anti-apoptotic protein depending on environmental stimuli, and this is governed by PP2A (Andrabi *et al.* 2007). The specific PP2A regulatory subunits controlling this apparent switch remain undefined; however, this study reinforces the importance of understanding PP2A regulated cell signaling in a context dependent manner.

6.2.3 PP2A and Wnt/β-catenin signaling

The function of PP2A in Wnt/β-catenin signaling is similar to its role in the MAPK pathway, with individual PP2A subunits exerting either positive or negative effects (Fig. 3). B56

family members associate with APC (Seeling *et al.* 1999; Yamamoto *et al.* 2001) and axin (Hsu *et al.* 1999; Li *et al.* 2001) to impair Wnt signaling; a function that is critical for normal dorsal/ventral axis formation in Xenopus development (Li *et al.* 2001). Further studies demonstrate that association of the PP2A PR72 subunit with Naked cuticle is critical for the inhibitory function of this protein on the Wnt pathway (Fig. 3A) (Creyghton *et al.* 2005).
PP2A is also an important positive regulator of Wnt signaling (Bajpai *et al.* 2004; Gotz *et al.* 2000; Ratcliffe *et al.* 2000; Willert *et al.* 1999). Loss of function analysis suggests that B56ε is required for Wnt-mediated development in Xenopus embryogenesis (Yang *et al.* 2003). Purified B55α-containing PP2A holoenzymes directly dephosphorylate β-catenin *in vitro*. Accordingly, specific knockdown of B55α in SW480 colon cancer cells significantly elevates β-catenin phosphorylation, which induces protein degradation and inhibits the Wnt pathway (Zhang *et al.* 2009). Surprisingly, PR130 opposes the action of PR72 and modulates Wnt signal transduction by restricting the ability of Naked to function as a Wnt inhibitor (Fig. 4B) (Creyghton *et al.* 2006). These studies illustrate an excellent example whereby specific PP2A regulatory subunits determine holoenzyme function and provide the fine control on important cellular processes.

6.2.4 PP2A and p53 regulation

The tumor suppressor, p53, plays a critical role in mediating cellular responses to various types of stress, such as DNA damage, by inducing growth arrest or programmed cell death. The stability and activity of p53 is regulated by phosphorylation which, under normal cellular growth conditions, targets the protein for proteasome-mediated degradation (Vogelstein *et al.* 2000). PP2A B56γ holoenzymes dephosphorylate p53 on Ser37 (Dohoney *et al.* 2004) and Thr55 (Li *et al.* 2007) following γ radiation; an event which stabilises p53 in response to DNA damage and contributes to apoptosis in mammalian cells. Furthermore, ataxia-telangiectasia mutated (ATM) directly phosphorylates and specifically regulates B56γ and B56δ. Phosphorylation of B56γ3 at Ser510 after DNA damage increases B56γ-PP2A complexes, and directs PP2A phosphatase activity toward p53, activating its tumor-suppressive functions (Shouse *et al.* 2010). Conversely, RNAi knockdown of B56γ reduces p53 stability and inhibits cell death (Li *et al.* 2007). B56ε also regulates the p53-dependent apoptotic pathway by controlling the stability of p53 protein (Jin *et al.* 2010).
Other findings implicate an important role for B56α-containing PP2A complexes in p53 degradation. One target of p53, cyclin G, recruits B56α into a quaternary complex with the E3 ubiquitin ligase, mouse double minute 2 (Mdm2) (Okamoto *et al.* 1996; Okamoto *et al.* 2002). The subsequent dephosphorylation and activation of Mdm2 leads to ubiquitination and degradation of p53 (Haupt *et al.* 1997), thus allowing the cell to proliferate. In this context, PP2A serves as a negative regulator.

6.2.5 PP2A and c-Myc regulation

PP2A also plays a prominent role in controlling the accumulation of the proto-oncoprotein, c-Myc (Yeh *et al.* 2004). Aberrant regulation of c-Myc has been linked to transformation in up to 70% of human tumors; therefore tight control of this protein is crucial for maintaining cellular homeostasis (Nesbit *et al.* 1999). c-Myc stability is regulated, in part, through phosphorylation at two residues, Ser62 and Thr58 (Sears *et al.* 2000). Whilst ERK-mediated phosphorylation at Ser62 stabilises c-Myc, specific B56α-containing PP2A complexes reverse these effects, leading to destabilisation and ubiquitin-mediated degradation (Arnold and

Sears 2006). In addition, a novel PP2A-interacting protein, designated cancerous inhibitor of PP2A (CIP2A), was found to selectively target the catalytic activity of PP2A-B56α associated with c-Myc, and protect c-Myc from Ser62 dephosphorylation. Accordingly, depletion of CIP2A results in significantly increased PP2A activity measured from c-Myc immunoprecipitates and correlates with c-Myc destabilisation (Junttila *et al.* 2007).
Collectively, these results illustrate the dynamic interaction of the PP2A holoenzyme with signaling cascades involved in fundamental cellular processes such as proliferation, survival and development. The fact that PP2A is involved in both the negative and positive regulation of these pathways highlights the exquisite nature of PP2A modulation and underscores the importance of investigating specific complexes when determining PP2A function. Identification of critical subunits that are aberrantly regulated during transformation may ultimately lead to the development of novel treatments for cancer patients.

6.3 PP2A as a tumor suppressor

The fundamental evidence that implicated PP2A as a tumor suppressor was the discovery that okadaic acid, a tumor promoter (Fujiki and Suganuma 2009; Suganuma *et al.* 1988), potently inhibits the phosphatase activity of PP2A (Bialojan and Takai 1988; Haystead *et al.* 1989). In addition, the oncogenic polyomavirus middle and small tumor (ST) antigens, along with the simian virus 40 (SV40) ST antigen, transforms mammalian cells by inhibiting PP2A (Pallas *et al.* 1990). Transformation of the normal human fibroblast kidney epithelial cell line, HEK293, required several key genetic elements; human telomerase catalytic subunit, an oncogenic allele of H-Ras, and the SV40 large T (LT) and ST antigens (HEK-TER) (Hahn *et al.* 1999). Whilst expression of LT enables the cells to bypass senescence, complete tumor formation requires the addition of ST and thus inhibition of PP2A (Yu *et al.* 2001). Accordingly, ST mutants lacking the PP2A binding domain fail to induce tumorigenic transformation of HEK-TER cells (Hahn *et al.* 2002). Structural insights reveal that ST interacts with the PP2A-A subunit which overlaps B56 subunit binding site and results in its displacement from the core enzyme. Functionally, expression of ST activates Akt signaling in human cells *in vitro* (Rodriguez-Viciana *et al.* 2006; Yuan *et al.* 2002; Zhao *et al.* 2003). Taken together, these observations indicate that complete transformation of human cells requires the perturbation of PP2A, for example by ST.
A somewhat confusing aspect of PP2A function in cancer arises because PP2A plays important roles in promoting cell cycle progression and cell survival (Li *et al.* 2002; Lin *et al.* 1998; Mayer-Jaekel *et al.* 1993), which are functions usually associated with tumor initiation and progression rather than suppression. Therefore, cellular transformation will most likely occur through the disruption of PP2A holoenzymes that normally exert negative regulation on oncogenic pathways.
Whilst some contradiction exists as to the importance of PP2A scaffolding subunits in cancer development, several mutations have been identified in spontaneously arising human cancers. Notably, somatic alterations of the gene encoding Aβ (PPP2R1B) have been detected in up to 8-15% of colon, 15% of lung and 13% of breast cancers (Calin *et al.* 2000; Takagi *et al.* 2000; Tamaki *et al.* 2004; Wang *et al.* 1998). Mutations of the more abundant Aα subunit have been observed, albeit at a lower frequency (Calin *et al.* 2000) and cancer-associated A subunit mutants exhibit differential defects in binding to the B and C subunits, which correlates with impaired PP2A activity (Chen *et al.* 2005; Ruediger *et al.* 2001a;

Ruediger *et al.* 2001b; Sablina *et al.* 2007). Even in the absence of mutations, reduced protein expression of Aα has been found in 25 out of 58 brain tumors (Colella *et al.* 2001). Decreased levels of Aβ have also been observed in 16 of 32 cancer cell lines derived from human lung, colon and breast cancer, as well as primary glioblastoma and B-CLL patient samples compared to normal tissue (Kalla *et al.* 2007; Suzuki and Takahashi 2003; Takagi *et al.* 2000; Zhou *et al.* 2003). Importantly, Ruediger *et al.*, recently generated knock-in mice with cancer associated Aα mutations, and Aα knockouts, both of which exhibited increased incidence of lung cancer when treated with benzopyrene, thus supporting the role of PP2A as a tumor suppressor (Ruediger *et al.* 2011).

Pivotal studies using the HEK-TER transformation model demonstrated that suppression of B56γ, but not B55α, functionally mimicked the introduction of ST and resulted in partial tumorigenic transformation (Chen *et al.* 2004; Moreno *et al.* 2004). Moreover, depletion of B56γ containing complexes leads to activation of the anti-apoptotic Akt pathway (Chen *et al.* 2005). These observations were the first to demonstrate that PP2A complexes containing B56γ modulate the phosphorylation of substrates associated with transformation. Loss of B56γ has been demonstrated in some human cancers. Decreased expression was identified in primary human melanoma samples compared to melanocytic nevi (Deichmann *et al.* 2001), and in human lung cancer cell lines where subsequent overexpression of B56γ reversed the tumorigenic phenotype (Chen *et al.* 2004). Reduced transcript levels of B56γ have also been documented in patients with aggressive B-CLL compared to those with stable disease (Falt *et al.* 2005). A mutation in B56γ has also been observed in lung cancer, and this was shown to disrupt the interaction of B56γ with p53 (Shouse *et al.* 2010). In contrast, higher expression levels of B56γ1 mRNA were reported in human melanoma cell lines compared to normal melanocytes (Francia *et al.* 1999).

Recently the HEK293T system was further utilised to systematically examine all PP2A regulatory subunits (Sablina *et al.* 2010). In addition to B56γ, suppression of B56α, PR72/PR130, and PTPA (protein phosphatase 2A activator), replaced the expression of ST in transformation. Interestingly, the effects on signaling pathways differed depending on the regulatory subunit suppressed. Knockdown of B56γ and PTPA, but not B56α or PR72/PR130, led to enhanced Akt phosphorylation, while knockdown of B56α, PR72/PR130, and PTPA, but not B56γ, resulted in increased c-Myc expression. Moreover, suppression of B56γ and PTPA led to increased β-catenin activity, whereas PR72/PR130 suppression decreased β-catenin activity (Sablina *et al.* 2010). Overexpression of CIP2A in the HEK-TER model can also replace ST in inducing transformation (Junttila *et al.* 2007), and increased CIP2A has been detected in myeloid leukemia patient samples (Wang and Li 2011), gastric and colon cancer samples (Khanna *et al.* 2009; Li *et al.* 2008; Soo Hoo *et al.* 2002)

6.4 PP2A in myeloid leukemias

An emerging body of evidence implicates PP2A as an important tumor suppressor in myeloid leukemias (Table 1). In particular, recent work from our laboratory and others has revealed a common theme in myeloid leukemias: inactivation of PP2A by leukemia associated tyrosine kinases (Fig. 3). Importantly, PP2A inhibition is essential for leukemias driven by these oncogenic tyrosine kinases, as re-activation of PP2A results in dephosphorylation, and thus deactivation, of the kinase and subsequent inhibition of leukemogenesis. Hence, re-activation of PP2A is an attractive strategy for leukemia therapy.

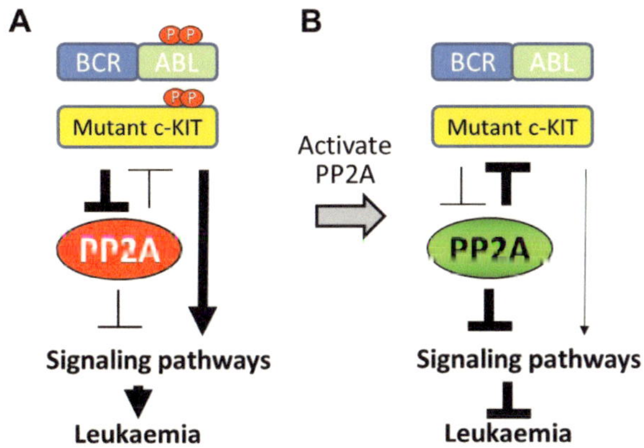

Fig. 3. Model of PP2A inhibition in myeloid leukemias. (A) PP2A activity is inhibited by BCR/ABL and oncogenic mutant c-KIT, enabling the activation of signaling pathways leading to leukemogenesis. (B) Pharmacological activation of PP2A induces de-activation (dephosphorylation) of BCR/ABL and c-KIT, and inhibition of downstream signaling pathways, leading to inhibition of leukemogenesis.

6.4.1 PP2A inhibition in CML

Functional inactivation of PP2A by BCR/ABL is essential for the development of CML-BC and Ph+ ALL, and is thought to result from upregulation of the endogenous PP2A inhibitor SET (I_2PP2A or TAF-1β) protein (Neviani *et al.* 2007; Neviani *et al.* 2005). Although its physiological function remains incompletely understood, abnormal expression of SET mRNA has been documented in solid tumors and haematological disorders (Carlson *et al.* 1998; Fornerod *et al.* 1995; Li *et al.* 1996). Expression of BCR/ABL in mouse myeloid precursor cells stimulates SET expression and correlates with a loss of PP2A activity (Neviani *et al.* 2005). Conversely, inhibition of BCR/ABL with imatinib treatment dramatically reduces SET expression, which results in the restoration of PP2A activity back to untransfected levels and results in the dephosphorylation of several substrates which are shared by BCR/ABL and PP2A (Neviani *et al.* 2005). These include STAT5, ERK1/2, Akt, BAD and JAK2 (Calabretta and Perrotti 2004; Janssens and Goris 2001). Importantly, molecular or pharmacological reactivation of PP2A resulted in growth suppression, enhanced apoptosis, restored differentiation, and decreased *in vivo* leukemogenesis of imatinib-sensitive and -resistant BCR/ABL+ cell lines and primary CML-BC cells. Furthermore, reactivation of PP2A, by overexpression of PP2AC or 1,9-dideoxyforskolin treatment (a cAMP-independent PP2A activator) (see section 6.5.1), reduced the activity and expression of BCR/ABL in both imatinib-sensitive and -resistant BCR/ABL cells, suggesting that BCR/ABL itself is a target for PP2A activity. Indeed, reactivation of PP2A results in PP2AC association with BCR/ABL via the SHP1 tyrosine phosphatase, BCR/ABL dephosphorylation, and proteasomal degradation (Neviani *et al.* 2005). These findings establish an important link between an oncogenic kinase and a tumor suppressing phosphatase, and indicate that pharmacologic enhancement of PP2A is a powerful therapeutic strategy for imatinib-resistant CML. Taken together, these results suggest that SET-dependent inhibition of PP2A is required for the transduction of aberrant mitogenic, survival and anti-differentiation signals that contribute to the development of CML from the chronic phase into blast crisis (Neviani *et al.* 2005).

Phosphatase	Leukaemia	Expression profile, prognosis, other	Reference
Ser/Thr PPs			
PP2A	CML	BCR/ABL inhibits PP2A activity via ↑ SET exp'n in CML-BC & BCR/ABL+ cell lines; Forskolin & FTY720 inhibit IM-sensitive and resistant BCR/ABL+ leukaemogenesis	(Neviani, Santhanam et al. 2005; Neviani, Santhanam et al. 2007; Samanta, Chakraborty et al. 2009; Salas, Ponnusamy et al. 2011)
	AML, APL	↑ exp'n regulatory subunits during differentiation of myeloid cell lines	(Uzunoglu, Uslu et al. 1999; Yuksel, Saydam et al. 2002)
	AML	SET translocations in AML	(Li, Makkinje et al. 1996)
		↓ activity in AML-M1	(Yamamoto, Suzuki et al. 1999)
		↓ activity in AML blasts	(Yang, Li et al.)
		↓ activity correlates with ↑ pAkt & poor prognosis/high risk karyotype patients	(Gallay, Dos Santos et al. 2009)
		↑ pY307-PP2A-C; ↓ subunit exp'n in AML blasts	(Cristobal, Garcia-Orti et al. 2011)
		Forskolin induced PP2A activation induces apoptosis in AML cell lines	(Cristobal, Garcia-Orti et al. 2011)
		↑ CIP2A in newly diagnosed & relapsed AML patients	(Wang, Li et al.)
		Mutant c-KIT inhibits activity & ↓ subunit exp'n; FTY720 inhibits leukaemogenesis	(Roberts KG 2010)
		↓ PP2A-B55α exp'n poor prognostic marker	(Ruvolo, Qui et al. 2011)
		↑ SETBP1 inhibits PP2A & associated with poor prognosis in elderly patients	(Cristobal, Blanco et al.)
		↓ activity associated with chemoresistance	(Jiffar, Kurinna et al. 2004)
		Antitumour agent, erucylphosphohomocholine, induces apoptosis via PP2A mediated ERK dephosphorylation in AML cell lines and primary cells	(Martelli, Papa et al.)
		↑ PP2A-B56γ exp'n in AML patients	(Zheng, Chen et al.)
		↓PP2A-Cα in del(5q) AML contributes to lanelomide sensitivity	(Wei, Chen et al. 2009)
		HRX fusion protein interacts with SET	(Adler, Nallaseth et al. 1997)
	T-ALL	PPP2R5E (B56ε) target for mir-19 in Notch-1 induced T-ALL	(Mavrakis, Wolfe et al. 2010)
		HOX11 interacts with PP2A & inhibits activity	(Kawabe, Muslin et al. 1997; Riz and Hawley 2005)
	B-ALL	Co-culture with stromal cells protects B-ALL cells from chemotherapeutics due to ↓ PP2A activity & ↑ pAkt	(Wang, Fortney et al. 2004)
	CLL	FTY720-induced PP2A activation inhibits leukaemogenesis	(Liu, Zhao et al. 2008)
		↓ exp'n & alternative splicing of PPP2R2B (Aβ) & ↓ activity	(Kalla, Scheuermann et al. 2007)
		PDE4 inhibitors apoptosis by activating PP2A	(Moon and Lerner 2003)
	APL	Altered PP2A activity & exp'n during differentiation of HL-60 cells	(Nishikawa, Omay et al. 1994; Bhoola and Hammond 2000; Luo, Huang et al. 2006; Ouyang, Xu et al. 2008; Xu, Ou-Yang et al. 2008)
PP1	APL, AML	Altered activity, subcellular distribution and gene exp'n during differentiation	(Omay, Ogasawara et al. 1995; Uzunoglu, Uslu et al. 1999; Bhoola and Hammond 2000; Luo, Huang et al. 2006)
	AML, ALL and B CLL	↓ activity in poorly differentiated AML-M1, ALL and B-CLL compared to blasts from more differentiated AML patients	(Yamamoto, Suzuki et al. 1999)
	T-ALL	HOX11 interacts & inhibits PP1	(Kawabe, Muslin et al. 1997; Riz and Hawley 2005)
PP2B	**AML**	**↑ activity in well differentiated AML blasts**	(Yamamoto, Suzuki et al. 1999)

Table 1. Ser/Thr Phosphatases in Leukaemia

6.4.2 PP2A inhibition in AML

Oncogenic c-KIT signaling also requires inhibition of PP2A for leukemogenesis (Roberts *et al.* 2010). c-KIT is a receptor tyrosine kinase that activates similar proliferation, differentiation and survival signaling pathways as BCR/ABL, such as the PI3K, ERK and JAK/STAT pathways (Linnekin 1999). Gain-of-function *c-KIT* mutations occur in a range of malignancies, including AML, systemic mastocytosis, testicular seminoma, gastrointestinal stromal tumors (GIST) and melanomas, making c-KIT an excellent target for anti-cancer therapies (Kitamura and Hirota 2004; Masson and Ronnstrand 2009). These mutants induce hyperphosphorylation of c-KIT and constitutive activation of downstream signaling pathways (Masson and Ronnstrand 2009). Activating c- KIT mutations occur in up to 48% of core binding factor-AML (CBF-AML) patients, and are associated with increased relapse and reduced survival (Muller *et al.* 2008). While imatinib has shown remarkable success in treating c-KIT+ GIST patients (Demetri *et al.* 2002), the majority of c-KIT mutations expressed in AML patients are intrinsically resistant to imatinib, and as such, many CBF-AML and systemic mastocytosis patients are unresponsive to imatinib therapy (Cairoli *et al.* 2005; Pardanani *et al.* 2003). Our laboratory has recently shown that myeloid precursor cells expressing oncogenic mutant c-KIT receptors display significantly reduced PP2A activity compared to c-KIT negative or WT-c-KIT expressing cells (Roberts *et al.* 2010). Inhibition of PP2A by mutant c-KIT is associated with reduced protein expression of PP2A subunits, together with altered expression of the endogenous PP2A inhibitory protein SET. Overexpression of PP2A-A caused growth inhibition and apoptosis, suggesting that PP2A inhibition is functionally important in c-KIT mediated leukemogenesis. Importantly, reactivation of PP2A resulted in dephosphorylation (and hence deactivation) of the mutant c-KIT receptor itself, as well as inactivation of downstream signaling proteins required for c-KIT induced leukemogenesis (e.g. Akt, ERK and STAT5) (Roberts *et al.* 2010). Furthermore, activation of PP2A by the pharmacological agent FTY720, inhibited leukemogenesis driven by mutant c-KIT (See section 6.5.2).

A number of recent studies further support a tumor suppressive role for PP2A in AML. Reduced expression of the PP2A-B55α subunit and increased Akt phophorylation in AML patient blasts was associated with shorter complete remission (Ruvolo *et al.* 2011). Hyperphosphorylation of PP2Ac, known to inhibit PP2A activity, has been observed in 78% of AML patients. This was associated with enhanced expression of PP2A inhibitors SET, CIP2A, and/or SET binding protein 1 (SETBP1) (Cristobal *et al.* 2011). Reduced expression of PP2A-A and a number of PP2A regulatory subunits was also observed in a number of patients. Increased expression of SETBP1 was also shown to be induced by a novel translocation t(12;18)(p13;q12) involving ETV6 in a patient with AML (Cristobal *et al.* 2010). SETBP1 overexpression protected SET from protease cleavage, leading to the formation of a SETBP1-SET-PP2A complex that results in PP2A inhibition, promoting proliferation of the leukemic cells. SETBP1 was further shown to be overexpressed in over 27% of AML patients and correlated with significantly shorter overall survival, in particular in patients over 60 years (Cristobal *et al.* 2010). Thus SETBP1 confers a negative prognostic impact and may be a predictive factor in any future clinical trials with PP2A activators. Increased expression of another PP2A inhibitory protein, CIP2A, has also been observed in diagnosis and relapse AML patients compared to patients in remission or healthy controls (Wang and Li 2011).

6.5 Targeting PP2A for anti-leukemia therapy

6.5.1 Forskolin

Forskolin, a diterpene isolated from the roots of *Coleus forskohlii*, is primarily known to stimulate the adenylate cyclase system, which results in elevated levels of cyclic AMP (cAMP) and subsequent activation of protein kinase A (PKA) (Seamon and Daly 1981; Seamon *et al.* 1981). The anticancer properties of this compound were initially demonstrated through potent inhibition of growth and tumor colonisation of the highly metastatic BL6 melanoma cell line (Agarwal and Parks 1983). Further studies indicated its potential use against ALL (Gutzkow *et al.* 2002) and CML cell lines (Taetle and Li-en 1984). However, more recent findings demonstrate that forskolin also activates PP2A (Feschenko *et al.* 2002); a mechanism which contributes to induction of apoptosis in B-CLL, CML-BC and AML patient samples (Cristobal *et al.* 2011; Moon and Lerner 2003; Neviani *et al.* 2005). Neviani *et al.*, was the first to highlight the therapeutic relevance of using PP2A-activators to specifically target leukemia cells (Neviani *et al.* 2005). Forskolin inhibited the *in vivo* leukemogenesis of imatinib sensitive and resistant BCR/ABL+ 32Dcl3 cells in mice, resulting in significantly prolonged survival. Furthermore, treatment with 1,9-dideoxy-forskolin, which lacks adenylate cyclase activity, impaired the clonogenic potential of BCR/ABL^{+} 32Dcl3 cells to a similar degree as forskolin, suggesting that the anti-leukaemic effects of forskolin and its derivative depends on the induction of PP2A activity rather than cAMP . Restoration of PP2A activity with forskolin was also found to inhibit Akt and ERK activity, block proliferation and induce caspase-dependant apoptosis in AML cell lines (Cristobal *et al.* 2011; Neviani *et al.* 2005). Furthermore, forskolin had an additive effect with common AML induction therapy drugs Idarubicin and Ara-c (Cristobal *et al.* 2011).

6.5.2 FTY720

FTY720 was first synthesised by structural modifications of myriocin (ISP-1), a fungal metabolite isolated from *Isaria sinclairii* culture broth (Fujita *et al.* 1994), and is structurally similar to sphingosine (Albert *et al.* 2005; Kiuchi *et al.* 2005). It is effectively phosphorylated *in vivo* by SphK2 to yield the biologically active FTY720-phosphate (FTY720-P) (Brinkmann *et al.* 2002; Zemann *et al.* 2006). Interaction of FTY720-P with one of the five known S1P receptors induces receptor internalisation and degradation (Graler and Goetzl 2004; Matloubian *et al.* 2004). The S1P signal is required for the migration of lymphocytes from secondary lymphoid tissues back into the efferent lymphatics and systemic circulation (Cyster 2005; Matloubian *et al.* 2004) and prolonged S1PR downregulation by FTY720-P inhibits the immune response by sequestering functional lymphocytes within secondary lymphoid organs (Brinkmann *et al.* 2002; Mandala *et al.* 2002). The use of FTY720 as an immunomodulator is currently being evaluated in Phase III trials for multiple sclerosis (Cohen *et al.* 2009; Takabe *et al.* 2008).

A more recent mechanism of action identified for FTY720 is its activation of purified PP2A trimers *in vitro* (Matsuoka *et al.* 2003) and as loss of PP2A phosphatase activity contributes to the pathophysiology of BCR/ABL-driven leukemias (Neviani *et al.* 2007) a logical prediction would be that restoration of PP2A levels reverses the leukaemic phenotype. Indeed, an extensive study has shown that pharmacological reactivation of PP2A with FTY720 inhibits the proliferation, enhances apoptosis, restores differentiation and impairs colony formation of imatinib-sensitive and –resistant BCR-ABL+ cell lines and CML-BC patient blasts (Neviani *et al.* 2007). Notably, FTY720 promotes BCR/ABL tyrosine dephosphorylation and proteolytic degradation, together with reduced phosphorylation of the PP2A targets Akt, ERK1/2 and STAT5 (Neviani *et al.* 2007). Co-treatment with okadaic acid or transduction of SV40 ST reverses the enhancement of PP2A activity and restores substrate phosphorylation, strongly indicating that FTY720 functions through a PP2A-dependent mechanism.

Importantly, the *in vitro* efficacy of FTY720 translated into an *in vivo* model markedly suppressing both imatinib-sensitive (WT) and –resistant (T315I) BCR/ABL^{+} leukemogenesis (Neviani *et al.* 2007). After 4 weeks of treatment, saline-treated mice contained a large number of undifferentiated myeloid cells within the peripheral circulation, representing an overt AML phenotype with extensive blast infiltration of distal organs. In contrast, FTY720-treated mice displayed undetectable levels of BCR/ABL^{+} cells in the systemic circulation and secondary organs. Accordingly, these effects were sustained long term with 80% and 50% of WT and T315I BCR/ABL^{+} FTY720-treated mice, respectively, still alive at 27 weeks

and showing no signs of leukemia. In contrast, all saline-treated mice were sacrificed 5 weeks post-tumor cell injection (Neviani *et al.* 2007). No toxic side effects were observed with administration of FTY720, highlighting the safety and therapeutic relevance of utilising PP2A-activating drugs in leukemia patients.
FTY720 also activates PP2A in mutant c-KIT myeloid cells, leading to growth inhibition and induction of apoptosis *in vitro* (Roberts *et al.* 2010). Activation of PP2A is required for the anti-leukaemic effects, as PP2A inhibition with okadaic acid inhibits these effects. FTY720-induced PP2A activity results in inhibition of c-KIT phosphorylation, and inactivation of downstream signaling proteins regulated by both c-KIT and PP2A. Importantly, FTY720 also inhibited the *in vivo* tumor growth of mutant c-KIT myeloid cells in a syngeneic mouse model (Roberts *et al.* 2010). Thus FTY720 may also be a useful therapeutic agent for CBF-AML patients harbouring activating c-KIT mutations.

7. Other serine/threonine phosphatases in myeloid leukemia

7.1 PP1

PP1 activity has been found to alter according to AML blast differentiation. Yamamoto *et al.*, found that AML patients with well differentiated leukemia had higher PP1 activity than patients with poorly differentiated AML-M1 (Yamamoto *et al.* 1999). AML blast PP1 activity also correlated with patient prognosis where individuals with significantly low PP1 activity had lower overall survival than those with high PP1 activity, with a median survival for each group of 8 and 27 months respectively (Nishikawa *et al.* 1994). Thus low PP1 activity may be a prognostic indicator of poor prognosis. The functional consequence of low PP1 activity in AML is not known, however PP1 was recently found to dephosphorylate Akt at T405, and PP1 overexpression induced Akt dephosphorylation, promoted cell survival and inhibited differentiation (Xiao *et al.* 2010). PP1 also promotes survival by negative regulation of p53 (Li *et al.* 2006), and is implicated in regulating Wnt/β-catenin (Jiang *et al.* 2009), TGF-β (Shi *et al.* 2004), and NF-κB (Li *et al.* 2008) signaling pathways. Luo *et al.*, showed that arsenic sulfide, a therapy historically used for treating CML in China, inhibited proliferation and induced differentiation of a human APL HL-60 cell line down a monocytic pathway. This correlated with increasing PP1 and PP2A activity, and co-treatment with a concentration of OA that inhibits both phosphatases suppressed the arsenic sulfide induced differentiation (Luo *et al.* 2006). Furthermore, while the mechanism was unknown at the time, other studies had previously shown similar effect in an APL NB4 cell model (Bai and Huang 1998; Lu and Wang 2002) and in chronic myeloid leukemia K562 cells (Yin *et al.* 2004). These studies suggest that PP1 plays a role in the growth inhibition and differentiation of AML, and may also provide a useful prognostic tool and/or therapy target.

7.2 PP2B

PP2B (calcineurin) is probably best known for its role in immunity where it is activated upon T cell receptor stimulation. Indeed, calcineurin is a well established target of prophylactic agents used in transplantation, such as Cyclosporin A and FK506, where calcineurin inhibition suppresses IL-2 production. Calcineurin was recently implicated as an important oncogene in lymphoid leukemias (Medyouf *et al.* 2007; Medyouf and Ghysdael 2008; Muller and Rao 2007). Sustained calcineurin activity was observed in human B- and T-cell lymphomas and in a range of mouse models of lymphoid malignancies. Moreover, expression of constitutively active mutant calcineurin favored leukemia progression, while treatment with Cyclosporin A or FK506 induced apoptosis of leukemic cells and rapid tumor clearance, and significantly improved mouse survival (Medyouf *et al.* 2007). Thus inhibiting calcineurin is a potential therapeutic strategy for lymphoid leukemias. In contrast, a specific role for calcineurin in myeloid leukemias has not been reported, however one study investigating its activity in AML patients of different FAB subtype found that calcineurin activity is relatively low in leukemic blasts arresting at the stage of early pluripotent stem cells, and increases during the course of myelomonocytic commitment and maturation (Yamamoto *et al.* 1999).

7.3 PP2C

Like PP2B, little information exists regarding the role of PP2C in myeloid leukemia. One study revealed it had low expression in AML patient blood cells and its activity and expression were relatively constant in various leukemic cell types from AML, ALL, and CLL patients (Yamamoto *et al.* 1999), suggesting it may not play a remarkable role in leukemogenesis.

8. Conclusions

There is no doubt that PP2A acts as a tumor suppressor in myeloid leukemias, and targeting its re-activation, either directly or via inhibition of an endogenous inhibitory protein such as SET, is a promising therapeutic strategy. Whether the pre-clinical promise will translate to improved survival of myeloid leukemia patients is currently unknown, but clinical trials of PP2A activators are eagerly awaited. Emerging studies indicate that other phosphatases may also play important roles in myeloid leukemias, and future studies aimed at deciphering the molecular mechanisms regulating these phosphatases and their downstream targets is sure to identify further targets for novel therapies.

9. Acknowledgements

This work was supported by grants from the Cancer Council NSW, the Anthony Rothe Memorial Foundation, and the Hunter Medical Research Institute (HMRI). AMS was supported by an Australian Postgraduate Award (APA) and an Arrow Bone Marrow Trust scholarship, KGR by an APA and Cancer Institute NSW scholarship, and NMV by a National Health and Medical Research Council (NHMRC) Peter Doherty Fellowship.

10. References

Abraham, D., K. Podar, et al. (2000). "Raf-1-associated protein phosphatase 2A as a positive regulator of kinase activation."*J Biol Chem,* 27529: 22300-22304 0021-9258 (Print).

Adams, D. G., R. L. Coffee, Jr., et al. (2005). "Positive regulation of Raf1-MEK1/2-ERK1/2 signaling by protein serine/threonine phosphatase 2A holoenzymes."*J Biol Chem,* 28052: 42644-42654 0021-9258 (Print).

Adler, H. T., F. S. Nallaseth, et al. (1997). "HRX leukemic fusion proteins form a heterocomplex with the leukemia-associated protein SET and protein phosphatase 2A."*J Biol Chem,* 27245: 28407-28414 0021-9258 (Print)

Agarwal, K. C. and R. E. Parks, Jr. (1983). "Forskolin: a potential antimetastatic agent."*Int J Cancer,* 326: 801-804 0020-7136 (Print).

Albert, R., K. Hinterding, et al. (2005). "Novel immunomodulator FTY720 is phosphorylated in rats and humans to form a single stereoisomer. Identification, chemical proof, and biological characterization of the biologically active species and its enantiomer."*J Med Chem,* 4816: 5373-5377 0022-2623 (Print).

Alessi, D. R., N. Gomez, et al. (1995). "Inactivation of p42 MAP kinase by protein phosphatase 2A and a protein tyrosine phosphatase, but not CL100, in various cell lines."*Curr Biol,* 53: 283-295.

Alonso, A., J. Sasin, et al. (2004). "Protein tyrosine phosphatases in the human genome."*Cell,* 1176: 699-711 0092-8674 (Print).

Andrabi, S., O. V. Gjoerup, et al. (2007). "Protein phosphatase 2A regulates life and death decisions via Akt in a context-dependent manner."*Proc Natl Acad Sci U S A,* 10448: 19011-19016.

Arino, J., C. W. Woon, et al. (1988). "Human liver phosphatase 2A: cDNA and amino acid sequence of two catalytic subunit isotypes."*Proc Natl Acad Sci U S A,* 8512: 4252-4256 0027-8424 (Print).

Arnold, H. K. and R. C. Sears (2006). "Protein phosphatase 2A regulatory subunit B56alpha associates with c-myc and negatively regulates c-myc accumulation."*Mol Cell Biol,* 267: 2832-2844.

Bai, Y. and S. Huang (1998). "[Studies on red orpiment induction of NB4 and HL-60 cell apoptosis]."*Zhonghua Xue Ye Xue Za Zhi,* 199: 477-480 0253-2727 (Print).

Bajpai, R., K. Makhijani, et al. (2004). "Drosophila Twins regulates Armadillo levels in response to Wg/Wnt signal."*Development,* 1315: 1007-1016 0950-1991 (Print).

Barford, D., A. K. Das, et al. (1998). "The structure and mechanism of protein phosphatases: insights into catalysis and regulation."*Annu Rev Biophys Biomol Struct,* 27: 133-164 1056-8700 (Print).

Begley, M. J. and J. E. Dixon (2005). "The structure and regulation of myotubularin phosphatases."*Curr Opin Struct Biol,* 156: 614-620 0959-440X (Print).

Bentires-Alj, M., J. G. Paez, et al. (2004). "Activating mutations of the noonan syndrome-associated SHP2/PTPN11 gene in human solid tumors and adult acute myelogenous leukemia."*Cancer Res,* 6424: 8816-8820 0008-5472 (Print).

Bhoola, R. and K. Hammond (2000). "Modulation of the rhythmic patterns of expression of phosphoprotein phosphatases in human leukaemia cells."*Cell Biol Int,* 248: 539-547 1065-6995 (Print).

Bialojan, C. and A. Takai (1988). "Inhibitory effect of a marine-sponge toxin, okadaic acid, on protein phosphatases. Specificity and kinetics."*Biochem J,* 2561: 283-290.

Borgatti, P., A. M. Martelli, et al. (2003). "Threonine 308 phosphorylated form of Akt translocates to the nucleus of PC12 cells under nerve growth factor stimulation and associates with the nuclear matrix protein nucleolin."*J Cell Physiol,* 1961: 79-88 0021-9541 (Print).

Brinkmann, V., M. D. Davis, et al. (2002). "The immune modulator FTY720 targets sphingosine 1-phosphate receptors."*J Biol Chem,* 27724: 21453-21457 0021-9258 (Print).

Bruecher-Encke, B., J. D. Griffin, et al. (2001). "Role of the tyrosine phosphatase SHP-1 in K562 cell differentiation."*Leukemia,* 159: 1424-1432 0887-6924 (Print).

Cairoli, R., A. Beghini, et al. (2005). "Imatinib mesylate in the treatment of Core Binding Factor leukemias with KIT mutations. A report of three cases."*Leuk Res,* 294: 397-400.

Calabretta, B. and D. Perrotti (2004). "The biology of CML blast crisis."*Blood,* 10311: 4010-4022.

Calin, G. A., M. G. di Iasio, et al. (2000). "Low frequency of alterations of the alpha (PPP2R1A) and beta (PPP2R1B) isoforms of the subunit A of the serine-threonine phosphatase 2A in human neoplasms."*Oncogene,* 199: 1191-1195 0950-9232 (Print).

Carlson, S. G., E. Eng, et al. (1998). "Expression of SET, an inhibitor of protein phosphatase 2A, in renal development and Wilms' tumor."*J Am Soc Nephrol,* 910: 1873-1880.

Chen, W., J. D. Arroyo, et al. (2005). "Cancer-associated PP2A Aalpha subunits induce functional haploinsufficiency and tumorigenicity."*Cancer Res,* 6518: 8183-8192 0008-5472 (Print).

Chen, W., R. Possemato, et al. (2004). "Identification of specific PP2A complexes involved in human cell transformation."*Cancer Cell,* 52: 127-136.

Chim, C. S., T. K. Fung, et al. (2004). "SOCS1 and SHP1 hypermethylation in multiple myeloma: implications for epigenetic activation of the Jak/STAT pathway."*Blood,* 10312: 4630-4635 0006-4971 (Print).

Cohen, J., J. Pelletier, et al. (2009). Oral Fingolimod (FTY720) Versus Interferon Beta-1a in RelapsingRemitting Multiple Sclerosis: Results from a Phase III Study (TRANSFORMS). *Proceedings of American Academy of Neurology*, Seattle, April 25 - May 2

Cohen, P. (1989). "The structure and regulation of protein phosphatases."*Annu Rev Biochem,* 58: 453-508 0066-4154 (Print).

Cohen, P. (2002). "Protein kinases--the major drug targets of the twenty-first century?"*Nat Rev Drug Discov,* 14: 309-315 1474-1776 (Print).

Colella, S., H. Ohgaki, et al. (2001). "Reduced expression of the Aalpha subunit of protein phosphatase 2A in human gliomas in the absence of mutations in the Aalpha and Abeta subunit genes."*Int J Cancer,* 936: 798-804.

Creyghton, M. P., G. Roel, et al. (2005). "PR72, a novel regulator of Wnt signaling required for Naked cuticle function."*Genes Dev,* 193: 376-386.

Creyghton, M. P., G. Roel, et al. (2006). "PR130 is a modulator of the Wnt-signaling cascade that counters repression of the antagonist Naked cuticle."*Proc Natl Acad Sci U S A,* 10314: 5397-5402.

Cristobal, I., F. J. Blanco, et al. (2010). "SETBP1 overexpression is a novel leukemogenic mechanism that predicts adverse outcome in elderly patients with acute myeloid leukemia."*Blood,* 1153: 615-625 1528-0020 (Electronic).

Cristobal, I., L. Garcia-Orti, et al. (2011). "PP2A impaired activity is a common event in acute myeloid leukemia and its activation by forskolin has a potent anti-leukemic effect."*Leukemia,* 254: 606-614 1476-5551 (Electronic).

Cyster, J. G. (2005). "Chemokines, sphingosine-1-phosphate, and cell migration in secondary lymphoid organs."*Annu Rev Immunol,* 23: 127-159 0732-0582 (Print).

Deichmann, M., M. Polychronidis, et al. (2001). "The protein phosphatase 2A subunit Bgamma gene is identified to be differentially expressed in malignant melanomas by subtractive suppression hybridization."*Melanoma Res,* 116: 577-585.

Demetri, G. D., M. von Mehren, et al. (2002). "Efficacy and safety of imatinib mesylate in advanced gastrointestinal stromal tumors."*N Engl J Med,* 3477: 472-480.

Dohoney, K. M., C. Guillerm, et al. (2004). "Phosphorylation of p53 at serine 37 is important for transcriptional activity and regulation in response to DNA damage."*Oncogene,* 231: 49-57 0950-9232 (Print).

Dougherty, M. K., J. Muller, et al. (2005). "Regulation of Raf-1 by direct feedback phosphorylation."*Mol Cell,* 172: 215-224.

Eichhorn, P. J., M. P. Creyghton, et al. (2009). "Protein phosphatase 2A regulatory subunits and cancer."*Biochim Biophys Acta,* 17951: 1-15 0006-3002 (Print).

Falt, S., M. Merup, et al. (2005). "Identification of progression markers in B-CLL by gene expression profiling."*Exp Hematol,* 338: 883-893 0301-472X (Print).

Feschenko, M. S., E. Stevenson, et al. (2002). "A novel cAMP-stimulated pathway in protein phosphatase 2A activation."*J Pharmacol Exp Ther,* 3021: 111-118 0022-3565 (Print).

Fornerod, M., J. Boer, et al. (1995). "Relocation of the carboxyterminal part of CAN from the nuclear envelope to the nucleus as a result of leukemia-specific chromosome rearrangements."*Oncogene,* 109: 1739-1748.

Foulkes, J. G. and P. Cohen (1980). "The regulation of glycogen metabolism. Purification and properties of protein phosphatase inhibitor-2 from rabbit skeletal muscle."*Eur J Biochem,* 1051: 195-203 0014-2956 (Print).

Francia, G., R. Poulsom, et al. (1999). "Identification by differential display of a protein phosphatase-2A regulatory subunit preferentially expressed in malignant melanoma cells."*Int J Cancer,* 825: 709-713.

Fujiki, H. and M. Suganuma (2009). "Carcinogenic aspects of protein phosphatase 1 and 2A inhibitors."*Prog Mol Subcell Biol,* 46: 221-254.

Fujita, T., K. Inoue, et al. (1994). "Fungal metabolites. Part 11. A potent immunosuppressive activity found in Isaria sinclairii metabolite."*J Antibiot (Tokyo),* 472: 208-215 0021-8820 (Print).

Gallay, N., C. Dos Santos, et al. (2009). "The level of AKT phosphorylation on threonine 308 but not on serine 473 is associated with high-risk cytogenetics and predicts poor overall survival in acute myeloid leukaemia."*Leukemia,* 236: 1029-1038 1476-5551 (Electronic).

Gallego, M. and D. M. Virshup (2005). "Protein serine/threonine phosphatases: life, death, and sleeping."*Curr Opin Cell Biol,* 172: 197-202 0955-0674 (Print).

Gotz, J., A. Probst, et al. (2000). "Distinct role of protein phosphatase 2A subunit Calpha in the regulation of E-cadherin and beta-catenin during development."*Mech Dev,* 931-2: 83-93.

Graler, M. H. and E. J. Goetzl (2004). "The immunosuppressant FTY720 down-regulates sphingosine 1-phosphate G-protein-coupled receptors."*Faseb J,* 183: 551-553 1530-6860 (Electronic).

Gutzkow, K. B., S. Naderi, et al. (2002). "Forskolin-mediated G1 arrest in acute lymphoblastic leukaemia cells: phosphorylated pRB sequesters E2Fs."*J Cell Sci,* 115Pt 5: 1073-1082 0021-9533 (Print).

Hahn, W. C., C. M. Counter, et al. (1999). "Creation of human tumour cells with defined genetic elements."*Nature,* 4006743: 464-468 0028-0836 (Print).

Hahn, W. C., S. K. Dessain, et al. (2002). "Enumeration of the simian virus 40 early region elements necessary for human cell transformation."*Mol Cell Biol,* 227: 2111-2123.

Haupt, Y., R. Maya, et al. (1997). "Mdm2 promotes the rapid degradation of p53."*Nature,* 3876630: 296-299 0028-0836 (Print).
Haystead, T. A., A. T. Sim, et al. (1989). "Effects of the tumour promoter okadaic acid on intracellular protein phosphorylation and metabolism."*Nature,* 3376202: 78-81 0028-0836 (Print).
Hemmings, B. A., C. Adams-Pearson, et al. (1990). "alpha- and beta-forms of the 65-kDa subunit of protein phosphatase 2A have a similar 39 amino acid repeating structure."*Biochemistry,* 2913: 3166-3173 0006-2960 (Print).
Hendrix, P., R. E. Mayer-Jackel, et al. (1993). "Structure and expression of a 72-kDa regulatory subunit of protein phosphatase 2A. Evidence for different size forms produced by alternative splicing."*J Biol Chem,* 26820: 15267-15276 0021-9258 (Print).
Heriche, J. K., F. Lebrin, et al. (1997). "Regulation of protein phosphatase 2A by direct interaction with casein kinase 2alpha."*Science,* 2765314: 952-955.
Hsu, W., L. Zeng, et al. (1999). "Identification of a domain of Axin that binds to the serine/threonine protein phosphatase 2A and a self-binding domain."*J Biol Chem,* 2746: 3439-3445.
Ingebritsen, T. S. and P. Cohen (1983a). "Protein phosphatases: properties and role in cellular regulation."*Science,* 2214608: 331-338 0036-8075 (Print).
Ingebritsen, T. S. and P. Cohen (1983b). "The protein phosphatases involved in cellular regulation. 1. Classification and substrate specificities."*Eur J Biochem,* 1322: 255-261 0014-2956 (Print).
Ivaska, J., L. Nissinen, et al. (2002). "Integrin alpha 2 beta 1 promotes activation of protein phosphatase 2A and dephosphorylation of Akt and glycogen synthase kinase 3 beta."*Mol Cell Biol,* 225: 1352-1359 0270-7306 (Print).
Janssens, V. and J. Goris (2001). "Protein phosphatase 2A: a highly regulated family of serine/threonine phosphatases implicated in cell growth and signalling."*Biochem J,* 353Pt 3: 417-439 0264-6021 (Print).
Janssens, V., S. Longin, et al. (2008). "PP2A holoenzyme assembly: in cauda venenum (the sting is in the tail)."*Trends Biochem Sci,* 333: 113-121 0968-0004 (Print).
Jaumot, M. and J. F. Hancock (2001). "Protein phosphatases 1 and 2A promote Raf-1 activation by regulating 14-3-3 interactions."*Oncogene,* 2030: 3949-3958 0950-9232 (Print).
Jiang, Y., W. Luo, et al. (2009). "Dab2 stabilizes Axin and attenuates Wnt/beta-catenin signaling by preventing protein phosphatase 1 (PP1)-Axin interactions."*Oncogene,* 2833: 2999-3007 1476-5594 (Electronic).
Jiang, Z. X. and Z. Y. Zhang (2008). "Targeting PTPs with small molecule inhibitors in cancer treatment."*Cancer Metastasis Rev,* 272: 263-272 0167-7659 (Print).
Jiffar, T., S. Kurinna, et al. (2004). "PKC alpha mediates chemoresistance in acute lymphoblastic leukemia through effects on Bcl2 phosphorylation."*Leukemia,* 183: 505-512 0887-6924 (Print).
Jin, Z., L. Wallace, et al. (2010). "PP2A:B56{epsilon}, a substrate of caspase-3, regulates p53-dependent and p53-independent apoptosis during development."*The Journal of biological chemistry,* 28545: 34493-34502 1083-351X (Electronic).
Johan, M. F., D. T. Bowen, et al. (2005). "Aberrant methylation of the negative regulators RASSFIA, SHP-1 and SOCS-1 in myelodysplastic syndromes and acute myeloid leukaemia."*Br J Haematol,* 1291: 60-65 0007-1048 (Print).

Julien, S. G., N. Dube, et al. (2011). "Inside the human cancer tyrosine phosphatome."*Nat Rev Cancer,* 111: 35-49 1474-1768 (Electronic)

Junttila, M. R., P. Puustinen, et al. (2007). "CIP2A inhibits PP2A in human malignancies."*Cell,* 1301: 51-62.

Kalla, C., M. O. Scheuermann, et al. (2007). "Analysis of 11q22-q23 deletion target genes in B-cell chronic lymphocytic leukaemia: evidence for a pathogenic role of NPAT, CUL5, and PPP2R1B."*Eur J Cancer,* 438: 1328-1335 0959-8049 (Print).

Kawabe, T., A. J. Muslin, et al. (1997). "HOX11 interacts with protein phosphatases PP2A and PP1 and disrupts a G2/M cell-cycle checkpoint."*Nature,* 3856615: 454-458 0028-0836 (Print).

Khanna, A., C. Bockelman, et al. (2009). "MYC-Dependent Regulation and Prognostic Role of CIP2A in Gastric Cancer."*J. Natl. Cancer Inst.,* 10111: 793-805.

Kitamura, Y. and S. Hirota (2004). "Kit as a human oncogenic tyrosine kinase."*Cell Mol Life Sci,* 6123: 2924-2931.

Kiuchi, M., K. Adachi, et al. (2005). "Asymmetric synthesis and biological evaluation of the enantiomeric isomers of the immunosuppressive FTY720-phosphate."*Bioorg Med Chem,* 132: 425-432 0968-0896 (Print).

Kubicek, M., M. Pacher, et al. (2002). "Dephosphorylation of Ser-259 regulates Raf-1 membrane association."*J Biol Chem,* 27710: 7913-7919 0021-9258 (Print).

Kuo, Y. C., K. Y. Huang, et al. (2008). "Regulation of phosphorylation of Thr-308 of Akt, cell proliferation, and survival by the B55alpha regulatory subunit targeting of the protein phosphatase 2A holoenzyme to Akt."*J Biol Chem,* 2834: 1882-1892.

Letourneux, C., G. Rocher, et al. (2006). "B56-containing PP2A dephosphorylate ERK and their activity is controlled by the early gene IEX-1 and ERK."*Embo J,* 254: 727-738.

Li, D. W., J. P. Liu, et al. (2006). "Protein serine/threonine phosphatase-1 dephosphorylates p53 at Ser-15 and Ser-37 to modulate its transcriptional and apoptotic activities."*Oncogene,* 2521: 3006-3022 0950-9232 (Print).

Li, H. H., X. Cai, et al. (2007). "A specific PP2A regulatory subunit, B56gamma, mediates DNA damage-induced dephosphorylation of p53 at Thr55."*Embo J,* 262: 402-411.

Li, H. Y., H. Liu, et al. (2008). "Deactivation of the kinase IKK by CUEDC2 through recruitment of the phosphatase PP1."*Nat Immunol,* 95: 533-541 1529-2916 (Electronic).

Li, M., A. Makkinje, et al. (1996). "The myeloid leukemia-associated protein SET is a potent inhibitor of protein phosphatase 2A."*J Biol Chem,* 27119: 11059-11062 0021-9258 (Print).

Li, W., Z. Ge, et al. (2008). "CIP2A Is Overexpressed in Gastric Cancer and Its Depletion Leads to Impaired Clonogenicity, Senescence, or Differentiation of Tumor Cells."*Clin Cancer Res,* 1412: 3722-3728.

Li, X., A. Scuderi, et al. (2002). "B56-associated protein phosphatase 2A is required for survival and protects from apoptosis in Drosophila melanogaster."*Mol Cell Biol,* 2211: 3674-3684.

Li, X., H. J. Yost, et al. (2001). "Protein phosphatase 2A and its B56 regulatory subunit inhibit Wnt signaling in Xenopus."*Embo J,* 2015: 4122-4131.

Lin, X. H., J. Walter, et al. (1998). "Protein phosphatase 2A is required for the initiation of chromosomal DNA replication."*Proc Natl Acad Sci U S A,* 9525: 14693-14698 0027-8424 (Print).

Linnekin, D. (1999). "Early signaling pathways activated by c-Kit in hematopoietic cells."*Int J Biochem Cell Biol,* 3110: 1053-1074.

Liu, Q., X. Zhao, et al. (2008). "FTY720 demonstrates promising preclinical activity for chronic lymphocytic leukemia and lymphoblastic leukemia/lymphoma."*Blood,* 111.

Lopez-Ruiz, P., J. Rodriguez-Ubreva, et al. (2011). "SHP-1 in cell-cycle regulation."*Anticancer Agents Med Chem,* 111: 89-98 1875-5992 (Electronic).

Lorenz, U., A. D. Bergemann, et al. (1996). "Genetic analysis reveals cell type-specific regulation of receptor tyrosine kinase c-Kit by the protein tyrosine phosphatase SHP1."*J Exp Med,* 1843: 1111-1126 0022-1007 (Print).

Lu, D. P. and Q. Wang (2002). "Current study of APL treatment in China."*Int J Hematol,* 76 Suppl 1: 316-318 0925-5710 (Print).

Luo, L. Y., J. Huang, et al. (2006). "Induction of human promyelocytic leukemia HL-60 cell differentiation into monocytes by arsenic sulphide: involvement of serine/threonine protein phosphatases."*Leuk Res,* 3011: 1399-1405 0145-2126 (Print).

Mandala, S., R. Hajdu, et al. (2002). "Alteration of lymphocyte trafficking by sphingosine-1-phosphate receptor agonists."*Science,* 2965566: 346-349 1095-9203 (Electronic).

Manning, G., D. B. Whyte, et al. (2002). "The protein kinase complement of the human genome."*Science,* 2985600: 1912-1934 1095-9203 (Electronic).

Martelli, A. M., V. Papa, et al. (2010). "Erucylphosphohomocholine, the first intravenously applicable alkylphosphocholine, is cytotoxic to acute myelogenous leukemia cells through JNK- and PP2A-dependent mechanisms."*Leukemia,* 244: 687-698 1476-5551 (Electronic).

Masson, K. and L. Ronnstrand (2009). "Oncogenic signaling from the hematopoietic growth factor receptors c-Kit and Flt3."*Cell Signal,* 2112: 1717-1726.

Matloubian, M., C. G. Lo, et al. (2004). "Lymphocyte egress from thymus and peripheral lymphoid organs is dependent on S1P receptor 1."*Nature,* 4276972: 355-360.

Matsuoka, Y., Y. Nagahara, et al. (2003). "A novel immunosuppressive agent FTY720 induced Akt dephosphorylation in leukemia cells."*Br J Pharmacol,* 1387: 1303-1312 0007-1188 (Print).

Mavrakis, K. J., A. L. Wolfe, et al. (2010). "Genome-wide RNA-mediated interference screen identifies miR-19 targets in Notch-induced T-cell acute lymphoblastic leukaemia."*Nat Cell Biol,* 124: 372-379 1476-4679 (Electronic).

Mayer-Jaekel, R. E., H. Ohkura, et al. (1993). "The 55 kd regulatory subunit of Drosophila protein phosphatase 2A is required for anaphase."*Cell,* 724: 621-633 0092-8674 (Print).

Mayer, R. E., P. Hendrix, et al. (1991). "Structure of the 55-kDa regulatory subunit of protein phosphatase 2A: evidence for a neuronal-specific isoform."*Biochemistry,* 3015: 3589-3597 0006-2960 (Print).

McCright, B., A. M. Rivers, et al. (1996). "The B56 family of protein phosphatase 2A (PP2A) regulatory subunits encodes differentiation-induced phosphoproteins that target PP2A to both nucleus and cytoplasm."*J Biol Chem,* 27136: 22081-22089 0021-9258 (Print).

McCright, B. and D. M. Virshup (1995). "Identification of a new family of protein phosphatase 2A regulatory subunits."*J Biol Chem,* 27044: 26123-26128 0021-9258 (Print).

Medyouf, H., H. Alcalde, et al. (2007). "Targeting calcineurin activation as a therapeutic strategy for T-cell acute lymphoblastic leukemia."*Nat Med,* 136: 736-741 1078-8956 (Print).

Medyouf, H. and J. Ghysdael (2008). "The calcineurin/NFAT signaling pathway: a novel therapeutic target in leukemia and solid tumors."*Cell Cycle,* 73: 297-303 1551-4005 (Electronic).

Moon, E. Y. and A. Lerner (2003). "PDE4 inhibitors activate a mitochondrial apoptotic pathway in chronic lymphocytic leukemia cells that is regulated by protein phosphatase 2A."*Blood,* 10110: 4122-4130 0006-4971 (Print).

Moorhead, G. B., L. Trinkle-Mulcahy, et al. (2007). "Emerging roles of nuclear protein phosphatases."*Nat Rev Mol Cell Biol,* 83: 234-244 1471-0072 (Print).

Moreno, C. S., S. Ramachandran, et al. (2004). "Signaling and transcriptional changes critical for transformation of human cells by simian virus 40 small tumor antigen or protein phosphatase 2A B56gamma knockdown."*Cancer Res,* 6419: 6978-6988.

Muller, A. M., J. Duque, et al. (2008). "Complementing mutations in core binding factor leukemias: from mouse models to clinical applications."*Oncogene,* 2744: 5759-5773.

Muller, M. R. and A. Rao (2007). "Linking calcineurin activity to leukemogenesis."*Nat Med,* 136: 669-671 1078-8956 (Print).

Neel, B. G., H. Gu, et al. (2003). "The 'Shp'ing news: SH2 domain-containing tyrosine phosphatases in cell signaling."*Trends Biochem Sci,* 286: 284-293 0968-0004 (Print).

Nesbit, C. E., J. M. Tersak, et al. (1999). "MYC oncogenes and human neoplastic disease."*Oncogene,* 1819: 3004-3016.

Neviani, P., R. Santhanam, et al. (2007). "FTY720, a new alternative for treating blast crisis chronic myelogenous leukemia and Philadelphia chromosome-positive acute lymphocytic leukemia."*J Clin Invest,* 1179: 2408-2421 0021-9738 (Print).

Neviani, P., R. Santhanam, et al. (2005). "The tumor suppressor PP2A is functionally inactivated in blast crisis CML through the inhibitory activity of the BCR/ABL-regulated SET protein."*Cancer Cell,* 85: 355-368 1535-6108 (Print).

Nimmo, G. A. and P. Cohen (1978). "The regulation of glycogen metabolism. Phosphorylation of inhibitor-1 from rabbit skeletal muscle, and its interaction with protein phosphatases-III and -II."*Eur J Biochem,* 872: 353-365 0014-2956 (Print).

Nishikawa, M., S. B. Omay, et al. (1994). "Expression of the catalytic and regulatory subunits of protein phosphatase type 2A may be differentially modulated during retinoic acid-induced granulocytic differentiation of HL-60 cells."*Cancer Res,* 5418: 4879-4884 0008-5472 (Print).

Oka, T., M. Ouchida, et al. (2002). "Gene silencing of the tyrosine phosphatase SHP1 gene by aberrant methylation in leukemias/lymphomas."*Cancer Res,* 6222: 6390-6394 0008-5472 (Print).

Okamoto, K., C. Kamibayashi, et al. (1996). "p53-dependent association between cyclin G and the B' subunit of protein phosphatase 2A."*Mol Cell Biol,* 1611: 6593-6602.

Okamoto, K., H. Li, et al. (2002). "Cyclin G recruits PP2A to dephosphorylate Mdm2."*Mol Cell,* 94: 761-771.

Olsen, J. V., B. Blagoev, et al. (2006). "Global, in vivo, and site-specific phosphorylation dynamics in signaling networks."*Cell,* 1273: 635-648 0092-8674 (Print).

Omay, S. B., H. Ogasawara, et al. (1995). "Translocation of protein phosphatase 1 catalytic subunits during 1,25-dihydroxyvitamin D3-induced monocytic differentiation of HL-60 cells."*Cancer Res,* 554: 774-780 0008-5472 (Print).

Ory, S., M. Zhou, et al. (2003). "Protein phosphatase 2A positively regulates Ras signaling by dephosphorylating KSR1 and Raf-1 on critical 14-3-3 binding sites."*Curr Biol,* 1316: 1356-1364.

Ouyang, J., X. H. Xu, et al. (2008). "Involvement of protein phosphatase 2A in arsenic trioxide-induced differentiation and apoptosis of NB4 cells."*Methods Find Exp Clin Pharmacol,* 306: 411-419 0379-0355 (Print).

Pallas, D. C., L. K. Shahrik, et al. (1990). "Polyoma small and middle T antigens and SV40 small t antigen form stable complexes with protein phosphatase 2A."*Cell,* 601: 167-176.

Pardanani, A., M. Elliott, et al. (2003). "Imatinib for systemic mast-cell disease."*Lancet,* 3629383: 535-536.

Ratcliffe, M. J., K. Itoh, et al. (2000). "A positive role for the PP2A catalytic subunit in Wnt signal transduction."*J Biol Chem,* 27546: 35680-35683.

Resjo, S., O. Goransson, et al. (2002). "Protein phosphatase 2A is the main phosphatase involved in the regulation of protein kinase B in rat adipocytes."*Cell Signal,* 143: 231-238 0898-6568 (Print).

Riz, I. and R. G. Hawley (2005). "G1/S transcriptional networks modulated by the HOX11/TLX1 oncogene of T-cell acute lymphoblastic leukemia."*Oncogene,* 2436: 5561-5575 0950-9232 (Print).

Roberts, K. G., A. M. Smith, et al. (2010). "Essential requirement for PP2A inhibition by the oncogenic receptor c-KIT suggests PP2A reactivation as a strategy to treat c-KIT+ cancers."*Cancer Res,* 7013: 9.

Rodriguez-Viciana, P., C. Collins, et al. (2006). "Polyoma and SV40 proteins differentially regulate PP2A to activate distinct cellular signaling pathways involved in growth control."*Proc Natl Acad Sci U S A,* 10351: 19290-19295.

Ruediger, R., H. T. Pham, et al. (2001a). "Alterations in protein phosphatase 2A subunit interaction in human carcinomas of the lung and colon with mutations in the A beta subunit gene."*Oncogene,* 2015: 1892-1899.

Ruediger, R., H. T. Pham, et al. (2001b). "Disruption of protein phosphatase 2A subunit interaction in human cancers with mutations in the A alpha subunit gene."*Oncogene,* 201: 10-15.

Ruediger, R., J. Ruiz, et al. (2011). "Human Cancer-Associated Mutations in A{alpha} Subunit of Protein Phosphatase 2A Increase Lung Cancer Incidence in A{alpha} Knock-in and Knockout Mice."*Molecular and cellular biology,* 1098-5549 (Electronic).

Ruela-de-Sousa, R. R., K. C. Queiroz, et al. (2011). "Reversible phosphorylation in haematological malignancies: potential role for protein tyrosine phosphatases in treatment?"*Biochim Biophys Acta,* 18062: 287-303 0006-3002 (Print).

Ruvolo, P. P., Y. H. Qui, et al. (2011). "Low expression of PP2A regulatory subunit B55alpha is associated with T308 phosphorylation of AKT and shorter complete remission duration in acute myeloid leukemia patients."*Leukemia,* 1476-5551 (Electronic).

Sablina, A. A., W. Chen, et al. (2007). "The tumor suppressor PP2A Abeta regulates the RalA GTPase."*Cell,* 1295: 969-982 0092-8674 (Print).

Sablina, A. A. and W. C. Hahn (2008). "SV40 small T antigen and PP2A phosphatase in cell transformation."*Cancer Metastasis Rev,* 272: 137-146 0167-7659 (Print).

Sablina, A. A., M. Hector, et al. (2010). "Identification of PP2A complexes and pathways involved in cell transformation."*Cancer Res,* 7024: 10474-10484 1538-7445 (Electronic).

Salas, A., S. Ponnusamy, et al. (2011). "Sphingosine kinase-1 and sphingosine 1-phosphate receptor 2 mediate Bcr-Abl1 stability and drug resistance by modulation of protein phosphatase 2A."*Blood,* 11722: 5941-5952 1528-0020 (Electronic).

Samanta, A. K., S. N. Chakraborty, et al. (2009). "Jak2 inhibition deactivates Lyn kinase through the SET-PP2A-SHP1 pathway, causing apoptosis in drug-resistant cells from chronic myelogenous leukemia patients."*Oncogene,* 2814: 1669-1681 1476-5594 (Electronic).

Sarbassov, D. D., D. A. Guertin, et al. (2005). "Phosphorylation and regulation of Akt/PKB by the rictor-mTOR complex."*Science,* 3075712: 1098-1101 1095-9203 (Electronic).

Seamon, K. and J. W. Daly (1981). "Activation of adenylate cyclase by the diterpene forskolin does not require the guanine nucleotide regulatory protein."*J Biol Chem,* 25619: 9799-9801 0021-9258 (Print).

Seamon, K. B., W. Padgett, et al. (1981). "Forskolin: unique diterpene activator of adenylate cyclase in membranes and in intact cells."*Proc Natl Acad Sci U S A,* 786: 3363-3367 0027-8424 (Print).

Sears, R., F. Nuckolls, et al. (2000). "Multiple Ras-dependent phosphorylation pathways regulate Myc protein stability."*Genes Dev,* 1419: 2501-2514 0890-9369 (Print).

Seeling, J. M., J. R. Miller, et al. (1999). "Regulation of beta-catenin signaling by the B56 subunit of protein phosphatase 2A."*Science,* 2835410: 2089-2091.

Shi, W., C. Sun, et al. (2004). "GADD34-PP1c recruited by Smad7 dephosphorylates TGFbeta type I receptor."*J Cell Biol,* 1642: 291-300 0021-9525 (Print).

Shouse, G. P., Y. Nobumori, et al. (2010). "A B56gamma mutation in lung cancer disrupts the p53-dependent tumor-suppressor function of protein phosphatase 2A."*Oncogene,* 2927: 3933-3941 1476-5594 (Electronic).

Sontag, E., S. Fedorov, et al. (1993). "The interaction of SV40 small tumor antigen with protein phosphatase 2A stimulates the map kinase pathway and induces cell proliferation."*Cell,* 755: 887-897 0092-8674 (Print).

Soo Hoo, L., J. Y. Zhang, et al. (2002). "Cloning and characterization of a novel 90 kDa 'companion' auto-antigen of p62 overexpressed in cancer."*Oncogene,* 2132: 5006-5015.

Stevens, I., V. Janssens, et al. (2003). "Identification and characterization of B"-subunits of protein phosphatase 2 A in Xenopus laevis oocytes and adult tissues."*Eur J Biochem,* 2702: 376-387 0014-2956 (Print).

Strack, S., D. Chang, et al. (1999). "Cloning and characterization of B delta, a novel regulatory subunit of protein phosphatase 2A."*FEBS Lett,* 4603: 462-466 0014-5793 (Print).

Strack, S., J. T. Cribbs, et al. (2004). "Critical role for protein phosphatase 2A heterotrimers in mammalian cell survival."*J Biol Chem,* 27946: 47732-47739 0021-9258 (Print).

Suganuma, M., H. Fujiki, et al. (1988). "Okadaic acid: an additional non-phorbol-12-tetradecanoate-13-acetate-type tumor promoter."*Proc Natl Acad Sci U S A,* 856: 1768-1771 0027-8424 (Print).

Suzuki, K. and K. Takahashi (2003). "Reduced expression of the regulatory A subunit of serine/threonine protein phosphatase 2A in human breast cancer MCF-7 cells."*Int J Oncol,* 235: 1263-1268 1019-6439 (Print).

Taetle, R. and S. Li-en (1984). "Further studies on mechanisms of abnormal prostaglandin response by chronic myelogenous leukaemia granulocyte/macrophage progenitors."*Leuk Res,* 85: 833-842 0145-2126 (Print).

Takabe, K., S. W. Paugh, et al. (2008). ""Inside-Out" Signaling of Sphingosine-1-Phosphate: Therapeutic Targets."*Pharmacol Rev,* 602: 181-195.

Takagi, Y., M. Futamura, et al. (2000). "Alterations of the PPP2R1B gene located at 11q23 in human colorectal cancers."*Gut,* 472: 268-271.

Tamaki, M., T. Goi, et al. (2004). "PPP2R1B gene alterations inhibit interaction of PP2A-Abeta and PP2A-C proteins in colorectal cancers."*Oncol Rep,* 113: 655-659.

Tartaglia, M. and B. D. Gelb (2005). "Germ-line and somatic PTPN11 mutations in human disease."*Eur J Med Genet,* 482: 81-96 1769-7212 (Print).

Tartaglia, M., S. Martinelli, et al. (2004). "Genetic evidence for lineage-related and differentiation stage-related contribution of somatic PTPN11 mutations to leukemogenesis in childhood acute leukemia."*Blood,* 1042: 307-313 0006-4971 (Print).

Tartaglia, M., S. Martinelli, et al. (2005). "Somatic PTPN11 mutations in childhood acute myeloid leukaemia."*Br J Haematol,* 1293: 333-339 0007-1048 (Print).

Tartaglia, M., C. M. Niemeyer, et al. (2003). "Somatic mutations in PTPN11 in juvenile myelomonocytic leukemia, myelodysplastic syndromes and acute myeloid leukemia."*Nat Genet,* 342: 148-150 1061-4036 (Print).

Uzunoglu, S., R. Uslu, et al. (1999). "Augmentation of methylprednisolone-induced differentiation of myeloid leukemia cells by serine/threonine protein phosphatase inhibitors."*Leuk Res,* 235: 507-512 0145-2126 (Print).

Vanhaesebroeck, B. and D. R. Alessi (2000). "The PI3K-PDK1 connection: more than just a road to PKB."*Biochem J,* 346 Pt 3: 561-576 0264-6021 (Print).

Vogelstein, B., D. Lane, et al. (2000). "Surfing the p53 network."*Nature,* 4086810: 307-310 0028-0836 (Print).

Wang, J. and W. Li, Li, L., Yu, X., Jia, J., Chen, C. (2011). "CIP2A is over-expressed in acute myeloid leukaemia and associated with HL60 cells proliferation and differentiation."*Int J Lab Hematol,* 333: 290-298 1751-553X (Electronic).

Wang, L., J. E. Fortney, et al. (2004). "Stromal cell protection of B-lineage acute lymphoblastic leukemic cells during chemotherapy requires active Akt."*Leuk Res,* 287: 733-742 0145-2126 (Print).

Wang, P. Y., P. Liu, et al. (2003). "A cholesterol-regulated PP2A/HePTP complex with dual specificity ERK1/2 phosphatase activity."*Embo J,* 2211: 2658-2667.

Wang, S. S., E. D. Esplin, et al. (1998). "Alterations of the PPP2R1B gene in human lung and colon cancer."*Science,* 2825387: 284-287.

Wei, S., X. Chen, et al. (2009). "A critical role for phosphatase haplodeficiency in the selective suppression of deletion 5q MDS by lenalidomide."*Proc Natl Acad Sci U S A,* 10631: 12974-12979 1091-6490 (Electronic).

Willert, K., C. Y. Logan, et al. (1999). "A Drosophila Axin homolog, Daxin, inhibits Wnt signaling."*Development,* 12618: 4165-4173 0950-1991 (Print).

Xiao, L., L. L. Gong, et al. (2010). "Protein phosphatase-1 regulates Akt1 signal transduction pathway to control gene expression, cell survival and differentiation."*Cell Death Differ,* 179: 1448-1462 1476-5403 (Electronic).

Xu, X. H., J. Ou-Yang, et al. (2008). "[Effect of okadaic acid on differentiation of NB4 and MR2 cells induced by all-trans retinoic acid]."*Zhonghua Xue Ye Xue Za Zhi,* 296: 379-383 0253-2727 (Print).

Yamamoto, H., T. Hinoi, et al. (2001). "Inhibition of the Wnt signaling pathway by the PR61 subunit of protein phosphatase 2A."*J Biol Chem,* 27629: 26875-26882.

Yamamoto, M., Y. Suzuki, et al. (1999). "Expressions of four major protein Ser/Thr phosphatases in human primary leukemic cells."*Leukemia,* 134: 595-600 0887-6924 (Print).

Yan, Z., S. A. Fedorov, et al. (2000). "PR48, a novel regulatory subunit of protein phosphatase 2A, interacts with Cdc6 and modulates DNA replication in human cells."*Mol Cell Biol,* 203: 1021-1029 0270-7306 (Print).

Yang, J., J. Wu, et al. (2003). "PP2A:B56epsilon is required for Wnt/beta-catenin signaling during embryonic development."*Development,* 13023: 5569-5578.

Yang, Y., X. Q. Li, et al. (2011). "[Influence of PP2A Activator on Proliferation of HL-60 Cells and Analysis of PP2A Activity Changes in Patients with Acute Myeloid Leukemia.]."*Zhongguo Shi Yan Xue Ye Xue Za Zhi,* 193: 594-597 1009-2137 (Print).

Yeh, E., M. Cunningham, et al. (2004). "A signalling pathway controlling c-Myc degradation that impacts oncogenic transformation of human cells."*Nat Cell Biol,* 64: 308-318.

Yin, T., Y. L. Wu, et al. (2004). "Combined effects of As4S4 and imatinib on chronic myeloid leukemia cells and BCR-ABL oncoprotein."*Blood,* 10413: 4219-4225 0006-4971 (Print).

Yu, J., A. Boyapati, et al. (2001). "Critical role for SV40 small-t antigen in human cell transformation."*Virology,* 2902: 192-198.

Yuan, H., T. Veldman, et al. (2002). "Simian virus 40 small tumor antigen activates AKT and telomerase and induces anchorage-independent growth of human epithelial cells."*J Virol,* 7621: 10685-10691.

Yuksel, S., G. Saydam, et al. (2002). "Arsenic trioxide and methylprednisolone use different signal transduction pathways in leukemic differentiation."*Leuk Res,* 264: 391-398 0145-2126 (Print).

Zemann, B., B. Kinzel, et al. (2006). "Sphingosine kinase type 2 is essential for lymphopenia induced by the immunomodulatory drug FTY720."*Blood,* 1074: 1454-1458 0006-4971 (Print).

Zhang, Q., P. N. Raghunath, et al. (2000). "Lack of phosphotyrosine phosphatase SHP-1 expression in malignant T-cell lymphoma cells results from methylation of the SHP-1 promoter."*Am J Pathol,* 1574: 1137-1146 0002-9440 (Print).

Zhang, W., J. Yang, et al. (2009). "PR55alpha, a regulatory subunit of PP2A, specifically regulates PP2A-mediated beta-catenin dephosphorylation."*J. Biol. Chem.*: M109.013698.

Zhao, J. J., O. V. Gjoerup, et al. (2003). "Human mammary epithelial cell transformation through the activation of phosphatidylinositol 3-kinase."*Cancer Cell,* 35: 483-495.

Zheng, H., Y. Chen, et al. (2011). "Expression and distribution of PPP2R5C gene in leukemia."*J Hematol Oncol,* 4: 21 1756-8722 (Electronic).

Zhou, B., Z. X. Wang, et al. (2002). "The specificity of extracellular signal-regulated kinase 2 dephosphorylation by protein phosphatases."*J Biol Chem,* 27735: 31818-31825 0021-9258 (Print).

Zhou, J., H. T. Pham, et al. (2003). "Characterization of the Aalpha and Abeta subunit isoforms of protein phosphatase 2A: differences in expression, subunit interaction, and evolution."*Biochem J,* 369Pt 2: 387-398.

Zolnierowicz, S., C. Csortos, et al. (1994). "Diversity in the regulatory B-subunits of protein phosphatase 2A: identification of a novel isoform highly expressed in brain."*Biochemistry,* 3339: 11858-11867 0006-2960 (Print).

8

Role of JAK2 Beyond Myeloproliferative Neoplasms (MPNs): Rationale for Targeting the JAK-STAT Pathway in Other Hematological Malignancies and Solid Tumors

Theresa M. McDevitt and Matthew V. Lorenzi
Oncology Drug Discovery,
Bristol-Myers Squibb
USA

1. Introduction

Janus kinases (JAKs) are a family of receptor-associated tyrosine kinases which are crucial for the survival and proliferation of immune and hematopoietic-derived cells. There are four mammalian JAKs identified to date: JAK1, JAK2, JAK3 and TYK2 (Lopez et al., 2010). JAKs are responsible for mediating the intracellular signaling of numerous growth factors and cytokines (Murray et al., 2007 & O'Shea et al., 2002). Once activated JAKs directly phosphorylate and activate the transcription factors signal transducers and activators of transcriptions (STATs) which transduce JAK signaling by translocating to the nucleus to modulate a subset of genes that are critical for cell proliferation and survival (Aaronson et al., 2002 & Levy et al., 2002). Dysregulated JAK signaling has been implicated in the pathogenesis of several blood-borne cancers but most notably in myeloproliferative neoplasms (MPNs) (Nelson et al., 2006; Lucia et al., 2011 & Patnaik et al., 2009). MPNs are hematological malignancies defined by the excessive proliferation of one or more myeloid-derived cells. MPNs are classified into two clinical categories either BCR-ABL-positive (BCR-ABL (+)) or BCR-ABL-negative (BCR-ABL (-)) based on the presence of the BCR-ABL fusion protein. The major BCR-ABL (-) MPNs include polycythemia vera (PV), essential thrombocythemia (ET) and myelofibrosis (MF). The specific pathogenic role that JAK2 has in driving some of these MPNs is highlighted by the recent seminal discovery of the $JAK2^{V617F}$ mutation (Baxter et al., 2005; James et al., 2005; Kralovics et al., 2005; & Levine et al., 2005). The $JAK2^{V617F}$ mutation is a somatic, gain-of function point mutation which leads to constitutive activation of JAK2 and subsequent downstream activation of STATs (Baxter et al., 2005 & James et al., 2005). Current data demonstrates that JAK2 is a disease associated gene involved in the pathogenesis of BCR-ABL (-) MPNs. However, it remains unclear if JAK2 pathway mutations are the primary drivers of sustained disease progression. New data is emerging that suggests that targeting the JAK-STAT pathway may have implications beyond the treatment of MPN and can be useful for the treatment of other hematological and non-hematological cancers. This review will summarize the pathogenic role of JAK-STAT signaling in BCR-ABL (-) MPNs and introduce the potential broader implications by which JAK-STAT pathway inhibition may have in treating hematological malignancies as well as solid tumors.

2. Janus Kinase Family (JAKs)

2.1 Function

Janus kinases are a family of cytoplasmic receptor associated tyrosine kinases responsible for integrating the signaling of numerous growth factors and cytokines that are critical for hematopoiesis and immune function. There are four JAK family members; JAK1, JAK2, JAK3 and TYK2. JAK1, JAK2 and TYK2 are ubiquitously expressed while JAK3 expression is restricted to myeloid and lymphoid tissue (Valentino et al., 2006 & Ward et al., 2000). Various cytokines and growth factor receptors rely on JAKs to propagate their intracellular signaling cascades since many of these receptors lack intrinsic kinase activity. JAKs can be differentially or coordinately activated in response to various growth factor or cytokine stimuli (Murray, 2007). Targeted disruption of individual JAKs have been generated in an effort to better understand the biological non-redundant roles that JAKs have in development. JAK1 knock-out mice have been generated and present with a perinatal lethal phenotype that is characterized by severe defects in lymphopoiesis and neuronal development (Rodig et al., 1998). JAK3 mutations in humans have been described in patients with severe combined immunodeficiency (SCID), an immune disorder where major defects in T- and B- cell development are observed. This clinical phenotype is recapitulated in JAK3 knock-out models where these mice manifest with SCID-like features characterized by impaired lymphocyte production (Nosaka et al., 1995 & Park et al., 2000). TYK2 deficiencies although rare have been reported, and these patients usually present with severe dermatitis and hyper-IgE syndrome-like symptoms (HIES). Genetic disruption studies involving TYK2 have presented with severe defects in IL-12 signaling and impaired Th1 and Th2 mediated immune responses (Karaghiosoff et al., 2003). Genetic inactivation of JAK2 in mice is embryonically lethal due to severe anemia, confirming the critical role that JAK2 is thought to have in erythropoiesis (Parganas et al., 1998).

2.2 Structure

JAK proteins share seven homologous structural domains (JH1-JH7) each of which elicit distinct functional features within JAK proteins. The JAK homology domains consist of the C-terminus JH1 domain which is the kinase-active domain, the auto-regulatory JH2 pseudokinase domain, the SH2-like JH3 domain and the N-terminus FERM (four-point-one, ezrin, radixin, and moesin) domain (JH4-JH7). Although the JH3 domain possesses a SH2-like sequence it is unable to bind and interact with phospho-tyrosine residues and therefore its precise function remains unclear while the FERM domain is responsible for mediating the interactions of JAKs with their cognate receptors (Huang et al., 2001 & Radtke et al., 2005). The JH2 pseudokinase domain is a unique structural feature of the JAKs that is otherwise absent in other kinase families. The JH2 pseudokinase domain bears high sequence identity to the JH1 kinase domain but is devoid of any catalytic activity and is thought to act as a regulatory domain through catalytic auto-inhbition (Saharinen et al., 2000). Moreover, key activating point mutations have been identified in the JH2 pseudokinase domain of JAK2 that are critically involved in the pathogenesis of some myeloproliferative neoplasms (MPNs).

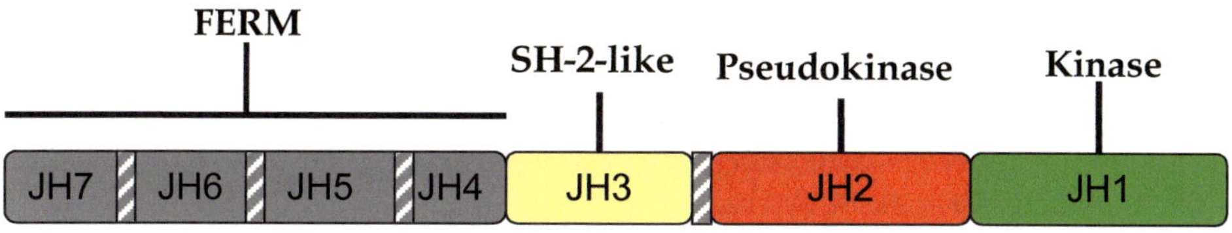

Fig. 1. **JAK Protein Domain Structure.** The seven homologous JAK domains (JH1-JH7) conserved throughout the JAK kinase family.

2.3 JAK-STAT signaling

In the absence of ligand, JAKs are pre-associated with receptor monomers, upon ligand binding receptor dimerzation ensues leading to trans-phosphorylation and auto-activation of JAKs. Once activated, JAKs proceed to phosphorylate specific tyrosine residues within the cytoplasmic domains of growth factor receptors creating docking sites for downstream mediators of JAK signaling. JAKs can activate classical signaling pathways such as PI-3-kinase and MAPK but JAKs also directly activate STATs as described above. STATs are latent transcription factors that are activated and phosphorylated by JAKs at specific tyrosine residues (Darnell J, 1997 & Benekli et al., 2003). Once phosphorylated, STAT monomers can then homo/hetero-dimerize through reciprocal Src homology 2 (SH2) interactions and translocate to the nucleus to modulate the transcription of key genes which promote cell growth and survival.

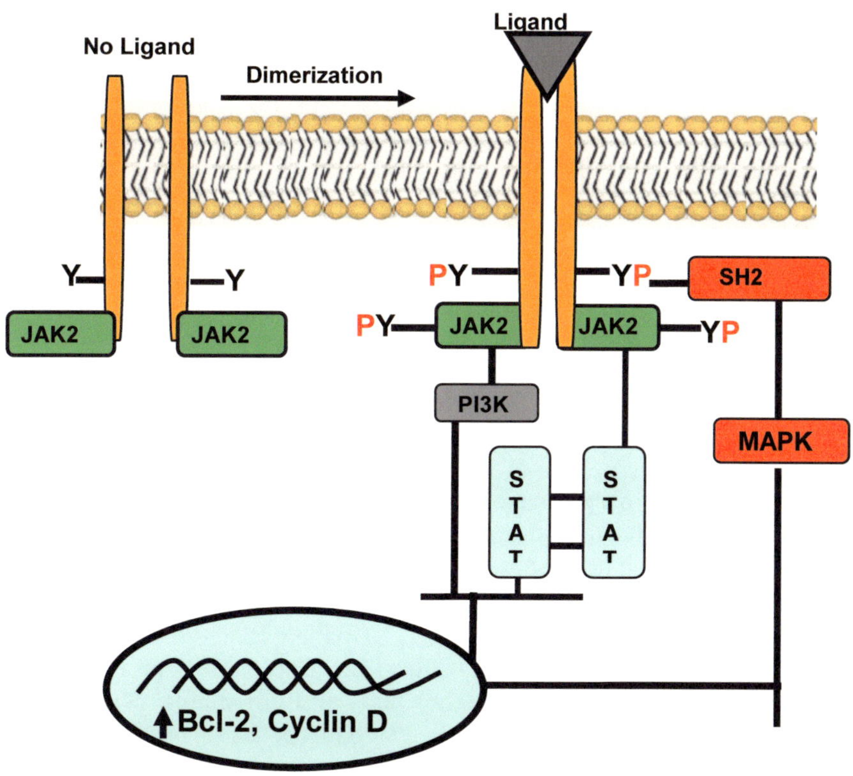

Fig. 2. Ligand-Induced JAK-STAT Activation

3. Myeloproliferative Neoplasms (MPNs)

3.1 Clinical biology

MPNs are hematopoietic malignancies characterized by excessive growth of one or more myeloid derived cell lineages such as erythrocytes, platelets and/or granulocytes. MPNs are clinically grouped into either BCR-ABL (+) or BCR-ABL (-) based on the presence of the BCR-ABL protein, as seen in CML patients. Dysregulated JAK-STAT signaling has been implicated in the pathogenesis of these BCR-ABL (-) MPNs. The three most common BCR-ABL (-) MPNs include polycythemia vera (PV), essential thrombocythemia (ET) and idiopathic myelofibrosis (IMF) with an estimated annual cumulative incidence of 130,000 patients in the United States which translates into an estimated prevalence of 6.2 per 100,000 cases (Ma et al., 2008; Mesa et al., 1999 & Ania B et al., 1994). The major clinical features of PV include uncontrolled growth of multiple myeloid-derived lineages with the dominating lineage being erythrocytes which is often reflected by an increased hematocrit and splenomegaly, while minor features include trilineage myeloproliferation of the bone marrow (Wadleigh & Tefferi, 2010). ET is characterized by an increase in both platelet size and number while hematocrit is unchanged. IMF is the most severe of the three MPNs and the major clinical criteria for diagnosis usually includes megakaryocytic proliferation accompanied by severe fibrosis of the bone marrow or hypercellularity of the bone marrow that is characterized by granulocyte proliferation (Wadleigh & Tefferi, 2010). IMF can manifest on its own or it can be preceded by PV or ET, post-PV or post-ET IMF has a variable evolution rate of roughly 25 evolutions per 1000 patients ET/PV patients (Passamonti et al., 2008 & Gangat et al., 2007). Furthermore, each one of these MPNs has the potential to progress to acute myelogenous leukemia (AML). In an unselected BCR-ABL (-) MPN population the overall leukemic transformation (LT) rate registered at 4.0% with MF having the highest transformation rate: 11.4%-MF, 4.3%-PV & 1.75% for ET (Cervantes et al., 1991). Aberrant tyrosine kinase signaling has been implicated in the pathogenesis in the majority of MPNs, most notably with CML where the product of a chromosomal translocation results in the production of constitutively active tyrosine kinase known as the BCR-ABL (Druker et al., 1996). The discovery of the BCR-ABL tyrosine kinase led to the development of the clinically successful small molecule inhibitor, imatinib, which predominately targets BCR-ABL in addition to PDGF-R and KIT kinases (O'Brien et al., 2003). The initial observation that altered tyrosine kinase signaling could single-handedly drive the entire pathogenesis of a disease as seen with BCR-ABL and CML hinted at the possibility that other altered tyrosine kinase signaling could be involved in the pathogenesis of these BCR-ABL (-) MPNs.

3.2 Pathogenic role of JAK2 in BCR-ABL-negative MPNs

Mutations in JAK2 have been implicated as a key genetic factor responsible for driving BCR-ABL (-) MPNs and several lines of evidence highlight this finding. The major hematopoietic growth factors erythropoietin (Epo) and thrombopoietin (Tpo) that give rise to the myeloid derived cells that often over-populate PV and ET patients such as erythrocytes and platelets signal exclusively through JAK2. Loss of heterozygosity (LOH) on chromosome 9, where JAK2 is localized is observed in roughly 30% of PV patients (Kralovics et al., 2002), moreover, progenitor cells isolated from PV patients have routinely demonstrated an increased sensitivity to hematopoietic growth factors such as Epo and Tpo in ex vivo colony growth assays. Additionally, multiple animal models involving targeting expression of

JAK2 including transgenic and retroviral transduction methods leads to a MPN-like phenotype *in vivo*, further supporting a causal role for JAK2 in the pathogenesis of these diseases (Wernig et al., 2006)

3.3 V617F and other JAK2-associated mutations in MPNs

In 2005, several independent laboratories identified a unique somatic activating point mutation in the JAK2 gene (^{V617F}). The JAK2^{V617F} mutation occurs in the JH2 pseudokinase domain of JAK2 in exon 14 at position 617 where a valine is replaced with a phenylalanine which leads to constitutive activation of JAK2. The mechanism of activation of the V617F mutation is believed to be due to the removal of the auto-inhibitory function of the JH2 pseudokinase domain present in JAK2. The incidence of the JAK2^{V617F} mutation is highly prevalent within the BCR-ABL (-) MPN patient population particularly within PV cohorts where more than 95% (Wernig et al., 2006) of PV patients are positive for it while 50% of ET and IMF patients are positive for it (Pikman et al, 2006). Although the JAK2^{V617F} mutation represents a major genetic event underlying the pathogenesis of these MPNs there is still a fraction of PV patients (~5%) and ET/IMF patients (~50%) that present with these MPNs but yet are negative for the V617F JAK2 mutation. The existence of V617F-negative MPNs highlights the need to identify additional JAK2 signaling components that may be involved in the pathogenesis of these V617F-independent MPNs. Several gain-of-function mutations comprised of deletions, insertions and frame-shifts have been indentified in exon 12 of JAK2 in a small subset of V617-negative PV patients (~3%) (Scott et al., 2007). Interestingly, exon 12 JAK2 mutations are mutually exclusive from V617F JAK2 mutations and to date have only been described in V617F-negative PV patients. Expression of exon 12 JAK2 mutations results in a PV-like phenotype *in vivo* that is characterized by erythrocytosis. Alternatively, activating point mutations in the thrombopoietin receptor (Tpo-R/c-MPL) have been identified in a subset of V617F-negative ET and IMF patients (5-10%). The mechanism of action for the MPLW515L mutation is similar to that of the V617F mutation since it also results in the removal of an auto-inhibitory sequence thought to be located within the transmembrane region of the Tpo receptor which causes spontaneous activation of downstream JAK2-STAT signaling (Pikman et al., 2006). The relative frequencies of these JAK-related mutations are summarized in figure 3 (Paradanani et al, 2011). The oncogenic potential of these mutations in MPN is further highlighted by their ability to induce MPN-like phenotypes in murine bone marrow reconstitution studies. JAK2^{V617F} expression induces a PV-like phenotype that presents with erythrocytosis and splenomegaly while (Wernig et al., 2006) MPLW515L promotes a more aggressive MF-like phenotype characterized by marked thrombocytopenia and severe fibrosis of the bone marrow (Pikman et al., 2006). Collectively, these results highlight a strong selective pressure to activate JAK-STAT signaling in BCR-ABL-(-) MPNs and thus therapies designed to target the JAK-STAT signaling may be beneficial for the treatment of MPN.

4. JAK inhibitors in clinical development

Since the discovery of the JAK2V617F mutation in 2004 remarkable scientific progress has been made from bench to beside with the first JAK inhibitors being tested in humans by mid 2007. Currently there are 36 clinical trials in the US underway evaluating various treatments for MPNs or investigating the molecular pathobiology underlying MPNs. The current JAK inhibitors are typically small molecule ATP competitive inhibitors of both wild-type and

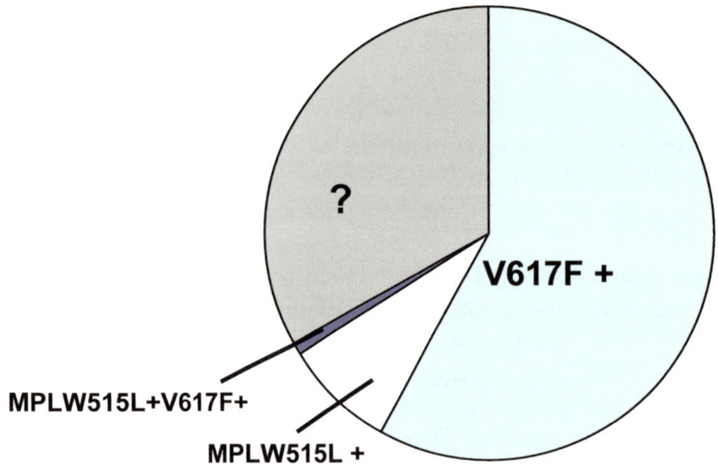

Fig. 3. **Allele Frequency in IMF Cohort,** adapted from Chaligne R, et al. *Leukemia* (2008). Relative mutation frequency in a IMF cohort (n =603), V617F; 58%, MPLW515L; 8.1% and MPLW515L/V617F <1%

mutant JAK enzymes that can be either selective JAK2 inhibitors or non-selective JAK2 inhibitors with the latter having additional activity against other kinases besides JAK2. Initial clinical trials with JAK inhibitors were designed to recruit only IMF patients based on the biological severity of IMF compared to ET or PV, however more recently, clinical trials have expanded to include testing of JAK inhibitors in both PV and ET cohorts. The most advanced JAK inhibitor in the clinic to date is ruxolitinib (INCB018424), a pan-JAK inhibitor which demonstrates potent activity against JAK2 and JAK1 (Quintas-Cardama et al., 2010). A recent phase I/II trial (n=153) has commenced evaluating ruxolitinib for the treatment of IMF. While on ruxolitinib, a significant number of patients demonstrated a favorable clinical response including a reduction in spleen size, improvement in constitutional symptoms and normalization of pro-inflammatory cytokine levels. The suppression of inflammatory cytokines is thought to be linked to the pan inhibitory effects of ruxolitinib on both JAK1 and JAK2 (Verstovsek et al., 2010). Given the clinical response of ruxolitinib in the treatment of IMF, trials have begun to evaluate the safety and efficacy of ruxolitinib in the treatment of PV and ET. Interestingly, these clinical responses did not correlate with JAK2V617F status and molecular remission of the mutant allele was absent even after two years of continued therapy (Verstovsek et al., 2008). The lack of effect on mutant allele burden could be due to direct loss of the mutant allele itself also known as "V617F-independence" that is reported to occur in some patients throughout the evolution of MPN (Passamonti et al., 2010). TG101348 is small molecule inhibitor of JAK 2 in clinical development. Results from a phase I/II multicenter study in IMF patients revealed that >45% of patients on TG101348 observed a >50% reduction in spleen size which was evident by five months but could be detected early two months and more than 70% of patients that presented with elevated white blood cell counts prior to treatment normalized (Pardanani et al., 2009). Unlike ruxolinitib, there was no significant decrease in serum levels of inflammatory cytokines while on therapy although the majority of patients did report a resolution of IMF-associated constitutional symptoms.

Compound	Company	Indication	Phase	NCT Trial #
INCB18424	Incyte	PV/ET/MF	I/II/III	NCT01445769
TG101348	TargeGen	MF	I/II	NCT00631462
SB1518	S*BIO	PV/ET/MF	I/II	NCT00745550
CYT387	YM BIOSCIENCES	MF	I/II	NCT00935987
AZD1480	Astra Zeneca	MF	I/II	NCT00910728
LY2784544	Eli Lilly	PV/ET/MF	I	NCT01134120
BMS-911543	Bristol Myers-Squibb	MF	I	NCT01236352

Table 1. Current JAK Inhibitors in the Clinic

5. Implications for targeting JAK-STAT signaling in additional hematological cancers and solid tumors

Activating mutations in JAK2 (V617F and exon 12) in BCR-ABL (-) MPNs appear to be the primary mechanism by which these cells preferentially activate JAK-STAT signaling, however there are additional mechanisms available for cells to activate JAKs. Cells can also undergo chromosomal rearrangements which also lead to constitutive activation of JAKs. Chromosomal translocations activate JAKs by causing constitutive dimerization through replacement of amino terminal sequences with a fusion partner. In non-MPN hematological malignancies such as acute leukemias and lymphomas chromosomal rearrangements involving JAK2 represent another mechanism for activating JAK2. There have been seven fusion partners identified for JAK2, most of which lead to constitutive activation of JAK2 signaling, these are summarized in table 2.

Fusion Partner	Cancer	Oncogenic	Reference
TEL (ETV6)	T-ALL, aCML,B-ALL	Yes	Lacronique, 1997
PCM1	ALL, aCML	Yes	Reiter, 2005
BCR	aCML	Yes	Greisinger, 2005
SSBP2	B-ALL	Yes	Poitras, 2008
STRN3	ALL	Yes	Mullighan, 2009
PAX5	ALL	No	Bousquet, 2007
SEC31-A	cHL	Yes	VanRoosbroeck, 2011

Table 2. **Summary of JAK2 fusion partners due to chromosomal translocations involving chromosome 9p24**. Abbreviations include-: T-ALL = T-cell acute lymphoblastic leukemia, aCML= atypical chronic myelogenous leukemia, B-ALL = B-cell acute lymphoblastic leukemia, ALL = acute lymphoblastic leukemia and cHL = classic Hodgkin lymphoma.

5.1 Role of JAK-STAT signaling in non-MPN hematological malignancies

Evidence is accumulating indicating dysregulated JAK-STAT signaling in various types of lymphomas. In classical Hodgkin lymphoma (cHL) and primary mediastinal B cell lymphoma (PMBL) several different mechanisms appear to be involved in the preferential activation of the JAK-STAT signaling network. An estimated 30% cHL patients and 35%-45% of PMBL patients (Joos et al., 2003, 2000; Meier et al.,2009) present with genetic gains in chromosome band 9p24, the region where JAK2 is localized. Recently, several tumorgenic functions have been associated with this amplicon including JAK2-mediated increases in programmed cell death 1 ligand 1 (PD-L1) expression. PD-L1 is also localized to band 9p24 and therefore cells positive for this genetic gain can also demonstrate increased PD-L1 expression in addition to elevated JAK 2 content. PD-L1 inhibits antitumor cytotoxic T lymphocyte (CTL) responses by activating its cognate inhibitor PD-1 receptor located on T-cells, therefore PD-L1-/PD-1 interactions can promote tumorgenesis by mediating tumor evasiveness. A recent study showed elevated expression of PD-L1 and JAK2 in a subset of cHL and PMBL cell lines that were positive for the 9p24 amplicon and went on to show that PD-L1 expression could be augmented upon JAK2 inhibition suggesting a regulatory role for JAK2 in PD-L1 expression (Green et al., 2010 & Rui et al., 2010). In another study, alternative oncogenic functions were implicated for the 9p24 amplicon based on STAT-independent epigenetic functions of JAK2. In this study, JAK2 was shown to cooperate with the epigenetic modifier JMJDC2 in several lymphoma cell lines positive for the 9p24 gain to induce epigenetic remodeling of the oncogene MYC locus leading to altered expression of MYC (Rui et al., 2010). The cooperative interplay between JAK2 and JMJDC2 was further demonstrated when the anti-proliferative effects induced by loss of JMJD2C were exaggerated upon JAK inhibition. In addition, inactivating mutations in SOCS-1, a negative regulator of JAK-STAT signaling are observed in 40% of cHL patients (Weniger et al., 2006 & Mottok et al., 2007). Increased expression of activated STATs, namely STAT 3 and STAT6 are often observed in cHL patients and this is thought to be due to sustained signaling loops perpetuated by chronic IL-13 stimulation (Skinnider et al., 2002) furthermore, loss of STAT3 or STAT6 in cHL cell lines results in diminished proliferative capacity and induction of apoptosis (Baus, 2009 & Kube et al., 2005). To further validate a role for abnormal JAK-STAT signaling in lymphoma-type cancers is the more recent study in which an inverse relationship between the inhibitory microRNA-135a and JAK2 was observed in cHL patients. Interestingly, low levels of miR-135a expression were strongly correlated with disease relapse and shorter disease-free survival in a cohort of cHL patients. The regulatory role of miR-135a on JAK2 was confirmed when over- expression of miR-135a led to an increase in JAK2 expression (25%-55%) in lymphoma cell lines (Navarro et al., 2009).

5.2 Role of dysregulated JAK-STAT signaling in multiple myeloma

Altered JAK-STAT signaling has also been implicated in the progression of multiple myeloma (MM). MM is an aggressive hematological malignancy characterized by excessive proliferation of clonal plasma B-cells that accumulate in the bone marrow (Anderson et al., 1999). The maintenance of MM is highly dependent on the interaction of myeloma cells with resident bone marrow stromal cells (BMSC) both of which secrete various cytokines and growth factors that promote myeloma cell growth. IL-6 is recognized as a critical cytokine that's essential for the survival and proliferation of myeloma cells (Bommert et al., 2006). Elevated serum levels of IL-6 are frequently observed in MM patients who fail to respond to conventional chemotherapies and IL-6 levels also correlate with poor prognosis of MM (Niesvizky et al., 1995). IL-6 signals through JAK1/JAK2/TYK2 leading to downstream activation of STAT3 to promote proliferation and survival of myeloma cells (Murray et al., 2007). Interestingly, elevated levels of activated STAT3 have been observed in more than 50% of myeloma patient samples (Bharti AC et al., 2004). Pre-clinical studies have shown that JAK inhibition can induce apoptosis, inhibit proliferation and block constitutive and IL-6 induced activation of STAT3 in several MM cell-based models. Furthermore, JAK inhibition also enhanced the anti-tumorgenic effects of bortezomib, a current therapy available for MM, in tumor models of myeloma. In summary, JAK inhibition may not be sufficient as a mono-therapy for the treatment of MM but studies that combine JAK inhibitors with the current treatments available for MM like bortezomib may prove beneficial for MM patients. Of note, the pan-JAK inhibitor, INCB18424, currently being tested for the treatment of MPN is also being evaluated in a phase I study for the treatment of MM.

5.3 Implications for abnormal JAK-STAT signaling in solid tumors

Dysregulated JAK-STAT signaling has also been implicated in the pathogenesis of solid tumors primarily due to elevated levels of constitutively activated STATs. Among the STATs, STAT3 and STAT5 are the most studied and well characterized regarding their oncogenic potential. Activated STATs possess multiple oncogenic traits which promote tumorgenesis including tumor cell proliferation, induction of anti-apoptotic and immune cell responses. A defined role has been established for STAT5 in driving some hematological malignancies, including some MPNs where STAT5 expression leads to a MPN-like phenotype, while STAT3 appears to be more involved in solid tumor progression (Germain, 2007). In solid tumors, increased STAT activation is thought to be due to sustained cytokine stimulation via autocrine/paracrine signaling loops rather than increased activity in upstream activators of STATs such as JAKs. Elevated levels of activated STAT3 are observed in multiple solid tumors including breast, prostate, colon, pancreatic, head and neck and ovarian cancers (Song et al, 2006 & Frank., 2003) Recently, an extensive profiling study was done that identified a subset of solid tumor cell lines that expressed high levels of constitutive and IL-6 inducible activated STAT3 and when these cells were treated with specific JAK inhibitors both constitutive and inducible STAT3 activation was suppressed (Hedvat et al., 2009). In a panel of pancreatic cell lines, elevated activated STAT3 levels were found to correlate with gp130 expression, an IL-6 receptor, reinforcing the idea that STAT activation in solid tumors is related to sustained cytokine stimulation (Corcoran et al., 2011)

6. Conclusion

Emerging clinical data on a variety of JAK2 inhibitors support a role of these agents in the symptomatic relief of MPN patients. However, there are still unresolved issues associated with these inhibitors including the inability of most inhibitors to reduce the amount of mutant allele burden. The numerous mechanisms that blood-derived cancer cells have acquired to preferentially activate JAK-STAT signaling (point mutations, translocations & chromosomal gains) demonstrates the importance of this pathway in promoting hematological malignancies. The use of JAK inhibitors for the treatment of other non-MPN hematological cancers such as lymphomas and multiple myelomas are intriguing but require additional pre-clinical studies to determine which JAKs underlie these findings. In this regard, lymphomas with a high frequency of the 9p24 gain (30%) coupled with the recent identification of the novel JAK2-SEC31-A fusion protein implicates a preference for these cells to also activate JAK-STAT signaling. In multiple myeloma, a reliance of these cells on IL-6 for their survival and growth suggests that these patients could benefit from JAK inhibition therapies. For the role of JAK2-STAT signaling in solid tumors, it remains unclear of the potential of pathway inhibition but is likely to require rational combination strategies with other agents in clinical development to unmask the full therapeutic potential of JAK inhibitors.

7. Conflict of Interest

Matthew Lorenzi & Theresa McDevitt are employees of Bristol-Myers Squibb.

8. References

Aaronson, D & Horvath C. (2002). A road map for those who don't know JAK-STAT. Science. 296: 1653-1655.

Adams, H., Obermann, E.C., Dirnhofer, S et al. (2011) Targetable molecular pathways in classical Hodgkin's lymphoma. Expert Opinion Investigative Drugs. 20(2):141-151.

Anderson, K & Lust, J. (1999). Role of cytokines in multiple myeloma. Seminars in Hematology. 36(1Supp3): 14-20.

Ania B., Suman V., & Sobell, J. (1994). Trends in the incidence of polycythemia vera among Olmsted county Minnesota residents, 1935-1989. American Journal of Hematology. 47:89-93.

Apostolidou, E., Kantarjian, H.M. & Verstovsek. (2009). JAK 2 Inhibtors: A Reality? A Hope?. Clinical Lymphoma, Myeloma & Leukemia Supplement (9):3 S340-S345.

Baus, D., Nonnenmacher, F & Jankowski, S et al. (2009). STAT6 and STAT1 are essential antagonistic regulators of cell survival in classic Hodgkin lymphoma cell line. Leukemia. (23): 1885-1893.

Baxter E, J., Scott, L., & Campbell P. (2005). Acquired mutation of the tyrosine kinase JAK2 in human myeloproliferative disorders. Lancet. 365: 1054-1061.

Benekli, M., Baer M., Baumann H et al. (2003). Signal transducer and activator of transcription proteins in leukemias. Blood, 101(8), 2940-2954.

Beer, P., Delhommeau, F & LeCouedic et al. (2010) tow routes of leukemic transformation after a JAK2 mutation-positive myeloproliferative neoplasm.

Blood. 115(14): 2891-2900.

Benekli M., Baumann, H & Wetzler M. (2009). Targeting signal transducer and activator of transcription signaling pathway in leukemias. Journal of Clinical Oncology. (27): 4422-4432.

Bharti, A., Shishodia, S & Reuben J, et al. (2004). Nuclear factor-kappa B and Stat3 are constitutively active in CD138+ cells derived from multiple myeloma patients, and suppression of these factors leads to apoptosis. Blood. 103(8):3175-3184.

Bommert, K., Bargou R & Stuhmer, T. (2006). Signaling and survival pathways in myeloma. Eur J. Cancer. 42:1574-1580.

Bousquet, M., Broccardo, C & Quelen C et al. (2007) A novel PAX5-ELN fusion protein identified in B-cell acute lymphoblastic leukemia acts as a dominant negative on wild-type PAX5. Blood. 109(8):3417-3423.

Chaligne R, Tonetti C & Besancenot R et al (2008). New mutations of MPL in primitive myelofibrosis; only MPLW515L mutations promote a G1/S phase transition. Leukemia. 22: 1557-1566.

Corcoran, R., Contino, G & Deshpande et al. (2011). STAT3 plays a critical role in KRAS-induced pancreatic tumorgenesis. Cancer Research. 71(14): 5020-5029.

Darnell, JE. (1997). STATs and gene regulation. Science, 277: 1630-1635.

Druker, B., Tamura, S & Buchdunger et al. (1996). Effects of a selective inhibitor of the Abl tyrosine kinase on the growth of Bcr-Abl positive cells. Nature Medicine. 2:561-566.

Frank, DA. (2003) STAT signaling in cancer: insights into pathogenesis and treatment strategies. Cancer Treatment Research. 115: 267-291.

Gangat N., Strand J & Li, C et al. (2007) Leucocytosis in polycythaemia predicts both inferior survival and leukaemic transformation. Br. J Haematol. 138(3):354-358.

Gangat, N., Wolanskyj, A & McClure R eta l. (2007). Risk stratification for survival and leukemic transformation in essential thrombocythemia: a single institutional study of 605 patients. Leukemia. 21(2):270-275.

Germain, D & Frank, D. (2007) Targeting the cytoplasmic and nuclear functions of STAT3. Clinical Cancer Research. 13:(19) 5665-5669.

Green, M., Monti, S & Rodig, S. et al. (2010). Integrative analysis reveals selective 9p24.1 amplification, increased PD-1 ligand expression, and further induction via JAK2 in nodular sclerosing Hodgkin lymphoma and primary mediastinal large B-cell lymphoma. Blood. (116) 17: 3268-3277.

Griesinger, F., Henning, H & Hillmer, F et al. (2005) A BCR-JAK2 fusion gene as the result of a t(9;22)(p24;q11.2) translocation in a patient with a clinically typical chronic myeloid leukemia. Genes Chromosomes Cancer 44(3):329-333.

Hedvat,. M., Huszar, D & Herrmann, A. et al. (2009) The JAK2 inhibitor AZD1480 potently blocks stat3 signaling and oncogenesis in solid tumors. Cancer Cell(16): 487-497.

Huang, L., Constantinescu, S & Lodish, H. (2001). The N-terminal domain of Janus Kinase 2 is required for Golgi processing and cell surface expression of erythropoietin receptor. Molecular Cell. 8: 1327-1338.

James, C., Ugo, V & LeCouedic J et al. (2005). A unique clonal mutation leading to constituitive signaling causes polycythemia vera (PV). Nature. 434:(7037) 1144-1148.

Joos, S., Kupper, M & Ohl, S, et al. (2000). Genomic imbalances including amplification of the tyrosine kinase gene JAK2 in CD30+ Hodgkin cells. Cancer Research. 60(3):549-552.

Joos, S, Granzow M, Holtgreve-Grez, H, et al. (2003). Hodgkin's lymphoma cell lines are characterized by frequent aberrations on chromosomes 2p and 9p including REL and JAK2. International Journal of Cancer. 103(4):489-495.

Karaghiosoff, M., Steinborn, R & Kovarik, P. (2003). Central role for type I interferons and Tyk2 in lipopolysaccharide-induced endotoxin shock. Nature Immunnology. 4: 471-477.

Kota J., Caceres N. & Constantinescu S. (2008). Aberrant signal transduction pathways in myleoproliferative neoplasm. Leukemia. 22: 1828-1840.

Kralovics, R., Guan, Y., & Prchal, J et al. (2002). Acquired uniparental disomy of chromosome 9p is a frequent stem cell defect in polycythemia vera. Experimental Haematology. 3:229-236.

Kralovics, R., Passamonti, F., & Buser A et al. (2005). A gain-of-function mutation of JAK2 in myeloproliferative disorders. New England Journal of Medicine. 352(17): 1779-1790.

Kube, D., Holtick U & Vockerodt, M et al. (2001). Stat3 is constitutively activated in Hodgkin cell lines. Blood. 98(3): 762-770.

Lacronique, V, Boureux, A, Valle, VD et al (1997) A TEL-JAK2 fusion protein with constitutive kinase activity in human leukemia. *Science*. 278 (5341): 1309-1312.

Levine, R., Wadleigh, M & Cools J et al. (2005). Activating mutation in the tyrosine kinase JAK2 in polycythemia vera, essential thrombocythemia and myeloid metaplasia with myelofibrosis. Cancer Cell. 7(4): 387-397.

Levy, D & Darnell J. (2002). Stats: transcriptional control and biological control. Nature Reviews of Molecular & Cell Biology. 3: 651-662.

Li W. (2008). Canonical and non-canonical JAK-STAT signaling. Trends in Cell Biology. 18(11) 545-551.

Lopez A.., Hercus T & Ekert P. et al. (2010) Molecular Basis of Cytokine Receptor Activation. IUBMB Life 62(7): 509-518.

Lucia. E., Recchia, A & Gentile, M. et al. (2011). Janus kinase 2 inhibitors in myeloproliferative disorders. Expert Opinion Investigative Drugs. (20):1.

Meier C., Hoellar S & Bourgau C, et al. (2009). Recurrent numerical aberrations of JAK2 and deregulation of JAK-STAT cascade in lymphomas. Modern Pathology. 22(3):476-487.

Mesa, r., Silverstein, M & Jacobse, S. et al. (1999). Population-based incidence and survival figures in essential thrombocytothemia and agnogenic myeloid metaplasia: an Olmstead County Study 1976-1995. American Journal of Hematology. 61(1): 10-15.

Mesa., R. (2010). New Drugs for the Treatment of Myelofibrosis. (2010). Current Hematologic Malignancy Reports. 5(1):15-21.

Mottok, A., Renne, C., Willenbrock K. et al. (2007). Somatic hypermutation of SOCS1 in lymphocyte-predominant Hodgkin lymphoma is accompanied by high JAK2 expression and activation of STAT6. Blood. 110 (9) :3387-3390.

Mullighan, C, Morin, R & Zhang J et al. Next Generation Transcriptomic Resequencing Identifies Novel Genetic Alterations in High Risk (HR) Childhood Acute Lymphoblastic Leukemia (ALL): A Report from the Children's Oncology Group (COG) HR ALL Target Project (Abstract 704). Blood (ASH Annual Meeting Abstracts) 23(1): 293-294.

Murray PJ. (2007). The JAK-STAT signaling pathway: input and output integration. The Journal of Immunology 178: 2623-2629.

Navarro A, Diaz T & Martinez A et al. (2009). Regulation of JAK2 by miR-135a: prognostic impact in classic Hodgkin lymphoma. Blood. 114(14):2945-2951.

Nebral, K, Denk, D & Attarbaschi A et al. (2009) Incidence and diversity of PAX5 fusion genes in childhood acute lymphoblastic leukemia. Leukemia. 23(1):134-143.

Nelson, M & Steennsma D. (2006) JAK2 V617F in myeloid disorders: What do we know now, and where are we headed? Leukemia & Lymphoma. 47:177-194.

Niesvizky, R., Siegel R., Busquets, X. et al (1995). Hypercalcaemia and increased serum IL-6 levels induced by all-trans retinoic acid in patients with multiple myeloma . British Journal Haematology. 89(1):217-218.

Nosaka, T., van Deursen, J & Tripp, R et al. (1995). Defective lymphoid signaling inmice lacking JAK3. Science. 270, 800-802.

O'Brien, S., Guilhot, F & Larson R etal. (2003). Imatinib compared with interferon and low dose cytarabine for newly diagnosed chronic phase chronic myeloid leukemia. N. ENG. J Med. 348: 994-1004.

O'Shea J, Gadina, M. & Schreiber R. (2002). Cytokine Signaling in 2002: new surprises in the Jak/STAT pathway. Cell. 109: S121-131

Paradanani, D., Gotlib, J & Jamieson C et al. (2009). A phase I evaluation of TG101348, a selective JAK2 inhibitor, in MF: clinical response is accompanied by significant reduction in JAK2V617F allele burden. Blood (Abstract-ASH conference) 114:755.

Pardanani A. (2008) JAK 2 inhibitor therapy in myeloproliferative disorders: rationale, preclinical studies and ongoing clinical trials. Leukemia. (22): 23-30.

Pardanani. A, Guglielmelli P, Lasho TL. (2011). Primary myelofibrosis with or without mutant MPL: comparison of survival and clinical features involving 603 patients. Leukemia 1-6.

Parganas, E., Wang, D & Stravopodis D et al. (1998). Jak2 is essential for signaling through a variety of cytokine receptors. Cell. 93(3):385-393.

Park, C., Li, S & Schindler C. (2000). Immune response in STAT2 knock-out mice. Immunity. 13(6): 795-804.

Passamonti, F., Rumi, E & Arcaini, L et al. (2005). Leukemic transformation of polycytehemia vera: a single center study of 23 patients. Cancer. 104(5):1032-1036.

Passamonti, F., Rumi, E & Caramella, M et al (2008). A dynamic prognostic marker to predict survival in post-cytothemia vera myelofibrosis. Blood. 111(7):3383-3387.

Patnaik, M & Tefferi A. (2009). Molecular diagnosis of myeloproliferative neoplasms. Expert Review of Molecular Diagnostics. 9(5):481-492.

Peeters, A., Raynaud S., Cools, J et al. (1997) Fusion of TEL, the ETS-variant gene 6 (ETV6), to the receptor associated kinase JAK2 as a aresult of t(9;12) in a luymphoid and t(9;15;12) in a myeloid leukemia. Blood. 90(7): 2535-2540.

Pikman Y., Lee, b & Mercher, T et al. (2006). MPLW515L is a novel somatic activating mutation in myelofibrosis with myeloid metaplasia. PLoS Med. 3:1140-1151.

Poitras, J., Dal Cin P & Aster, J et al. (2008). Novel SSBP2-JAK2 fusion gene resulting from a t(5;9)(q14.1;p24.1) in pre-B acute lymphocytic leukemia. Genes Chromosomes Cancer, 47(10):884-889.

Quintas-Cardama, A., Vaddi K & Liu, P et al. (2010). Pre-clinical characterization of a selective JAK1/2 inhibitor INCB018424: therapeutic implications for the treatment of MPNs. Blood. 115:3109-3117.

Radtke, S., Haan, S & Jorissen, A et al. (2005). The Jak1 SH2 domain does not fulfill a classical SH2 function in Jak/Stat signaling but plays a structural role for receptor interaction and up-regulation of receptor surface expression. Journal of Biological Chemistry. 280(27):25760-25768.

Reiter, A., Walz, C & Watmore, A et al. (2005) The t(8;9)(p22;p24) is recurrent abnormality in chronic and acute leukemia that fuses PCM1 to JAK2. Cancer Research 65(7): 2662-2667.

Rodig, S., Meraz, M & White, J et al. (1998). Disruption of the JAK1 gene demonstrates obligatory and non-redundant roles of the JAKs in cytokine-induced biologic responses. Cell. 93(3): 373-383.

Rui, L., Emre, T & Kruhlak M et al. (2010). Cooperative epigenetic modulation by cancer amplicon genes. Cancer Cell. 18(6): 590-605.

Saharinen, P., Takaluoma K & Silvennoinen, O, et al. (2000). Regulation of JAK2 tyrosine kinase by its pseudokinase domain. Molecular and Cellular Biology. 20(10): 3387-3395.

Santos P.S. & Vertosvek S. (2011). JAK2 inhibitors: What's the true therapeutic potential? Blood Reviews. 25:53-63.

Scott, L., Tong, W & Levine R et al. (2007). JAK2 exon 12 mutations in PV and idiopathic erythrocytosis. N Engl. J Med, 356(5): 459-468.

Skinnider B., Elia, A & Gascoyne L et al. (2002) Signal transducer an activator of transcription 6 is frequently in Hodgkin and Reed-Sternberg cells of Hodgkin lymphoma. Blood 99(2): 618-626.

Song, L., Bhattacharya S & Yunus A et al. (2006). Stat1 and SUMO modification. Blood. 108(10) 3237:3244.

Valentino, L & Pierre J. (2006). JAK/STAT signal transduction: regulators and implication in hematological malignancies. Biochemical Pharmacology. 71(6): 713-721.

Van Roosbroeck, K., Cox, L & Tousseyn T et al. (2011). JAK2 rearrangements, including the novel SEC31-A-JAK2 fusion, are recurrent in classical Hodgkin lymphoma. Blood. 117(15):4056-4064.

Verstovsek, S., Kantajian, H & Pardanani, A et al. (2008) Characterization of allele JAK2V617F allele burden in advanced myelofibrosis patients: no change in V617F:WT JAK2 ratio in patients with high allele burdens despite profound clinical improvement following treatment with the JAK inhibitor. Blood (Abstract) 112: 2802.

Verstovsek, S., Kantarjian, H & Mesa, R et al. (2010). Safety and Efficacy of INCB018424, a JAK1 and JAK2 inhibitor in myelofibrosis. New England Journal of Medicine. 363: 1117-1127.

Wadleigh, M & Tefferi A. (2010). Classification and diagnosis of myeloproliferation neoplasms according to the 2008 World Health Organization criteria. International Journal of Hematology. 91:174-179.

Ward, A., Touw, I & Yoshimura, A. (2000). The JAK-Stat pathway in normal and perturbed hematopoiesis. Blood. 95(1):19-29

Weniger, M., Melzner, C & Menz S et al. (2006). Mutations of the suppressor gene SOCS-1 in classical Hodgkin lymphoma are frequent and associated with nuclear phospho-STAT5 accumulation. Oncogene. (25):2679-2684.

Wernig G., Mercher, T & Okabe R et al. (2006). Expression of JAKV617F causes a polycytothemia vera–like disease associated with myelofibrosis in a murine bone marrow transplant model. Blood. 107(11):4274-4281.

9

Genetic Alterations and Their Clinical Implications in Acute Myeloid Leukemia

Hsin-An Hou, Wen-Chien Chou and Hwei-Fang Tien
Division of Hematology, Department of Internal Medicine, National Taiwan University Hospital, College of Medicine, National Taiwan University, Taipei, Taiwan

1. Introduction

Acute myeloid leukemia (AML) is a hematologic malignancy with great variability in the pathogenesis, clinical features, and treatment outcomes. Advances in molecular research have greatly improved our understanding of the leukemogenesis in AML. A two-hit model proposes that the development of AML requires the cooperation between at least two classes of gene mutations.(Frohling, *et al* 2005, Gilliland 2002) Class I mutations, such as *RAS, FLT3, KIT, PTPN11* and *JAK2* mutations, involve genes in the kinase signaling pathways leading to cell survival and proliferation and Class II mutations, such as t(15;17)/*PML-RARA*, inv(16)/*CBFB-MYH11* and t(8;21)/*RUNX1-RUNX1T1* fusions, and *MLL*/PTD, and *CEBPA* and *AML1/RUNX1* mutations, involve transcription factors or cofactors resulting in impaired hematopoietic differentiation. In addition to genetic abnormalities, increasing evidences show that epigenetic deregulations are also critical to the pathogenesis of AML.(Chen, *et al* 2010) Compatible with these findings, several novel mutations involving genes related to epigenetic modifications, such as *isocitrate dehydrogenase 1* (*IDH1*), *IDH2, ten-eleven translocation* 2 (*TET2*), *additional sex comb-like 1* (*ASXL1*), and DNA methyltransferase 3A *(DNMT3A)* were detected in AML recently.(Chou, *et al* 2010b, Delhommeau, *et al* 2009, Gelsi-Boyer, *et al* 2009, Ley, *et al* 2010, Mardis, *et al* 2009, Metzeler, *et al* 2011)

Risk-adapted treatment may not only improve the prognosis, but also reduce the toxicity from the therapy in patients with AML. In addition to the conventional risk factors, such as age, white blood cell (WBC) counts and cytogenetics, molecular genetic alterations, such as mutations of *NPM1, CEBPA, AML1/RUNX1, WT1, FLT3, TET2*, and *DNMT3A* etc., are also important prognostic factors in AML patients. Furthermore, the gene mutations which are stable during treatment courses can also be used as biomarkers to monitor minimal residual disease (MRD). Herein, we will review the gene mutations in AML and discuss their clinical implications.

2. Class I mutations that lead to cell survival and proliferation

2.1 *FLT3* mutations

FMS-like tyrosine kinase 3 (FLT3), mapped at 13q12, encodes a receptor tyrosine kinase.(Kiyoi, *et al* 1998) *FLT3*-internal tandem duplication (*FLT3*-ITD) mutation, one of the most common mutations in AML, was found by Nakao et al in 1996.(Nakao, *et al* 1996) The mutation occurs as a duplication of nucleotide sequences of variable lengths in exons 14 and 15, leading to addition of repeated peptide in the juxtamembrane domain in the cytoplasm. Another activating *FLT3* mutation occurs in tyrosine kinase domain (*FLT3*-TKD), causing point mutations, small deletions or insertions mainly at codon 835 or 836 within the activation loop of the second kinase domain.(Bacher, *et al* 2008, Yamamoto, *et al* 2001) The FLT3 mutant protein constitutively activates the cascade of FLT3 signaling in the absence of FLT3 ligand promoting cell proliferation and decreased apoptosis.

FLT3-ITD occurs in about 25% of adult AML and shows association with normal karyotype and *NPM1* mutation. The patients with this mutation have higher WBC counts, shorter disease-free survival (DFS) and overall survival (OS), and increased relapse rate.(Kottaridis, *et al* 2001, Kottaridis, *et al* 2002) While mutant size may not be related to prognosis, higher mutant levels are associated with higher relapse rate and shorter survival.(Gale, *et al* 2008) Absence of *FLT3*-ITD combined with *NPM1* mutation is regarded as a favorable prognostic genotype.(Gale, *et al* 2008, Schlenk, *et al* 2008) Up to one third of AML patients with *FLT3*-ITD can lose the mutation at disease relapse, indicating that this mutation is much less stable than *NPM1* mutation, and is not a good marker for disease monitoring.(Chou, *et al* 2011b, Kottaridis, *et al* 2002, Palmisano, *et al* 2007, Shih, *et al* 2002) *FLT3*-TKD occurred in about 4%-10% of AML patients.(Yamamoto, *et al* 2001, Bacher, *et al* 2008) AML with this mutation also shows specific clinical and biologic features, such as elevated WBC counts at diagnosis, higher frequency of normal karyotype and mutations in *NPM1*, *CEBPA*, and *NRAS*. However, the prognostic significance is still inconclusive.(Bacher, *et al* 2008, Whitman, *et al* 2008)

2.2 *RAS* mutations

The RAS proteins are a large superfamily of low molecular-weight guanine nucleotide-binding proteins, which are activated by cytokine receptors in response to ligand stimulation and therefore control cell proliferation and survival of hematopoietic progenitors.(Downward 2003, Reuther and Der 2000, Shields, *et al* 2000, Wittinghofer 1998) Three members of the RAS family, HRAS, KRAS and NRAS, are found to be activated by mutations in human cancers.(Bos 1989, Downward 2003) Almost all RAS mutations occur by single nucleotide substitutions in codons 12, 13 and 61.(Bos, *et al* 1987, Farr, *et al* 1988, Senn, *et al* 1988, Toksoz, *et al* 1989) *NRAS* and *KRAS* mutations are found in approximately 12-30% and 9-14%, respectively, of AML patients. In a large cohort study of 2502 AML patients, the mutations were found much prevalent in patients with inv(16)/t(16;16) and inv(3)/t(3;3), but seldom found in those with t(15;17) and complex karyotype.(Bacher, *et al* 2006)

The prognostic relevance of *RAS* mutation in AML has not been firmly established. Some studies showed *RAS* mutation predicted poor prognosis(De Melo, *et al* 1997, Kiyoi, *et al* 1999, Meshinchi, *et al* 2003), some showed no impact on clinical outcome,(Bacher, *et al* 2006, Bowen, *et al* 2005, Radich, *et al* 1990, Ritter, *et al* 2004) whereas others found *RAS* mutations were associated with a favorable prognosis.(Coghlan, *et al* 1994, Neubauer, *et al* 1994) However, higher dose of cytarabine may decrease the relapse rate in *RAS*-mutated AML patients.(Neubauer, *et al* 2008)

2.3 *KIT* mutations

KIT, a member of type III receptor tyrosine kinase family, is important for the development of hematopoietic progenitor cells and also crucial in leukemogenesis.(Blume-Jensen and

Hunter 2001, Bowen, *et al* 2005, Radich, *et al* 1990) High expression of *KIT* (CD117) is a common finding in AML,(Ikeda, *et al* 1991, Reuss-Borst, *et al* 1994) and activation mutations of *KIT*, most commonly affecting exons 8 and 17 can be identified in 20–45% of AML with inv (16) and 12.8–46.8% of AML with t(8;21), but infrequently found in other AML types.(Beghini, *et al* 2000, Beghini, *et al* 2004, Care, *et al* 2003) Most, though not all, studies,(Boissel, *et al* 2006, Care, *et al* 2003, Schnittger, *et al* 2006) showed *KIT* mutation was associated with inferior outcome in the core binding factor (CBF) AML, especially *KIT*-D816 mutations in t(8;21)/*RUNX1-RUNX1T1*-positive AML.

2.4 *JAK2* mutations

JAK2 is a nonreceptor tyrosine kinase. The *JAK2* V617F mutation induces the activation of JAK2-STAT5 signal transduction pathway and then substantially alters the proliferation and self-renewal of hematopoietic precursors.(Liu, *et al* 1999, Walz, *et al* 2006) Although the *JAK2* V617F mutation is a common genetic event in the patients with myeloproliferative neoplasms (MPN),(Baxter, *et al* 2005, Goldman 2005, Kralovics, *et al* 2005, Levine, *et al* 2005b) it is seldom found (<1%-2%) in *de novo* AML patients.(Frohling, *et al* 2006, Illmer, *et al* 2007, Lee, *et al* 2006, Levine, *et al* 2005a) Illmer et al showed 3.6% of patients with CBF AML had *JAK2* V617F mutation and these patients had an aggressive clinical course and poor outcome.(Illmer, *et al* 2007)

2.5 *PTPN 11* mutations

SHP-2 is encoded by *PTPN11* which is located on chromosome 12q24. The protein is a non-receptor tyrosine phosphatase participating in intracellular signaling elicited by a number of growth factors, cytokines, hormones and adhesion molecules.(Neel, *et al* 2003, Tartaglia, *et al* 2004) Germline *PTPN11* mutations were first reported by Tartaglia *et al* in patients afflicted with Noonan syndrome.(Tartaglia, *et al* 2002, Tartaglia, *et al* 2001) Subsequently, somatic *PTPN11* mutations were also found in patients with juvenile myelomonocytic leukemia, and myelodysplastic syndrome (MDS).(Chen, *et al* 2006, Loh, *et al* 2004b, Tartaglia, *et al* 2003) The *PTPN11* mutation is not a frequent molecular event (4-5%) in AML.(Hou, *et al* 2008, Loh, *et al* 2004a, Tartaglia, *et al* 2005) In a study of 272 primary AML patients, we found this gene mutation was closely associated with older age, French-American-British (FAB) M4/M5 subtype, CD14 expression, normal karyotype and *NPM1* mutation.(Hou, *et al* 2008) Loh *et al* and Tartaglia *et al* revealed that the *PTPN11* mutation had no prognostic implication for pediatric patients with AML;(Loh, *et al* 2004a, Tartaglia, *et al* 2005) however, this mutation may be a poor-risk factor for OS in adult AML patients without *NPM1* mutations.(Hou, *et al* 2008)

3. Class II mutations that impair hematopoietic differentiation

3.1 *CEBPA* mutations

CCAAT/enhancer binding protein α (C/EBPα) is a 42-kDa transcription factor that possesses a DNA-binding basic leucine zipper domain (bZIP) in the COOH terminus and two transactivation domains TAD 1 and TAD 2 in the NH2 terminus.(Friedman and McKnight 1990) As a transcription factor, it plays a crucial role in granulocytic differentiation and diminished C/EBPα activity contributes to myeloid progenitor transformation.(Cammenga, *et al* 2003, Oelgeschlager, *et al* 1996, Smith, *et al* 1996) *CEBPA* mutations are observed in 7% to 18% of patients with AML.(Frohling, *et al* 2004, Lin, *et al* 2005, Pabst, *et al* 2001b, Preudhomme, *et al* 2002) Two major types of *CEBPA* mutations have been identified; one alters COOH terminal bZIP of *CEBPA*, resulting in decreased DNA-binding and/or dimerization activity and the other disrupts translation of the C/EBPα NH2 terminus, thereby up-regulates an alternative 30-kDa isoform with dominant-negative effect on the full-length wild-type C/EBPα.(Koschmieder, *et al* 2009, Lin, *et al* 1993, Pabst, *et al* 2001b) Most patients with *CEBPA* mutations harbored biallelic mutations involving both the NH2-terminal TAD region and the COOH-terminal bZIP domain.(Hou, *et al* 2009, Lin, *et al* 2005, Pabst, *et al* 2009, Renneville, *et al* 2009a) *CEBPA* mutations occur most frequently in patients with FAB subtype M2, and are closely associated with CD7, CD15, CD34, and HLA-DR expression on the leukemic cells, higher circulatory blasts and normal cytogenetics.(Frohling, *et al* 2004, Lin, *et al* 2005, Pabst, *et al* 2001a, Zhang, *et al* 1997) This mutation seems quite stable during AML evolution and may be a potential marker to monitor MRD. The fact that none of the AML patients who do not have *CEBPA* mutations at diagnosis acquire the mutation at relapse suggests that this mutation may not play a major role in the progression of AML.(Lin, *et al* 2005, Tiesmeier, *et al* 2003) Several studies have shown mutant *CEBPA* predicts favorable outcome in AML patients with intermediate or normal cytogenetics.(Barjesteh van Waalwijk van Doorn-Khosrovani, *et al* 2003, Bienz, *et al* 2005, Frohling, *et al* 2004, Preudhomme, *et al* 2002) The favorable impact of *CEBPA* mutations in the AML patients is only observed in the absence of *FLT3*/ITD or other associated cytogenetic abnormalities.(Renneville, *et al* 2009a) Moreover, only double *CEBPA* mutations, but not single *CEBPA* mutation, are associated with better prognosis and define a distinct genetic entity.(Dufour, *et al* 2010, Hou, *et al* 2009, Pabst, *et al* 2009, Wouters, *et al* 2009)

3.2 *MLL* -PTD

The *MLL* partial tandem duplication (*MLL*-PTD) most commonly results from a duplication of a genomic region encompassing exon 5 through exon 11/12 and insertion of the duplicated segment into intron 4 of the full-length *MLL* gene.(Caligiuri, *et al* 1994, Schichman, *et al* 1994, Whitman, *et al* 2005) The duplication involves a portion of the gene corresponding to the amino terminus of the MLL protein which contains the AT hook and a region of homology to DNA methyltransferase motifs.(Schichman, *et al* 1995) The mechanism by which *MLL*-PTD contributes to leukemic phenotype is not clear, but may be through silencing of the wild-type *MLL* by epigenetic mechanisms.(Dimartino and Cleary 1999, Whitman, *et al* 2005) This mutation is found in 5-12% of patients with cytogenetically normal AML (CN-AML),(Dohner, *et al* 2002, Munoz, *et al* 2003, Schnittger, *et al* 2000, Shiah, *et al* 2002) and up to 54% of AML patients with trisomy 11.(Rege-Cambrin, *et al* 2005) Compared with patients without *MLL*-PTD, patients with this mutation more often have FAB M2 subtype, CD11b expression, wild-type *NPM1* and high *BAALC* expression, but lower WBC counts, less frequently extramedullary involvement and FAB M4/M5 subtype at diagnosis.(Shiah, *et al* 2002, Whitman, *et al* 2007) The presence of *MLL*-PTD predicts shorter remission duration and worse OS;(Dohner, *et al* 2002, Munoz, *et al* 2003, Shiah, *et al* 2002) however, more intensive consolidation therapy that includes hematopoietic stem cell transplantation (HSCT) during first complete remission (CR) may reverse the poor prognosis conferred by this mutation.(Whitman, *et al* 2007)

3.3 *AML1/RUNX1*

The *AML1/RUNX1* gene(Ito 2008), consisting of 10 exons (exons 1-6, 7A, 7B, 7C and 8), is one of the most frequently deregulated genes in leukemia through chromosomal translocations and point mutations.(Friedman 2009, Niebuhr, *et al* 2008, Osato 2004, Yamagata, *et al* 2005) Monoallelic germ-line mutation of the *RUNX1* gene occurs in rare cases of familial platelet disorder with predisposition to AML (FPD/AML).(Michaud, *et al* 2002) Acquired *RUNX1* mutation was frequently reported in therapy-related MDS or MDS/AML.(Harada, *et al* 2004) The incidence of *RUNX1* mutation in AML varies from 2.9% to 46% depending on the population selected, the regions of *RUNX1* screened, and the methods used.(Dicker, *et al* 2007, Preudhomme, *et al* 2000, Tang, *et al* 2009) In a large cohort study of 470 adult patients with *de novo* non-M3 AML, we detected *RUNX1* mutation in 13.2% of cases. The *RUNX1* mutation is closely associated with older age, immature FAB subtypes (M0/M1) and specific cytogenetic abnormalities such as trisomy 8 (+8), +13, or +21.(Dicker, *et al* 2007, Schnittger, *et al* 2011, Tang, *et al* 2009) None of the patients with t(8;21), inv(16), t(15;17) or 11q23 translocation shows *RUNX1* mutation.(Tang, *et al* 2009) One half of *RUNX1*-mutated patients have concurrently other gene mutations, mostly (83.9%) Class I mutations, especially *FLT3/*ITD, *FLT3/*TKD and *N-RAS* mutations(Tang, *et al* 2009) which all result in hyperactivation of the receptor tyrosine kinase (RTK)-RAS signalling pathways.(Niimi, *et al* 2006) This finding is consistent with the two-hit model of leukemogenesis.(Frohling, *et al* 2005, Gilliland 2002) Further, the *RUNX1* mutation is mutually exclusive with *CEBPA* and *NPM1* mutations, but closely associated with *MLL/*PTD.(Schnittger, *et al* 2011, Tang, *et al* 2009) The mutation may be lost at relapse in *RUNX1*-mutated patients, but none of the patients who do not harbor *RUNX1* mutation at diagnosis acquire novel mutation at relapse.(Tang, *et al* 2009) *RUNX1* mutation is an independent poor-risk factor for DFS and OS in *de novo* AML patients.(Gaidzik, *et al* 2011, Schnittger, *et al* 2011, Tang, *et al* 2009) In addition, HSCT seems to ameliorate the poor survival impact of *RUNX1* mutations.(Gaidzik, *et al* 2011, Tang, *et al* 2009)

4. Other mutations

4.1 *NPM1* mutations

NPM1 mutation in AML was first identified by Dr. Falini's group, who noticed that some AML patients' leukemia cells exhibited aberrant cytoplasmic localization of NPM1 protein, which normally located in nucleoli in non-mitotic cells.(Falini, *et al* 2005) Subsequent investigation revealed a tetra-nucleotide insertion near the C-terminal end of the coding sequence of *NPM1*. The most frequent form of mutation is duplication of TCTG (type A, c.860_863dupTCTG), resulting in alteration of the peptide sequence from DLWQWRKSL* to DLCL AVEEVSLRK*. *NPM1* mutation occurs in about 30% of AML, more frequently in elder patients,(Falini, *et al* 2011, Falini, *et al* 2005) and is highly associated with normal karyotype, and *FLT3*/ITD, but significantly exclusive with *CEBPA* mutation, favorable karyotype, and expression of CD34 and HLA-DR.(Boissel, *et al* 2005, Chou, *et al* 2006, Dohner, *et al* 2005, Falini, *et al* 2005, Schnittger, *et al* 2005, Suzuki, *et al* 2005, Verhaak, *et al* 2005) *NPM1* mutation generally renders better prognosis,(Falini, *et al* 2005) especially when *FLT3*-ITD is absent.(Schlenk, *et al* 2008, Thiede, *et al* 2006) Further refinement of patient groups disclosed 3 groups with distinct prognosis: good ($NPM1^{+}$/*FLT3*-ITD^{-}), intermediate ($NPM1^{+}$/*FLT3*-ITD^{+} or $NPM1^{-}$/*FLT3*-ITD^{-}), and poor ($NPM1^{-}$/*FLT3*-ITD^{+}).(Gale, *et al* 2008) *NPM1* mutation seems quite consistent with disease status.(Chou, *et al* 2007, Schnittger, *et al*

2009) Serial analyses of *NPM1* mutations showed the mutation disappeared at CR, but the same mutation usually reappeared at relapse. This feature makes *NPM1* mutation an ideal marker for MRD monitoring. Studies have shown *NPM1* mutant levels reflect disease status, predict impending relapse, and bring prognostic implication.(Chou, *et al* 2007, Gorello, *et al* 2006, Kronke, *et al* 2011, Schnittger, *et al* 2009)

4.2 *WT1* mutations

The *Wilms' Tumor 1* (*WT1*) gene, encoding a zinc-finger transcription factor, is physiologically expressed in hematopoietic stem cells and involved in regulation of cellular growth and differentiation.(Baird and Simmons 1997, Ellisen, *et al* 2001) *WT1* was initially identified as a tumor suppressor gene,(Haber, *et al* 1990) but was later found to be overexpressed in AML as well as other cancers and thus was suggested to be an oncogene.(Bergmann, *et al* 1997, King-Underwood, *et al* 1996, Miwa, *et al* 1992) Mutations in *WT1* gene are found in about 7-13% of CN-AML patients with hotspots in the four Cys-His zinc finger domains on exons 7 and 9.(Gaidzik, *et al* 2009, Hou, *et al* 2010, King-Underwood, *et al* 1996, Paschka, *et al* 2008, Virappane, *et al* 2008) The precise role of WT1 mutations in the leukemogenesis remains to be defined. The majority of *WT1* mutations are frame-shift mutations occurring in exon 7, followed by single amino acid substitutions in exon 9; whereas frame-shift mutations in exon 9 are rare. *WT1* mutations occur with similar frequencies in patients with normal karyotype and those with abnormal cytogenetics.(Hou, *et al* 2010) Chromosomal abnormality t(7;11)(p15;15), a translocation resulting in *NUP98/HOXA9* fusion, is closely associated with *WT1* mutation.(Hou, *et al* 2010) *WT1* mutations are positively associated with *FLT3*/ITD and *CEBPA* mutations.(Gaidzik, *et al* 2009, Renneville, *et al* 2009b) Paschka *et al* showed patients with *WT1* mutations had higher expression of *ERG* and *BAALC* than patients without.(Paschka, *et al* 2008) *WT1* mutation is an independent poor prognostic factor in CN-AML as well as total AML patients.(Hou, *et al* 2010, Paschka, *et al* 2008, Renneville, *et al* 2009b, Virappane, *et al* 2008), though different results have been reported.(Gaidzik, *et al* 2009, Santamaria, *et al* 2009)

5. Mutations of genes that involve epigenetic modifications

Different from genetic abnormalities which result in DNA sequence changes, epigenetic dysregulation causes aberrant gene expression without alteration of gene sequences.(Baylin and Ohm 2006, Chen, *et al* 2010, Jones and Baylin 2002) Epigenetic regulation includes DNA methylation, histone modifications, such as methylation, acetylation and phosphorylation, etc, and microRNA expression. (Baylin and Ohm 2006, Chen, *et al* 2010, Jones and Baylin 2002) The recent findings that mutations of genes related to epigenetic modifications, such as *IDH1, IDH2, TET2, ASXL1* and *DNMT3A*, are detected in AML patients provide new insights into mechanisms of epigenetic deregulation in the leukemogenesis.

5.1 *TET2* mutations

TET2 protein can catalyze the conversion of 5-methylcytosine (5-mC) of DNA to 5-hydroxymethylcytosine (5-hmC), with ferrous iron and α-ketoglutarate (α-KG) as cofactors, indicating a role of TET2 in DNA methylation.(Ito, *et al* 2010) Mutations of *TET2* result in global DNA hypermethylation.(Figueroa, *et al* 2010) *TET2* mutation was originally identified in myeloid malignancies via single nucleotide polymorphism and comparative genomic-hybridization array, which revealed common deletion of this gene in chromosome 4q.(Delhommeau, *et al* 2009) Subsequent studies confirmed this mutation in MDS, MPN, MDS/MPN, and secondary AML, with frequencies around 10% to 26%, 7% to 13%, 22% to 58% and 24% to 32%, respectively.(Bacher, *et al* 2010, Couronne, *et al* 2010, Flach, *et al* 2010, Jankowska, *et al* 2009, Kosmider, *et al* 2009a, Kosmider, *et al* 2009b, Langemeijer, *et al* 2009, Saint-Martin, *et al* 2009, Schaub, *et al* 2010, Smith, *et al* 2010, Tefferi, *et al* 2009a, Tefferi, *et al* 2009b) *TET2* mutation occurs in 18.0% to 23% of CN-AML patients.(Chou, *et al* 2011a, Metzeler, *et al* 2011) It is closely associated with older age, higher WBC count, but mutually exclusive with *IDH* mutation.(Chou, *et al* 2011a, Metzeler, *et al* 2011) In our study of AML patients with and without chromosomal abnormalities, *TET2* mutation was also found to be positively associated with normal karyotype, intermediate-risk cytogenetics, isolated trisomy 8, *NPM1* mutation, and *ASXL1* mutation.(Chou, *et al* 2011a) In European LeukemiaNet (ELN) favorable-risk group (patients with CN-AML with mutated *CEBPA* and/or mutated *NPM1* without *FLT3*-ITD),(Dohner, *et al* 2010) but not intermediate-1 risk group (CN-AML with wild-type *CEBPA* and wild-type *NPM1* and/or FLT3-ITD), *TET2*-mutated patients were found to have a lower CR rate, shorter DFS and OS, compared with *TET2*-wild type patients.(Metzeler, *et al* 2011) However, we did not have the same finding, but found that *TET2* mutation was an unfavorable prognostic factor in patients with intermediate-risk cytogenetics, and its negative impact was further enhanced when the mutation was combined with *FLT3*-ITD, *NPM1*-wild, or unfavorable genotypes (other than ELN favorable-risk group).(Chou, *et al* 2011a) More studies are needed to clarify the prognostic implication of *TET2* mutations in AML.

5.2 *IDH* mutations

IDH1 and *IDH2* genes encode two isoforms of isocitrate dehydrogenase which catalyzes the carboxylation of isocitrate to α-KG. *IDH1* and *IDH2* mutations were first detected in patients with brain tumors.(Parsons, *et al* 2008) Later, *IDH1* mutations (Mardis, *et al* 2009) and then *IDH2* mutations were discovered in AML patients, too.(Abbas, *et al* 2010, Marcucci, *et al* 2010, Ward, *et al* 2010) *IDH1* mutations affect arginine residue in position 132 (R132) and *IDH2* mutations, in R140 and R172 of exon 4. *IDH* mutations occur at low frequencies (3.6% to 5%) in MDS,(Kosmider, *et al* 2010) and in chronic-phase MPN (about 1.8%)(Pardanani, *et al* 2010), but obviously increased as these diseases progress to AML (7.5% to 21%),(Kosmider, *et al* 2010, Pardanani, *et al* 2010) indicating a role of *IDH* mutations in leukemogenesis. In *de novo* AML, *IDH2* mutations occur more frequently than *IDH1* mutations, with frequencies of 11% vs. 6% in patients younger than 60 years,(Abbas, *et al* 2010) 15.4% vs. 7.7% in total patients,(Ward, *et al* 2010) and 19% vs. 14% in adults with normal karyotype.(Marcucci, *et al* 2010) The underlying mechanism of *IDH* mutations in the leukemogenesis of AML remains to be determined, but several implications of *IDH1/2* mutations in AML have been generated. First, *IDH* mutations are loss-of-function mutations, as mutant IDH proteins show decreased enzyme activities,(Zhao, *et al* 2009) and have dominant-negative effects on wild type IDH upon homodimerization.(Zhao, *et al* 2009) Secondly, *IDH* mutations are also gain-of-function mutations because the mutant proteins can convert α-KG to 2-hydroxyglutarate (2-HG), a metabolite that may contribute to tumor growth through activating hypoxia-inducing factor-1α (HIF-1α).(Dang, *et al* 2009, Reitman, *et al* 2010, Ward, *et al* 2010) Thirdly, *IDH* mutations reduce production of α-KG, a cofactor of TET2, thus impair catalytic function of TET2 resulting in global DNA hypermethylation, similar to the effect of *TET2* mutations. 2-HG converted from α-KG in *IDH*-mutated cells is also shown to inhibit TET2-mediated hydroxymethylation of cytosine, indicating overlapping effects of these two mutations.(Xu, *et al* 2011) Compatible with this, *IDH* and *TET2* mutations are mutually exclusive in AML patients.(Figueroa, *et al* 2010, Metzeler, *et al* 2011)

Studies have shown similar clinical features between AML with *IDH1* and *IDH2* mutations, including strong association of both mutations with normal karyotype and isolated monosomy 8, but inverse correlation with expression of HLA-DR. However, some differences exist. *IDH1* mutation shows strong correlation with *NPM1* mutation, and FAB M1 subtype, but is inversely associated with FAB M4 subtype and expression of CD13 and CD14. On the other hand, mutation of *IDH2* is associated with higher platelet counts, but is inversely correlated with expression of CD34, CD15, CD7, and CD56, and is mutually exclusive with *WT1* mutation and chromosomal translocations involving CBF. While there is no impact of *IDH1* mutation on patient survival, multivariate analysis reveals *IDH2* mutation as an independent favorable prognostic factor,(Chou, *et al* 2010a, Chou, *et al* 2011c,) but different results have also been reported.(Marcucci, *et al* 2010, Thol, *et al* 2010) More intriguing are the differences of clinical presentations between patients with R140 and R172 mutations. Compared with *IDH2* R140 mutation, *IDH2* R172 mutation is associated with younger age, lower WBC count and LDH level, and is mutually exclusive with *NPM1* mutation. Recent studies also reported worse prognosis in AML patients bearing *IDH2* R172Q,(Boissel, *et al* 2010, Marcucci, *et al* 2010) while *IDH2* R140Q, in the contrary, conferred a better prognosis.(Green, *et al* 2010) Why mutations in different isoforms or loci of the same gene render distinct clinical and prognostic features remains to be investigated. Serial analyses of *IDH1/2* mutations at both diagnosis and relapse confirmed high stability of these two mutations.(Chou, *et al* 2010a, Chou, *et al* 2011c)

5.3 *ASXL1* mutations

Recently, mutations in exon 12 of *Additional sex comb-like 1* (*ASXL1*) gene were found in various types of myeloid malignances, including MDS, MPN, MDS/MPN, and AML.(Abdel-Wahab, *et al* 2010, Boultwood, *et al* 2010, Carbuccia, *et al* 2009, Carbuccia, *et al* 2010, Gelsi-Boyer, *et al* 2009) *ASXL1*, a human homologue of the *Additional sex combs* (*Asx*) gene of *Drosophila*, mapped to chromosome 20q11, a region commonly involved in cancers.(Fisher, *et al* 2003) It consists of an N-terminal *ASX* Homology (ASXH) domain and a C-terminal plant homeodomain (PHD) zinc finger region.(Fisher, *et al* 2003, Fisher, *et al* 2006) In human, the exact function of *ASXL1* mutation remains to be defined, but it is involved in regulation of histone methylation by cooperation with heterochromatin protein-1 (HP1) to modulate the activity of LSD1, a histone demethylase for H3K4 and H3K9.(Dange and Colman 2010, Wang, *et al* 2009) *ASXL1* mutations in exon 12 are found with an incidence of 10.8%, 8.9% and 12.9% among total cohort of patients with *de novo* AML, those with normal karyotype and abnormal cytogenetics, respectively.(Chou, *et al* 2010b) Most of the mutations appear to be either non-sense or frame-shift mutations, leading to disruption of the plant hoemodomain (PHD) at the C terminal of ASXL1, which is well conserved among different species and can recognize methylated H3K4.(Abdel-Wahab, *et al* 2010, Fisher, *et al* 2003, Pena, *et al* 2006, Shi, *et al* 2006, Wysocka, *et al* 2006) Up to two thirds of mutations occurred at c.1934dupG (an extra G after 1934th nucleotide of the coding sequence of *ASXL1*) causing G646WfsX12 (change of glycine to tryptophan at amino acid 646, with a premature stop codon after another 11 amino acid).(Chou, *et al* 2010b) The mutation was closely associated with older age, male gender, isolated trisomy 8, *RUNX1* mutation, and expression of HLA-DR and CD34, but inversely associated with t(15;17), complex cytogenetics, *FLT3*-ITD, *NPM1* mutations, *WT1* mutations, and expression of CD33 and CD15.(Chou, *et al* 2010b) Patients with *ASXL1* mutations had a shorter OS than those without, but the mutation was not an independent adverse prognostic factor in multivariate analysis. Sequential analyses showed that the original *ASXL1* mutations could disappear at relapse and/or refractory status in some patients. Moreover, two out of the 109 *ASXL1*-wild patients acquired a novel *ASXL1* mutation at relapse.(Chou, *et al* 2010b) Thus, the *ASXL1* mutation status can change during disease evolution in a few patients.

5.4 *DNMT3A* mutations

By whole genome sequencing on a single patient with normal cytogenetics, Ley and his colleagues found a mutation in *DNMT3A* gene, which encodes the enzyme DNA methyltransferase 3A which belongs to the family of DNMTs that catalyze the addition of methyl group to cytosine of CpG dinucleotide.(Ley, *et al* 2010) In this seminal study, *DNMT3A* mutation was detected in 22.1% of AML patients. Most of the mutations occurred at R882 amino acid. Others included mis-sense, non-sense and frame-shift mutations. Although DNMT3A is directly related to DNA methylation, the real significance of this mutation to leukemogenesis remains unknown. First, the wide spreading of mutation spots in *DNMT3A* suggests a loss-of-function mutation, but the remarkable aggregate of mutation at R882 implies a gain of function. Reduction of DNA methylation in 182 genomic areas was noted in R882 mutation-harboring AML cells, however, the methylation patterns of vast majority of cytosine methylation regions are the same as wild type.(Ley, *et al* 2010)

DNMT3A mutations are associated with intermediate or normal cytogenetics, higher WBC counts, FAB M4/M5 subtypes, and *FLT3*-ITD, *NPM1*, and *IDH1* mutations but mutually exclusive with favorable karyotypes.(Ley, *et al* 2010, Thol, *et al* 2011) In our study of 500 AML patients, *DNMT3A* mutations were identified in 14% of total patients and 22.9% of patients with CN-AML. (Hou, *et al* 2011) In addition to the findings shown in previous reports, (Ley, *et al* 2010, Thol, *et al* 2011) we for the first time identified the *DNMT3A* mutation was positively associated with *PTPN11* and *IDH2* mutations, but negatively associated with *CEBPA* mutation.(Hou, *et al* 2011) Intriguingly, the majority (97.1%) of the *DNMT3A*-mutated patients showed additional molecular alterations at diagnosis. This mutation renders poor OS among all AML patients, patients with a normal karyotype, and those with *FLT3*-ITD.(Hou, *et al* 2011, Ley, *et al* 2010, Thol, *et al* 2011) Importantly, *DNMT3A* mutation is an independent poor prognostic factor. Further, *DNMT3A* mutation is rather stable during disease progression and can be a potential biomarker for monitoring of MRD.(Hou, *et al* 2011)

6. Gene mutations as markers to monitor Minimal Residual Disease (MRD)

Since gene mutations are theoretically absent in healthy people and restricted in leukemia cells, it is reasonably to monitor MRD by detection of gene mutations. This is an advantage of leukemia over solid tumors in that leukemia cells are indigenous to blood and marrow, which are easy for access. There are two critical considerations of MRD monitoring by gene mutations: one is the stability of the mutations, and the other is the pattern of mutation. An ideal MRD marker should be very consistent with disease status, while those that may disappear after disease evolution are not suitable for this purpose. Also, if the mutation appears as a point mutation, probably only qualitative rather than absolute quantitative measurement can be achieved because of inevitable background signals due to minimal sequence differences between wild-type and mutant alleles. Moreover, if the mutation occurs sporadically across the whole coding sequence without a hot spot, the absolute quantification techniques (usually fluorescence-based real-time PCR) would become very cumbersome.

Among the mutations in AML, *NPM1* mutation is perhaps the most useful and intensively studied marker of MRD because this mutation is quite stable, relatively prevalent, highly concentrated at a hot spot, and has 4 nucleotide insertion, which can be clearly discriminated from the wild-type allele in quantitative real-time PCR.(Chou, *et al* 2007, Schnittger, *et al* 2009) Studies have shown *NPM1* mutant levels reflect disease status, predict impending relapse, and bring prognostic implication.(Chou, *et al* 2007, Gorello, *et al* 2006, Kronke, *et al* 2011, Schnittger, *et al* 2009) Another stable marker is *IDH* mutation. *IDH1* and *IDH2* mutations are stable and highly consistent with disease status.(Chou, *et al* 2010a, Chou, *et al* 2011c) We have developed a single-tube, highly sensitive and specific PCR method to detect all *IDH1* mutations at R132 residue.(Chou, *et al* 2010c) However, the *IDH* mutation is not a good marker for MRD monitoring because the minimal difference between the point mutation and normal allele.

Other gene mutations are not readily applicable in MRD monitoring. *FLT3*-ITD is not stable. This mutation can disappear at disease relapse in a significant proportion of patients,(Chou, *et al* 2011b, Shih, *et al* 2002) although this length mutation can be readily and sensitively detected by GeneScan-based method.(Stirewalt and Radich 2003) *DNMT3A* mutation at R882, which occurs at a frequency of up to 60% of all *DNMT3A* mutation, can be a potential marker for qualitative assessment of MRD, but awaits for further testing.(Ley, *et al* 2010, Thol, *et al* 2011, Hou, *et al* 2011) *ASXL1* and *TET2* mutations do not have hot spots and are not stable during AML evolution. Other mutations have lower incidences and have not been well investigated in MRD monitoring.

7. Risk-adapted treatment according to gene mutations in AML patients

The ultimate goal of risk stratification according to molecular alterations is to explore personalized therapy, thereby reduce the risk of relapse and treatment-related side effects. How to integrate gene mutations into clinical management is a crucial issue. The choice between high-dose Cytarabine (HDAC) and allogeneic HSCT as the post-remission therapy is traditionally based on the cytogenetic risks and the patients' condition. The meta-analysis showed that allogeneic HSCT resulted in better clinical outcome in younger AML patients with intermediate- and unfavorable-risk cytogenetics in first CR.(Cornelissen, *et al* 2007, Koreth, *et al* 2009) Although allogeneic HSCT reduces the risk of relapse and is a curative approach for AML patients, the higher rate of transplantation related morbidity and mortality counterbalances its beneficial effect. Thus, allogeneic HSCT is currently recommended only in those patients with acceptable benefit-risk ratio. Given that AML is a heterogenous disease especially in intermediate-risk cytogenetics and CN-AML, increasing understanding of novel molecular genetic markers in AML leukemogenesis can further help to reassess the value of HSCT in different prognostic groups.

Recently, ELN proposed a new classification to stratify AML patients into different risk groups according to cytogenetics and genetic alterations.(Dohner, *et al* 2010) In addition to CBF AML, CN-AML with mutated *NPM1* without *FLT3*-ITD and those with mutated *CEBPA* are categorized as favorable-risk groups; the regimen using repetitive cycles of HDAC as postremission therapy is considered beneficial for this group of patients. Allogeneic HSCT in first CR is not beneficial for CN-AML patients with mutated *NPM1* without *FLT3*-ITD,(Schlenk, *et al* 2008) and probably neither for those with mutated *CEBPA*. Allogeneic HSCT is generally not considered in patients with CBF AML in first CR, but may be indicated in those who harbor *KIT* mutations because such patients did poorly with chemotherapy. For the patients with adverse-risk genotype (other than mutated *NPM1* without *FLT3*/ITD or mutated *CEBPA*), an allogeneic HSCT from a matched related donor or even unrelated donor in first CR is suggested.(Basara, *et al* 2009, Cornelissen, *et al* 2007, Slovak, *et al* 2000, Suciu, *et al* 2003, Tallman, *et al* 2007) Recent studies showed that allogeneic HSCT may be considered in patients with *FLT3*-ITD even if definite results of prospective trials are not available.(Bornhauser, *et al* 2007, Gale, *et al* 2005, Schlenk, *et al* 2008) Besides, allogeneic HSCT also ameliorates the poor survival impact of *RUNX1* mutations on AML patients.(Gaidzik, *et al* 2011, Tang, *et al* 2009) The treatment of choice for patients with other recently documented poor-risk mutations, such as *WT1*, *TET2* and *DNMT3A* mutations is currently unclear.

In addition to chemotherapy and transplantation, targeted therapies aiming to specific molecular pathway are evolving as an adjunctive treatment in AML patients. *FLT3*/ITD and *FLT3*/TKD occur in about 20-35% of AML patients. Since FLT3 is a receptor tyrosine kinase and promote cancer phenotypes, it is an ideal target for therapy. Several FLT3 inhibitors, such as sorafenib, PKC-412 (midostaurin), sunitinib, semaxanib, tandutinib, AC220, KW-2449, and CEP701 (lestaurtinib) have been used in clinical trials and some effects were noticed in relapse/refractory setting.(Levis, *et al* 2002, Metzelder, *et al* 2009, Stone, *et al* 2005, Zhang, *et al* 2008) An ongoing international intergroup trial (10603 RATIFY), incorporating midostaurin into induction, consolidation or maintenance setting is currently underway. All-trans retinoic acid in combination with chemotherapy was found to be beneficial for *NPM1*-mutated patients (Burnett, *et al* 2010); however this preliminary result was not confirmed by the other study done on younger patients.(Schlenk, *et al* 2009) Tyrosine kinase inhibitor, such as imatinib, might be of clinical value in treatment of patients with *KIT* mutations.(Kindler, *et al* 2004, Kindler, *et al* 2003, Kohl, *et al* 2005) Epigenetic modification through demethylation agent azacitidine or decitibine may play a role in the treatment of patients with *MLL* rearrangement,(Altucci and Minucci 2009) and those with genetic alterations relating to epigenetic changes, such as *TET2* mutations.(Itzykson, *et al* 2011) Besides, recent report demonstrated that inhibition of glutaminase preferentially killed *IDH1*-mutated glial cells, which were more dependent on glutaminolysis pathway to supply α-KG, so glutaminase itself could be a potential therapeutical target.(Seltzer, *et al* 2010) Eventually, it may be reasonable to use combinations of molecularly targeted therapies and chemotherapy to improve the clinical outcome in AML patients.

8. Acknowledgment

This work was partially sponsored by grants from the National Science Council (NSC 97-2314-B002-015-MY3, 98-2314-B-002-033-MY3, 100-2325-B-002-032, 100-2325-B-002-033 and 100-2628-B-002-003-MY3), National Health Research Institute (NHRI-EX97-9731BI),

Department of Health (DOH100-TD-C-111-001), and Department of Medical Research (NTUH.99P14), National Taiwan University Hospital, Taiwan, Republic of China

9. References

Abbas, S., et al. (2010) Acquired mutations in the genes encoding IDH1 and IDH2 both are recurrent aberrations in acute myeloid leukemia: prevalence and prognostic value. *Blood,* 116, 2122-2126.

Abdel-Wahab, O., et al. (2010) Genetic analysis of transforming events that convert chronic myeloproliferative neoplasms to leukemias. *Cancer Res,* 70, 447-452.

Altucci, L. & Minucci, S. (2009) Epigenetic therapies in haematological malignancies: searching for true targets. *Eur J Cancer,* 45, 1137-1145.

Bacher, U., et al. (2006) Implications of NRAS mutations in AML: a study of 2502 patients. *Blood,* 107, 3847-3853.

Bacher, U., et al. (2008) Prognostic relevance of FLT3-TKD mutations in AML: the combination matters--an analysis of 3082 patients. *Blood,* 111, 2527-2537.

Bacher, U., et al. (2010) Mutations of the TET2 and CBL genes: novel molecular markers in myeloid malignancies. *Ann Hematol,* 89, 643-652.

Baird, P.N. & Simmons, P.J. (1997) Expression of the Wilms' tumor gene (WT1) in normal hemopoiesis. *Exp Hematol,* 25, 312-320.

Barjesteh van Waalwijk van Doorn-Khosrovani, S., et al. (2003) Biallelic mutations in the CEBPA gene and low CEBPA expression levels as prognostic markers in intermediate-risk AML. *Hematol J,* 4, 31-40.

Basara, N., et al. (2009) Early related or unrelated haematopoietic cell transplantation results in higher overall survival and leukaemia-free survival compared with conventional chemotherapy in high-risk acute myeloid leukaemia patients in first complete remission. *Leukemia,* 23, 635-640.

Baxter, E.J., et al. (2005) Acquired mutation of the tyrosine kinase JAK2 in human myeloproliferative disorders. *Lancet,* 365, 1054-1061.

Baylin, S.B. & Ohm, J.E. (2006) Epigenetic gene silencing in cancer - a mechanism for early oncogenic pathway addiction? *Nat Rev Cancer,* 6, 107-116.

Beghini, A., et al. (2000) C-kit mutations in core binding factor leukemias. *Blood,* 95, 726-727.

Beghini, A., et al. (2004) KIT activating mutations: incidence in adult and pediatric acute myeloid leukemia, and identification of an internal tandem duplication. *Haematologica,* 89, 920-925.

Bergmann, L., et al. (1997) High levels of Wilms' tumor gene (wt1) mRNA in acute myeloid leukemias are associated with a worse long-term outcome. *Blood,* 90, 1217-1225.

Bienz, M., et al. (2005) Risk assessment in patients with acute myeloid leukemia and a normal karyotype. *Clin Cancer Res,* 11, 1416-1424.

Blume-Jensen, P. & Hunter, T. (2001) Oncogenic kinase signalling. *Nature,* 411, 355-365.

Boissel, N., et al. (2005) Prevalence, clinical profile, and prognosis of NPM mutations in AML with normal karyotype. *Blood,* 106, 3618-3620.

Boissel, N., et al. (2006) Incidence and prognostic impact of c-Kit, FLT3, and Ras gene mutations in core binding factor acute myeloid leukemia (CBF-AML). *Leukemia,* 20, 965-970.

Boissel, N., et al. (2010) Prognostic impact of isocitrate dehydrogenase enzyme isoforms 1 and 2 mutations in acute myeloid leukemia: a study by the Acute Leukemia French Association group. *J Clin Oncol,* 28, 3717-3723.

Bornhauser, M., et al. (2007) Improved outcome after stem-cell transplantation in FLT3/ITD-positive AML. *Blood,* 109, 2264-2265; author reply 2265.

Bos, J.L., et al. (1987) Mutations in N-ras predominate in acute myeloid leukemia. *Blood,* 69, 1237-1241.

Bos, J.L. (1989) ras oncogenes in human cancer: a review. *Cancer Res,* 49, 4682-4689.

Boultwood, J., et al. (2010) Frequent mutation of the polycomb-associated gene ASXL1 in the myelodysplastic syndromes and in acute myeloid leukemia. *Leukemia,* 24, 1062-1065.

Bowen, D.T., et al. (2005) RAS mutation in acute myeloid leukemia is associated with distinct cytogenetic subgroups but does not influence outcome in patients younger than 60 years. *Blood,* 106, 2113-2119.

Burnett, A.K., et al. (2010) The impact on outcome of the addition of all-trans retinoic acid to intensive chemotherapy in younger patients with nonacute promyelocytic acute myeloid leukemia: overall results and results in genotypic subgroups defined by mutations in NPM1, FLT3, and CEBPA. *Blood,* 115, 948-956.

Caligiuri, M.A., et al. (1994) Molecular rearrangement of the ALL-1 gene in acute myeloid leukemia without cytogenetic evidence of 11q23 chromosomal translocations. *Cancer Res,* 54, 370-373.

Cammenga, J., et al. (2003) Induction of C/EBPalpha activity alters gene expression and differentiation of human CD34+ cells. *Blood,* 101, 2206-2214.

Carbuccia, N., et al. (2009) Mutations of ASXL1 gene in myeloproliferative neoplasms. *Leukemia,* 23, 2183-2186.

Carbuccia, N., et al. (2010) Mutual exclusion of ASXL1 and NPM1 mutations in a series of acute myeloid leukemias. *Leukemia,* 24, 469-473.

Care, R.S., et al. (2003) Incidence and prognosis of c-KIT and FLT3 mutations in core binding factor (CBF) acute myeloid leukaemias. *Br J Haematol,* 121, 775-777.

Chen, C.Y., et al. (2006) Acquisition of JAK2, PTPN11, and RAS mutations during disease progression in primary myelodysplastic syndrome. *Leukemia,* 20, 1155-1158.

Chen, J., et al. (2010) Leukaemogenesis: more than mutant genes. *Nat Rev Cancer,* 10, 23-36.

Chou, W.C., et al. (2006) Nucleophosmin mutations in de novo acute myeloid leukemia: the age-dependent incidences and the stability during disease evolution. *Cancer Res,* 66, 3310-3316.

Chou, W.C., et al. (2007) Clinical implications of minimal residual disease monitoring by quantitative polymerase chain reaction in acute myeloid leukemia patients bearing nucleophosmin (NPM1) mutations. *Leukemia,* 21, 998-1004.

Chou, W.C., et al. (2010a) Distinct clinical and biologic characteristics in adult acute myeloid leukemia bearing the isocitrate dehydrogenase 1 mutation. *Blood,* 115, 2749-2754.

Chou, W.C., et al. (2010b) Distinct clinical and biological features of de novo acute myeloid leukemia with additional sex comb-like 1 (ASXL1) mutations. *Blood,* 116, 4086-4094.

Chou, W.C., et al. (2010c) A single-tube, sensitive multiplex method for screening of isocitrate dehydrogenase 1 (IDH1) mutations. *Blood,* 116, 495-496.

Chou, W.C., et al. (2011a) TET2 mutation is an unfavorable prognostic factor in acute myeloid leukemia patients with intermediate-risk cytogenetics. *Blood.*

Chou, W.C., et al. (2011b) Sensitive measurement of quantity dynamics of FLT3 internal tandem duplication at early time points provides prognostic information. *Ann Oncol*, 22, 696-704.

Chou, W.C., et al. (2011c) The prognostic impact and stability of Isocitrate dehydrogenase 2 mutation in adult patients with acute myeloid leukemia. *Leukemia*, 25, 246-253.

Coghlan, D.W., et al. (1994) The incidence and prognostic significance of mutations in codon 13 of the N-ras gene in acute myeloid leukemia. *Leukemia*, 8, 1682-1687.

Cornelissen, J.J., et al. (2007) Results of a HOVON/SAKK donor versus no-donor analysis of myeloablative HLA-identical sibling stem cell transplantation in first remission acute myeloid leukemia in young and middle-aged adults: benefits for whom? *Blood*, 109, 3658-3666.

Couronne, L., et al. (2010) Analyses of TET2 mutations in post-myeloproliferative neoplasm acute myeloid leukemias. *Leukemia*, 24, 201-203.

Dang, L., et al. (2009) Cancer-associated IDH1 mutations produce 2-hydroxyglutarate. *Nature*, 462, 739-744.

Dange, M. & Colman, R.F. (2010) Each conserved active site Tyr in the three subunits of human isocitrate dehydrogenase has a different function. *J Biol Chem*.

De Melo, M.B., et al. (1997) N-ras gene point mutations in Brazilian acute myelogenous leukemia patients correlate with a poor prognosis. *Leuk Lymphoma*, 24, 309-317.

Delhommeau, F., et al. (2009) Mutation in TET2 in myeloid cancers. *N Engl J Med*, 360, 2289-2301.

Dicker, F., et al. (2007) Trisomy 13 is strongly associated with AML1/RUNX1 mutations and increased FLT3 expression in acute myeloid leukemia. *Blood*, 110, 1308-1316.

Dimartino, J.F. & Cleary, M.L. (1999) Mll rearrangements in haematological malignancies: lessons from clinical and biological studies. *Br J Haematol*, 106, 614-626.

Dohner, H., et al. (2010) Diagnosis and management of acute myeloid leukemia in adults: recommendations from an international expert panel, on behalf of the European LeukemiaNet. *Blood*, 115, 453-474.

Dohner, K., et al. (2002) Prognostic significance of partial tandem duplications of the MLL gene in adult patients 16 to 60 years old with acute myeloid leukemia and normal cytogenetics: a study of the Acute Myeloid Leukemia Study Group Ulm. *J Clin Oncol*, 20, 3254-3261.

Dohner, K., et al. (2005) Mutant nucleophosmin (NPM1) predicts favorable prognosis in younger adults with acute myeloid leukemia and normal cytogenetics: interaction with other gene mutations. *Blood*, 106, 3740-3746.

Downward, J. (2003) Targeting RAS signalling pathways in cancer therapy. *Nat Rev Cancer*, 3, 11-22.

Dufour, A., et al. (2010) Acute myeloid leukemia with biallelic CEBPA gene mutations and normal karyotype represents a distinct genetic entity associated with a favorable clinical outcome. *J Clin Oncol*, 28, 570-577.

Ellisen, L.W., et al. (2001) The Wilms tumor suppressor WT1 directs stage-specific quiescence and differentiation of human hematopoietic progenitor cells. *Embo J*, 20, 1897-1909.

Falini, B., et al. (2005) Cytoplasmic nucleophosmin in acute myelogenous leukemia with a normal karyotype. *N Engl J Med*, 352, 254-266.

Falini, B., et al. (2011) Acute myeloid leukemia with mutated nucleophosmin (NPM1): is it a distinct entity? *Blood*, 117, 1109-1120.

Farr, C.J., et al. (1988) Analysis of RAS gene mutations in acute myeloid leukemia by polymerase chain reaction and oligonucleotide probes. *Proc Natl Acad Sci U S A,* 85, 1629-1633.

Figueroa, M.E., et al. (2010) Leukemic IDH1 and IDH2 mutations result in a hypermethylation phenotype, disrupt TET2 function, and impair hematopoietic differentiation. *Cancer Cell,* 18, 553-567.

Fisher, C.L., et al. (2003) A human homolog of Additional sex combs, ADDITIONAL SEX COMBS-LIKE 1, maps to chromosome 20q11. *Gene,* 306, 115-126.

Fisher, C.L., et al. (2006) Characterization of Asxl1, a murine homolog of Additional sex combs, and analysis of the Asx-like gene family. *Gene,* 369, 109-118.

Flach, J., et al. (2010) Mutations of JAK2 and TET2, but not CBL are detectable in a high portion of patients with refractory anemia with ring sideroblasts and thrombocytosis. *Haematologica,* 95, 518-519.

Friedman, A.D. (2009) Cell cycle and developmental control of hematopoiesis by Runx1. *J Cell Physiol,* 219, 520-524.

Friedman, A.D. & McKnight, S.L. (1990) Identification of two polypeptide segments of CCAAT/enhancer-binding protein required for transcriptional activation of the serum albumin gene. *Genes Dev,* 4, 1416-1426.

Frohling, S., et al. (2004) CEBPA mutations in younger adults with acute myeloid leukemia and normal cytogenetics: prognostic relevance and analysis of cooperating mutations. *J Clin Oncol,* 22, 624-633.

Frohling, S., et al. (2005) Genetics of myeloid malignancies: pathogenetic and clinical implications. *J Clin Oncol,* 23, 6285-6295.

Frohling, S., et al. (2006) Rare occurrence of the JAK2 V617F mutation in AML subtypes M5, M6, and M7. *Blood,* 107, 1242-1243.

Gaidzik, V.I., et al. (2009) Prognostic impact of WT1 mutations in cytogenetically normal acute myeloid leukemia: a study of the German-Austrian AML Study Group. *Blood,* 113, 4505-4511.

Gaidzik, V.I., et al. (2011) RUNX1 mutations in acute myeloid leukemia: results from a comprehensive genetic and clinical analysis from the AML study group. *J Clin Oncol,* 29, 1364-1372.

Gale, R.E., et al. (2005) No evidence that FLT3 status should be considered as an indicator for transplantation in acute myeloid leukemia (AML): an analysis of 1135 patients, excluding acute promyelocytic leukemia, from the UK MRC AML10 and 12 trials. *Blood,* 106, 3658-3665.

Gale, R.E., et al. (2008) The impact of FLT3 internal tandem duplication mutant level, number, size, and interaction with NPM1 mutations in a large cohort of young adult patients with acute myeloid leukemia. *Blood,* 111, 2776-2784.

Gelsi-Boyer, V., et al. (2009) Mutations of polycomb-associated gene ASXL1 in myelodysplastic syndromes and chronic myelomonocytic leukaemia. *Br J Haematol,* 145, 788-800.

Gilliland, D.G. (2002) Molecular genetics of human leukemias: new insights into therapy. *Semin Hematol,* 39, 6-11.

Goldman, J.M. (2005) A unifying mutation in chronic myeloproliferative disorders. *N Engl J Med,* 352, 1744-1746.

Gorello, P., et al. (2006) Quantitative assessment of minimal residual disease in acute myeloid leukemia carrying nucleophosmin (NPM1) gene mutations. *Leukemia,* 20, 1103-1108.

Green, C.L., et al. (2010) The prognostic significance of IDH1 mutations in younger adult patients with acute myeloid leukemia is dependent on FLT3/ITD status. *Blood,* 116, 2779-2782.

Haber, D.A., et al. (1990) An internal deletion within an 11p13 zinc finger gene contributes to the development of Wilms' tumor. *Cell,* 61, 1257-1269.

Harada, H., et al. (2004) High incidence of somatic mutations in the AML1/RUNX1 gene in myelodysplastic syndrome and low blast percentage myeloid leukemia with myelodysplasia. *Blood,* 103, 2316-2324.

Hou, H.A., et al. (2008) Characterization of acute myeloid leukemia with PTPN11 mutation: the mutation is closely associated with NPM1 mutation but inversely related to FLT3/ITD. *Leukemia,* 22, 1075-1078.

Hou, H.A., et al. (2009) Reply to 'Heterogeneity within AML with CEBPA mutations; only CEBPA double mutations, but not single CEBPA mutations are associated with favorable prognosis'. *Br J Cancer,* 101, 738-740.

Hou, H.A., et al. (2010) WT1 mutation in 470 adult patients with acute myeloid leukemia: stability during disease evolution and implication of its incorporation into a survival scoring system. *Blood,* 115, 5222-5231.

Hou, H.A., et al. (2011) DNMT3A Mutations in Acute Myeloid Leukemia-Stability during Disease Evolution and the Clinical Implication. *Blood, in revision.*

Ikeda, H., et al. (1991) Expression and functional role of the proto-oncogene c-kit in acute myeloblastic leukemia cells. *Blood,* 78, 2962-2968.

Illmer, T., et al. (2007) Tyrosine kinase mutations of JAK2 are rare events in AML but influence prognosis of patients with CBF-leukemias. *Haematologica,* 92, 137-138.

Ito, S., et al. (2010) Role of Tet proteins in 5mC to 5hmC conversion, ES-cell self-renewal and inner cell mass specification. *Nature,* 466, 1129-1133.

Ito, Y. (2008) RUNX genes in development and cancer: regulation of viral gene expression and the discovery of RUNX family genes. *Adv Cancer Res,* 99, 33-76.

Itzykson, R., et al. (2011) Impact of TET2 mutations on response rate to azacitidine in myelodysplastic syndromes and low blast count acute myeloid leukemias. *Leukemia,* 25, 1147-1152.

Jankowska, A.M., et al. (2009) Loss of heterozygosity 4q24 and TET2 mutations associated with myelodysplastic/myeloproliferative neoplasms. *Blood,* 113, 6403-6410.

Jones, P.A. & Baylin, S.B. (2002) The fundamental role of epigenetic events in cancer. *Nat Rev Genet,* 3, 415-428.

Kindler, T., et al. (2003) Sustained complete hematologic remission after administration of the tyrosine kinase inhibitor imatinib mesylate in a patient with refractory, secondary AML. *Blood,* 101, 2960-2962.

Kindler, T., et al. (2004) Efficacy and safety of imatinib in adult patients with c-kit-positive acute myeloid leukemia. *Blood,* 103, 3644-3654.

King-Underwood, L., et al. (1996) Mutations in the Wilms' tumor gene WT1 in leukemias. *Blood,* 87, 2171-2179.

Kiyoi, H., et al. (1998) Internal tandem duplication of the FLT3 gene is a novel modality of elongation mutation which causes constitutive activation of the product. *Leukemia,* 12, 1333-1337.

Kiyoi, H., et al. (1999) Prognostic implication of FLT3 and N-RAS gene mutations in acute myeloid leukemia. *Blood,* 93, 3074-3080.

Kohl, T.M., et al. (2005) KIT exon 8 mutations associated with core-binding factor (CBF)-acute myeloid leukemia (AML) cause hyperactivation of the receptor in response to stem cell factor. *Blood,* 105, 3319-3321.

Koreth, J., et al. (2009) Allogeneic stem cell transplantation for acute myeloid leukemia in first complete remission: systematic review and meta-analysis of prospective clinical trials. *JAMA,* 301, 2349-2361.

Koschmieder, S., et al. (2009) Dysregulation of the C/EBPalpha differentiation pathway in human cancer. *J Clin Oncol,* 27, 619-628.

Kosmider, O., et al. (2009a) TET2 mutation is an independent favorable prognostic factor in myelodysplastic syndromes (MDSs). *Blood,* 114, 3285-3291.

Kosmider, O., et al. (2009b) TET2 gene mutation is a frequent and adverse event in chronic myelomonocytic leukemia. *Haematologica,* 94, 1676-1681.

Kosmider, O., et al. (2010) Mutations of IDH1 and IDH2 genes in early and accelerated phases of myelodysplastic syndromes and MDS/myeloproliferative neoplasms. *Leukemia,* 24, 1094-1096.

Kottaridis, P.D., et al. (2001) The presence of a FLT3 internal tandem duplication in patients with acute myeloid leukemia (AML) adds important prognostic information to cytogenetic risk group and response to the first cycle of chemotherapy: analysis of 854 patients from the United Kingdom Medical Research Council AML 10 and 12 trials. *Blood,* 98, 1752-1759.

Kottaridis, P.D., et al. (2002) Studies of FLT3 mutations in paired presentation and relapse samples from patients with acute myeloid leukemia: implications for the role of FLT3 mutations in leukemogenesis, minimal residual disease detection, and possible therapy with FLT3 inhibitors. *Blood,* 100, 2393-2398.

Kralovics, R., et al. (2005) A gain-of-function mutation of JAK2 in myeloproliferative disorders. *N Engl J Med,* 352, 1779-1790.

Kronke, J., et al. (2011) Monitoring of Minimal Residual Disease in NPM1-Mutated Acute Myeloid Leukemia: A Study From the German-Austrian Acute Myeloid Leukemia Study Group. *J Clin Oncol,* 29, 2709-2716.

Langemeijer, S.M., et al. (2009) Acquired mutations in TET2 are common in myelodysplastic syndromes. *Nat Genet,* 41, 838-842.

Lee, J.W., et al. (2006) The JAK2 V617F mutation in de novo acute myelogenous leukemias. *Oncogene,* 25, 1434-1436.

Levine, R.L., et al. (2005a) The JAK2V617F activating mutation occurs in chronic myelomonocytic leukemia and acute myeloid leukemia, but not in acute lymphoblastic leukemia or chronic lymphocytic leukemia. *Blood,* 106, 3377-3379.

Levine, R.L., et al. (2005b) Activating mutation in the tyrosine kinase JAK2 in polycythemia vera, essential thrombocythemia, and myeloid metaplasia with myelofibrosis. *Cancer Cell,* 7, 387-397.

Levis, M., et al. (2002) A FLT3-targeted tyrosine kinase inhibitor is cytotoxic to leukemia cells in vitro and in vivo. *Blood,* 99, 3885-3891.

Ley, T.J., et al. (2010) DNMT3A mutations in acute myeloid leukemia. *N Engl J Med,* 363, 2424-2433.

Lin, F.T., et al. (1993) A 30-kDa alternative translation product of the CCAAT/enhancer binding protein alpha message: transcriptional activator lacking antimitotic activity. *Proc Natl Acad Sci U S A*, 90, 9606-9610.

Lin, L.I., et al. (2005) Characterization of CEBPA mutations in acute myeloid leukemia: most patients with CEBPA mutations have biallelic mutations and show a distinct immunophenotype of the leukemic cells. *Clin Cancer Res*, 11, 1372-1379.

Liu, R.Y., et al. (1999) Constitutive activation of the JAK2/STAT5 signal transduction pathway correlates with growth factor independence of megakaryocytic leukemic cell lines. *Blood*, 93, 2369-2379.

Loh, M.L., et al. (2004a) PTPN11 mutations in pediatric patients with acute myeloid leukemia: results from the Children's Cancer Group. *Leukemia*, 18, 1831-1834.

Loh, M.L., et al. (2004b) Mutations in PTPN11 implicate the SHP-2 phosphatase in leukemogenesis. *Blood*, 103, 2325-2331.

Marcucci, G., et al. (2010) IDH1 and IDH2 gene mutations identify novel molecular subsets within de novo cytogenetically normal acute myeloid leukemia: a Cancer and Leukemia Group B study. *J Clin Oncol*, 28, 2348-2355.

Mardis, E.R., et al. (2009) Recurring mutations found by sequencing an acute myeloid leukemia genome. *N Engl J Med*, 361, 1058-1066.

Meshinchi, S., et al. (2003) Activating mutations of RTK/ras signal transduction pathway in pediatric acute myeloid leukemia. *Blood*, 102, 1474-1479.

Metzelder, S., et al. (2009) Compassionate use of sorafenib in FLT3-ITD-positive acute myeloid leukemia: sustained regression before and after allogeneic stem cell transplantation. *Blood*, 113, 6567-6571.

Metzeler, K.H., et al. (2011) TET2 mutations improve the new European LeukemiaNet risk classification of acute myeloid leukemia: a Cancer and Leukemia Group B study. *J Clin Oncol*, 29, 1373-1381.

Michaud, J., et al. (2002) In vitro analyses of known and novel RUNX1/AML1 mutations in dominant familial platelet disorder with predisposition to acute myelogenous leukemia: implications for mechanisms of pathogenesis. *Blood*, 99, 1364-1372.

Miwa, H., et al. (1992) Expression of the Wilms' tumor gene (WT1) in human leukemias. *Leukemia*, 6, 405-409.

Munoz, L., et al. (2003) Acute myeloid leukemia with MLL rearrangements: clinicobiological features, prognostic impact and value of flow cytometry in the detection of residual leukemic cells. *Leukemia*, 17, 76-82.

Nakao, M., et al. (1996) Internal tandem duplication of the flt3 gene found in acute myeloid leukemia. *Leukemia*, 10, 1911-1918.

Neel, B.G., et al. (2003) The 'Shp'ing news: SH2 domain-containing tyrosine phosphatases in cell signaling. *Trends Biochem Sci*, 28, 284-293.

Neubauer, A., et al. (1994) Prognostic importance of mutations in the ras proto-oncogenes in de novo acute myeloid leukemia. *Blood*, 83, 1603-1611.

Neubauer, A., et al. (2008) Patients with acute myeloid leukemia and RAS mutations benefit most from postremission high-dose cytarabine: a Cancer and Leukemia Group B study. *J Clin Oncol*, 26, 4603-4609.

Niebuhr, B., et al. (2008) Gatekeeper function of the RUNX1 transcription factor in acute leukemia. *Blood Cells Mol Dis*, 40, 211-218.

Niimi, H., et al. (2006) Hyperactivation of the RAS signaling pathway in myelodysplastic syndrome with AML1/RUNX1 point mutations. *Leukemia*, 20, 635-644.

Oelgeschlager, M., et al. (1996) C/EBP, c-Myb, and PU.1 cooperate to regulate the neutrophil elastase promoter. *Mol Cell Biol,* 16, 4717-4725.

Osato, M. (2004) Point mutations in the RUNX1/AML1 gene: another actor in RUNX leukemia. *Oncogene,* 23, 4284-4296.

Pabst, T., et al. (2001a) AML1-ETO downregulates the granulocytic differentiation factor C/EBPalpha in t(8;21) myeloid leukemia. *Nat Med,* 7, 444-451.

Pabst, T., et al. (2001b) Dominant-negative mutations of CEBPA, encoding CCAAT/enhancer binding protein-alpha (C/EBPalpha), in acute myeloid leukemia. *Nat Genet,* 27, 263-270.

Pabst, T., et al. (2009) Heterogeneity within AML with CEBPA mutations; only CEBPA double mutations, but not single CEBPA mutations are associated with favourable prognosis. *Br J Cancer,* 100, 1343-1346.

Palmisano, M., et al. (2007) NPM1 mutations are more stable than FLT3 mutations during the course of disease in patients with acute myeloid leukemia. *Haematologica,* 92, 1268-1269.

Pardanani, A., et al. (2010) IDH1 and IDH2 mutation analysis in chronic- and blast-phase myeloproliferative neoplasms. *Leukemia,* 24, 1146-1151.

Parsons, D.W., et al. (2008) An integrated genomic analysis of human glioblastoma multiforme. *Science,* 321, 1807-1812.

Paschka, P., et al. (2008) Wilms' tumor 1 gene mutations independently predict poor outcome in adults with cytogenetically normal acute myeloid leukemia: a cancer and leukemia group B study. *J Clin Oncol,* 26, 4595-4602.

Pena, P.V., et al. (2006) Molecular mechanism of histone H3K4me3 recognition by plant homeodomain of ING2. *Nature,* 442, 100-103.

Preudhomme, C., et al. (2000) High incidence of biallelic point mutations in the Runt domain of the AML1/PEBP2 alpha B gene in Mo acute myeloid leukemia and in myeloid malignancies with acquired trisomy 21. *Blood,* 96, 2862-2869.

Preudhomme, C., et al. (2002) Favorable prognostic significance of CEBPA mutations in patients with de novo acute myeloid leukemia: a study from the Acute Leukemia French Association (ALFA). *Blood,* 100, 2717-2723.

Radich, J.P., et al. (1990) N-ras mutations in adult de novo acute myelogenous leukemia: prevalence and clinical significance. *Blood,* 76, 801-807.

Rege-Cambrin, G., et al. (2005) Trisomy 11 in myeloid malignancies is associated with internal tandem duplication of both MLL and FLT3 genes. *Haematologica,* 90, 262-264.

Reitman, Z.J., et al. (2010) IDH1 and IDH2: not your typical oncogenes. *Cancer Cell,* 17, 215-216.

Renneville, A., et al. (2009a) The favorable impact of CEBPA mutations in patients with acute myeloid leukemia is only observed in the absence of associated cytogenetic abnormalities and FLT3 internal duplication. *Blood,* 113, 5090-5093.

Renneville, A., et al. (2009b) Wilms tumor 1 gene mutations are associated with a higher risk of recurrence in young adults with acute myeloid leukemia: a study from the Acute Leukemia French Association. *Cancer,* 115, 3719-3727.

Reuss-Borst, M.A., et al. (1994) AML: immunophenotypic heterogeneity and prognostic significance of c-kit expression. *Leukemia,* 8, 258-263.

Reuther, G.W. & Der, C.J. (2000) The Ras branch of small GTPases: Ras family members don't fall far from the tree. *Curr Opin Cell Biol,* 12, 157-165.

Ritter, M., et al. (2004) Prognostic significance of N-RAS and K-RAS mutations in 232 patients with acute myeloid leukemia. *Haematologica,* 89, 1397-1399.

Saint-Martin, C., et al. (2009) Analysis of the ten-eleven translocation 2 (TET2) gene in familial myeloproliferative neoplasms. *Blood,* 114, 1628-1632.

Santamaria, C.M., et al. (2009) Molecular stratification model for prognosis in cytogenetically normal acute myeloid leukemia. *Blood,* 114, 148-152.

Schaub, F.X., et al. (2010) Clonal analysis of TET2 and JAK2 mutations suggests that TET2 can be a late event in the progression of myeloproliferative neoplasms. *Blood,* 115, 2003-2007.

Schichman, S.A., et al. (1994) ALL-1 partial duplication in acute leukemia. *Proc Natl Acad Sci U S A,* 91, 6236-6239.

Schichman, S.A., et al. (1995) Self-fusion of the ALL1 gene. A new genetic mechanism for acute leukemia. *JAMA,* 273, 571-576.

Schlenk, R.F., et al. (2008) Mutations and treatment outcome in cytogenetically normal acute myeloid leukemia. *N Engl J Med,* 358, 1909-1918.

Schlenk, R.F., et al. (2009) Gene mutations and response to treatment with all-trans retinoic acid in elderly patients with acute myeloid leukemia. Results from the AMLSG Trial AML HD98B. *Haematologica,* 94, 54-60.

Schnittger, S., et al. (2000) Screening for MLL tandem duplication in 387 unselected patients with AML identify a prognostically unfavorable subset of AML. *Leukemia,* 14, 796-804.

Schnittger, S., et al. (2005) Nucleophosmin gene mutations are predictors of favorable prognosis in acute myelogenous leukemia with a normal karyotype. *Blood,* 106, 3733-3739.

Schnittger, S., et al. (2006) KIT-D816 mutations in AML1-ETO-positive AML are associated with impaired event-free and overall survival. *Blood,* 107, 1791-1799.

Schnittger, S., et al. (2009) Minimal residual disease levels assessed by NPM1 mutation-specific RQ-PCR provide important prognostic information in AML. *Blood,* 114, 2220-2231.

Schnittger, S., et al. (2011) RUNX1 mutations are frequent in de novo AML with noncomplex karyotype and confer an unfavorable prognosis. *Blood,* 117, 2348-2357.

Seltzer, M.J., et al. (2010) Inhibition of glutaminase preferentially slows growth of glioma cells with mutant IDH1. *Cancer Res,* 70, 8981-8987.

Senn, H.P., et al. (1988) Mutation analysis of the N-ras proto-oncogene in active and remission phase of human acute leukemias. *Int J Cancer,* 41, 59-64.

Shi, X., et al. (2006) ING2 PHD domain links histone H3 lysine 4 methylation to active gene repression. *Nature,* 442, 96-99.

Shiah, H.S., et al. (2002) Clinical and biological implications of partial tandem duplication of the MLL gene in acute myeloid leukemia without chromosomal abnormalities at 11q23. *Leukemia,* 16, 196-202.

Shields, J.M., et al. (2000) Understanding Ras: 'it ain't over 'til it's over'. *Trends Cell Biol,* 10, 147-154.

Shih, L.Y., et al. (2002) Internal tandem duplication of FLT3 in relapsed acute myeloid leukemia: a comparative analysis of bone marrow samples from 108 adult patients at diagnosis and relapse. *Blood,* 100, 2387-2392.

Slovak, M.L., et al. (2000) Karyotypic analysis predicts outcome of preremission and postremission therapy in adult acute myeloid leukemia: a Southwest Oncology Group/Eastern Cooperative Oncology Group Study. *Blood,* 96, 4075-4083.

Smith, A.E., et al. (2010) Next-generation sequencing of the TET2 gene in 355 MDS and CMML patients reveals low-abundance mutant clones with early origins, but indicates no definite prognostic value. *Blood,* 116, 3923-3932.

Smith, L.T., et al. (1996) PU.1 (Spi-1) and C/EBP alpha regulate the granulocyte colony-stimulating factor receptor promoter in myeloid cells. *Blood,* 88, 1234-1247.

Stirewalt, D.L. & Radich, J.P. (2003) The role of FLT3 in haematopoietic malignancies. *Nat Rev Cancer,* 3, 650-665.

Stone, R.M., et al. (2005) Patients with acute myeloid leukemia and an activating mutation in FLT3 respond to a small-molecule FLT3 tyrosine kinase inhibitor, PKC412. *Blood,* 105, 54-60.

Suciu, S., et al. (2003) Allogeneic compared with autologous stem cell transplantation in the treatment of patients younger than 46 years with acute myeloid leukemia (AML) in first complete remission (CR1): an intention-to-treat analysis of the EORTC/GIMEMAAML-10 trial. *Blood,* 102, 1232-1240.

Suzuki, T., et al. (2005) Clinical characteristics and prognostic implications of NPM1 mutations in acute myeloid leukemia. *Blood,* 106, 2854-2861.

Tallman, M.S., et al. (2007) Impact of cytogenetics on outcome of matched unrelated donor hematopoietic stem cell transplantation for acute myeloid leukemia in first or second complete remission. *Blood,* 110, 409-417.

Tang, J.L., et al. (2009) AML1/RUNX1 mutations in 470 adult patients with de novo acute myeloid leukemia: prognostic implication and interaction with other gene alterations. *Blood,* 114, 5352-5361.

Tartaglia, M., et al. (2001) Mutations in PTPN11, encoding the protein tyrosine phosphatase SHP-2, cause Noonan syndrome. *Nat Genet,* 29, 465-468.

Tartaglia, M., et al. (2002) PTPN11 mutations in Noonan syndrome: molecular spectrum, genotype-phenotype correlation, and phenotypic heterogeneity. *Am J Hum Genet,* 70, 1555-1563.

Tartaglia, M., et al. (2003) Somatic mutations in PTPN11 in juvenile myelomonocytic leukemia, myelodysplastic syndromes and acute myeloid leukemia. *Nat Genet,* 34, 148-150.

Tartaglia, M., et al. (2004) SHP-2 and myeloid malignancies. *Curr Opin Hematol,* 11, 44-50.

Tartaglia, M., et al. (2005) Somatic PTPN11 mutations in childhood acute myeloid leukaemia. *Br J Haematol,* 129, 333-339.

Tefferi, A., et al. (2009a) Detection of mutant TET2 in myeloid malignancies other than myeloproliferative neoplasms: CMML, MDS, MDS/MPN and AML. *Leukemia,* 23, 1343-1345.

Tefferi, A., et al. (2009b) Mutation in TET2 in myeloid cancers. *N Engl J Med,* 361, 1117; author reply 1117-1118.

Thiede, C., et al. (2006) Prevalence and prognostic impact of NPM1 mutations in 1485 adult patients with acute myeloid leukemia (AML). *Blood,* 107, 4011-4020.

Thol, F., et al. (2010) Prognostic impact of IDH2 mutations in cytogenetically normal acute myeloid leukemia. *Blood,* 116, 614-616.

Thol, F., et al. (2011) Incidence and Prognostic Influence of DNMT3A Mutations in Acute Myeloid Leukemia. *J Clin Oncol.*

Tiesmeier, J., et al. (2003) Evidence for allelic evolution of C/EBPalpha mutations in acute myeloid leukaemia. *Br J Haematol,* 123, 413-419.

Toksoz, D., et al. (1989) Ras genes and acute myeloid leukaemia. *Br J Haematol,* 71, 1-6.

Verhaak, R.G., et al. (2005) Mutations in nucleophosmin (NPM1) in acute myeloid leukemia (AML): association with other gene abnormalities and previously established gene expression signatures and their favorable prognostic significance. *Blood,* 106, 3747-3754.

Virappane, P., et al. (2008) Mutation of the Wilms' tumor 1 gene is a poor prognostic factor associated with chemotherapy resistance in normal karyotype acute myeloid leukemia: the United Kingdom Medical Research Council Adult Leukaemia Working Party. *J Clin Oncol,* 26, 5429-5435.

Walz, C., et al. (2006) Activated Jak2 with the V617F point mutation promotes G1/S phase transition. *J Biol Chem,* 281, 18177-18183.

Wang, J., et al. (2009) The lysine demethylase LSD1 (KDM1) is required for maintenance of global DNA methylation. *Nat Genet,* 41, 125-129.

Ward, P.S., et al. (2010) The common feature of leukemia-associated IDH1 and IDH2 mutations is a neomorphic enzyme activity converting alpha-ketoglutarate to 2-hydroxyglutarate. *Cancer Cell,* 17, 225-234.

Whitman, S.P., et al. (2005) The MLL partial tandem duplication: evidence for recessive gain-of-function in acute myeloid leukemia identifies a novel patient subgroup for molecular-targeted therapy. *Blood,* 106, 345-352.

Whitman, S.P., et al. (2007) Long-term disease-free survivors with cytogenetically normal acute myeloid leukemia and MLL partial tandem duplication: a Cancer and Leukemia Group B study. *Blood,* 109, 5164-5167.

Whitman, S.P., et al. (2008) FLT3 D835/I836 mutations are associated with poor disease-free survival and a distinct gene-expression signature among younger adults with de novo cytogenetically normal acute myeloid leukemia lacking FLT3 internal tandem duplications. *Blood,* 111, 1552-1559.

Wittinghofer, A. (1998) Signal transduction via Ras. *Biol Chem,* 379, 933-937.

Wouters, B.J., et al. (2009) Double CEBPA mutations, but not single CEBPA mutations, define a subgroup of acute myeloid leukemia with a distinctive gene expression profile that is uniquely associated with a favorable outcome. *Blood,* 113, 3088-3091.

Wysocka, J., et al. (2006) A PHD finger of NURF couples histone H3 lysine 4 trimethylation with chromatin remodelling. *Nature,* 442, 86-90.

Xu, W., et al. (2011) Oncometabolite 2-hydroxyglutarate is a competitive inhibitor of alpha-ketoglutarate-dependent dioxygenases. *Cancer Cell,* 19, 17-30.

Yamagata, T., et al. (2005) Runx1/AML1 in normal and abnormal hematopoiesis. *Int J Hematol,* 82, 1-8.

Yamamoto, Y., et al. (2001) Activating mutation of D835 within the activation loop of FLT3 in human hematologic malignancies. *Blood,* 97, 2434-2439.

Zhang, D.E., et al. (1997) Absence of granulocyte colony-stimulating factor signaling and neutrophil development in CCAAT enhancer binding protein alpha-deficient mice. *Proc Natl Acad Sci U S A,* 94, 569-574.

Zhang, W., et al. (2008) Mutant FLT3: a direct target of sorafenib in acute myelogenous leukemia. *J Natl Cancer Inst,* 100, 184-198.

Zhao, S., et al. (2009) Glioma-derived mutations in IDH1 dominantly inhibit IDH1 catalytic activity and induce HIF-1alpha. *Science,* 324, 261-265.

10

Bone Marrow Microenvironment in the Pathogenesis of AML

Olga Blau
Charité University School of Medicine
Germany

1. Introduction

Acute myeloid leukemia (AML) arises from a series of genetic abnormalities in a stem or progenitor cell that lead to uncontrolled growth. Data from the past few decades have implicated the hematopoietic microenvironment (HM) in the pathogenesis of hematologic malignancies (Ramakrishnan et al., 2009). Hematopoietic stem cells (HSCs) live in a highly specialized complex microenvironment, also known as a niche (Scadden et al., 2007; Konopleva et al., 2009). Two distinct microenvironmental niches defined: "osteoblastic (endosteal)" and "vascular" niches (Perry and Li, 2007). Recent studies suggest that these niches work together. Coordination between the osteoblastic and vascular niches regulates HSC selfrenewal, proliferation, differentiation and mobilization in and out of the bone marrow (BM). HSCs leave the osteoblastic niche, mobilize to the vascular niche, and enter the blood vessel. They subsequently may undergo transendothelial migration from the peripheral circulation and return first to the vascular niche and then to the osteoblastic niche (Lapidot et al., 2005; Cancelas and Williams, 2006). Within the niche, there are critical bidirectional signals that ensure the regulation of normal HSCs (Calvi et al., 2003) and maintenance of the quiescent long-term HSC pool (Fleming et al., 2008). The quiescent fraction of immunophenotypically defined HSCs has been previously demonstrated to correlate with long-term repopulating ability of BM (Passegue et al., 2005) and loss of this fraction is associated with inability to sustain serial transplantation, the most stringent *in vivo* assay of self-renewal (Fleming et al., 2008).

The HM consists of a complex structure of both non-hematopoietic and hematopoietic cells, extracellular matrix as well as soluble and membrane bound factors that cooperate to support normal hematopoiesis. It was known as early as the 1960s, based on experiments on mice, that normal hematopoiesis could not occur without a supportive environment (Russell et al., 1979). In vitro studies of the HM over the last several decades have mostly relied on the long-term marrow culture system, first reported by Dexter (1977).

The key component of the HM is mesenchymal stromal cells (MSC). These plastic-adherent cells currently described as mesenchymal stem cells are termed multipotent mesenchymal stromal cells, while the term mesenchymal stem cell should be reserved for a subset of these cells that demonstrate stem cell activity by clearly stated criteria (Horowitz et al., 2005). MSCs are primitive cells originating from the mesodermal germ layer and were classically described to give rise to connective tissues, skeletal muscle cells, and cells of the vascular system. Friedenstein and colleagues (1974) first described MSC as fibroblast-like cells that could be isolated from BM via inherent adherence to plastic in culture. He defined a population of cells as multipotential stromal precursor cells that were spindle-shaped and clonogenic in culture conditions, defining them as colony-forming unit fibroblasts. MSCs, in the traditional view, should refer to stem cells that are also capable of producing blood cells; however, blood cells are actually derived from a distinct cell population called the hematopoietic stem cells. This allows classified MSC as nonhematopoietic, multipotential stem cells that are capable of differentiating into mesenchymal and non-mesenchymal cell lineages (Chamberlain et al., 2007). These cells were able to differentiate into adipocytes, chondrocytes, osteocytes, and myoblasts, both in vitro and in vivo. In addition, it has also been demonstrated that MSCs are capable of differentiating into cardiomyocytes, neurons, and astrocytes in vitro and in vivo (Pittenger et al., 1999; Jori et al., 2005; Beyer Nardi et al., 2006; Tokcaer-Keskin et al., 2009). By generating functionally distinct cell types and structures, MSC play a crucial role in supporting hematopoiesis as key components of the HM (Sacchetti et al., 2007).

Phenotypically MSCs express a number of markers, none of which are specific only to MSCs. It is generally agreed that adult human MSCs do not express the hematopoietic markers CD45, CD34, CD14, or CD11. They also do not express the costimulatory molecules CD80, CD86, or CD40 or the adhesion molecules CD31, CD18, or CD56, but they can express CD105 (SH2), CD73 (SH3/4), CD44, CD90 (Thy-1), CD71, and Stro-1 as well as the adhesion molecules CD106, CD166, intercellular adhesion molecule, and CD29 (Sordi et al., 2005; Chamberlain et al., 2007). Although there are no unique cell surface markers for the identification of MSCs, minimal criteria to define human MSC have been published. According to such criteria, MSC must be plastic-adherent; and have to express CD105, CD90 and CD73; they must lack expression of CD45, CD34 and CD14; and they must show in vitro differentiation capabilities into osteoblasts, adipocytes and chondroblasts (Horowitz et al., 2005; Chamberlain et al., 2007). This *in vitro* system has allowed for the dissection of the components of the microenvironment and the study of the complex contact dependent and contact independent interactions that occur between the stromal compartment and hematopoietic stem cells that regulate stem cell fate decisions.

Normal hematopoiesis requires complex bidirectional interactions between the HM and HSCs. The HM can regulate hematopoiesis by interacting directly with HC and/or by secreting regulatory molecules that exert a positive or negative influence on the growth of HC. These interactions influence HSC self-renewal. HM controls the formation of blood cells through the production and secretion of cytokines, chemokines, and intracellular signals initiated by cellular adhesion (Konopleva et al., 2009). Chemokines are a large superfamily of small glycoproteins that are required in a various series of biological processes, including leukocyte trafficking, hematopoiesis, angiogenesis, and organogenesis. MSCs have the ability to migrate into tissues from the circulation, possibly in response to signals that are upregulated under injury conditions. Although the mechanisms by which MSCs are recruited to tissues and cross the endothelial cell layer are not yet fully understood, it is probable that chemokines and their receptors are involved, as they are important factors known to control cell migration (Chamberlain et al., 2007).

CXCL12/stromal cell-derived factor-1alpha (SDF-1α) and its receptor CXCR4 are involved in homing of HSC into BM (Abkowitz et al., 2003; Broxmeyer et al., 2005; Morrison and Spradling, 2008). Perivascular reticular cells secrete much higher levels of CXCL12 than other constitutive sources of CXCL12, such as osteoblasts, fibroblasts, and endothelial cells

(Sugiyama et al. 2006). These reticular cells, defined as CXCL12-abundant reticular cells, may serve as a transit pathway for shuttling HSC between the osteoblastic and vascular niches, where essential but different maintenance signals are provided (Perry and Li, 2007).
The molecular interactions between HC and MSC involve ligand-receptor relationship between adhesion molecules on the surface of HC and stromal cells or between such molecules on the cells surface with specific domains within certain extracellular matrix molecules. BM engraftment involves subsequent cell-to-cell interactions through the MSC-produced complex extracellular matrix (ECM) (Zuckerman and Wicha, 1983; Wight et al., 1986). Vascular cell-adhesion molecule-1 (VCAM-1) or fibronectin is critical for adhesion to the MSC (Miyake et al., 1991; Garcia-Gila et al., 2002). One very important type of interaction between the MSC and the HSC is the synthesis and presentation by MSC of hematopoietic growth factors. Interactions of HSC with stromal elements of BM play a role in the egress of mature blood cells from the BM (Chamberlain et al., 2007).
Whether MSC alterations influence hematological disorders and how such alterations contribute to the progression of the disease remains controversial. The molecular mechanisms for maintaining quiescence of normal stem cells may also facilitate leukemia stem cells (LSC) survival. Whereas LSC share certain features of self-renewal and differentiation with HSC, LSC differ in their deregulated proliferation and ability to invade and spread. LSC exhibit the capacity for long-term self-renewal (Holyoake et al., 2002; Warner et al., 2004; Liesveld et al., 2004) within the BM microenvironment, which is required for maintenance of the malignant clone (Braun and Shannon, 2008). LSCs are able to generate leukemic blasts, and the leukemic clone is organized as a hierarchy (Zhang et al., 2003). LSCs may steal the homeostatic mechanisms, take refuge within the HM during chemotherapy, and consequently contribute to eventual disease relapse (Warner et al., 2004; Lane et al., 2009). Consecutively, LSC are believed to arise through transforming events targeting HSC, which allow growth-independent survival and proliferation. MSC are capable of promoting the growth, survival and drug resistance of leukemic cells by providing the necessary cytokines and cell contact-mediated signals to LSC (Dazzi et al., 2006; Ramasamy et al., 2007). There is increasing evidence that microenvironment alterations may be important and pathogenic in leukemia leading to enhanced stem cell mobilization and the creation of alternate niches (Lataillade et al., 2008). Recent data indicate that, in parallel with leukemogenic events in the hematopoietic system, the niche is converted into an environment with dominant signals favoring cell proliferation and growth. In some cases, a combination of these events may be required (Li and Neaves, 2006). Therefore, LSC may receive the support of a BM niche for their survival and may in turn influence deregulation of the BM niche by their dominant proliferation-promoting signals.
AML may arise in an abnormal HM, resulting in the generation of multiple populations with varying initiation events. Ninomiya et al. (2007) modeled the homing, proliferation, and survival sites of human leukemia cells and of cord blood CD34+ cells. The transplanted leukemia cells initially localized on the surface of osteoblasts in the epiphysial region and then expanded to the inner vascular and diaphysial regions. 8 weeks after transplantation, the number of leukemia cells transiently increased by as much as 50%, predominantly in the epiphysial region. After administration of high-dose cytarabine, residual leukemia cells clustered and adhered to the blood vessels as well as to the endosteum, suggesting that leukemia cells receive anti-apoptotic signals not only from osteoblasts but also from vascular endothelium (Ninomiya et al., 2007).

Several studies have proposed that important quantitative and functional alterations occur in MSCs of patients with different hematological disorders (Borojevic et al., 2004; Flores-Figueroa et al., 2008). In some disorders, such as multiple myeloma, MSC show alterations in the expression of some cell adhesion molecules and cytokines, and reduced immunosuppressive efficiency (Wallace et al., 2001; Arnulf et al., 2007; Corre et al., 2007). Neoplastic plasma cells communicate with the environment through cell/cell contact as well cytokines to induce functional changes that support the malignant population (Mitsiades et al., 2006; Podar et al., 2007). In myeloproliferative disorders, has been shown, that megakaryocytes and macrophages play a principle role in the pathogenesis of the fibrotic reaction by secreting PDGF, FGF and TGFα cytokines (Chagraoui et al., 2006). In chronic myeloid leukemia (CML), Bhatia (1995) showed that MSC did not provide optimal support for normal hematopoietic cells. In contrast, growth of CML cells on CML-derived stroma was significantly better, suggesting that the microenvironment in CML was more supportive for the malignant clone. Using fluorescent activated cell sorting (FACS) and fluorescent in situ hybridization (FISH), it was determined that stromal macrophages were all bcr-abl positive and were directly responsible for the selective advantage of clonal bcr-abl cells to proliferate through a contact-dependent mechanism (Bhatia et al. 1995). Interestingly, other researches estimated that CML-derived MSC do not express the bcr-abl gene (Zhao et al., 2006; Jootar et al., 2006). In myelodysplastic syndrome (MDS) MSC show alterations in the levels of TNFα (Deeg et al., 2000). Furthermore, the MDS-derived monocytes respond abnormally to stromal signals, MDS monocytes fail to upregulate matrix metalloproteinase-9 (MMP-9) expression when exposed to stromal signals (Iwata et al., 2007). MMP-9 has been implicated in the cleavage of SDF1 from the microenvironment and may facilitate the egress of HCs from the BM to the peripheral blood (Heissig et al., 2002). In the solid tumors, tumor-derived MSC shown acquire aberrant methylation patterns due either to direct contact with or via factors secreted by the malignant cells (Hanson et al., 2006; Fiegl et al., 2006).

Dysfunction of a BM niche may contribute to leukemogenesis by supplying abundant growth factors that promote proliferation and/or inhibit apoptosis (Jones and Wagers, 2008). MSCs seem to have a relevant role in AML as they prevent spontaneous and induced apoptosis and may attenuate chemotherapy-induced cell death. This possibility has been confirmed by the finding that co-cultivation of a leukemic cell line with the murine stroma cell line MS-5 can block apoptosis (Konopleva et al., 2002).

The significance role of the HM in initiation of leukemia has been suggested by studies with mice deficient in phosphatase and tensin homolog (PTEN) (Yilmaz et al., 2006). PTEN deficiency in both HSC and the HM resulted in myeloproliferation that progressed to overt leukemia/lymphoma. However, inducible PTEN deletion in HSC in the presence of a wild type HM promoted HSC depletion without evidence of myeloproliferation or leukemic development. These results suggest that PTEN deficiency in HSC alone is not sufficient for malignant transformation. Rupec et al. (2005) reported that activation of NF-kB in myelopoietic cells and the absence of its inhibitor IκBα are not sufficient for induction of hypergranulopoiesis, but these changes in the non-hematopoietic compartment, such as fetal liver, resulted in increased numbers of dysplastic hematopoietic cells with progression into secondary AML. These results indicate that non-hematopoietic cells with inactive IκBα can initiate premalignant hematopoietic disorder, conceivably via activation of the Notch pathway. Additional studies indicate the role of Notch signaling in the interactions of HSC and the HM (Matsuoka et al., 2008) demonstrated that the tumor suppressor Fbxw7, which negatively regulates cyclin E, Notch, and c-Myc protein levels, plays a role in maintaining HSC quiescence and repressing potential oncogenic activity of HSC. Notably, Notch ligand Jagged is expressed by the HSC niche, and Jagged/Notch activation results in increased HSC number and niche expansion (Calvi et al., 2003).

Evidence from research conducted over the last few decades has clearly implicated abnormalities of the marrow microenvironment in the pathophysiology of hematologic malignancies. Marcondes et al. (2008) demonstrated that MSC derived from patients with MDS, in contrast to that from more advanced stages of MDS expressed 14- to 17-fold higher levels of IL-32 mRNA than healthy controls, and this constitutive IL-32 expression promoted apoptosis in MDS cells, reproducing the inefficient hematopoiesis and extensive apoptosis in MDS marrow. These findings indicate that stroma-produced IL-32 could contribute to the pathophysiology of MDS, and serve as a therapeutic target. Furthermore, this modified microenvironment phenotype was reproduced when the MSC were exposed to TNFα, known to be produced at high levels by MDS cells.

There are significant data to support mechanism, in which the malignant hematopoietic clone induces reversible functional changes in the HM that result in improved growth conditions for the malignant cells. Gene expression changes occurred in the stroma cell lines, HS5 and HS27a, derived from normal marrow in response to TNFα exposure (Stirewalt et al., 2008), known to be up-regulated in the bone marrow of patients with MDS. Previous experiments showed that interactions between MSC and HSC were required for TNFα to trigger apoptosis in hematopoietic cells (Goda et al., 2006).

Recent discoveries utilizing mouse models have provided the first experimental evidence for genetic changes in the HM contributing to or required for leukemogenesis. Raaijmakers et al. (2010) using transgenic mice showed that genetic alteration of HM can induce MDS with ineffective hematopoiesis and dysmorphic HCs, and with occasional transformation to AML. The authors used *Dicer1* deletion as a means of altering several gene products in subsets of mesenchymal osteolineage cells. *Dicer1* is an RNase III endonuclease essential for microRNA biogenesis (Bartel, 2004) and RNA processing (Krol et al., 2007), that regulates haematopoietic cell fate (Lu et al., 2008). Global repression of microRNA maturation by *Dicer1* deletion promotes cellular transformation and tumorigenesis (Kumar et al., 2007). Raaijmakers et al. (2010) show that deletion of *Dicer1* in HM cells of mouse may be sufficient to initiate a complex change of homeostasis with similarities to myelodysplasia. The authors demonstrated that the ability of HM abnormality to result in the emergence of a clonal neoplasm in a cell type of clearly distinct lineage with distinct secondary genetic changes (Raaijmakers et al., 2010).

Previously, Walkley et al (2007a, 2007b) demonstrated that conditional deletion of the Retinoblastoma gene (RB) in the BM microenvironment can contribute to the development of pre-leukemic myeloproliferative disease in mice. They showed that this was a result of interactions between myeloid cells and the microenvironment. The defect had to be present in both hematopoietic cells and the microenvironment to initiate disease. Widespread inactivation of RB, a central regulator of the cell cycle and a tumor suppressor, resulted in extramedullary hematopoiesis and myeloproliferative disease in the murine hematopoietic system. However, myeloid-specific loss of RB did not induce myeloproliferative disease or HSC abnormalities. Therefore, the myeloproliferative-like disorder in the RB mutants is the result of perturbed interactions between hematopoietic cells and the BM microenvironment

(Walkley et al., 2007a). The final model, reported by the same group, may be the most compelling. In this report, deletion of the Retinoic Acid Receptor γ (RARγ) in mice resulted in a chronic myeloproliferative disorder. Transplant studies revealed that RARγ-hematopoietic cells functioned normally when transplanted into normal mice. However, transplantation of normal hematopoietic cells into the RARγ-microenvironment resulted in a myeloproliferative disorder in the transplanted cells. TNFα was implicated in the pathogenesis of this MPD as the disorder was partially abrogated when TNFα null stem cells were transplanted into the RARγ-microenvironment (Walkley et al., 2007b). These studies showed that a defect in HM could be sufficient to generate a myeloproliferative disorder.

Until recently, there has been little evidence to support the role of primary stromal abnormalities in the pathogenesis of hematologic neoplasms. Some independent studies have documented the existence of genomic alterations in the stroma of leukemia patients (Flores-Figueroa et al., 2005; Blau et al., 2007; Lopez-Villar et al., 2009; Klaus et al., 2010). Different groups have shown the extensive variability of the aberrations, such as hypodiploidy, balanced and unbalanced translocations, whole chromosome gains, and deletions. All cytogenetic markers in MSCs never repeated aberrations identified in HCs. Since there were no associations between chromosomal aberrations in HCs and MSCs, we can state that MSCs were devoid of residue HCs. These findings suggest enhanced genetic instability of MSC in leukemia, and indicate the potential involvement of MSC in the pathophysiology of these conditions (Blau et al., 2007). Recently, Lopez-Villar et al. (2009) reported the presence of cytogenetic aberrations on MSC from MDS patients by array-based comparative genomic hybridization and fluorescence in situ hybridization, some of them specially linked to a particular MDS subtype, the 5q-syndrome.

These date indicate that there are significant functional abnormalities, genetic aberrations, and epigenetic changes in MSC in leukemia patients. Also of interest are the recent reports of abnormalities in the stroma that lead to malignancies of the hematopoietic compartment. Although historically, hematologic malignancies are thought to arise from a stem or progenitor cell abnormality, there may be groups of patients that have a primary stromal defect leading to the hematologic malignancy. Moreover, although a series of genetic and epigenetic events in a single cell may be necessary for oncogenesis, they may not be sufficient, and a permissive microenvironment has been suggested to be required for frank malignancy to emerge (Hanahan and Weinberg, 2007).

It is known that even years after allogeneic stem cell transplantation (alloSCT), and despite successful engraftment of donor-derived hematopoiesis, MSC are in general of host origin (Rieger et al., 2005). Some patients after alloSCT do not recover their stem cells despite receiving high levels of CD34+ progenitor cells. The presumed basis for this is that the preparation regimen has in some way affected the niche, so it no longer has the same nurturing capability. It was shown that transplanted HSCs migrate to the endosteal surfaces of bone within hours of intravenous injection (Nilsson et al., 1997). Endochondral ossification has been shown to be an essential prerequisite for the development of normal haematopoiesis in the BM (Zhou et al., 1995), indicating a possible fundamental interrelationship of ossification to the mature haematopoietic process in mammals. Recent reports have identified that a key cellular component of the HSC niche is cells of the osteoblast lineage, the cell type responsible for the formation of bone (Calvi et al., 2003; Zhang et al., 2003). Additionally, these studies raise the issue that under transplant conditions, there may be agents that rather than drive hematopoiesis, might affect the osteoblast component.

Understanding the niche has ramifications beyond simple biological interest. Niche biology and function has relevance not only in bone marrow transplantation, but in developing agents that may impact on the ability to generate a larger number of stem cells or increase the efficiency of stem cells to engraft in the transplant setting. By elucidating the role of the BM microenvironment in the pathogenesis of hematologic tumors, recent studies have provided the framework for identifying and validating novel therapies that target both leukemic cells and cells in their surrounding microenvironment (Konopleva et al., 2009). Thus in general, treatment strategies have been focused on the eradication of the stem or progenitor cell from which the malignancy arose. However, recent evidence suggests that focusing therapeutic strategies on the microenvironmental abnormalities can be extremely effective. The Imid family of agents has changed the treatment paradigm in diseases such as myeloma and MDS and highlighted the importance of targeting the microenvironment (Sokol et al., 2007; Melchert and List, 2007).

If primary stromal defects are identified in humans and implicated in the initiation of malignancy, this clearly will have great impact on the treatment strategies offered to patients. By explanation the role of the MSC in the pathogenesis of AML, recent studies have provided novel therapies that target both leukemic cells and cells of microenvironment. Studies of MSC can also aid in potentially modifying the relative abundance of normal versus malignant cells in the context of the post chemotherapy setting in AML. The underlying molecular mechanisms implicated in stem cell activation and homing to the niche will provide important insight into the precise mechanisms involved in interactions between leukemic and normal cells that contribute to drug resistance. This understanding will provide a framework for the rational combination of agents in clinical trials to overcome drug resistance and improve patient outcomes. Detection of alterations in MSCs suggests that unstable MSCs may facilitate the expansion of malignant cells. In view of these data, alterations in MSCs may be a particular mechanism of leukemogenesis. Especially, further understanding of the contribution of the BM niche to the process of leukemogenesis may provide new targets aimed at destroying LSC without adversely affecting normal stem cell self-renewal.

2. References

Abkowitz JL, Robinson AE, Kale S, Long MW, Chen J. Mobilization of hematopoietic stem cells during homeostasis and after cytokine exposure. *Blood* 2003;102:1249–1253.

Arnulf B, Lecourt S, Soulier J et al. Phenotypic and functional characterization of bone marrow mesenchymal stem cells derived from patients with multiple myeloma. *Leukemia* 2007;21:158–63.

Bartel DP. MicroRNAs: genomics, biogenesis, mechanism, and function. *Cell* 2004;116:281–297.

Beyer Nardi N, da Silva Meirelles L. Mesenchymal stem cells: Isolation, in vitro expansion and characterization. *Handb Exp Pharmacol* 2006:249–282.

Bhatia R, McGlave PB, Dewald GW et al. Abnormal function of the bone marrow microenvironment in chronic myelogenous leukemia: Role of malignant stromal macrophages. *Blood* 1995;85:3636–3645.

Blau O, Hofmann WK, Baldus CD et al. Chromosomal aberrations in bone marrow mesenchymal stroma cells from patients with myelodysplastic syndrome and acute myeloblastic leukemia. *Exp Hematol* 2007;35(2):221-229.

Borojevic R, Roela R, Rodarte R et al. Bone marrow stroma in childhood myelodysplastic syndrome: composition, ability to sustain hematopoiesis in vitro, and altered gene expression. *Leuk Res* 2004;28(8):831-844.

Braun BS, Shannon K. Targeting Ras in myeloid leukemias. *Clin Cancer Res* 2008;14:2249–2252.

Broxmeyer HE., Orschell CM, Clapp DW et al. Rapid mobilization of murine and human hematopoietic stem and progenitor cells with AMD3100, a CXCR4 antagonist. *J Exp Med* 2005;201:1307–1318.

Calvi LM, Adams GB, Weibrecht KW et al. Osteoblastic cells regulate the haematopoietic stem cell niche. *Nature* 2003;425:841-846.

Cancelas JA, Williams DA. Stem cell mobilization by beta2-agonists. *Nat Med* 2006;12:278–279.

Chagraoui H, Wendling F, Vainchenker W. Pathogenesis of myelofibrosis with myeloid metaplasia: Insight from mouse models (Review). *Best Pract Res Clin Haematol* 2006;19:399–412.

Chamberlain G, Fox J, Ashton B, Middleton J. Concise Review: Mesenchymal Stem Cells: Their Phenotype, Differentiation Capacity, Immunological Features, and Potential for Homing. *Stem Cells* 2007;25:2739–2749.

Corre J, Mahtouk K, Attal M et al. Bone marrow mesenchymal stem cells are abnormal in multiple myeloma. *Leukemia* 2007;21:1079–1088.

Dazzi F, Ramasamy R, Glennie S, Jones SP, Roberts I. The role of mesenchymal stem cells in haemopoiesis. *Blood Rev* 2006;20:161–171.

Deeg HJ, Beckham C, Loken MR et al. Negative regulators of hemopoiesis and stroma function in patients with myelodysplastic syndrome. *Leuk Lymphoma* 2000;37:405–414.

Dexter TM, Allen TD, Lajtha LG. Conditions controlling the proliferation of haemopoietic stem cells in vitro. *J Cell Physiol* 1977;91:335–344.

Fiegl H, Millinger S, Goebel G et al. Breast cancer DNA methylation profiles in cancer cells and tumor stroma: association with HER-2/neu status in primary breast cancer. *Cancer Res* 2006;66:29–33.

Fleming HE, Janzen V, Lo Celso C et al. Wnt signaling in the niche enforces hematopoietic stem cell quiescence and is necessary to preserve self-renewal in vivo. *Cell Stem Cell* 2008;2:274-283.

Flores-Figueroa E, Arana-Trejo RM, Gutiérrez-Espíndola G, Pérez-Cabrera A, Mayani H. Mesenchymal stem cells in myelodysplastic syndromes: phenotypic and cytogenetic characterization. *Leuk Res* 2005;29(2):215-224.

Flores-Figueroa E, Montesinos JJ, Flores-Guzman P et al. Functional analysis of myelodysplastic syndromes-derived mesenchymal stem cells. *Leuk Res* 2008;32:1407–1416.

Friedenstein AJ, Chailakhyan RK, Latsinik NV et al. Stromal cells responsible for transferring the microenvironment of the hemopoietic tissues. Cloning in vitro and retransplantation in vivo. *Transplantation* 1974;17:33-40.

Garcia-Gila M, Lopez-Martin EM, Garcia-Pardo A. Adhesion to fibronectin via alpha4 integrin (CD49d) protects B cells from apoptosis induced by serum deprivation but not via IgM or Fas/Apo-1 receptors. *Clin Exp Immunol* 2002;127:455–462.

Goda C, Kanaji T, Kanaji S et al. Involvement of IL-32 in activation-induced cell death in T cells. *Int Immunol* 2006;18:233–240.

Hanahan D, Weinberg RA. The hallmarks of cancer. *Cell* 2000;100:57–70.

Hanson JA, Gillespie JW, Grover A et al. Gene promoter methylation in prostate tumor-associated stromal cells. *J Natl Cancer Inst* 2006;98:255–261.

Heissig B, Hattori K, Dias S et al. Recruitment of stem and progenitor cells from the bone marrow niche requires MMP-9 mediated release of kit-ligand. *Cell* 2002;109:625–637.

Holyoake TL, Jiang X, Drummond MW, Eaves AC, Eaves CJ. Elucidating critical mechanisms of deregulated stem cell turnover in the chronic phase of chronic myeloid leukemia. *Leukemia* 2002;16:549–558.

Horwitz EM, Le Blanc K, Dominici M et al. Clarification of the nomenclature for MSC: The International Society for Cellular Therapy position statement. *Cytotherapy* 2005;5;393-395.

Iwata M, Pillai M, Ramakrishnan A et al. Reduced expression of inducible gelatinase B/matrix metalloproteinase-9 in monocytes from patients with myelodysplastic syndrome: correlation of inducible levels with the percentage of cytogenetically marked cells and with marrow cellularity. *Blood* 2007;109:85–92.

Jones DL, Wagers AJ. No place like home: anatomy and function of the stem cell niche. *Nat Rev Mol Cell Biol* 2008;9:11–21.

Jootar S, Pornprasertsud N, Petvises S et al. Bone marrowderived mesenchymal stem cells from chronic myeloid leukemia t(9;22) patients are devoid of Philadelphia chromosome and support cord blood stem cell expansion. *Leuk Res* 2006;30:1493–1498.

Jori FP, Napolitano MA, Melone MA et al. Molecular pathways involved in neural in vitro differentiation of marrow stromal stem cells. *J Cell Biochem* 2005;94:645–655.

Klaus M, Stavroulaki E, Kastrinaki MC et al. Reserves, Functional, Immunoregulatory, and Cytogenetic Properties of Bone Marrow Mesenchymal Stem Cells in Patients with Myelodysplastic Syndromes. *Stem Cells Dev* 2010;19(7):1043-1055.

Konopleva M, Tabe Y, Zeng Z, Andreeff M. Therapeutic targeting of microenvironmental interactions in leukemia: mechanisms and approaches. *Drug Resist Updat* 2009;12(4):103-113.

Konopleva M, Konoplev S, Hu W et al. Stromal cells prevent apoptosis of AML cells by up-regulation of antiapoptotic proteins. Leukemia 2002;16:1713–1724.

Krol J, Fiszer A, Mykowska A et al. Ribonuclease dicer cleaves triplet repeat hairpins into shorter repeats that silence specific targets. *Mol Cell* 2007;25:575–586.

Kumar MS, Lu J, Mercer KL, Golub TR, Jacks T. Impaired microRNA processing enhances cellular transformation and tumorigenesis. *Nature Genet.* 2007;39:673–677.

Lane SW, Scadden DT, Gilliland DG. The leukemic stem cell niche: current concepts and therapeutic opportunities. *Blood* 2009 114:1150-1157.

Lapidot T, Dar A, Kollet O. How do stem cells find their way home? *Blood* 2005;106:1901–1910.

Lataillade JJ, Pierre-Louis O, Hasselbalch HC et al. Does primary myelofibrosis involve a defective stem cell niche? From concept to evidence. *Blood* 2008;112:3026-3035.

Li L, Neaves WB. Normal stem cells and cancer stem cells: the niche matters. *Cancer Res* 2006;66:4553–4557.

Liesveld JL, Jordan CT, Phillips II GL. The hematopoietic stem cell in myelodysplasia. *Stem Cells* 2004;22:590–599.

Lopez-Villar O, Garcia JL, Sancez-Guijo FM et al. Both expanded and uncultured mesenchymal stem cells from MDS patients are genomically abnormal, showing a specific genetic profile for the 5q- syndrome. *Leukemia* 2009;23:664-672.

Lu J, Guo S, Ebert BL et al. MicroRNA-mediated control of cell fate in megakaryocyte-erythrocyte progenitors. *Dev Cell* 2008;14:843–853.

Marcondes AM, Mhyre AJ, Stirewalt DL et al. Dysregulation of IL-32 in myelodysplastic syndrome and chronic myelomonocytic leukemia modulates apoptosis and impairs NK function. Proc Natl Acad Sci USA 2008;105:2865–2870.

Matsuoka S, Oike Y, Onoyama I et al. Fbxw7 acts as a critical fail-safe against premature loss of hematopoietic stem cells and development of T-ALL. *Genes Dev* 2008;22:986–991.

Melchert M, List A. The thalidomide saga (Review). Int J Biochem Cell Biol 2007;39:1489–99.

Mitsiades CS, Mitsiades NS, Munshi NC et al. The role of the bone microenvironment in the pathophysiology and therapeutic management of multiple myeloma: interplay of growth factors, their receptors and stromal interactions (Review). *Eur J Cancer* 2006;42:1564–73.

Miyake K, Medina K, Ishihara K et al. A VCAM-like adhesion molecule on murine bone marrow stromal cells mediates binding of lymphocyte precursors in culture. *J Cell Biol* 1991;114:557–565.

Morrison SJ, Spradling AC. Stem cells and niches: mechanisms that promote stem cell maintenance throughout life. Cell 2008;132:598–611.

Nilsson SK, Johnston HM, Coverdale JA. Spatial localization of transplanted hemopoietic stem cells: inferences for the localization of stem cell niches. *Blood* 1997;2293–2299.

Ninomiya M, Abe A, Katsumi A et al. Homing, proliferation and survival sites of human leukemia cells in vivo in immunodeficient mice. *Leukemia* 2007;21:136–142.

Passegue E, Wagers AJ, Giuriato S, Anderson WC, Weissman IL. Global analysis of proliferation and cell cycle gene expression in the regulation of hematopoietic stem and progenitor cell fates. *J Exp Med* 2005;202:1599-1611.

Perry JM, Li L. Disrupting the stem cell niche: good seeds in bad soil. *Cell* 2007;129:1045–1047.

Pittenger MF, Mackay AM, Beck SC et al. Multilineage potential of adult human mesenchymal stem cells. *Science* 1999;284:143–147.

Podar K, Richardson PG, Hideshima T et al. The malignant clone and the bone marrow environment (Review). *Best Pract Res Clin Haematol* 2007;20:597–612.

Raaijmakers MH, Mukherjee S, Guo S et al. Bone progenitor dysfunction induces myelodysplasia and secondary leukemia. *Nature* 2010;464:852-857.

Ramakrishnan A, Deeg HJ. A Novel Role for the Marrow Microenvironment in Initiating and Sustaining Hematopoietic Disease. Expert *Opin Biol Ther* 2009;9(1):21–28.

Ramasamy R, Lam EW, Soeiro I et al. Mesenchymal stem cells inhibit proliferation and apoptosis of tumor cells: impact on in vivo tumor growth. Leukemia 2007;21:304–310.

Rieger K, Marinets O, Fietz T, Körper S, Sommer D, Mücke C, Reufi B, Blau WI, Thiel E, Knauf WU. Mesenchymal stem cells remain of host origin even a long time after allogeneic peripheral blood stem cell or bone marrow transplantation. *Exp Hematol* 2005;33:605-11.

Rupec RA, Jundt F, Rebholz B et al. Stroma-mediated dysregulation of myelopoiesis in mice lacking I kappa B alpha. *Immunity* 2005;22:479-491.

Russell ES. Hereditary anemias of the mouse: a review for geneticists (Review). *Adv Genetics* 1979;20:357-459.

Sacchetti B, Funari A, Michienzi S et al. Self-renewing osteoprogenitors in bone marrow sinusoids can organize a hematopoietic microenvironment. *Cell* 2007;131:324-336.

Scadden DT. The stem cell niche in health and leukemic disease. *Best Pract Res Clin Haematol* 2007;20(1):19-27.

Sokol L, List AF. Immunomodulatory therapy for myelodysplastic syndromes. *Int J Hematol* 2007;86:301-305.

Sordi V, Malosio ML, Marchesi F et al. Bone marrow mesenchymal stem cells express a restricted set of functionally active chemokine receptors capable of promoting migration to pancreatic islets. *Blood* 2005;106:419 - 427.

Stirewalt DL, Mhyre AJ, Marcondes M et al. Tumour necrosis factor-induced gene expression in human marrow stroma: clues to the pathophysiology of MDS? *Br J Haematol* 2008;140:444-453.

Sugiyama T, Kohara H, Noda M, Nagasawa T. Maintenance of the hematopoietic stem cell pool by CXCL12-CXCR4 chemokine signaling in bone marrow stromal cell niches. *Immunity* 2006;25:977-988.

Tokcaer-Keskin Z, Akar AR, Ayaloglu-Butun F et al. Timing of induction of cardiomyocyte differentiation for in vitro cultured mes- enchymal stem cells: A perspective for emergencies. *Can J Physiol Pharmacol* 2009;87:143-150.

Walkley CR, Shea JM, Sims NA et al. Rb regulates interactions between hematopoietic stem cells and their bone marrow microenvironment. *Cell* 2007a;129:1081-1095.

Walkley CR, Olsen GH, Dworkin S et al. A microenvironment-induced myeloproliferative syndrome caused by retinoic acid receptor gamma deficiency. *Cell* 2007b;129:1097-1110.

Wallace SR, Oken MM, Lunetta KL, Panoskaltsis-Mortari A, Masellis AM. Abnormalities of bone marrow mesenchymal cells in multiple myeloma patients. *Cancer* 2001;91:1219-30.

Warner JK, Wang JC, Hope KJ, Jin L, Dick JE. Concepts of human leukemic development. *Oncogene* 2004;23:7164-7177.

Wight TN, Kinsella MG, Keating A, Singer JW. Proteoglycans in human long-term bone marrow cultures: biochemical and ultrastructural analyses. *Blood* 1986;67:1333-1343.

Yilmaz OH, Valdez R, Theisen BK et al. Pten dependence distinguishes haematopoietic stem cells from leukaemia-initiating cells. *Nature* 2006;44: 475-482.

Zhang J, Niu C, Ye L et al. Identification of the haematopoietic stem cell niche and control of the niche size. *Nature* 2003;425:836-841.

Zhao Z, Tang X, You Y et al. Assessment of bone marrow mesenchymal stem cell biological characteristics and support hematopoiesis function in patients with chronic myeloid leukemia. *Leuk Res* 2006;30:993-1003.

Zhou H, Choong PFM, Henderson S et al. Marrow development and its relationship to bone formation *in vivo*: a histological study using an implantable titanium device in rabbits. *Bone* 1995; 17:407–415.

Zuckerman KS, Wicha MS. Extracellular matrix production by the adherent cells of long-term murine bone marrow cultures. *Blood* 1983;61:540–547.

11

Distinct Inhibitory Effect of TGFβ on the Growth of Human Myeloid Leukemia Cells

Xiao Tang Hu
Department of Biology, College of Arts & Sciences, Barry University, Miami Shores, FL, USA

1. Introduction

Hematopoiesis is the formation and development of blood cells. In a healthy adult person, approximately 10^{11}–10^{12} new blood cells are produced daily in order to maintain steady state levels in the peripheral circulation. Disruption of the steady state may cause the development of hematological diseases, such as acute (AML) or chronic myelogenous leukemia (CML). All mature blood cells ultimately originate from a rare population of primitive pluripotent (multipotential) stem cells. The pluripotent stem cells possess self-renewal and multi-lineage differentiation potential. The latter process leads to two major multipotent progenitors: myeloid progenitors and lymphoid progenitors. The myeloid progenitors have the ability to differentiate into mature white cells, erythrocytes, megakaryocytes/platelets and mast cells; whereas the lymphoid progenitors cells mainly produce mature T, NK, and B lymphocytes. Production of myeloid lineage cells is a highly complex process involving the balance between cell proliferation and differentiation, which is regulated by growth stimulating or inhibiting signals. Transforming Growth Factor-beta (TGFβ) is a pleiotropic growth factor and is one of the major regulators of hematopoiesis (Fortunel NO et al. 2000). A major effect of TGFβ on hematopoietic cells is inhibitory (Hu X et al 1999, Batard P et al. 2000, Ducos K et al. 2000, Fortunel NO 2000) although its stimulatory effect has also been observed in some types of blood cells (Keller JR 1990, 1992). Due to its importance in the understanding human diseases including leukemia, over past 20 years, the mechanisms responsible for TGFβ-induced growth inhibition or stimulation have been a major area of investigation and considerable insights into its action mechanisms have been learned. This review highlights recent progress in understanding regulatory role of TGFβ and its signaling pathways in various types of cells with a focus on human myeloid leukemia cells.

2. Myeloid leukemia and myelogenous leukemia cell lines

Myeloid leukemia is a type of blood and bone marrow cancers, which includes AML and CML. AML is a characterized by the rapid accumulation of abnormal, immature white blood cells in both borrow and blood, which is caused by defects in the progenitors and/or stem cells population. Unlike AML, myeloid cell differentiation is preserved during the chronic phase of CML, a disease which originates from the presence of a genetic abnormality in stem cells/progenitors and the nuclei show an abnormal chromosome called the Philadelphia chromosome. In a healthy person, bone marrow makes the blood stem cells and progenitors that mature into mature white blood cells, red blood cells and blood platelets.

In order to simplify the study of leukemia and basic research, a number of human AML cell lines were established. These lines provide model systems to study the control of proliferation and differentiation in human myelogenous leukemia and, in a broader framework, the controls of normal myeloid development. More than 10 leukemic cell lines have been used in our lab to study Transforming Growth Factor-β (TGFβ)-mediated cell cycle control and transformed events, among which K562 is the first myelogenous leukemia cell line established. The cell line was isolated from a 53 year old female CML patient in blast crisis (Lozzio CB and Lozzio BB 1975). K652 composed of undifferentiated blast cells that are rich in glycophorin and may be induced to produce fetal and embryonic hemoglobin in the presence of hemin. The rest nine cell lines were isolated from AML patients as described below. MV4-11 cell line was derived from blast cells of a 10-year-old male with biphenotypic myelomonocytic leukemia (Lange B et al. 1987). This cell line expresses mutated FLT3, a member of the type III receptor tyrosine kinase (RTK) family (Quentmeier 2003). KG-1 cell line is composed predominantly of myeloblasts and promyelocytes (Koeffler HP et al. 1978). Recent studies identified a fusion of two genes encoding fibroblast growth factor receptors, making this cell line is a good model for studying gene fusion-linked leukemia (Gu TL et al. 2006). KG-1a (Koeffler HP et al. 1980) is a subline isolated from KG-1. TF-1 is a growth factor-dependent human cell line that was originally isolated from the bone marrow cells of a patient with erythroleukemia (Kitamura T et al. 1989). TF-1 cells express a wide range of cytokine receptors and respond to a variety of cytokines. Thus, this cell line is a useful tool for studying cytokine signaling network (Rosas M et al 2005). TF-1a (Hu X et al. 1998) is growth factor-independent subline isolated from TF-1. A unique characteristic of the KG-1 and TF-1 cells is their dependence on colony-stimulating factor (CSF) or GM-CSF/IL-3 for proliferation, respectively, whereas KG-1a and TF-1a are factor-independent cell lines for their growth, although TF-1a retains its ability to respond to several growth factors. HL-60 is a promyelocytic cell line derived from peripheral blood leukocytes from a female patient with acute promyelocytic leukemia, which can be induced into granulocytes in the presence of DMSO (Gallagher R et al.1979). HL-60 cells differentiate into mononuclear phagocytes when exposed to phorbol esters (Xu YZ et al. 2011). HEL is an erythroleukemia cell line isolated from the bone marrow cells of a patient (Martin P and Papayannopoulou 1982). A mutation in *Janus kinase 2* gene (JAK2) in HEL cells was identified in 2006 (Quentmeier H et al 2006). Mo7e (Avancd GC et al. 1988) is a subline of the M-07 human megakaryoblastic leukemia cell line. The cells express platelet glycoprotein-2b-3a. The growth of Mo7e is dependent on IL-3 or GM-CSF. U937 is a cell line established from a diffuse histiocytic lymphoma of 37 year old male patient (Sundstrom C et al. 1976). A histocyte is a cell that is part of the mononuclear phagocytic system that takes part in the immune responses. Since U937 displays many monocytic characteristics and has thus served as a model for the differentiation of monocytes and macrophage in vitro (Aida J, et al. 2011). This cell line is also a good model for induction of apoptosis (Piedfer M et al. 2011).

3. Effect of TGFβ on the growth of human myeloid leukemia cell lines in culture

Transforming Growth Factor-β (TGFβ) has three isoforms in mammals: TGFβ1, TGFβ2, and TGFβ3. The β1 isoform is the most abundant, universally expressed, which has been intensively studied. This review focuses on TGFβ1 unless indicated otherwise. The TGFβ-induced biological activities are achieved through the binding of the ligand to its cell surface receptor, a serine-threonine kinase complex, known as type I, II, and III (adaptor) receptors. TGFβ binds to and activates the type II receptor. Then the type II receptor recruits and phosphorylates the type I receptor, which in turn activates Smad family proteins that carry signals from the receptors to the nucleus to control transcription of target genes. These gene products may stimulate or inhibit cell cycle progression. TGFβ plays an essential regulatory role in the control of hematopoiesis (Fortunel NO et al. 2000). First, the development of hematopoietic cells from mesoderm in embryos is regulated by TGFβ signaling. Park et al (Park C et al. 2004) demonstrated that BMP-4, a member of TGFβ superfamily, is able to induce hematopoietic differentiation from mouse embryonic stem cells. The differentiated cells contain all types of myeloid and lymphoid progeny (Olsen AL et al. 2006). Similar roles of TGFβ in human hematopoietic stem cells have been reported (Kaufman DS et al. 2001, Chadwick K et al. 2003, Cerdan C et al. 2004). Second, it has also been found that TGFβ is required for maintaining hematopoietic stem/progenitor cells in quiescent states (Batard P et al. 2000); in contrast, application of anti-endogenous TGFβ antibody induces release of these cells from G1 phase (Ducos K et al. 2000). In TGFβ$^{-/-}$ mice, enhanced numbers of circulating granulocytes, monocytes, platelets, as well as colony forming units, were observed (Kulkarni AB et al 1993, Shull MM et al 1992). In addition, inactivation of the TGFβ signaling pathway leads to malignant transformation of early hematopoietic cells (Le Bousse-Kerdiles MC et al. 1996). These data indicate that TGFβ is inhibitory to hematopoietic cells. However, studies from several groups suggest that the response of myeloid stem/progenitor cells to the inhibitory effect of TGFβ appears to be inversely correlated with their maturation stage (Sing GK 1988, Keller JR 1990, Ottmann OG & Pellus LM 1991, Snoeck H-W 1996). Long-term repopulating stem cells, CD34+ or CD34+/CD38- stem/progenitor cells, early myeloid and erythroid progenitors are markedly inhibited in the presence of TGFβ, whereas more differentiated myeloid progenitors forming granulocyte-macrophage colonies, and late erythroid progenitors forming CFU-e are less inhibited or even stimulated by TGFβ (Keller JR 1990, 1992, 1994, Fortunel NO 2000, Ruscetti FW 2005, Sitnicka E 1996, McNiece IK 1992, Goey H 1989, Morita N 2003, Classen S 2007). The inhibitory or stimulatory role by TGFβ in some cases seems to correlate with the cytokines used to promote cell growth. TGFβ inhibits SCF-, IL-3- and CSF-1-induced colony formation from mouse and human hematopoietic progenitors (McNiece IK 1992, Sitnicka E et al 1996). In contrast, TGFβ enhances GM-CSF-induced colony formation derived from normal bone marrow cells and Lin^{-} progenitors (Keller JR 1991).

For leukemia cells, both inhibitory and stimulatory effects have been reported (Tessier N & Hoang T 1988, Otten J 2011, Aglietta M 1989, Cashman JD 1992). TGFβ has been shown to inhibit the growth of clonogenic blast cells from patients with acute myeloblastic leukemia (AML) (Tessier N & Hoang T 1988). Mutations in the components of TGFβ signal pathways may relate to the disease development (Imai Y et al. 2001). In contrast, high expression of ALK-1 and ALK-5, two members of TGFβ type I receptors, was reported to be associated with AML (Otten J 2011). An inhibitory effect of TGFβ was suggested by the finding of low levels of TGFβ type II receptors in CML (Rooke HM 1999) and lymphoid neoplasms (Inman GJ et al 2000); whereas, by using TGFβ inhibitors, Naka et al found that TGFβ signal is required for maintaining Leukemia Initiating Cells (LIC) by controlling nuclear localization of transcription factor, FOXO, in a CML mouse model (Naka K et al. 2010).

The data described above suggest that TGFβ has both negative and positive effects on the proliferation of normal hematopoietic and leukemia cells. However, some of the data appear discordant, which may be due to the complexity of the network in vivo. In the presence of other growth factors, TGFβ-induced stimulation or inhibition could be an indirect result or affected by other factors. Therefore, using a cell line as a research model may provide a direct effect of TGFβ and produce more consistent results. A TGFβ knock out hematopoietic cell line exhibited increased colony formation in response to IL-3, IL-6, and G-CSF (Kim S-J & Letterio J 2003), suggesting that TGFβ is inhibitory to the cells. TGFβ has been reported to inhibit proliferation of mouse myeloid leukemic M1 cells and induce adherence of M1 myeloid leukemia cells to plastic dishes (Okabe-Kado J 1989). In Josk-1 monoblastic leukemia cells, dephosphorylation of pRb and inhibition of c-myc were responsible for TGFβ1-induced G1 arrest (Furukawa Y 1992). In U937 cells, it identified that the inhibition of the cells by TGFβ1 was linked to low levels of transcription factors, C-jun, C-fos and Jun B (Kanatni Y 1996). In order to delineate the effect of TGFβ on more myeloid leukemia cell lines and to reach a general conclusion, we examined more than 10 human myeloid leukemia cell lines, among which MV4-11 and TF-1a are factor-independent but response cell lines; TF-1 and Mo7e are factor-dependent cell lines; and KG-1, KG-1a, K562, U937, HL60, and HEL are factor-independent and insensitive to any growth factors. We demonstrated that TGFβ is inhibitory for all these human myeloid leukemia cell lines in culture, with heterogeneous inhibitory responses being observed (Hu X et al 1999, Hu X & Zuckerman KS 2000). Inhibition of TF-1, KG-1, and K562, Mo7e, and HEL by TGFβ has also been reported by other groups recently (Moller GM et al. 2007, Koutoulaki A et al 2010, Fukuchi Y et al 2001, Kalina U et al. 2001). Our data and some recent discoveries, clearly indicate that the responses of the cell lines to TGFβ are not related to the apparent differentiation stages of the cells (Hu X et al 1999) but could result from differences in the amount of TGFβ receptors expressed or the degrees of the mutations (Quentmeier et al. 2003, 2006, Gu TL et al. 2006) in TGFβ signal components in these cells. The mechanisms by which TGFβ inhibits hematopoietic cells involves in the regulation of pRb pocket proteins-E2F complexes, downregulation of a number of cell cycle regulatory molecules, and upregulation of p21 (Ducos K et al 2000) and p57 (Scandura JM et al 2004) as described in following sections.

4. Regulation of pRb-E2F complexes in human myeloid leukemia cells

pRb acts as a signal transducer collecting signals from cell cycle regulatory molecules to transcriptional machinery. G1 protein kinases have been reported to modify pRb by phosphorylation, thereby promoting cell cycle progression toward DNA replication (Suryadinata R et al. 2011, Takaki T et al. 2004). The growth inhibition of human myeloid leukemia cells by TGFβ is linked to suppression of pRb phosphorylation on multiple serine and threonine residues, including Ser249/Thr252, Thr373, Ser780, Ser795, and Ser807/811 (Chen P et al. 1989, Mihara K et al. 1989, Hu X et al. 1999). Dephosphorylated pRb interacts with E2F transcription factors. E2F-binding sites have been found in the promoters of many genes that control cell cycle progression and cell proliferation, thereby E2Fs play a critical role in cell growth control (Iaquinta PJ et al. 2007). Previous studies identified that E2F binds to the pocket domain of pRB. In E2F1, the pRB-binding domain interacts with the C-terminus of the E2F molecule. As a consequence of the pRB-E2F interaction, E2F activity is repressed. pRB, therefore, exerts its growth suppression function mainly through its sequestration of E2F activity. However, one recent report suggests that E2F-1 binding affinity for pRb is not the only determinant of the E2F1 activity (Sahin F and Sladek TL 2010a). Of the seven E2Fs well documented, E2F1, E2F2, and E2F3 are considered as "activator" E2Fs, whereas, E2F4, E2F5, E2F6, and E2F7 are considered to be "repressor" E2Fs (Attwooll C et al. 2004, Sahin F and Sladek TL 2010b). pRb and two pRb-related proteins, p107 and p130, show a common structure, which are collectively termed the "pocket proteins". E2F1-3 bind to pRb, and E2F5 binds to p130. E2F4 can interact with the all three pocket proteins.

Dephosphorylated pRb preferentially interacts with E2F1-3 (Weinberg RA et al. 1995), and the pRb/E2F complexes are found primarily during the G1 phase of the cell cycle (Shirodkar S et al. 1992, Schwarz JK et al. 1993), during which time E2F-responsive promoters are repressed. The dissociation of the pRb/E2F-repressor complex and liberation of free E2F allows for the activation of these promoters (Hiebert SW et al. 1993, Qin X-Q et al. 1995, Helin K et al. 1993). It was demonstrated that E2F-1 responsive gene activation was inhibited by overexpression of wild-type pRb, but not by a mutant pRb, whereas transactivation mediated by mutants of E2F1, which do not bind to pRb, was not affected by overexpression of wild-type pRb. Loss of E2F1-3 resulted in an acute cell cycle arrest (Wu L et al. 2001). It has been found that Rb gene was often mutated in patients with various cancers, whereas p107 and p130 genes appear to be less frequently mutated in human cancers, suggesting that pRb is a tumor suppressor, whereas p107 and p130 are not. However, recent studies from several labs have shown that p130 and p107 also actively involved in E2F-dependent transcription activities. For example, the major E2F complexes in quiescent fibroblasts were E2F4-p130. As cells enter the cell cycle, E2F4-p130 was replaced by E2F4-p107 and E2F4-pRb (Ikeda M et al. 1996, Moberg K et al. 1996). Subsequent investigators, by performing chromatin immunoprecipitation (ChIP) experiments, were able to locate E2F complexes in a gene promoter. They have demonstrated that in serum-deprived cells, predominantly E2F4, p130, and a histone deacetylase (HDAC) are found to bind to corresponding E2F-responsive promoters (Rayman JB et al. 2002, Ren B et al. 2002, Takahashi Y et al. 2000). Since histones are generally hypoacetylated when a gene is turned off, which is regulated by HDAC, the results described above suggest that p130-E2F4 DNA binding activity is required for the gene inactivity and for arresting cells in quiescent state. As cells progress through mid-G1, E2F4 and p130 are replaced by activators E2F1, 2, and 3. Unexpectedly, loss of pRB had no effect on HDAC recruitment to the promoter or pRb was not detectable in the promoters containing the E2F responsive site in quiescent cells (Rayman JB et al. 2002, Takahashi Y et al. 2000). Thus, these data suggest that pRb may not be a primary negative regulator of E2F activity in control of cell cycle progression in these cells.

As indicated in the previous section, TGFβ dramatically inhibits the growth of several human myeloid leukemia cell lines in culture with a maximal growth inhibition being observed in MV4-11 cells. We asked how pRb-E2F complexes were regulated in MV4-11 cells. We found that in actively proliferating MV4-11 cells, p130 and pRb were expressed as peptides that migrated in multiple bands in SDS-PAGE, whereas in the cells treated with TGFβ, p130 and pRb were dephosphorylated. However, TGFβ did not dephosphrylate p107 but inhibited expression of the molecule (Hu X et al. 2000). Subsequently, we found that TGFβ-treated MV4-11 cells had very low levels of pRb-associated E2F1 and E2F3. The low levels of pRb-E2Fs are resulted from a low expression of E2F1 and E2F3 in response to TGFβ that arrested cells in G1 phase. Unexpectedly, proliferating cells without TGFβ contained substantial quantities of pRb-E2F1 and pRb-E2F3 complexes. In contrast, the cells treated with TGFβ (i.e. G1 cells) showed increased levels of pRb-E2F4 and p130-E2F4 and low level of p107-E2F4, as detected by immunoprecipitation and Western blotting. Since TGFβ treatment inhibited the expression p107 but not E2F4, thus, the low level of p107-E2F4 complexes is a result of the inhibition of p107. Our data indicate that E2F4 was switched from p107 to pRb and p130 when p107 was inhibited in response to TGFβ treatment. By performing electrophoretic gel mobility shift assay (EMSA), we were not able to detect pRb-E2F4 DNA binding activities either in proliferating cells or in G1 cells but exhibited the existence of p107-E2F4 and p130-E2F4 DNA binding complexes in G1 cells. which is consistent with the reports from the ChIP experiments described above. Taking together, our data suggest that p107 and p130, but not pRb, and the repressor E2F, but not activator E2Fs, play a critical role in regulating E2F-responsive gene expression in TGFβ-mediated cell cycle control in human myeloid leukemia cells. This conclusion is consistent with several studies that have failed to detect pRb at E2F-responsive genes, whereas p107 and p130 are readily detectable (Aslanian A 2004, Rayman JB 2002, Takahashi Y 2000, Wells J 2000). In addition, many cell cycle-regulated E2F targets are depressed in p107-/- and p130-/- cells but are not depressed in Rb-/- cells (Herrera RE 1996, Hurford Jr RK 1997, Mulligan GJ 1998). It is not clear if traditional activator E2Fs have any significant impact on cell cycle progression of MV4-11 cells, because pRb-E2F1 and pRb-E2F3 complexes have been found in the proliferating but not in G1 phase cells. Previous studies suggest that pRb may bind other regulatory regions of DNA or uses other mechanisms (Sun H et al. 2011), directly or indirectly, for its inhibitory function as a tumor repressor. pRb may also have both positive or negative role on cell growth, depending on the transcription factors it interacted (Calo E et al. 2010).

5. TGFβ inhibits both G1 and G2 protein kinases in human myeloid leukemia cells

In mammalian cells, the cell cycle progression is regulated by a group of cyclin dependent kinases (cdks) and their regulatory subunits in sequential order: cyclin D-cdk4/cdk6 and cyclin E-cdk2 complexes act on G1 and G1-S transition, respectively, followed by cyclin A-cdk2 on S and cyclin B-cdc2 at G2-M transition. TGFβ is well known to be a negative regulator of G_1 cyclin/cdk activity in many types of cells. This has been reported to be a major mechanism that is responsible for TGFβ-induced growth inhibition of cells. In epithelial and fibroblasts, the negative role of TGFβ includes inhibition of cdk4 and disruption of cyclin E-cdk2 assembly (Ewen ME et al. 1993, Koff A et al 1993). Although TGFβ is known to be a G1 cdk inhibitor, studies from several groups suggest potential effect of TGFβ on G2 checkpoint kinase. For instance, the mouse epithelial cells treated with TGFβ expressed a lower level of cdc2 as compared with the cells without TGFβ (Fautsch MP et al 1995); in a hepatoma cell line, TGFβ activates cdc2 and cdk2 followed by phosphorylation of pRb which in turn triggers apoptosis of the cells (Choi KS et al 1999). A new report published in 2008 presented evidence that disruption of Smad 3, a key component of TGFβ-induced signal pathway, elevated cdk 1(cdc2) activity via upregulating the expression of cyclin B. As a result, the uncontrolled cdk1 delayed mitotic progression (Fujita T 2008). In human myeloid leukemia cells, we found that inhibition of multiple cdks including cdc2 and cdc25C is a dominant event in TGFβ-induced growth inhibition of the cells (Hu X et al.

2001). Our recent studies, using TF-1 and MV4-11 human myeloid leukemia cells, demonstrated that TGFβ1-induced inhibition of leukemia cell growth is not due solely to downregulation of G_1 cyclins and cdks but also G2 check point kinases (Hu X 2007). In MV4-11 cells, TGFβ caused a rapid and transient dephosphorylation of cdc2 (Tyr15) and cdc25c (Ser216), with 60% and 70% inhibition of phosphorylation of the both proteins by 2-3 hours, respectively, followed by returning to near normal by 12 hours, and 70-100% inhibitions again by 24-72 hours, repectively. The dephosphorylation of cdc2 and cdc25c was followed by a dramatic decrease of total cdc25c (100% decrease at 48 and 72 hours) and cylcin B1 and cdc2 (70-90% reduction at 24 to 72 hours). Consistent with these data, cdc2 kinase activity, as determined by ability to phosphorylate histone H1 and GST-Rb in vitro, was markedly reduced in the leukemia cells treated with TGFβ for 24-48 h. Cyclin B1 and cdc25c were degraded in a ubiquitin/26S proteosome assay system in vitro, which suggests strongly that ubiquitination and proteasomal degradation may be the key mechanism of degradation that leads to block of G_2-M transition. The downregulation of cdc2, cdc25c, and cyclin B1 was not a result of G1 arrest but a direct effect of TGFβ, because the time required for the inhibition of the cells released from G2 is much shorter than the cells released from G1. Using immunoprecipitation and Western blotting we detected that the levels of cyclin B1-cdc2 complexes were much lower in extracts of TGFβ-treated cells than in control cells. Based on our data, we suggest that TGFβ suppresses growth of human myeloid leukemia cells through multiple pathways, by inhibiting both G1 and G2 checkpoint kinases. Since the G1 and G2 checkpoint kinases are able to phosphorylate pRb in proliferating cells, the down regulation of G1 and G2 checkpoint kinases would prevent pRb phospharylation, leading to G1 arrest. The data also suggest that cdc2, a traditional G2 regulator in mammalian cells, may participate in G1 regulation. Fig. 1 illustrates diagrammatically the negative roles of TGFβ in the cell cycle control in myeloid leukemic MV4-11 cells.

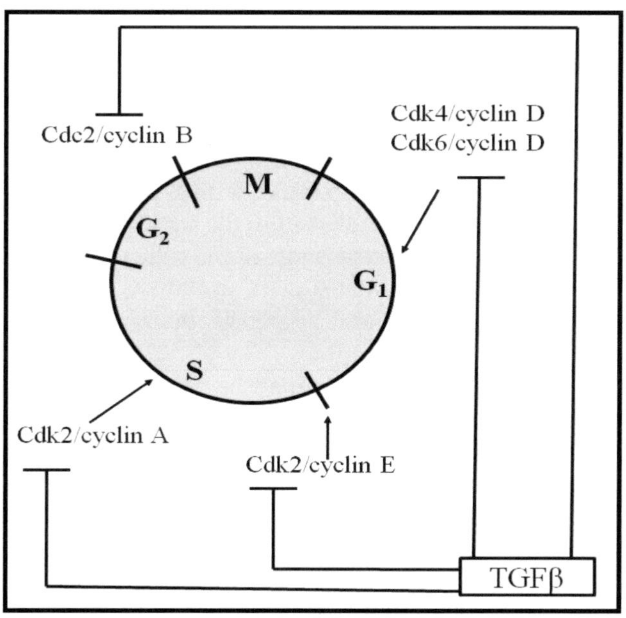

Fig. 1. TGFβ inhibits both G! and G@ cdks in MV4-11 cells

6. Dual roles of cdk inhibitors in human myeloid leukemia cells

It is well known that activity of cdks is counterbalanced by cdk inhibitors (ckis). The cdk inhibitors can be classified into two different families: Ink4 (p16, p15, p18 and p19) and cip/kip (p21, p27, and p57), based on their structure similarity. Among these cdk inhibitors, p27 and p21 have been intensively studied in various types of cells. In quiescent cells or cells treated with TGFβ show high level of p27, whereas proliferating cells or cells treated with mitogens express low level of p27 (Moller MB 2000). Overexpression of p27 in cultured cells arrests the cells in G1 phase and antisense inhibition of p27 reverses cell cycle arrest induced by p27 (Coats S et al 1996; Rivard N et al. 1996). In vivo, p27 is a critical regulator of cellular proliferation. Mice lacking p27 gene are 15–30% larger than their wild-type or hemizygous ($p27^{+/-}$) littermates (Fero et al. 1996; Kiyokawa et al. 1996). p27 was initially thought to interfere with the activities of cyclin D-, E-, and A-dependent kinases. The crystal structure of p27 bound to cyclin-cdk2 reveals that a p27 fragment inserts itself within the cdk2 catalytic site, blocking ATP access (Russo et al., 1996). These data lead to a popular model in which anti-proliferative stimuli up-regulate p27, followed by inhibition of cyclinD-cdk4, cyclinE-cdk2, cyclin A-cdk2 activities, and by G1 arrest/growth inhibition. Similar to p27, as a negative regulator of the cell cycle progression, p21 is thought to bind and inhibit cdk2/cyclin E and/or cdk4/cyclin D complexes, thereby arresting cells at the G1 phase. The induction of p21 is regulated by the tumor suppressor gene, p53, in response to DNA damage.

The traditional model of p27 or p21 as a cdk inhibitor has been challenged by a number of studies from several labs in which p21 or p27 were demonstrated to be required for a cdk/cyclin kinase activity or to be a dual player in cell cycle control (Zhang H et al 1994, LaBaer et al 1997). It was reported that p21, at low concentration, promotes the assembly of active kinase complexes, whereas a high concentration of p21 causes the opposite effect in SAOS-2 cells derived from osteosarcoma (LaBaer et al., 1997). In an animal model, it was found that low concentration of p21 could promote tumor progression in the presence of oncogenic factors (Jones JM 1999). Primary mouse fibroblasts that are p21-/- and p27-/- were failed to assemble cylcin D-CDK complexes and were unable to direct cyclin D nuclear translocation (Cheng M 1999). Consistent with this report, p27 was demonstrated to be essential for mouse mammary gland morphogenesis and function (Muraoka RS et al. 2001); an increased level of p21 was found to be parallel with S-phase entry of oligodendrocytes (Bansal R et al. 2005). In another report published in the same year, p27 in mouse T cells was found to acts as a promoter during the early stage of the cell cycle (Rowell EA et al 2005). In addition, it has been reported that in MCF-7 cells, cyclin D1 promotes cellular migration through inducing the expression of p27 and by physically associating with p27 to promote cellular migration (Li Z et al. 2006). These dual roles of p21 and p27 in non-hematopoietic cells are consistent with what we found in human hematopoietic cells a few years ago. By using several human myeloid leukemia cell lines as research models, we demonstrated that p27 has differential effect on cdk2 and cyclin E activities, which provides supplementary information to the evidence of p27 and p21 having dual roles in cell cycle control described above (Hu X et al. 2001). Although TGFβ greatly upregulated p27 in both cytosol and nucleus in MV4-11 cells, the association of p27 with cylcin E and cdk2 showed different patterns with increased amount of cyclin E-p27 and decreased levels of cdk2-p27 being detected by Western blot and immunoprecipitation. Surprised, a significant amount of p27 was found to associate with cdk2 in proliferating cells, which was downregulated in response to TGFβ. The downregulation is a result of inhibition of total cdk2 by TGFβ. However, TGFβ had no effect on the expression of cyclin E. By carrying out p27 immunodepletion and transfection experiments, we further demonstrated that that at least some cdk2 kinase activity is associated with p27 in MV4-11cells. Additional support for this possibility was the observation that cells transfected with anti-sense p27 cDNA but not empty plasmid, downregulated cdk2 kinase activity by more than 60%. Although p27 also may act as an adapter of cyclin E activity, as suggested by expression of cyclin E- p27 complexes in proliferating MV4 11 cells, p27 mainly acts as an inhibitor of cyclin E activity in response to TGFβ. This is indicated by the fact that TGFβ1 upregulated cyclin E-associated p27 and was accompanied by the inhibition of cyclin E-dependent kinase activity. Moreover, p27 immunodepletion dramatically upregulated cyclin E-dependent kinase activity in TGFβ1 treated cells. The effect of p27 on cyclin E-dependent kinase activity is dose-dependent, with only high concentrations of p27 being inhibitory to cyclin E activity. This may explain the observation that immunodepletion of p27 or anti-sense p27 cDNA did not significantly increase cyclin E-dependent kinase activity in proliferating MV4-11 cells. These results are against the notion that p27 is a negative regulator of cdk2 kinase *in vivo,* at least in these human myeloid leukemia cells. Our data are consistent with previous findings, in which cell cycle arrest mediated by TGFβ remained intact in p27-/- cells (Nakayama et al., 1996) and p21 and p27 has dual roles in cell cycle control (Rowell EA et al. 2005, LaBaer et al. 1997, Zhang H et al. 1994). The difference is that the negative or positive role of p27 in our model is related to the molecules p27 interacted but not the concentrations of p27 as reported in the case of p21 (Matsushime et al., 1992). Taken together, we interpret our results to suggest that in proliferating cells p27 is associated with cdk2 and cdk4 as an adapter. TGFβ1 downregulates cdk2, cdk4, and D-type cyclins, which leaves $p27^{kip1}$ free to bind and saturate cyclin E, inhibiting cyclin E-cdk2 assembly, rendering cyclin E-dependent kinase inactive. By using these two different regulatory mechanisms, TGFβ1 magnifies its cell cycle inhibitory efficiency in human myeloid leukemia cells (Hu X et al 2001).

7. Conclusion

New findings in recent years have provided insight into the complex roles and action mechanisms of TGFβ in various types of cells. TGFβ exhibits its distinct effect on the growth of human myeloid leukemia cells. Although both positive and negative roles of TGFβ in hematopoiesis have been reported, the major role of TGFβ appears to be inhibitory with heterogeneous responses being observed in human myeloid leukemia cells. The heterogeneous responses of the cells to TGFβ are not related to the apparent differentiation stages of the cells but could result from differences in the expression of TGFβ receptors or degrees of the mutations in the components of TGFβ signal pathways. TGFβ, a traditional G1 cdk inhibitor, represses not only G1 but also G2 protein kinases in human myeloid leukemia cells. pRb has been reported to be a tumor suppressor in various types of cells. The new studies suggest that p130, whose gene is less mutated in cancer patients, plays a critical role in maintaining cells in quiescent status and in TGFβ-mediated growth inhibition. Traditionally, p27 and p21 are G1 cdk inhibitors. However, new evidence suggests that p27 and p21 have both positive and negative effect on G1 cdk activities.

Based on the data described in this review, it is clear that TGFβ signals have a defined role in regulating normal hematopoiesis, and disruption of the signaling components could lead

to hematologic malignancies including myeloid leukemia. These are suggested by the observations described above: (1) The development of hematopoietic cells from mesoderm in embryos is regulated by TGFβ signaling; (2) inactivation of the TGFβ signaling pathway leads to malignant transformation of early hematopoietic cells; (3) abnormal expressions of the components of TGFβ signaling pathway have been found in AML and CML; and (4) a number of mutations of genes that encode TGFβ signaling components have been detected in several myeloid leukemia cell lines. Thus, the mutated components may be the targets for therapeutic strategy of myeloid leukemia in future.
Although new information on TGFβ and myeloid leukemia have been emerged at an incredibly rapid pace, it is unclear whether some information obtained from studies performed *in vitro* mimic a physiological status *in vivo*. In addition, the detail about dual role of cdk inhibitiors and the role of pRb in leukemia transformation are also need to be clarified in future.

8. References

Aglietta, M., Stacchini, A., Severino, A., Sanavio, F., Ferrando, M.L., Piacibello, W. (1989). Interaction of transforming growth factor-beta with hematopoietic growth factors in the regulation of human normal and leukemic myelopoiesis. *Exp Hematol,* 17 (3): 296-299.

Aida J, Higuchi S, Hasegawa Y, Nagano-Ito M, Hirabayashi Y, Banba A, Shimizu T, Kikuchi A, Saga M, Ichikawa S (2011). Up-regulation of ceramide glucosyltransferase during the differentiation of U937 cells. *J Biochem.* May 10. (ahead of print)

Aslanian A, Iaquinta PJ, Verona R, Lees JA (2004). Repression of the Arf tumor suppressor by E2F3 is required for normal cell cycle kinetics. *Genes Dev.* 18 (12):1413-22.

Attwooll, C., Denchi, E.L., Helin, K. (2004). The E2F family: specific functions and overlapping interests. EMBO J, 23 (24): 4709-4716.

Avancd GC, Lista P, Giovinazzo B, Miniero R, Saglio G, Benetton G, Coda R, Catoretti G and Pegoraro P. (1988). Selective growth response to IL-3 of a human leukemic cell line with megakaryoblastic features. *Br J Haematol* 69 (3): 359-366.

Bansal R, Marin-Husstege M, Bryant M, Casaccia-Bonnefil P. (2005). S-phase entry of oligodendrocyte lineage cells is associated with increased levels of p21Cip1. Neurosci Res. May 1; 80(3):360-368.

Batard P, Monier MN, Fortunel N, Ducos K, Sansilvestri-Morel P, Phan T Hatzfeld A, Hatzfeld JA. (2000). TGF-b1 maintains hematopoietic immaturity by a reversible negative control of cell cycle and induces CD34 antigen up-modulation. J Cell Sci 113: (Pt 3) 383–390.

Calo E, Quintero-Estades JA, Danielian PS, Nedelcu S, Berman SD, Lees JA (2010). Rb regulates fate choice and lineage commitment in vivo. Nature. Aug 26; 466 (7310):1110-1114.

Cashman, J.D., Eaves, A.C., Eaves, C.J. (1992). Granulocyte-macrophage colony-stimulating factor modulation of the inhibitory effect of transforming growth factor-beta on normal and leukemic human hematopoietic progenitor cells. *Leukemia,* Sep, 6 (9): 886-892.

Cerdan C, Rouleau A, Bhatia M. (2004) VEGF-A165 augments erythropoietic development from human embryonic stem cells. *Blood* 2004; April 1, 103(7):2504-2512.

Chadwick K, Wang L, Li L, Menendez P, Murdoch B, Rouleau A, Bhatia M (2003) Cytokines and BMP-4 promote hematopoietic differentiation of human embryonic stem cells. *Blood,* August 1, 102(3):906-915.

Chen, P., Scully, P.J., Shew, Y., Wang, J.Y., Lee, W.H. (1989). Phosphorylation of the retinoblastoma gene product is modulated during the cell cycle and cellula differentiation. *Cell,* Sep 22, 58 (6): 1193-1198.

Cheng, M., Olivier, P., Diehl, J.A., Fero, M., Roussel, M.F., Roberts, J.M., Sherr, C.J. (1999). The p21cip1 and p27kip1 'inhibitors' are essential activators of cyclin D-dependent kinases in murine fibroblasts. EMBO J, March 15, 18(6): 1571-1583.

Choi KS, Eom YW, Kang Y, Ha MJ, Rhee H, Yoon JW, Kim SJ. (1999) Cdc2 and Cdk2 kinase activated by transforming growth factor-beta1 trigger apoptosis through the phosphorylation of retinoblastoma protein in FaO hepatoma cells. *J Biol Chem.* Nov 5, 274(45):31775-83.

Classen, S., Zander, T., Eggle, D., Chemnitz, J.M., Brors, B., Büchmann, I., Popov, A., Beyer, M., Eils, R., Debey, S., Schultze, J.L. (2007). Human resting CD4+ T cells are constitutively inhibited by TGF beta under steady-state conditions. *J Immunol,* Jun 1, 178(11): 6931-6940.

Coats S, Flanagan WM, Nourse J, Roberts JM. (1996) Requirement of p27Kip1 for restriction point control of the fibroblast cell cycle. *Science,* May 10, 272(5263):877-880.

Ducos K, Panterne B, Fortunel N, Hatzfeld A, Monier MN, Hatzfeld J. (2000) p21(cip1) mRNA is controlled by endogenous transforming growth factor-b1 in quiescent human hematopoietic stem/progenitor cells. J Cell Physiol July, 184 (1): 80–85.

Ewen ME, Sluss HK, Whitehouse LL, Livingston DM (1993). TGF beta inhibition of cdk4 synthesis is linked to cell cycle arrest. *Cell,* Sep 24, 74 (6):1009-1020.

Fautsch MP, Eblen ST, Anders RA, Burnette RJ, Leof EB (1995). Differential regulation of p34cdc2 and p33cdk2 by transforming growth factor-beta 1 in murine mammary epithelial cells. *J Cell Biochem* August, 58 (4):517-526.

Fero M.L., Rivkin M., Tasch M., Porter P., Carow C.E., Firpo E., Polyak K., Tsai L.H., Broudy V., Perlmutter R.M. (1996). A syndrome of multiorgan hyperplasia with features of gigantism, tumorigenesis, and female in p27(Kip1)-deficient mice. *Cell,* May 31 85 (5) :733–744

Fortunel NO, Hatzfeld A, Hatzfeld JA. (2000). Transforming growth factor-b: pleiotropic role in the regulation of hematopoiesis. *Blood* Sep 15, 96(6): 2022–2036.

Fujita T, Epperly MW, Zou H, Greenberger JS, Wan Y. (2008) Regulation of the anaphase-promoting complex-separase cascade by transforming growth factor-beta modulates mitotic progression in bone marrow stromal cells. *Mol Biol Cell,* Dec., 19(12):5446-55.

Fukuchi Y, Kizaki M, Yamato K, Kawamura C, Umezawa A, Hata Ji, Nishihara T, Ikeda Y. (2001) Mcl-1, an early-induction molecule, modulates activin A-induced apoptosis and differentiation of CML cells. *Oncogene,* Feb 8, 20(6):704-713.

Furukawa, Y., Uenoyama, S., Ohta, M., Tsunoda, A., Griffin, J.D., Saito, M. (1992). Transforming growth factor-β inhibits phosphorylation of the retinoblastoma susceptibility gene product in human monocytic leukemia cell line JOSK-I. *J Bio Chem,* August 25, 267(24), 17121-17127.

Gallagher R, Collins S, Trujillo J, *et al.* (1979). Characterization of the continuous, differentiating myeloid cell line (HL-60) from a patient with acute promyelocytic leukemia. *Blood*, Sep., 54 (3): 713–733.

Goey, H., Keller, J.R., Back, T., Longo, D.L., Ruscetti, F.W., Wiltrout, R.H. (1989). Inhibition of early murine hematopoietic progenitor cell proliferation after in vivo localregional administration of transforming growth factor-β1. *J Immunol,* August 1, 143(3), 877-880.

Gu TL, Goss VL, Reeves C, Popova L, Nardone J, Macneill J, Walters DK, Wang Y, Rush J, Comb MJ, Druker BJ, Polakiewicz RD. (2006). Phosphotyrosine profiling identifies the KG-1 cell line as a model for the study of FGFR1 fusions in acute myeloid leukemia. *Blood,* Dec 15, 108(13):4202-4204.

Helin, K., Harlow, E., and Fattaey, A. (1993). Inhibtion of E2F-1 transactivation by direct binding of the retinoblastoma gene. *Mol cell Biol,* Oct, 13(10): 6501-6508.

Herrera, R.E., Sah, V.P., Williams, B.O., Makela, T.P., Weinberg, R.A., Jacks, T. (1996). Altered cell cycle kinetics, gene expression, and G1 restriction point regulation in Rb-deficient fibroblasts. *Mol. Cell Biol, May, 16(5), 2402-2407.*

Hiebert, S.W. (1993). Regions of the retinoblastoma gene product required for its interaction with the E2F transcription factor are necessary for E2F promoter repression and pRb-mediated growth suppression. Mol Cell Biol, Jun, 13(6): 3384-3391.

Hu, X., Cress, D.W., Zhong, Q., Zuckerman, K.S. (2000). Phosphorylation of pRB family and formation of pRb family/E2F-4 complexes are differentially regulated in proliferating cells and cells arrested in G1-phase by TGFβ1. *Biochem Biophys Res Commun,* Oct, 276(3): 930-939.

Hu X, Cui D, Moscinski LC, Zhang X, Maccachero V, Zuckerman KS. (2007) TGFbeta regulates the expression and activities of G2 checkpoint kinases in human myeloid leukemia cells. Cytokine, Feb, 37(2):155-162.

Hu X, Moscinski LC, Hill BJ, Fisher AB, and Zuckerman KS. (1998). Characterization of a unique factor-independent variant derived from human factor-dependent TF-1 cells: a transformed event. *Leukemia Res* Sep, 22(9): 817-826

Hu, X., Moscinski, L.C., Zuckerman, K.S. (1999). Transforming growth factor-β (TGFβ) inhibits growth of more differentiated myeloid leukemia cells and retinoblastoma protein phosphorylation at Ser795. *Exp Hematol,* Apr, 27(4), 605-614.

Hu, X., Zhang, X., Zhong, Q., Fisher, A.B., Bryington, M., Zuckerman. K.S. (2001). Differential effects of transforming growth factor on cell cycle regulatory molecules in human myeloid leukemia cells. *Oncogene,* Oct 18, 20(47): 6840-6850.

Hu X Zuckerman KS (2000) Cell cycle and transcriptional control of human myeloid leukemic cells by transforming growth factor beta. Leukemia and Lymphoma Jul, 38(3-4): 235-246.

Hurford, R.K. Jr., Cobrinik, D., Lee, M.H., Dyson, N. (1997). pRB and p107/p130 are required for the regulated expression of different sets of E2F responsive genes. *Genes Dev,* Jun 1, 11(11): 1447-1463.

Iaquinta PJ, Lees JA. (2007). Life and death decisions by the E2F transcription factors. Curr Opin Cell Biol. Dec, 19(6):649–657.

Ikeda, M.A., Jakoi, L., Nevins, J.R. (1996). A unique role for the Rb protein in controlling E2F accumulation during cell growth and differentiation. *Proc Natl Acad Sci U S A,* Apr 16, 93(8): 3215-3220.

Imai Y, Kurokawa M, Izutsu K, Hangaishi A, Maki K, Ogawa S, Chiba S, Mitani K, Hirai H. (2001). Mutations of the Smad4 gene in acute myelogeneous leukemia and their functional implications in leukemogenesis. *Oncogene*. Jan 4, 20(1): 88-96.

Inman GJ, Allday MJ. (2000). Resistance to TGF-β1 correlates with a reduction of TGF-β type II receptor expression in Burkitt's pymphoma and Epsein-Barr virus-transformed B lymphoblastoid cell lines. *J Gen Virol,* Jun, 81(Pt 6): 1567-1578.

Inman GJ, Nicolás FJ, Callahan JF, Harling JD, Gaster LM, Reith AD, Laping NJ, Hill CS. (2002) SB-431542 is a potent and specific inhibitor of transforming growth factor-beta superfamily type I activin receptor-like kinase (ALK) receptors ALK4, ALK5, and ALK7. *Mol Pharmacol*. Jul, 62(1): 65-74.

Jones JM, Cui XS, Medina D, Donehower LA. (1999). Heterozygosity of p21WAF1/CIP1 enhances tumor cell proliferation and cyclin D1-associated kinase activity in a murine mammary cancer model. *Cell Growth Differ,* Apr,10(4):213-222.

Kanatni, Y., Kasukabe, T., Okabe-Kado, J., Hayashi, S.I., Yamamoto-Yamaguchi, Y., Motoyoshi, K., Nagata, N., Honma, Y. (1996). Transforming growth factor beta and dexamethasone cooperatively enhance c-jun gene expression and inhibit the growth of human monocytoid leukemia cells. *Cell Growth & Differ,* Feb, 7(2): 187-196.

Kalina U, Koschmieder S, Hofmann WK, Wagner S, Kauschat D, Hoelzer D, Ottmann OG. Transforming growth factor-beta1 interferes with thrombopoietin-induced signal transduction in megakaryoblastic and erythroleukemic cells.(2001). Exp Hematol May, 29(5): 602-608.

Kaufman DS, Hanson ET, Lewis RL, Auerbach R, Thomson JA. Hematopoietic colony-forming cells derived from human embryonic stem cells. *Proc Natl Acad Sci USA* 2001, Sep 11, 98(19):10716-10721.

Keller, J.R., Bartelmez, S.H., Sitnicka, E., Ruscetti, F.W., Ortiz, M., Gooya, J.M., Jacobsen, S.E.W. (1994). Distinct and overlapping direct effects of macrophage inflammatory protein-1 alpha and transforming growth factor beta on hematopoietic progenitor/stem cell growth. *Blood,* Oct 1, *84(7),* 2175-2181.

Keller, J.R., Jacobsen, S.E.W., Dubois, C.M., Hestda, I.K., Ruscetti, F.W. (1992). Transforming growth factor-beta: A bidirectional regulator of hematopoietic cell growth. *Int. J Cell Cloning,* Jan, *10(1)*:2-11.

Keller, J.R., Jacobsen, S.E.W., Sill, K., Ellingsworth, L., Ruscetti, F.W. (1991). Stimulation of granulopoiesis by transforming growth factor β: Synergy with granulocyte-macrophage colony-stimulating factor. *Proc Natl Acad Sci USA,* Aug 15, 88(16): 7190-7194

Keller, J.R., McNiece, I.M., Sill, K.T., Ellingsworth, L.R., Quesenberry, P.J., Sing, G.K., Ruscetti, F.W. (1990). Transforming growth factor-β directly regulates primitive murine hematopoietic cell proliferation. *Blood,* Feb 1, 75(3): 596-602.

Kim SJ, Letterio J. (2003). Transforming growth factor-β signaling in normal and malignant hematopoiesis. *Leukemia,* Sep, 17(9): 1731-1737.

Kitamura T, Tange T, Terasawa T, Chiba S, Kuwaki T, Miyagawa K, Piao Y-F, Miyazonno K, Urabe A and Takaku F. (1989). Establishment and characterization of a unique human cell line that proliferates dependently on GM-CSF, IL-3, or erythropoietin. *J Cell Physiol* Aug, 140(2): 323-334.

Kiyokawa H., Kineman R.D., Manova-Todorova K.O., Soares V.C., Hoffman E.S., Ono M., Khanam D., Hayday A.C., Frohman L.A., Koff A (1996). Enhanced growth of mice lacking the cyclin-dependent kinase inhibitor function of p27(Kip1) *Cell.* May 31, 85(5):721-732

Koeffler HP, Billing R, Lusis AJ, Sparkes R and Golde DW. (1980). An undifferentiated variant derived from the human acute myelogenous leukemia cell line (KG-1). *Blood* Aug, 56(2): 265-273

Koeffler HP and Golde DW. (1978). Acute myelogenous leukemia: a human cell line responsive to colony-stimulating activity. *Science,* Jun 9, 200(4346): 1153-1154

Koff A, Ohtsuki M, Polyak K, Roberts JM, Massague J (1993). Negative regulation of G1 in mammalian cells: inhibition of cyclin E-dependent kinase by TGF-beta. Science Apr 23, 260(5107): 536-539.

Koutoulaki A, Langley M, Sloan AJ, Aeschlimann D, Wei XQ. (2010). TNFalpha and TGF-beta1 influence IL-18-induced IFNgamma production through regulation of IL-18 receptor and T-bet expression. Cytokine, Feb, 49(2):177-184.

Kulkarni AB, Huh CG, Becker D, Geiser A, Lyght M, Flanders KC et al (1993). Transforming growth factor beta 1 null mutation in mice causes excessive inflammatory response and early death. Proc Natl Acad Sci USA, Jan 15, 90(2): 770–774.

LaBaer J, Garrett MD, Stevenson LF, Slingerland JM, Sandhu C, Chou HS, Fattaey A, Harlow E. (1997). New functional activities for the p21 family of CDK inhibitors. *Genes Dev,* Apr 1, 11(7):847-862.

Lange B, Valtieri M, Santoli D, Caracciolo D, Mavilio F, Gemperlein I, Griffin C, Emanuel B, Finan J, Nowell P, Rovera G. (1987). Growth factor requirements of childhood acute leukemia: establishment of GM-CSF-dependent cell lines. *Blood,* Jul, 70 (1): 192-199.

Le Bousse-Kerdiles MC, Chevillard S, Charpentier A, Romquin N, Clay D, Smadja-Joffe F, Praloran V, Dupriez B, Demory JL, Jasmin C, Martyré MC. (1996). Differential expression of transforming growth factor-b, basic fibroblast growth factor, and their receptors in CD34+ hematopoietic progenitor cells from patients with myelofibrosis and myeloid metaplasia. Blood. Dec 15, 88(12):4534-4546.

Li Z, Jiao X, Wang C, Ju X, Lu Y, Yuan L, Lisanti MP, Katiyar S, Pestell RG. (2006). Cyclin D1 induction of cellular migration requires p27(KIP1). *Cancer Res,* Oct 15, 66(20):9986-94.

Lozzio, C.B. Lozzio, B.B. (1975), "Human chronic myelogenous leukemia cell-line with positive Philadelphia chromosome", *Blood* Mar, 45(3): 321–334,

Martin P and Papayannopoulou T. (1982). HEL cells: a new human erythroleukemia cell line with spontaneous and induced globin expression. *Science,* Jun 11, 216(4551): 1233-1235.

McNiece, I.K., Bertoncello, I., Keller, J.R., Ruscetti, F.W., Hartley, C.A., Zsebo, K.M. (1992). Transforming growth factor □ inhibits the action of stem cell factor on mouse and human hematopoietic progenitors. *Int. J. Cell Cloning,* Mar, 10(2), 80-86.

Mihara, K., X.R. Cao, A. Yen, S. Chandler, B. Driscoll, AL. Murphree, A. Tang, and YK Fung. (1989). Cell cycle-dependent regulation of phosphorylation of the human retinoblastoma gene product. *Science,* Dec 8, 246(4935): 1300-1303

Moberg, K., Starz, M.A., Lees, J.A. (1996). E2F-4 switches from p130 to p107 and pRb in response to cell cycle reentry. Mol Cell Biol, Apr 16(4): 1436-1449.

Moller MB (2000). P27 in cell cycle control and cancer. Leukemia and Lymphoma, Sep, 39(1-2): 19-27.

Møller GM, Frost V, Melo JV, Chantry A. (2007) Upregulation of the TGFbeta signalling pathway by Bcr-Abl: implications for haemopoietic cell growth and chronic myeloid leukaemia. *FEBS Lett,* Apr 3, 581(7):1329-1334.

Morita, N., Yamamoto, M., Tanizawa, T. (2003). Correlation of c-kit expression and cell cycle regulation by transforming growth factor-beta in CD34+ CD38- human bone marrow cells. Eur J Haematol, Nov, 71(5), 351-358.

Mulligan, G.J., Wong, J., Jacks, T. (1998). p130 is dispensable in peripheral T lymphocytes: evidence for functional compensation by p107 and pRB. Mol Cell Biol, Jan, 18(1), 206-220.

Muraoka RS, Lenferink AE, Simpson J, Brantley DM, Roebuck LR, Yakes FM, Arteaga CL. (2001). Cyclin-dependent kinase inhibitor p27(Kip1) is required for mouse mammary gland morphogenesis and function. *J Cell Biol.* May 28, 153(5):917-932.

Naka K, Hoshii T, Muraguchi T, Tadokoro Y, Ooshio T, Kondo Y, Nakao S, Motoyama N, Hirao A. (2010). TGF-beta-FOXO signalling maintains leukaemia-initiating cells in chronic myeloid leukaemia. Nature, Feb 4, 463(7281):676-680.

Nakayama K, Ishida N, Shirane M, Inomata A, Inoue T, Shishido N, Horii I, Loh DY, Nakayama K. (1996) Mice lacking p27(Kip1) display increased body size, multiple organ hyperplasia, retinal dysplasia, and pituitary tumors. *Cell,* May 31, 85(5):707-720.

Okabe-Kado J, Honma Y, Hayashi M, Hozumi M. (1989). Inhibitory action of transforming growth factor-beta on induction of differentiation of myeloid leukemia cells. Jpn J Cancer Res. Mar, 80(3):228-232.

Olsen AL, Stachura DL, Weiss MJ. (2006). Designer blood: creating hematopoietic lineages from embryonic stem cells. *Blood*; Feb 15, 107(4):1265-1275.

Otten J, Schmitz L, Vettorazzi E, Schultze A, Marx AH, Simon R, Krauter J, Loges S, Sauter G, Bokemeyer C, Fiedler W. (2011). Expression of TGF-β receptor ALK-5 has a negative impact on outcome of patients with acute myeloid leukemia. *Leukemia.* Feb;25(2):375-379.

Ottmann, O.G. & Pelus, L.M. (1991). Differential proliferative effects of transforming growth factor-β on human hematopoietic progenitor cells. *J Immunol,* Apr 15, 140(8), 2661-2665.

Park C, Afrikanova I, Chung YS, Zhang WJ, Arentson E, Fong Gh G, Rosendahl A, Choi K. (2004). A hierarchical order of factors in the generation of FLK1- and SCL-expressing hematopoietic and endothelial progenitors from embryonic stem cells. *Development,* Jun, 131(11):2749-2762.

Piedfer M, Dauzonne D, Tang R, N'guyen J, Billard C, Bauvois B. Aminopeptidase-N/CD13 is a potential proapoptotic target in human myeloid tumor cells. FASEB J. 2011 May 12 (ahead of print).

Qin, X-Q., Livingston, D.M., Ewen, M., Sellers, W.R., Arany, Z., Kaelin, W.G. Jr. (1995). The transcription factor E2F1 is a downstream target of Rb action. *Mol Cell Biol,* Feb, 15(2), 742-755.

Quentmeier H, MacLeod RAF, Zaborski M and Drexler HG (2006) *JAK2* V617F tyrosine kinase mutation in cell lines derived from myeloproliferative disorders. *Leukemia,* Mar, 20(3) 471–476.

Quentmeier H, Reinhardt J, Zaborski M and Drexler HG (2003). FLT3 mutations in acute myeloid leukemia cell lines. *Leukemia,* Jan, 17(1), 120–124.

Rayman, J.B., Takahashi, Y., Indjeian, V.B., Dannenberg, J.H., Catchpoles, S., Watson, R.J., te Riele, H., Dynlacht, B.D. (2002). E2F mediates cell cycle-dependent transcriptional repression in vivo by recruitment of an HDAC1/mSin3B corepressor complex. *Genes Dev,* 16(8), 933-947.

Ren B, Cam H, Takahashi Y, Volkert T, Terragni J, Young RA, Dynlacht BD. (2002). E2F integrates cell cycle progression with DNA repair, replication, and G(2)/M checkpoints. Genes Dev. Jan 15, 16(2):245-56.

Reynisdottir, I. & Massague, J. (1997).The subcellular locations of p15ink4b and p27kip1 coordinate their inhibitory interactions with Cdk4 and cdk2. *Genes Dev,* Feb 15, 11(4): 492-503.

Rivard N, L'Allemain G, Bartek J, Pouysségur J. (1996). Abrogation of p27Kip1 by cDNA antisense suppresses quiescence (G0 state) in fibroblasts. *J Biol Chem.* Aug 2, 271(31):18337-18341.

Rooke HM, Vitas MR, Crosier PS, Crosier KE. (1999). The TGF-beta type II receptor in chronic myeloid leukemia: analysis of microsatellite regions and gene expression. *Leukemia.* Apr, 13(4):535-541.

Rosas M, Birkenkamp KU, Lammers JW, Koenderman L, Coffer PJ. (2005). Cytokine mediated suppression of TF-1 apoptosis requires PI3K activation and inhibition of Bim expression. *FEBS Lett.* Jan 3, 579(1):191-198.

Rowell EA, Walsh MC, Wells AD. (2005). Opposing Roles for the Cyclin-Dependent Kinase Inhibitor p27^{kip1} in the Control of CD4^{+} T Cell Proliferation and Effector Function. *The Journal of Immunology,* Mar 15, 174(6): 3359-3368.

Ruscetti, F.W., Akel, S., Bartelmez, S.H. (2005). Autocrine transforming growth factor-beta regulation of hematopoiesis: many outcomes that depend on the context. *Oncogene,* Aug 29, 24(37): 5751-5763.

Russo AA, Jeffrey PD, Patten AK, Massagué J, Pavletich NP. (1996). Crystal structure of the p27Kip1 cyclin-dependent-kinase inhibitor bound to the cyclin A-Cdk2 complex. *Nature.* Jul 25, 382(6589):325-331.

Sahin F and Sladek TL. (2010a). E2F-1 binding affinity for pRb is not the only determinant of the E2F-1 activity. , Jul 4, 6(4):382-395.

Sahin F and Sladek TL. (2010b). E2F-1 has dual roles depending on the cell cycle. *Int J Biol Sci.* Mar 3, 6(2):116-128.

Scandura JM, Boccuni P, Massagué J, Nimer SD (2004). Transforming growth factor beta-induced cell cycle arrest of human hematopoietic cells requires p57KIP2 up-regulation. Proc Natl Acad Sci U S A. Oct 19, 101(42):15231-15236.

Schwarz, J.K., Devoto, S.H., Smith, E.J., Chellappan, S.P., Jakoi, L., Nevins, J.R. (1993). Interactions of the p107 and Rb proteins with E2F during the cell proliferation response. *EMBO J*, Mar, 12(3): 1013-1020.

Shirodkar, S., Ewen, M., DeCaprio, J.A., Morgan, J., Livingston, D.M., Chittenden, T. (1992). The transcription factor E2F interacts with the retinoblastoma product and a p107-cyclin A complex in a cell cycle-regulated manner. *Cell*, Jan 10, 68(1): 157-166.

Shull MM, Ormsby I, Kier AB, Pawlowski S, Diebold RJ, Yin M Allen R, Sidman C, Proetzel G, Calvin D, Annunziata N, Doetschman T (1992). Targeted disruption of the mouse transforming growth factor-b1 gene results in multifocal inflammatory disease. *Nature*, Oct 22, 359(6397): 693–699.

Sing, G.K., Keller, J.R., Ellingsworth, L.R., Ruscetti, F.W. (1988). Transforming growth factor-β selectively inhibits normal and leukemic human bone marrow cell growth in vitro. *Blood*, Nov, 72(5): 1504-1511.

Sitnicka, E., Ruscetti, F.W., Priestley, G.V., Wolf, N.S., Bartelmez, S.H. (1996) Transforming growth factor β1 directly and reversibly inhibits the initial cell divisions of long-term repopulating hematopoietic stem cells. *Blood*, Jul 1, 88(1): 82-88

Snoeck, H-W., Weekx, S., Moulijn, A., Lardon, F., Lenjou, M., Nys, F., Van Ranst, P.C.F., Van Bockstaele, D.R., Berneman, Z.N. (1996). Tumor necrosis factor αis a potent synergistic factor for the proliferation of primitive human hematopoietic progenitor cells and induces resistance to transforming growth factor β but not to interferon γ. *J Exp Med*, Feb 1, 183(2): 705-710.

Sun H, Wang Y, Chinnam M, Zhang X, Hayward SW, Foster BA, Nikitin AY, Wills M, Goodrich DW. (2011) E2f binding-deficient Rb1 protein suppresses prostate tumor progression in vivo. *Proc Natl Acad Sci U S A*, Jan 11, 108(2):704-709.

Sundstrom C, Nilsson K. (1976). Establishment and characterization of a human histiocytic lymphoma cell line (U-937). *Int J Cancer*, May 15, 17(5): 565-77.

Suryadinata R, Sadowski M, Steel R, Sarcevic B (2011). Cyclin-dependent kinase-mediated phosphorylation of RBP1 and pRb promotes their dissociation to mediate release of the SAP30·mSin3·HDAC transcriptional repressor complex. *J Biol Chem*. Feb 18;286(7):5108-5118.

Takahashi, Y., Rayman, J.B., Dynlacht, B.D. (2000). Analysis of promoter binding by the E2F and pRB families in vivo: distinct E2F proteins mediate activation and repression. *Genes Dev*, Apr 1, 14(7), 804-816.

Takaki T, Fukasawa K, Suzuki-Takahashi I, Hirai H. (2004). Cdk-mediated phosphorylation of pRB regulates HDAC binding in vitro. *Biochem Biophys Res Commun*. Mar 26, 316(1):252-5.

Tessier, N. & Hoang, T. (1988). Transforming growth factor beta inhibits the proliferation of the blast cells of acute myeloblastic leukemia. *Blood*, Jul, 72(1): 159-164

Weinberg, R.A. (1995). The retinoblastoma protein and cell cycle control. Cell, May 5, 81(3): 323-330.

Wells J, Boyd KE, Fry CJ, Bartley SM, Farnham PJ. (2000). Target gene specificity of E2F and pocket protein family members in living cells , Aug, 20(16):5797-5807.

Wu, L., Timmers, C., Maiti, B., Saabedra, H.I., Sang, L., Chong, G.T., Nuckolls, F., Giangrande, P., Wright, F.A., Field, S.J., Greenberg, M.E., Orkin, S., Nevins, J.R., Robinson, M.L., Leone, G. (2001). The E2F1-3 transcription factors are essential for cellular proliferation. Nature, Nov 22, 414(6862): 457-462.

Xu YZ, Thuraisingam T, Marino R, Radzioch D. (2011). Recruitment of SWI/SNF Complex Is Required for Transcriptional Activation of the SLC11A1 Gene during Macrophage Differentiation of HL-60 Cells. *J Biol Chem,* Apr 15, 286(15):12839-12849.

Zhang H, Hannon GJ, Beach D (1994). p21-containing cyclin kinases exist in both active and inactive states. *Genes Dev.* Aug 1, 8(15):1750-1758.

12

Novel Targets in Myelogenous Leukemia: The Id Family of Proteins

Kimberly D. Klarmann[1], Ming Ji[1], Huajie Li[1], Ande Satyanarayana[2], Wonil Kim[1], Emily Bowers[2], Bjorg Gudmundsdottir[2] and Jonathan R. Keller[1]

[1]*Laboratory of Cancer Prevention, SAIC-Frederick, Inc., NCI-Frederick, Frederick, Maryland*

[2]*Laboratory of Cancer Prevention, Center for Cancer Research, National Cancer Institute, Frederick, Maryland*

USA

1. Introduction

1.1 Myelogenous leukemia and the need for novel drug targets

The successful treatment of myelogenous leukemia depends upon the continuing coordinate efforts of the medical and research communities and patients to understand the complex nature of leukemia development and progression, and to battle drug resistant cells. Novel drug therapies, like Imatinib, have been developed which target the mutant BCR-ABL (Breakpoint Cluster Region-Abelson Kinase) protein, and have significantly changed the treatment regimens for chronic myelogenous leukemia (CML). However, while Imatinib is frequently effective against the majority of the leukemic cells, and patients often undergo remission after treatment, these patients also relapse due to a leukemic drug-resistant population (Schemionek et al., 2010). In comparison to CML, the treatment for acute myelogenous leukemia (AML) is predominantly induction therapy using strong anti-mitotic agents, followed by consolidation therapy to kill residual diseased cells (Venditti et al., 2000). These therapies are not specifically targeted to mutated proteins in the cells, and therefore can be more toxic to the patient's normal cells. Researchers have attempted to target mutated proteins in AML. However, unlike BCR-ABL, targeting FLT3-ITD (FMS-like tyrosine kinase 3-Internal Tandem Duplication) and FLT3-TKD (FMS-like tyrosine kinase 3-Tyrosine Kinase Domain) mutations have not been as successful as CML-Imatinib therapy (Kindler et al., 2010). Therefore, challenges facing patients with AML remain significant, and drug-resistant relapses remain a threat.

1.2 Transcription factor deregulation in myelogenous leukemia

To identify novel drug targets, researchers will have to gain a better understanding of the molecular mechanisms that regulate normal hematopoietic development. Hematopoiesis depends upon the activity of transcription factors and their regulators to function at the correct time and place during differentiation. Failure to control these processes can lead to deregulated proliferation and impaired normal differentiation. Ultimately, these errors can lead to myeloproliferative diseases (MPD), myelodysplastic syndromes (MDS), and chronic or acute myelogenous leukemia (Rosenbauer et al., 2005). Current research efforts are focused on the molecular mechanism(s) that contribute to transcription factor deregulation with a goal of designing better, safer and less toxic therapies, to restore normal differentiation or initiate apoptosis of leukemic cell populations. Deregulation can result from many different types of mutations including translocations, deletions, and point mutations, which can result in loss of function, gain of function, overexpression or underexpression. The Id (Inhibitor of DNA Binding) proteins are key downstream transcriptional regulators of multiple neoplastic mutations and are deregulated (have increased expression) in many types of cancer, and therefore may be good therapeutic targets particularly for drug-resistant forms of leukemia.

2. Id proteins inhibit transcription factors that regulate cell cycle and differentiation

2.1 Tissue specific expression of Id proteins

The Id proteins belong to a subclass of the helix-loop-helix (HLH) family of proteins. There are four family members (Id1, Id2, Id3, Id4), which range in size from 13 to 20 kDa **(Figure 1)**. In normal tissues, Id1 and Id3 are ubiquitously expressed; they are detectable throughout embryonic development and are present in the bone marrow, testis, kidney, brain, liver and spleen. The expression of Id2 and Id4 are more restricted (Riechmann et al., 1994). Id2, is not detectable until day 13.5 of fetal liver development. Id2 is most highly expressed in the bone

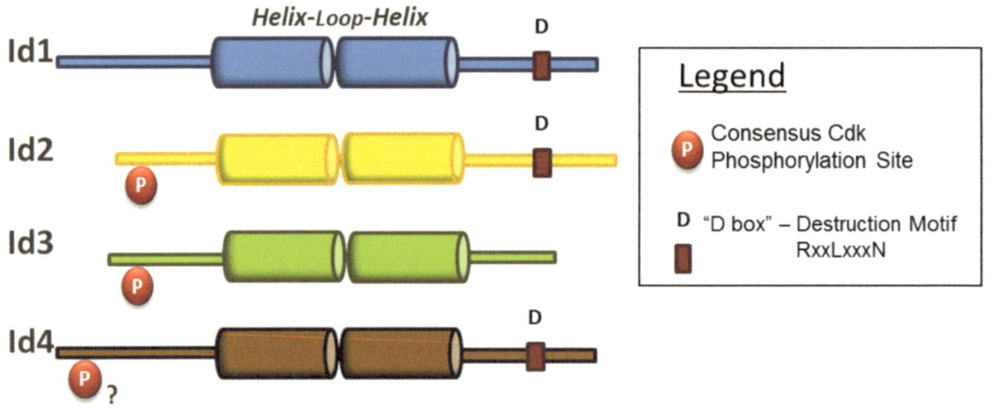

Fig. 1. Schematic representation of the Id family
Id2, Id3, and Id4 have Cdk2 phosphorylation sites, although only Id2 and Id3 are known to be phosphorylated by cyclinA/E-Cdk2. Cdk2-dependent phosphorylation of Id2 (Hara et al., 1997) and Id3 (Deed et al., 1997) inhibits binding to E proteins and Ets transcription factors. Id proteins are ubiquitinated and undergo rapid turnover during the cell cycle mediated by ubiquitination and proteosomal degredation, and two different targeting mechanisms have been reported. Id1, Id2, and Id4 have "D box" destruction motifs (RxxLxxxN) which is recognized by the anaphase promoting complex (APC) which targets the proteins for ubiquitination (Harper et al., 2002; Lasorella et al., 2006). Degradation of Id1 and Id3, is mediated by the COP9 signalosome (Berse et al., 2004).

marrow, testis and brain. Id4 is expressed during embryogenesis, but is not detectable in the fetal liver. Id4 expression is present in the adult bone marrow, testis, kidney, brain, and spleen. These data suggest that the Id proteins may be critical during development, as well as having important functions in the adult. In this regard, simultaneous deletion of any two Id gene family members results in early embryonic lethality, demonstrating that these genes are required for development (Fraidenraich et al., 2004). Therefore, in summary, as a family the Id proteins are present in many different tissues, and are expressed during early development as well as in adult tissues.

2.2 Id protein function: Regulation of transcription factors and cell cycle regulators

The Id proteins function by blocking the DNA binding activity of three types of essential transcription factors: **(1)** The basic Helix-Loop-Helix (bHLH) proteins (E proteins), **(2)** Helix-Turn-Helix ETS transcription factors, and **(3)** Pax transcription factors (Pax-5 in B cells) **(Figure 2)**. In addition, specific members of the Id family decrease the activity of Rb tumor suppressors (Iavarone et al., 1994; Lasorella et al., 1996).

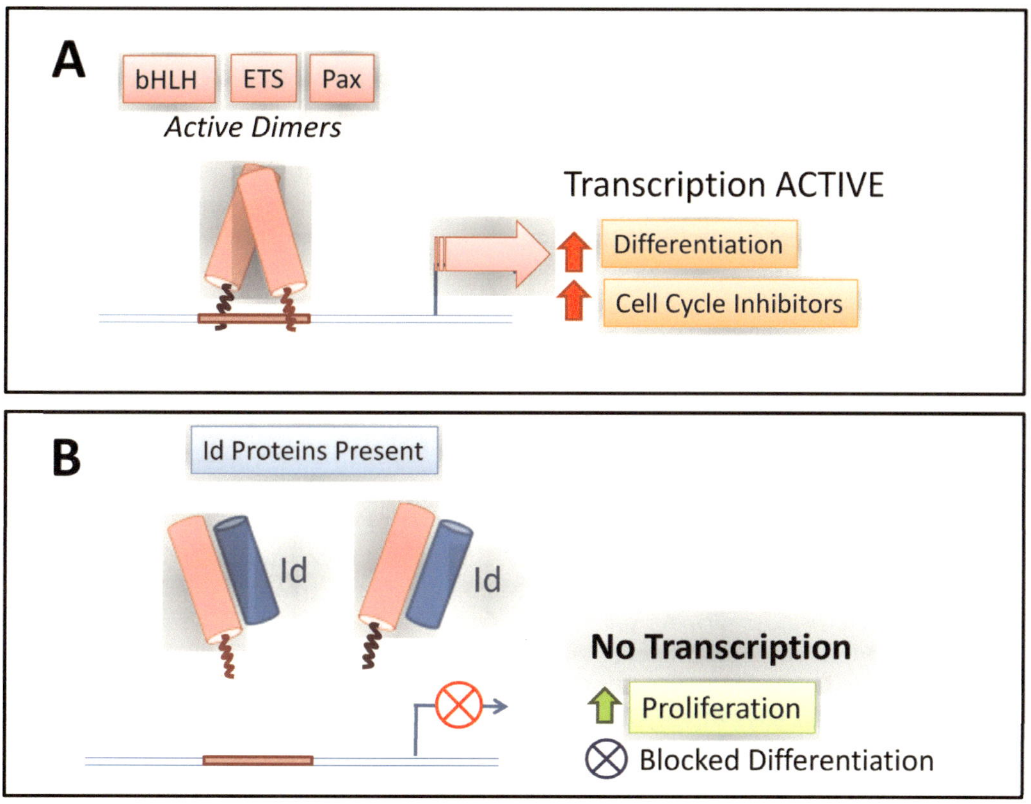

Fig. 2. Id proteins bind bHLH, ETS, and Pax transcription factors and block their function.
(A) bHLH, ETS, and Pax factors dimerize and bind to and activate the promoter regions of genes essential for differentiation and cell cycle arrest.
(B) When Id proteins are present, they bind to bHLH, ETS and Pax transcription factors, blocking their dimerization and inhibiting their ability to activate transcription.

E proteins and regulation of differentiation. The HLH transcription factors are essential for regulating the differentiation programs of multiple tissues types. The E proteins, also known as "Class A" HLH family members, include *E2A* (encoding E12 and E47 proteins), *HEB*, and *E2-2*. E proteins homodimerize or heterodimerize with "Class B" bHLH family members, tissue specific proteins such as SCL/tal1 (hematopoiesis), HAND, MyoD, myogenin (myogenesis), NeuroD/BETA2 (pancreatic development and neurogenesis), HES-1, and MASH-1 (neurogenesis). When dimerized, these bHLH proteins bind to E box consensus sequence (CANNTG, where "N" is any nucleotide) through their basic N-terminal regions. When Id proteins are present, they bind to the E proteins and disrupt their dimerization with the Class B binding partners (Langlands et al., 1997), and block the differentiation of muscle, neuronal, pancreatic and hematopoietic cells. The Id proteins homodimerize poorly with each other and preferentially bind to the Class A HLH factors (Sun et al., 1991). In summary, the effect of Id proteins, prevents or arrests differentiation by blocking the E protein transcription activating function in many different cell types.

E proteins and cell cycle control. The E proteins also induce the expression of cell cycle inhibitors, such as $p16^{INK4a}$ and $p21^{Cip1}$. The cell cycle inhibitors cyclin dependent kinases 4 and 6 (Cdk4, Cdk6), are necessary for the cell to progress to S phase. Therefore, Id proteins inhibit the transcriptional activity of the E proteins, which decrease the expression of cell cycle inhibitors, and ultimately results in increased cellular proliferation (Alani et al., 2001; Zheng et al., 2004; Prabhu et al., 1997). In support of this, when Id1 is knocked-out in mice, mouse embryo fibroblasts that lack Id1 (Id1-/-) undergo premature senescence, due in part to increased expression of $p16^{INK4a}$ (Alani et al., 2001). Thus, increased expression of Id1 proteins promotes cell proliferation by inhibiting the function of E protein transcriptional activity, by blocking their ability to induce the expression of key cell cycle inhibitors.

Regulation of ETS proteins by Ids. The Id proteins also regulate the activity of the ETS (E twenty-six) helix-turn-helix family of transcription factors. The ETS proteins comprise one of the largest families of transcription factors, and they bind the canonical sequence GGAA/T. The ETS proteins are characterized by the presence of the ETS DNA binding domain, and the family includes PU.1 (SPI1), Ets1, Ets2, TEL, and TEL2 as well as the ternary complex factors (TCF): Elk1, Elk3 (Net/SAP2), and Elk4 (SAP1). The Id family members interact with the ETS protein DNA binding domain, blocking the ability of the ETS proteins to bind DNA, and repressing their ability to activate transcription. Id1, Id2 and Id3 have all been shown to bind to the TCF proteins Elk-1 and Elk-4, and Id1 and Id3 both suppress the expression of the cell cycle inhibitor $p27^{Kip1}$ by blocking Elk-1's ability to activate transcription (Yates et al., 1999; Chassot et al., 2007). As previously described, Ids can decrease $p16^{INK4a}$ protein expression by repressing E protein activity, in addition, Id1 has also been shown to reduce $p16^{INK4a}$ expression by the inhibiting the activation of its expression by Ets1 and Ets2 (Ohtani et al., 2001). Interestingly, the ability of the Id proteins to bind to the ETS transcription factors can be inhibited by phosphorylation of the Ids. Within the Id family, only Id2 and Id3 undergo phosphorylation, and phosphorylation of these Ids by cyclin A/E-Cdk2 decreases their ability to bind to ETS proteins (specifically, Elk-1), resulting in cell cycle arrest (Stinson et al., 2003). This mechanism may compose part of a normal cell cycle regulatory feedback mechanism in cells that permits cell populations to expand and then return to a growth arrested state. In summary, Id proteins inhibit the function of the ETS proteins, blocking their ability to activate transcription of cell cycle inhibitors, which results in increased proliferation.

Retinoblastoma (Rb) and p53 tumor suppressors. The retinoblastoma protein (Rb), is an important part of normal cell cycle control. When Rb is hypo-phosphorylated, it is active and bound to E2F, causing cell cycle arrest by preventing E2F from inducing the expression of genes necessary for cell proliferation (Sherr and McCormick, 2002). When Rb is phosphorylated by the cyclin dependent kinases (Cdks), it dissociates from E2F, and this allows E2F to activate the expression of genes necessary for DNA replication. Rb is frequently mutated in many different malignancies, and finding ways to restore Rb function remains a goal in cancer research. Interestingly, Id2 alone of the Id family binds to the hypo-phosphorylated Rb, as well as related proteins p107 and p130 and inhibits their growth suppressive activities. The Id proteins do not affect the expression levels or phosphorylation state of Rb (Lasorella et al., 1996). However, when Id2 binds in the pocket-binding of Rb site it prevents it from arresting the cell cycle (Iavarone et al., 1994; Lasorella et al., 1996). There are also reports that Id1 can decrease p53 activity, although it is not known whether this is a direct or an indirect effect. The reduction of p53 activity results in decreased PTEN tumor suppressor expression, and ultimately results in increased cellular proliferation (Lee et al., 2009).

In summary, the Id family of proteins affects both differentiation and cell cycle progression by inhibiting the DNA binding activity of the E and ETS protein transcription factors, by binding to and disrupting the activity of Rb and related proteins, and by decreasing p53 activity.

3. The role of Id proteins in normal myelopoiesis

3.1 Id protein levels during myelopoiesis

Id proteins were first identified in a mouse leukemic cell line in the search for novel factors containing HLH domains. Benezra et al. identified the first Id protein in murine erythroleukemia (MEL) cells in 1990 (Benezra et al., 1990). They observed that Id1 was present in less-differentiated cell types, and found that Id expression decreased after differentiation was induced in erythroid, muscle, and endothelial cell lines. Subsequently, using a myeloid progenitor cell line, 32DCl3, it was found that endogenous Id1 expression rapidly decreased in cells induced to differentiate to neutrophilic granulocytes by granulocyte colony stimulating factor (G-CSF), then rose again during the later stages of differentiation. Id2 expression also decreased following G-CSF treatment of 32DCl3 cells (Leeanansaksiri et al., 2005), as well as in multiple other myeloid cell lines (Ishiguro et al., 1996). When Id1 concentration was artificially elevated in the 32DCl3 cells, the cells failed to differentiate in response to G-CSF (Kreider et al., 1992). Similarly, overexpression of Id1 in MEL cells also resulted in a block in differentiation (Shoji et al., 1994). Therefore, in normal cells, Id1 expression needs to decrease for a defined period after the induction of differentiation. If Id proteins are overexpressed during this phase, the cells do not differentiate in spite of the extracellular signals instructing them to mature.

In mouse bone marrow, moderate levels of Id1 are present in the hematopoietic stem cells (HSC) and common lymphoid progenitors (CLP). Id1 expression is increased in the more differentiated common myeloid progenitors (CMP), and further increased in the granulocyte macrophage progenitors (GMP), however Id1 levels do not increase in megakaryocyte erythroid progenitors (MEP). The dynamic levels of Id1 expression during these early stages of hematopoiesis suggest that Id1 may regulate cell fate decisions during myeloid, erythroid, and lymphoid development (Leeanansaksiri et al., 2005). In support of this hypothesis, culture of mouse bone marrow cells in the presence of interleukin-3 (IL-3) or IL-3 with stem cell factor (SCF), or GM-CSF, which promote granulocyte and macrophage development, all increased Id1 expression. Correspondingly, culture of human CD34+ bone marrow cells with myeloid growth factors SCF and IL-3, SCF and macrophage colony stimulating factor (M-CSF), SCF and granulocyte macrophage colony stimulating factor (GM-CSF), or with GM-CSF alone also induced Id1 expression (Suh et al., 2008). However, SCF alone, SCF and erythropoietin (EPO), or SCF and thrombopoietin (TPO), which promote erythroid and megakaryocyte development, did not induce Id1 expression in murine or human hematopoietic progenitors. Furthermore, initial reports showed that Id2 expression increases during differentiation of myeloid cells (Ishiguro et al., 1996), although the onset of its expression in myelopoiesis is later in hematopoietic development than Id1 (Cooper et al., 1997). In summary, in normal mouse and human progenitor cells, hematopoietic growth factors that promote granulocyte and macrophage development induce the expression of Id1.

3.2 Id protein levels rise in later stages of differentiation

The study by Kreider et al., which examined Id1 expression during induction of differentiation in 32DCl3 cells by G-CSF showed that Id1 levels also increased during terminal neutrophil differentiation of 32DCl3 (Kreider et al., 1992). In agreement with this, Shoji et al. demonstrated that if Id1 is overexpressed in later stages of myeloid differentiation, that Id1 did not block myeloid maturation, as in the early stages of myeloid differentiation (Shoji et al., 1994). These reports suggest that Id protein expression may have an additional role in terminal myeloid differentiation. This model is supported by studies in human CD34+ cord blood cells that show ectopic expression of Id1 can enhance neutrophil development; and expression of Id2 accelerates final maturation of eosinophils and neutrophils (Buitenhuis et al., 2005). In addition, restoring Id1 expression (along with C/EBPα expression) in cells isolated from patients with low-risk myelodysplastic syndrome (MDS) restores neutrophil maturation *in vitro* (Geest et al., 2009). Thus, the expression of the Id proteins is biphasic during normal hematopoietic development, appearing first in the stem and progenitor stages, decreases during the intermediate developmental stages, and then rises again during terminal differentiation.

3.3 Loss of Id proteins disrupts normal hematopoietic development

The Id proteins are necessary for proper hematopoietic development, including progenitor expansion and fate determination. While Id1 knockout mice are viable and show no overt developmental defects, several groups have reported that hematopoietic stem and progenitor cells in these mice show impaired development (Yan et al., 1997; Perry et al., 2007; Suh et al., 2009). Specifically, the hematopoietic stem cells responsible for long term engraftment and repopulation (LT-HSC) fail to compete against co-transplanted bone marrow cells as well as normal control bone marrow LT-HSC (Jankovic et al., 2007; Perry et al., 2007). However, four serial transplantations of Id1-/- bone marrow, without the addition of co-transplanted competitor bone marrow, supported equal engraftment and viability of the transplant recipients as wild type mouse bone marrow cells, suggesting the intrinsic loss of Id1 does not impair the fundamental long-term self-renewal ability of LT-HSC (Suh et al., 2009). In addition, these studies also showed that the loss of Id1 also significantly alters the bone marrow microenvironment, specifically the stromal cells and the hematopoietic growth factors they produce, reducing the amount of SCF and SDF produced, and increasing the amount of GM-CSF, G-CSF, and M-CSF produced by the stromal cells (Suh et al., 2009). These changes in the stromal microenvironment may explain the myeloid-priming effect reported in the Id1-null LT-HSC (Jankovic et al., 2007). In summary, the loss of Id1 can disrupt normal hematopoiesis, causing significant changes in the bone marrow microenvironment as well as in the hematopoietic stem and progenitor populations.

While Id1 expression is important for maintenance of the hematopoietic microenvironment, and affects the competitive repopulation ability of LT-HSC, Id2 is essential for normal hematopoietic development as demonstrated by deletion of Id2 in mouse models. Id2 knockout mouse models have defects in natural killer (NK) and dendritic cell development, as well as impaired lymphopoiesis and erythroid defects (Yokota et al., 1999). Id2 regulates fate determination in myeloid development by interaction with the ETS transcription factor PU.1. Id2 relieves PU.1 repression of the GATA-1 transcription factor, which shifts progenitor cell development from a monocyte/granulocyte differentiation program to an erythroid program (Ji et al., 2008). In summary, Id2 is essential for normal hematopoietic development and is a key regulatory factor in the fate determination of B and erythroid cell development.

In contrast to its family members Id1 and Id2, the normal physiological role of Id3 appears to be regulation of lymphoid development. Specifically Id3 has a major role in supporting the proper maturation of B cells, as mice that are Id3 null have defects in B cell proliferation and maturation (Pan et al., 1999; Rivera et al., 2000). However, Id3 is not normally expressed in myeloid development, nor is Id4 (Ishiguro et al., 1995; Ishiguro et al., 1996). The levels at which the Id proteins are expressed in the cells and the stage in differentiation at which they are expressed as well as the type of cell in which they are expressed affect how Id proteins function "normally" in the cells. Altogether, the Id family of proteins has two functions in normal cells: to regulate the process of fate determination and differentiation, and to control cell proliferation.

4. Id proteins and leukemia

4.1 Ids and leukemogenesis

Id proteins have oncogenic properties in myeloid cells. Overexpression of the Id genes is associated with malignancy and poor prognosis in many different tissues **(Table 1).** Whether increased expression of Id proteins are a by-product of deregulated growth or are causative is still under investigation. Id gene overexpression in cell lines results in hyperproliferation and blocked differentiation. For example, Shoji et al., demonstrated that Id1 overexpression inhibits differentiation of erythroleukemia cell lines (Shoji et al., 1994) and Kreider et al. demonstrated Id1 blocks 32DCl3 myeloid progenitor differentiation (Kreider et al., 1992).

When Id protein expression is deregulated, normal progenitor expansion and differentiation becomes unbalanced and shifts towards progenitor hyperproliferation. In the myeloid lineage, forced expression of Id1 or Id2 can impair monocyte, granulocyte, and erythroid maturation (Jen et al., 1996; Kreider et al., 1992; Leeanansaksiri et al., 2005; Lister et al., 1995). Furthermore, in mouse bone marrow cells, overexpression of either Id1 or Id3 can immortalize growth factor-dependent hematopoietic progenitors *in vitro*, resulting in cells with an AML-like morphology. Immunophenotypic and gene expression analyses of these

Id Family Member	Tumor Type	Reference
Id1, Id3	Glioblastoma, Medulloblastoma, Neuroblastoma	(Lyden et al., 1999)
Id1, Id2, Id3	Pancreatic Cancer	(Kleeff et al., 1998; Maruyama et al., 1999)
Id1, Id2, Id3, Id4	Testicular Seminoma	(Sablitzky et al., 1998)
Id1	Thyroid Cancer	(Kebebew et al., 2000, 2003)
Id1, Id2, Id3	Squamous Cell Carcinoma	(Hu et al., 2001; Langlands et al., 2000; Nishimine et al., 2003; Wang et al., 2002)
Id1	Breast Cancer	(Lin et al., 2000; Schoppmann et al., 2003)
Id1	Endometrial Cancer	(Takai et al., 2001)
Id1	Cervical Cancer	(Schindl et al., 2001)
Id1	Melanoma	(Polsky et al., 2001)
Id2	Neuroblastoma	(Lasorella et al., 2002; Lasorella et al., 2000)
Id2	Ewing Sarcoma	(Fukuma et al., 2003; Nishimori et al., 2002)
Id1, Id2, Id3	Astrocytic Tumor	(Vandeputte et al., 2002)
Id1	Basal Cell Carcinoma	(Chaturvedi et al., 2003)
Id1, Id2, Id3	Colorectal Carcinoma	(Norton, 2000; Wilson et al., 2001)
Id1	Hepatocellular Carcinoma	(Lee et al., 2003)
Id1	Kaposi's Sarcoma	(Tang et al., 2003)
Id1	Ovarian Cancer	(Schindl et al., 2003)
Id1	Prostate Cancer	(Ouyang et al., 2002)
Id1	AML subsets	(Suh et al., 2008; Tang et al., 2009)

Table 1. Id Protein Expression in Cancer

immortalized cells suggest they are developmentally arrested at the CMP/GMP phase of maturation (Suh et al., 2008). The bone marrow cells immortalized by Id1 overexpression showed decreased levels of $p15^{INK}$, $p16^{INK4a}$, $p19^{ARF}$ and $p21^{Cip1}$ during culture (Suh et al., 2008), indicating that Id1 expression reduced the expression of multiple cell cycle inhibitors to cause increased growth in deregulated myelopoiesis.

These results showed that overexpression of Id1 immortalized normal bone marrow cells *in vitro*, and led researchers to investigate if deregulated Id1 expression cells would cause a myeloproliferative disease *in vivo*. Transplantation of Id1 overexpressing mouse HSPC resulted in the development of a myeloproliferative disease in mice, causing the animals to become moribund within a year. Complete blood cell counts showed the mice had monocytosis, and low levels of hemoglobin and hematocrit, as well as the presence of cells with leukemic-blast morphology. Pathology revealed that the mice had myeloid and erythroid hyperplasia in their bone marrow and spleens which lead to splenomegaly (Suh et al., 2008). Therefore, overexpression of Id1 is sufficient to immortalize mouse progenitor cells *in vitro*, and leads to a lethal myeloproliferative disease *in vivo*.

Similar to Id1, overexpression of Id2 has also been shown to cause the development of leukemia in mouse models. Transgenic overexpression of Id2 in mouse models leads to a block in lymphoid differentiation, aberrant apoptosis, and development of T cell lymphoma (Morrow et al., 1999). Id2 also blocks differentiation in human cells, specifically, ectopic expression of Id2 in human CD34+ myeloid progenitor cells inhibits the acquisition of monocyte characteristics, suggesting that Id2 can block myeloid as well as lymphoid differentiation (Heinz et al., 2006). It is important to note, that the effects of Id1 or Id2 overexpression depend upon the developmental stage and lineage in which overexpression occurs. In summary, overexpression of both Id1 and Id2 can block differentiation, over-ride senescence, and lead to the development of myelo- and lymphoproliferative disease, and ultimately leukemogenesis.

Increased Id1 and Id2 expression is associated with human AML. The finding that Ids immortalize primary mouse bone marrow cells *in vitro*, and promote MPD *in vivo*, led investigators to ask if Id expression levels are elevated in myelogenous leukemia. A microarray performed on 285 AML patient samples demonstrated an increase in Id1 and Id2 in AML subsets (Suh et al., 2008). Specifically, 17.5% of the mRNA samples from AML patients had increased Id1 expression, and 19.2% had increased Id2 mRNA levels. Surprisingly, most of the patients with elevated Id1 and Id2 levels had a normal karyotype, and were evenly distributed across the French-American-British (FAB) subtype classifications: M0-M6. 61% and 50% of patients with 5q and/or 7q deletion and 28 and 22%of patients with t(15;17) showed increased expression of Id1 and Id2, suggesting that elevated Id expression levels contribute to a block in granulocyte development. Seventy-eight patients had high levels of FLT3-ITD mutations, and 23 of those (29%) had elevated levels of Id1 expression. Twenty-three patients had EVI1 deregulation, of which 8 patients (35%) had increased Id1 expression. Id2 expression was found in patients with deregulated NRAS (30%), KRAS (44%), C/EBPα (6%) and EVI1 (30%) expression. Altogether, the analysis suggests that Id gene expression may be induced downstream of multiple signal transduction pathways of activated oncogenes. A separate analysis of a different cohort of AML samples showed that patients with the highest levels of Id1 had a poor prognosis compared to those with lower levels of Id1 (Tang et al., 2009). The causes of Id1 and Id2 overexpression in AML are still under investigation. Thus, elevated levels of Id gene expression could be used diagnostically to elucidate the severity and prognosis of AML patients.

Expression of Id1 and Id2 are increased by known leukemic oncogenes. It is possible that in many cases Id1 and Id2 mRNA levels increase due to mutations in upstream regulatory pathways. Id1 is a downstream target of multiple leukemia-associated oncogenic tyrosine kinases, including BCR-ABL and FLT3-ITD (Tam et al., 2008). In addition, the JAK2V617F—STAT5, and AML-ETO mutations can also increase Id1 expression (Cammenga et al., 2003; Wood et al., 2009). PLZF and the PLZF translocation products, associated with APL (acute promyelocytic leukemia), activate Id1 and Id3 expression (Bernardo et al., 2007; Doulatov et al., 2009; Rice et al., 2009). In addition, overexpression of HOXA9 and HOXA10, both of which are associated with myeloid hyperplasia, directly activate expression of Id2 (Nagel et al., 2010). Furthermore, viruses also induce Id expression, for example, Id1 is upregulated by Epstein-Barr viral protein LMP1 (NH) (Li et al., 2004). Therefore, the Id proteins are likely to be part of the mechanism by which several of the known oncogenic mutations impair growth control.

Id2 has both oncogenic and tumor suppressor properties. Interestingly, although Id2 has been shown to be upregulated in AML patient samples (as described above), Id2 may have have both oncogenic and tumor suppressor properties. Specifically, there are data demonstrating that the loss of Id2 *in vivo* results in the development of a lethal myeloproliferative disorder (Ko et al., 2008). This effect was seen in Id2 knockout mice backcrossed onto a C57Bl/6 background, but not in 129/sv Id2 knockout, although the reasons for this difference are not yet known. Altogether, the data suggest that Id2 is important for functional hematopoiesis, but that its function as an oncogene or as a tumor suppressor depend upon the cellular environment in which it is expressed.

Id1 causes genomic instability. Of the Id family of proteins, overexpression of Id1 is most consistently reported as associated with oncogenesis. A possible explanation for this may be that Id1 has been associated with genomic instability. Interestingly, it was shown that Id1 contributes to the acquisition of secondary mutations by causing centrosome abnormalities. One mechanism by which this been shown to occur is by Id1 binding to the S5A protein. Loss of S5A has been associated with mitotic defects resulting in abnormal chromosome segregation (Szlanka et al., 2003). When Id1 is overexpressed it interacts with S5A, and this interaction causes overduplication of the centrosomes (Hasskarl et al., 2004; Hasskarl et al., 2008). Leukemogenic translocation mutations such as BCR-ABL can induce genomic instability (Dierov et al., 2009). Based on the data showing that BCR-ABL can induce expression of Id1, it is possible that part of the mechanism by which BCR-ABL causes genomic instability is by inducing overexpression of Id1 (Dierov et al., 2009). Thus, the presence of overexpressed Id1 can not only block differentiation and override senescence; it can actively contribute to the acquisition of additional mutations.

Id family overexpression is associated with disruption of apoptosis. In addition to causing genomic instability, another mechanism by which cancer cells survive is by avoiding programmed cell death. Multiple reports have shown that Id1, Id2, and Id3 can influence apoptosis. However, whether the Id proteins behave as pro-apoptotic or anti-apoptotic factors depends upon the the cell context. Transgenic expression of Id1 in developing T cells in a mouse model resulted in a large percentage of the developing thymocytes to undergo apoptosis. The authors of the study speculated that this was because the thymocytes were blocked in maturation and apoptosis was initiated during the process of V(D)J recombination (Kim et al., 1999). Interestingly, lymphomas developed from the surviving thymocytes, suggesting that overexpression of Id1 alone did not drive apoptosis. In addition, Id1 overexpression in prostate cancer cells actually protects malignant cells from apoptosis (Ling et al., 2003; Wong et al., 2004). Furthermore, decreasing the activity of the Id proteins promotes cell cycle arrest and apoptosis in both breast and ovarian cancer cells (Mern et al., 2010a; Mern et al., 2010b). In summary, the Id proteins can have variable affects on apoptosis, depending upon the developmental stage and microenvironment of the cell.

Id4 functions as a tumor suppressor in myeloid leukemia. Id4 is interesting because of reports that suggest it may function *not* as an oncogene, but as a tumor suppressor in leukemia (in contrast to its siblings). Methylation of the Id4 promoter is associated with poor prognosis in high risk MDS patients, who have a greater probability of developing leukemia (Wang et al., 2010b). In addition, high risk myelodysplastic patients whose Id4 promoters are methylated have an increased risk of leukemic transformation, an obersvation which would support for the use of demethylating agents in MDS/AML treatment (Chen et al., 2011; Wang et al., 2010b). Id4 methylation also correlates with CML progression. Specifically, Id4 is un-methylated in the chronic phase of CML, but is frequently methylated in patients in the accelerated and blast crisis stages (Wang et al., 2010a).

Reports also show that Id4 promoter is methylated in AML cell lines and in AML primary patient samples (Yu et al., 2005). This study also demonstrated that Id4 promoter methylation resulted in decreased Id4 mRNA expression. At the same time, the role of Id4 as a tumor suppressor in myelodysplasia appears to be cell type specific, as Id4 overexpression increases the proliferation of other cell types (breast cancer) (Dell'Orso et al., 2010). Therefore, of all of the Id family members, Id4 is the only one that is consistently reported to be a tumor suppressor in myeloid cells, although how it functions mechanistically in that role is not yet understood.

4.2 Ids and drug resistance in leukemia

Altogether, the reports described above suggest a strong link between Id expression levels and malignancy. It is possible, therefore, that Ids may be part of a mechanism that helps the malignant cells evade standard chemotherapeutic treatments. A search of the Gene Expression Omnibus (GEO; (Barrett and Edgar, 2006)) database reveals studies, which show a correlation between increased Id expression and drug resistance in AML and CML cell lines. Specifically, these analyses show that Id1 expression is increased in cytarabine resistant AML cell lines **(Figure 3A)**(GDS 1907), and that Id1 is also increased in cyclophosphamide resistant CML **(Figure 3B)** (GDS2729) (Bao et al., 2007). In addition, Id3 mRNA levels are increased in cyclophosphamide resistant CML lines **(Figure 3C)** (GDS2729) (Bao et al., 2007). Altogether, these analyses indicate that high levels of Id1 and/or Id3 expression may correlate with a drug resistant phenotype in myelogenous leukemia.

These analyses agree with many other studies that show Id1 functions as an anti-apoptotic factor in cancerous cells from non-hematopoietic tissues. Id1 expression has been shown to prevent malignant cells from undergoing programmed cell death when treated with chemotherapeutic agents (Summarized in (Zhang et al., 2007)). Decreasing Id1 expression with Id1-targeted siRNA restored drug sensitivity in many of these malignant cell lines, however, it has not yet been tested in hematopoietic cells (Zhang et al., 2007). In summary, the data from these studies suggest that high levels of Id1 expression may be indicative of drug resistance in leukemic cells, or may possibly be part of the mechanism underlying drug resistance, which will likely be a focus of future studies with both AML and CML.

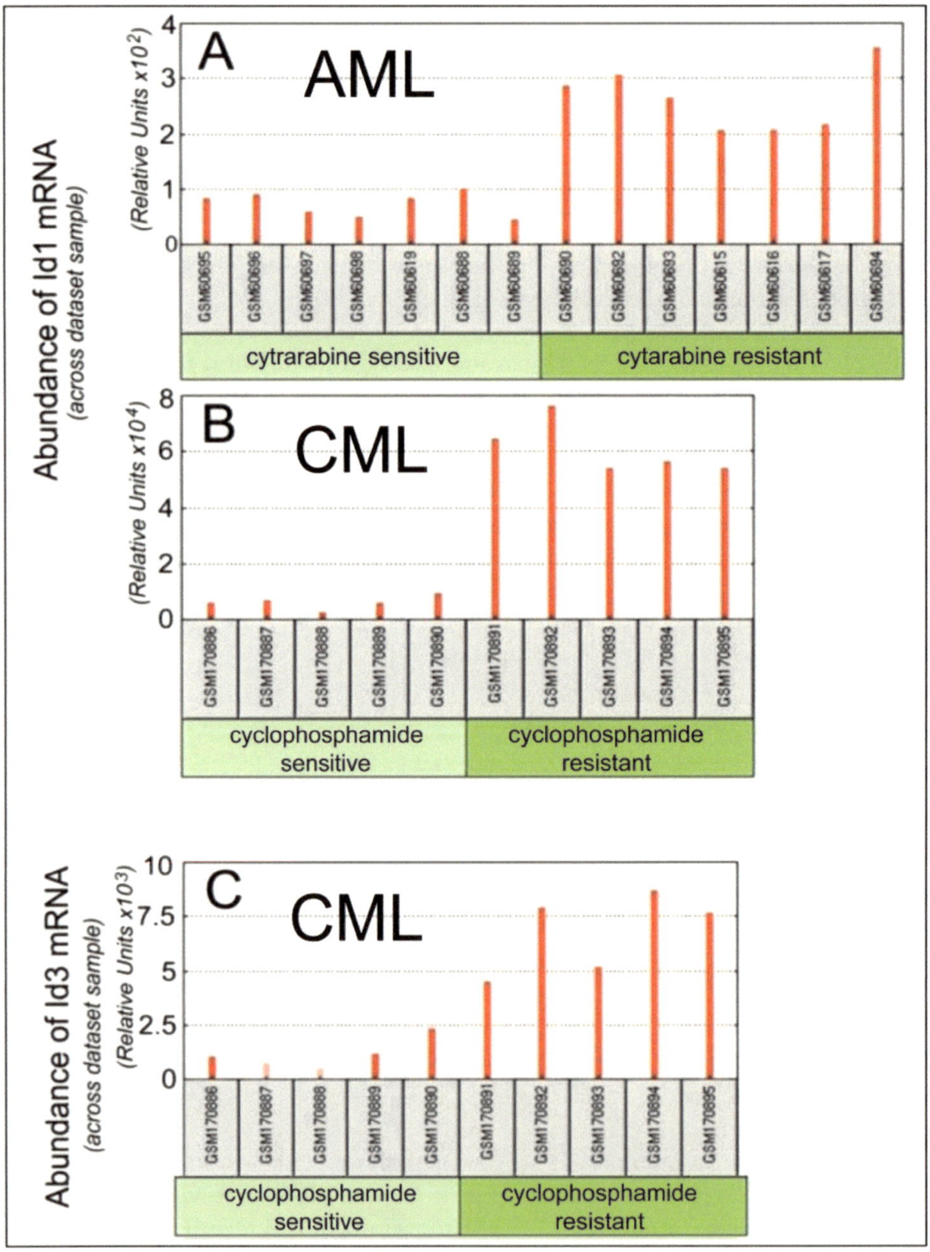

Fig. 3. Increased Id levels associated with drug resistance in leukemic cell lines
(A) Id1 mRNA expression is increased in cytarabine resistant AML cell lines (GDS 1907); **(B)** Id1 is also increased in cyclophosphamide resistant CML (GDS2729), and **(C)** Id3 mRNA is increased in cyclophosphamide resistant CML lines (GDS2729)

4.3 Ids and Leukemia Initiating Cells

The results shown above lead to the question of whether or not the Ids might be expressed in the "Leukemia Initiating Cell" (LIC) population that is resistant to drug treatment. These quiescent leukemic stem cells have been termed the "Holy Grail of Leukemia Therapy" (Misaghian et al., 2009). However, identifying and understanding the regulation of these cells depends on a better understanding of normal transcription factors in stem cells; and how they may be deregulated, and become leukemia stem cells (Rosenbauer et al. 2005).

The process of normal stem-cell self-renewal must be tightly regulated to prevent the creation of leukemic stem cells. Therefore, the proteins that regulate the HSC self-renewal process are currently under intense investigation. E proteins maintain the stem cell pool and promote myeloid progenitor differentiation, and because Id proteins control E protein function, variations in Id protein levels can significantly affect HSC self-renewal (Semerad et al., 2009). In support of this concept, Id proteins were shown to have a role in maintaining the self-renewal capacity of stem cells. Specifically, BMP induction of Id proteins suppresses differentiation and sustains ES cell self-renewal in collaboration with STAT3 (Ying et al., 2003). In addition, in glioma cancer stem cells, decreasing expression of Id1 and Id3 effectively targeted and reduced the malignant stem cell population (Anido et al., 2010). There are also reports that loss of Id1 significantly decreases hematopoietic stem cell function, although reports vary on whether this is an environmental effect or a result of changes in the bone marrow microenvironment (Jankovic et al., 2007; Perry et al., 2007; Suh et al., 2009). In addition, it has been observed that loss of Id2 significantly decreases the long-term self-renewal capacity of hematopoietic stem cells (Ming Ji et al., unpublished). All of these studies suggest that Id genes contribute to the control of self-renewal of normal HSC and deregulation of the Id proteins may contribute to the generation of leukemic stem cells. Future studies will likely focus on this important aspect of Id protein function, as they may provide a novel approach to target leukemic stem cells.

5. Id proteins and the bone marrow microenvironment

Chemotherapy-resistant human leukemia stem cells home to and engraft within the bone-marrow endosteal region (Ishikawa et al., 2007), and reports indicate that the Id proteins may also have an effect on this microenvironment. As previously described, the loss of Id1 in the bone marrow niche leads to increased progenitor cycling caused by a change in the cytokine milieu (Suh et al., 2009). Thus, Id genes may additionally contribute to the initiation or progression of AML by affecting the stromal cells that constitute the hematopoietic niche.

Interestingly, in addition to affecting the local cytokine milieu, the Ids regulate the fundamental structure of the bones by controlling osteoblast and osteoclast activity. For example, ectopic Id4 expression promotes osteoblast differentiation and was suggested as a possible preventative treatment for senile osteoporosis (Tokuzawa et al., 2010). Id1, Id2, and Id3 are all upregulated in response to BMP9 treatment of mesenchymal progenitor cells (via Smad4), which results in increased proliferation and a block in differentiation of osteogenic progenitors (Peng et al., 2004). In addition, Id proteins have been shown to regulate osteogenic transcription factor activity (Ogata and Noda, 1991; Tamura and Noda, 1994; Zhang et al., 2008). Id2, and Id4 genes also regulate adipogenesis by regulating the proliferation pre-adipoctye progenitors and their ability to undergo differentiation (Murad et al., 2010; Park et al., 2008). Altogether, these results suggest that the Id family members not only regulate hematopoietic growth factor expression, but the fundamental structure of the niche itself.

6. Targeting Id proteins

The identification of Id1 as a common downstream effector of oncogenic mutations such as BCR-ABL and FLT3-ITD in CML and AML, as well as their upreglation in multiple types of cancer, suggest that the Id proteins represent potential targets for therapeutic intervention (Suh et al., 2008; Tam et al., 2008). Inhibiting Id1 protein expression in human induced pluripotential stem cells using with small inhibitory RNAs (siRNA) increases differentiation into committed progenitors suggesting that decreasing Id expression can support cell maturation (Hong et al., 2011). To date, there are three novel inhibitors of Id function currently under investigation.

6.1 Peptide conjugated antisense oligonucleotides

Henke et al. generated an anti-sense oligonucleotide that is covalently coupled to an "address-peptide," Id1-PCAO (peptide-conjugated anti-sense oligonucleotide) (Henke et al., 2008). The peptide used in this study was designed specifically to target endothelial cells; however, other targeting peptides are available and could be linked to the Id1 anti-sense molecule to direct the anti-sense molecule to hematopoietic cells. While the Id1-PCAO strategy has not been tested in hematopoietic cells, it is a feasible approach for use in the hematopoietic malignancies. Targeting peptides have been identified which home to bone marrow and bind primitive hematopoietic stem cells (Nowakowski et al., 2004). The benefit of this procedure would be that it does not require the use of any viral transduction procedures, and the targeting peptide should limit potential toxicity by localizing the anti-sense molecule to the diseased area.

6.2 Peptide aptamer

Another small molecule which has recently been developed is a peptide that binds both Id1 and Id3. Mern et al. identified a peptide aptamer (a short peptide), Id1/Id3-PA7, from a randomized combinatorial expression library using yeast and mammalian two-hybrid systems. When the aptamer is fused to a "cell-penetrating protein transduction domain" or PTD (truncated VP22 ORF), and tested on ovarian cancer cell lines, it causes increased expression of $p16^{INK4a}$, and it induced apoptosis (as indicated by PARP cleavage) (Mern et al., 2010a). The aptamer colocalized with Id1 and Id3 staining based on immunohistochemistry, suggesting that its effects result from its direct interaction with Id1 and/or Id3. To date, the authors have tested this molecule on ovarian and breast cancer cell lines *in vitro* and demonstrated growth inhibition, but have not yet examined its effects on normal cells nor in hematopoiesis (Mern et al., 2010a; Mern et al., 2010b).

6.3 Dominant interfering molecule 13I

In an effort to better understand the rules of HLH protein interaction, Ciarapica and collegues screened a phage display library to identify and isolate mutant domains with could interfere with HLH domain interactions. They discovered a dominant interfering HLH domain, 13I, which selectively binds to Ids (Id1, Id2, Id3) as opposed to their E protein HLH binding partners, and also impairs complex formation with Rb (Id2). Expression of 13I in a human embryonic kidney cell line (293) and in neuroblastoma cell lines restored the ability of the E protein E47 to bind and activate the promoters of cell cycle inhibitors. In addition, 13I was also able to induce differentiation in neuroblastoma cells suggesting it can over-ride both the cell cycle promotion and differentiation blocking functions of the Id proteins (Ciarapica et al., 2009). To date, 13I has not yet been tested on normal or hematopoietic cells.

Each of these inhibitors represents a hopeful step forward to reducing aberrant Id levels and restoring proper differentiation to hyperproliferative cells. The attractive feature of the Ids as potential therapeutic targets is that their expression does not need to be completely reduced, just suppressed to low enough levels to restore differentiation, as seen in normal tissues.

7. Summary

In summary, the Id proteins are potential targets in myelogenous leukemia. Much of the work that has gone into characterizing this family of small proteins indicates that if the expression of Id1, Id2, and Id3 is maintained at high levels in progenitor cells, and if their expression is not reduced at the correct time during maturation or differentiation that this could contribute to hyperplasia or neoplasia. Currently there are three targeting molecules available that are undergoing testing at the basic research level.

The discovery of novel mediators of oncogenesis, and biomarkers for disease identification and progression, such as the Id family of proteins, will contribute to the design of better drugs and more effective therapies for myelogenous leukemia.

8. Acknowledgements

This project has been funded in whole or in part with federal funds from the National Cancer Institute, National Institutes of Health, under contract HHSN26120080001E. The content of this publication does not necessarily reflect the views or policies of the Department of Health and Human Services, nor does mention of trade names, commercial products, or organizations imply endorsement by the U.S. Government. This Research was supported [in part] by the Intramural Research Program of the NIH, National Cancer Institute, Center for Cancer Research.

9. References

Alani, R.M., Young, A.Z., and Shifflett, C.B. (2001). Id1 regulation of cellular senescence through transcriptional repression of p16/Ink4a. Proceedings of the National Academy of Sciences of the United States of America *98*, 7812-7816.

Anido, J., Saez-Borderias, A., Gonzalez-Junca, A., Rodon, L., Folch, G., Carmona, M.A., Prieto-Sanchez, R.M., Barba, I., Martinez-Saez, E., Prudkin, L., *et al.* (2010). TGF-beta Receptor Inhibitors Target the CD44(high)/Id1(high) Glioma-Initiating Cell Population in Human Glioblastoma. Cancer cell *18*, 655-668.

Bao, F., Polk, P., Nordberg, M.L., Veillon, D.M., Sun, A., Deininger, M., Murray, D., Andersson, B.S., and Munker, R. (2007). Comparative gene expression analysis of a chronic myelogenous leukemia cell line resistant to cyclophosphamide using oligonucleotide arrays and response to tyrosine kinase inhibitors. Leukemia research *31*, 1511-1520.

Barrett, T., and Edgar, R. (2006). Gene expression omnibus: microarray data storage, submission, retrieval, and analysis. Methods in enzymology *411*, 352-369.

Benezra, R., Davis, R.L., Lockshon, D., Turner, D.L., and Weintraub, H. (1990). The protein Id: a negative regulator of helix-loop-helix DNA binding proteins. Cell *61*, 49-59.

Bernardo, M.V., Yelo, E., Gimeno, L., Campillo, J.A., and Parrado, A. (2007). Identification of apoptosis-related PLZF target genes. Biochemical and biophysical research communications *359*, 317-322.

Berse, M., Bounpheng, M., Huang, X., Christy, B., Pollmann, C., and Dubiel, W. (2004). Ubiquitin-dependent degradation of Id1 and Id3 is mediated by the COP9 signalosome. Journal of molecular biology *343*, 361-370.

Buitenhuis, M., van Deutekom, H.W., Verhagen, L.P., Castor, A., Jacobsen, S.E., Lammers, J.W., Koenderman, L., and Coffer, P.J. (2005). Differential regulation of granulopoiesis by the basic helix-loop-helix transcriptional inhibitors Id1 and Id2. Blood *105*, 4272-4281.

Cammenga, J., Mulloy, J.C., Berguido, F.J., MacGrogan, D., Viale, A., and Nimer, S.D. (2003). Induction of C/EBPalpha activity alters gene expression and differentiation of human CD34+ cells. Blood *101*, 2206-2214.

Chassot, A.A., Turchi, L., Virolle, T., Fitsialos, G., Batoz, M., Deckert, M., Dulic, V., Meneguzzi, G., Busca, R., and Ponzio, G. (2007). Id3 is a novel regulator of p27kip1 mRNA in early G1 phase and is required for cell-cycle progression. Oncogene *26*, 5772-5783.

Chaturvedi, V., Bonish, B., Bacon, P., Qin, J.Z., Denning, M.F., Foreman, K., Diaz, M.O., Robinson, J., and Nickoloff, B.J. (2003). Role for Id-1 in immunobiology of normal keratinocytes and in basal cell carcinoma. Experimental dermatology *12*, 255-260.

Chen, Z., Liu, S., Sumida, T., Sun, S., Wei, Y., Liu, M., Dong, Z., Zhang, F., Hamakawa, H., and Wei, F. (2011). Silencing id-1 with RNA interference inhibits adenoid cystic carcinoma in mice. The Journal of surgical research *169*, 57-66.

Ciarapica, R., Annibali, D., Raimondi, L., Savino, M., Nasi, S., and Rota, R. (2009). Targeting Id protein interactions by an engineered HLH domain induces human neuroblastoma cell differentiation. Oncogene *28*, 1881-1891.

Cooper, C.L., Brady, G., Bilia, F., Iscove, N.N., and Quesenberry, P.J. (1997). Expression of the Id family helix-loop-helix regulators during growth and development in the hematopoietic system. Blood *89*, 3155-3165.

Deed, R.W., Hara, E., Atherton, G.T., Peters, G., and Norton, J.D. (1997). Regulation of Id3 cell cycle function by Cdk-2-dependent phosphorylation. Molecular and cellular biology *17*, 6815-6821.

Dell'Orso, S., Ganci, F., Strano, S., Blandino, G., and Fontemaggi, G. (2010). ID4: a new player in the cancer arena. Oncotarget *1*, 48-58.

Dierov, J., Sanchez, P.V., Burke, B.A., Padilla-Nash, H., Putt, M.E., Ried, T., and Carroll, M. (2009). BCR/ABL induces chromosomal instability after genotoxic stress and alters the cell death threshold. Leukemia : official journal of the Leukemia Society of America, Leukemia Research Fund, UK *23*, 279-286.

Doulatov, S., Notta, F., Rice, K.L., Howell, L., Zelent, A., Licht, J.D., and Dick, J.E. (2009). PLZF is a regulator of homeostatic and cytokine-induced myeloid development. Genes & development *23*, 2076-2087.

Fraidenraich, D., Stillwell, E., Romero, E., Wilkes, D., Manova, K., Basson, C.T., and Benezra, R. (2004). Rescue of cardiac defects in id knockout embryos by injection of embryonic stem cells. Science *306*, 247-252.

Fukuma, M., Okita, H., Hata, J., and Umezawa, A. (2003). Upregulation of Id2, an oncogenic helix-loop-helix protein, is mediated by the chimeric EWS/ets protein in Ewing sarcoma. Oncogene *22*, 1-9.

Geest, C.R., Buitenhuis, M., Vellenga, E., and Coffer, P.J. (2009). Ectopic expression of C/EBPalpha and ID1 is sufficient to restore defective neutrophil development in low-risk myelodysplasia. Haematologica *94*, 1075-1084.

Hara, E., Hall, M., and Peters, G. (1997). Cdk2-dependent phosphorylation of Id2 modulates activity of E2A-related transcription factors. The EMBO journal *16*, 332-342.

Harper, J.W., Burton, J.L., and Solomon, M.J. (2002). The anaphase-promoting complex: it's not just for mitosis any more. Genes & development *16*, 2179-2206.

Hasskarl, J., Duensing, S., Manuel, E., and Munger, K. (2004). The helix-loop-helix protein ID1 localizes to centrosomes and rapidly induces abnormal centrosome numbers. Oncogene *23*, 1930-1938.

Hasskarl, J., Mern, D.S., and Munger, K. (2008). Interference of the dominant negative helix-loop-helix protein ID1 with the proteasomal subunit S5A causes centrosomal abnormalities. Oncogene *27*, 1657-1664.

Heinz, L.X., Platzer, B., Reisner, P.M., Jorgl, A., Taschner, S., Gobel, F., and Strobl, H. (2006). Differential involvement of PU.1 and Id2 downstream of TGF-beta1 during Langerhans-cell commitment. Blood *107*, 1445-1453.

Henke, E., Perk, J., Vider, J., de Candia, P., Chin, Y., Solit, D.B., Ponomarev, V., Cartegni, L., Manova, K., Rosen, N., *et al.* (2008). Peptide-conjugated antisense oligonucleotides for targeted inhibition of a transcriptional regulator in vivo. Nature biotechnology *26*, 91-100.

Hong, S.H., Lee, J.H., Lee, J.B., Ji, J., and Bhatia, M. (2011). ID1 and ID3 represent conserved negative regulators of human embryonic and induced pluripotent stem cell hematopoiesis. Journal of cell science *124*, 1445-1452.

Hu, Y.C., Lam, K.Y., Law, S., Wong, J., and Srivastava, G. (2001). Identification of differentially expressed genes in esophageal squamous cell carcinoma (ESCC) by cDNA expression array: overexpression of Fra-1, Neogenin, Id-1, and CDC25B genes in ESCC. Clinical cancer research : an official journal of the American Association for Cancer Research *7*, 2213-2221.

Iavarone, A., Garg, P., Lasorella, A., Hsu, J., and Israel, M.A. (1994). The helix-loop-helix protein Id-2 enhances cell proliferation and binds to the retinoblastoma protein. Genes & development *8*, 1270-1284.

Ishiguro, A., Spirin, K., Shiohara, M., Tobler, A., Norton, J.D., Rigolet, M., Shimbo, T., and Koeffler, H.P. (1995). Expression of Id2 and Id3 mRNA in human lymphocytes. Leukemia research *19*, 989-996.

Ishiguro, A., Spirin, K.S., Shiohara, M., Tobler, A., Gombart, A.F., Israel, M.A., Norton, J.D., and Koeffler, H.P. (1996). Id2 expression increases with differentiation of human myeloid cells. Blood *87*, 5225-5231.

Ishikawa, F., Yoshida, S., Saito, Y., Hijikata, A., Kitamura, H., Tanaka, S., Nakamura, R., Tanaka, T., Tomiyama, H., Saito, N., *et al.* (2007). Chemotherapy-resistant human AML stem cells home to and engraft within the bone-marrow endosteal region. Nature biotechnology *25*, 1315-1321.

Jankovic, V., Ciarrocchi, A., Boccuni, P., DeBlasio, T., Benezra, R., and Nimer, S.D. (2007). Id1 restrains myeloid commitment, maintaining the self-renewal capacity of hematopoietic stem cells. Proceedings of the National Academy of Sciences of the United States of America *104*, 1260-1265.

Jen, Y., Manova, K., and Benezra, R. (1996). Expression patterns of Id1, Id2, and Id3 are highly related but distinct from that of Id4 during mouse embryogenesis. Developmental dynamics : an official publication of the American Association of Anatomists *207*, 235-252.

Ji, M., Li, H., Suh, H.C., Klarmann, K.D., Yokota, Y., and Keller, J.R. (2008). Id2 intrinsically regulates lymphoid and erythroid development via interaction with different target proteins. Blood *112*, 1068-1077.

Kebebew, E., Treseler, P.A., Duh, Q.Y., and Clark, O.H. (2000). The helix-loop-helix transcription factor, Id-1, is overexpressed in medullary thyroid cancer. Surgery *128*, 952-957.

Kebebew, E., Treseler, P.A., Duh, Q.Y., and Clark, O.H. (2003). The helix-loop-helix protein, Id-1, is overexpressed and regulates growth in papillary thyroid cancer. Surgery *134*, 235-241.

Kim, D., Peng, X.C., and Sun, X.H. (1999). Massive apoptosis of thymocytes in T-cell-deficient Id1 transgenic mice. Molecular and cellular biology *19*, 8240-8253.

Kindler, T., Lipka, D.B., and Fischer, T. (2010). FLT3 as a therapeutic target in AML: still challenging after all these years. Blood *116*, 5089-5102.

Kleeff, J., Ishiwata, T., Friess, H., Buchler, M.W., Israel, M.A., and Korc, M. (1998). The helix-loop-helix protein Id2 is overexpressed in human pancreatic cancer. Cancer research *58*, 3769-3772.

Ko, J., Patel, N., Ikawa, T., Kawamoto, H., Frank, O., Rivera, R.R., Van Etten, R.A., and Murre, C. (2008). Suppression of E-protein activity interferes with the development of BCR-ABL-mediated myeloproliferative disease. Proceedings of the National Academy of Sciences of the United States of America *105*, 12967-12972.

Kreider, B.L., Benezra, R., Rovera, G., and Kadesch, T. (1992). Inhibition of myeloid differentiation by the helix-loop-helix protein Id. Science *255*, 1700-1702.

Langlands, K., Down, G.A., and Kealey, T. (2000). Id proteins are dynamically expressed in normal epidermis and dysregulated in squamous cell carcinoma. Cancer research *60*, 5929-5933.

Langlands, K., Yin, X., Anand, G., and Prochownik, E.V. (1997). Differential interactions of Id proteins with basic-helix-loop-helix transcription factors. The Journal of biological chemistry *272*, 19785-19793.

Lasorella, A., Boldrini, R., Dominici, C., Donfrancesco, A., Yokota, Y., Inserra, A., and Iavarone, A. (2002). Id2 is critical for cellular proliferation and is the oncogenic effector of N-myc in human neuroblastoma. Cancer research *62*, 301-306.

Lasorella, A., Iavarone, A., and Israel, M.A. (1996). Id2 specifically alters regulation of the cell cycle by tumor suppressor proteins. Molecular and cellular biology *16*, 2570-2578.

Lasorella, A., Noseda, M., Beyna, M., Yokota, Y., and Iavarone, A. (2000). Id2 is a retinoblastoma protein target and mediates signalling by Myc oncoproteins. Nature *407*, 592-598.

Lasorella, A., Stegmuller, J., Guardavaccaro, D., Liu, G., Carro, M.S., Rothschild, G., de la Torre-Ubieta, L., Pagano, M., Bonni, A., and Iavarone, A. (2006). Degradation of Id2 by the anaphase-promoting complex couples cell cycle exit and axonal growth. Nature *442*, 471-474.

Lee, J.Y., Kang, M.B., Jang, S.H., Qian, T., Kim, H.J., Kim, C.H., Kim, Y., and Kong, G. (2009). Id-1 activates Akt-mediated Wnt signaling and p27(Kip1) phosphorylation through PTEN inhibition. Oncogene *28*, 824-831.

Lee, T.K., Man, K., Ling, M.T., Wang, X.H., Wong, Y.C., Lo, C.M., Poon, R.T., Ng, I.O., and Fan, S.T. (2003). Over-expression of Id-1 induces cell proliferation in hepatocellular carcinoma through inactivation of p16INK4a/RB pathway. Carcinogenesis *24*, 1729-1736.

Leeanansaksiri, W., Wang, H., Gooya, J.M., Renn, K., Abshari, M., Tsai, S., and Keller, J.R. (2005). IL-3 induces inhibitor of DNA-binding protein-1 in hemopoietic progenitor cells and promotes myeloid cell development. J Immunol *174*, 7014-7021.

Li, H.M., Zhuang, Z.H., Wang, Q., Pang, J.C., Wang, X.H., Wong, H.L., Feng, H.C., Jin, D.Y., Ling, M.T., Wong, Y.C., *et al.* (2004). Epstein-Barr virus latent membrane protein 1 (LMP1) upregulates Id1 expression in nasopharyngeal epithelial cells. Oncogene *23*, 4488-4494.

Lin, C.Q., Singh, J., Murata, K., Itahana, Y., Parrinello, S., Liang, S.H., Gillett, C.E., Campisi, J., and Desprez, P.Y. (2000). A role for Id-1 in the aggressive phenotype and steroid hormone response of human breast cancer cells. Cancer research *60*, 1332-1340.

Ling, M.T., Wang, X., Ouyang, X.S., Xu, K., Tsao, S.W., and Wong, Y.C. (2003). Id-1 expression promotes cell survival through activation of NF-kappaB signalling pathway in prostate cancer cells. Oncogene *22*, 4498-4508.

Lister, J., Forrester, W.C., and Baron, M.H. (1995). Inhibition of an erythroid differentiation switch by the helix-loop-helix protein Id1. The Journal of biological chemistry *270*, 17939-17946.

Lyden, D., Young, A.Z., Zagzag, D., Yan, W., Gerald, W., O'Reilly, R., Bader, B.L., Hynes, R.O., Zhuang, Y., Manova, K., *et al.* (1999). Id1 and Id3 are required for neurogenesis, angiogenesis and vascularization of tumour xenografts. Nature *401*, 670-677.

Maruyama, H., Kleeff, J., Wildi, S., Friess, H., Buchler, M.W., Israel, M.A., and Korc, M. (1999). Id-1 and Id-2 are overexpressed in pancreatic cancer and in dysplastic lesions in chronic pancreatitis. The American journal of pathology *155*, 815-822.

Mern, D.S., Hasskarl, J., and Burwinkel, B. (2010a). Inhibition of Id proteins by a peptide aptamer induces cell-cycle arrest and apoptosis in ovarian cancer cells. British journal of cancer *103*, 1237-1244.

Mern, D.S., Hoppe-Seyler, K., Hoppe-Seyler, F., Hasskarl, J., and Burwinkel, B. (2010b). Targeting Id1 and Id3 by a specific peptide aptamer induces E-box promoter activity, cell cycle arrest, and apoptosis in breast cancer cells. Breast cancer research and treatment *124*, 623-633.

Misaghian, N., Ligresti, G., Steelman, L.S., Bertrand, F.E., Basecke, J., Libra, M., Nicoletti, F., Stivala, F., Milella, M., Tafuri, A., *et al.* (2009). Targeting the leukemic stem cell: the

Holy Grail of leukemia therapy. Leukemia : official journal of the Leukemia Society of America, Leukemia Research Fund, UK *23*, 25-42.

Morrow, M.A., Mayer, E.W., Perez, C.A., Adlam, M., and Siu, G. (1999). Overexpression of the Helix-Loop-Helix protein Id2 blocks T cell development at multiple stages. Molecular immunology *36*, 491-503.

Murad, J.M., Place, C.S., Ran, C., Hekmatyar, S.K., Watson, N.P., Kauppinen, R.A., and Israel, M.A. (2010). Inhibitor of DNA binding 4 (ID4) regulation of adipocyte differentiation and adipose tissue formation in mice. The Journal of biological chemistry *285*, 24164-24173.

Nagel, S., Venturini, L., Marquez, V.E., Meyer, C., Kaufmann, M., Scherr, M., MacLeod, R.A., and Drexler, H.G. (2010). Polycomb repressor complex 2 regulates HOXA9 and HOXA10, activating ID2 in NK/T-cell lines. Molecular cancer *9*, 151.

Nishimine, M., Nakamura, M., Mishima, K., Kishi, M., Kirita, T., Sugimura, M., and Konishi, N. (2003). Id proteins are overexpressed in human oral squamous cell carcinomas. Journal of oral pathology & medicine : official publication of the International Association of Oral Pathologists and the American Academy of Oral Pathology *32*, 350-357.

Nishimori, H., Sasaki, Y., Yoshida, K., Irifune, H., Zembutsu, H., Tanaka, T., Aoyama, T., Hosaka, T., Kawaguchi, S., Wada, T., *et al.* (2002). The Id2 gene is a novel target of transcriptional activation by EWS-ETS fusion proteins in Ewing family tumors. Oncogene *21*, 8302-8309.

Norton, J.D. (2000). ID helix-loop-helix proteins in cell growth, differentiation and tumorigenesis. Journal of cell science *113 (Pt 22)*, 3897-3905.

Nowakowski, G.S., Dooner, M.S., Valinski, H.M., Mihaliak, A.M., Quesenberry, P.J., and Becker, P.S. (2004). A specific heptapeptide from a phage display peptide library homes to bone marrow and binds to primitive hematopoietic stem cells. Stem Cells *22*, 1030-1038.

Ogata, T., and Noda, M. (1991). Expression of Id, a negative regulator of helix-loop-helix DNA binding proteins, is down-regulated at confluence and enhanced by dexamethasone in a mouse osteoblastic cell line, MC3T3E1. Biochemical and biophysical research communications *180*, 1194-1199.

Ohtani, N., Zebedee, Z., Huot, T.J., Stinson, J.A., Sugimoto, M., Ohashi, Y., Sharrocks, A.D., Peters, G., and Hara, E. (2001). Opposing effects of Ets and Id proteins on p16INK4a expression during cellular senescence. Nature *409*, 1067-1070.

Ouyang, X.S., Wang, X., Lee, D.T., Tsao, S.W., and Wong, Y.C. (2002). Over expression of ID-1 in prostate cancer. The Journal of urology *167*, 2598-2602.

Pan, L., Sato, S., Frederick, J.P., Sun, X.H., and Zhuang, Y. (1999). Impaired immune responses and B-cell proliferation in mice lacking the Id3 gene. Molecular and cellular biology *19*, 5969-5980.

Park, K.W., Waki, H., Villanueva, C.J., Monticelli, L.A., Hong, C., Kang, S., MacDougald, O.A., Goldrath, A.W., and Tontonoz, P. (2008). Inhibitor of DNA binding 2 is a small molecule-inducible modulator of peroxisome proliferator-activated receptor-gamma expression and adipocyte differentiation. Mol Endocrinol *22*, 2038-2048.

Peng, Y., Kang, Q., Luo, Q., Jiang, W., Si, W., Liu, B.A., Luu, H.H., Park, J.K., Li, X., Luo, J., *et al.* (2004). Inhibitor of DNA binding/differentiation helix-loop-helix proteins mediate bone morphogenetic protein-induced osteoblast differentiation of mesenchymal stem cells. The Journal of biological chemistry *279*, 32941-32949.

Perry, S.S., Zhao, Y., Nie, L., Cochrane, S.W., Huang, Z., and Sun, X.H. (2007). Id1, but not Id3, directs long-term repopulating hematopoietic stem-cell maintenance. Blood *110*, 2351-2360.

Polsky, D., Bastian, B.C., Hazan, C., Melzer, K., Pack, J., Houghton, A., Busam, K., Cordon-Cardo, C., and Osman, I. (2001). HDM2 protein overexpression, but not gene amplification, is related to tumorigenesis of cutaneous melanoma. Cancer research *61*, 7642-7646.

Prabhu, S., Ignatova, A., Park, S.T., and Sun, X.H. (1997). Regulation of the expression of cyclin-dependent kinase inhibitor p21 by E2A and Id proteins. Molecular and cellular biology *17*, 5888-5896.

Rice, K.L., Hormaeche, I., Doulatov, S., Flatow, J.M., Grimwade, D., Mills, K.I., Leiva, M., Ablain, J., Ambardekar, C., McConnell, M.J., *et al.* (2009). Comprehensive genomic screens identify a role for PLZF-RARalpha as a positive regulator of cell proliferation via direct regulation of c-MYC. Blood *114*, 5499-5511.

Riechmann, V., van Cruchten, I., and Sablitzky, F. (1994). The expression pattern of Id4, a novel dominant negative helix-loop-helix protein, is distinct from Id1, Id2 and Id3. Nucleic acids research *22*, 749-755.

Rivera, R.R., Johns, C.P., Quan, J., Johnson, R.S., and Murre, C. (2000). Thymocyte selection is regulated by the helix-loop-helix inhibitor protein, Id3. Immunity *12*, 17-26.

Rosenbauer, F., Koschmieder, S., Steidl, U., and Tenen, D.G. (2005). Effect of transcription-factor concentrations on leukemic stem cells. Blood *106*, 1519-1524.

Sablitzky, F., Moore, A., Bromley, M., Deed, R.W., Newton, J.S., and Norton, J.D. (1998). Stage- and subcellular-specific expression of Id proteins in male germ and Sertoli cells implicates distinctive regulatory roles for Id proteins during meiosis, spermatogenesis, and Sertoli cell function. Cell growth & differentiation : the molecular biology journal of the American Association for Cancer Research *9*, 1015-1024.

Schemionek, M., Elling, C., Steidl, U., Baumer, N., Hamilton, A., Spieker, T., Gothert, J.R., Stehling, M., Wagers, A., Huettner, C.S., *et al.* (2010). BCR-ABL enhances differentiation of long-term repopulating hematopoietic stem cells. Blood *115*, 3185-3195.

Schindl, M., Oberhuber, G., Obermair, A., Schoppmann, S.F., Karner, B., and Birner, P. (2001). Overexpression of Id-1 protein is a marker for unfavorable prognosis in early-stage cervical cancer. Cancer research *61*, 5703-5706.

Schindl, M., Schoppmann, S.F., Strobel, T., Heinzl, H., Leisser, C., Horvat, R., and Birner, P. (2003). Level of Id-1 protein expression correlates with poor differentiation, enhanced malignant potential, and more aggressive clinical behavior of epithelial ovarian tumors. Clinical cancer research : an official journal of the American Association for Cancer Research *9*, 779-785.

Schoppmann, S.F., Schindl, M., Bayer, G., Aumayr, K., Dienes, J., Horvat, R., Rudas, M., Gnant, M., Jakesz, R., and Birner, P. (2003). Overexpression of Id-1 is associated with poor clinical outcome in node negative breast cancer. International journal of cancer Journal international du cancer *104*, 677-682.

Semerad, C.L., Mercer, E.M., Inlay, M.A., Weissman, I.L., and Murre, C. (2009). E2A proteins maintain the hematopoietic stem cell pool and promote the maturation of myelolymphoid and myeloerythroid progenitors. Proceedings of the National Academy of Sciences of the United States of America *106*, 1930-1935.

Sherr, C.J., and McCormick, F. (2002). The RB and p53 pathways in cancer. Cancer cell *2*, 103-112.

Shoji, W., Yamamoto, T., and Obinata, M. (1994). The helix-loop-helix protein Id inhibits differentiation of murine erythroleukemia cells. The Journal of biological chemistry *269*, 5078-5084.

Stinson, J., Inoue, T., Yates, P., Clancy, A., Norton, J.D., and Sharrocks, A.D. (2003). Regulation of TCF ETS-domain transcription factors by helix-loop-helix motifs. Nucleic acids research *31*, 4717-4728.

Suh, H.C., Ji, M., Gooya, J., Lee, M., Klarmann, K.D., and Keller, J.R. (2009). Cell-nonautonomous function of Id1 in the hematopoietic progenitor cell niche. Blood *114*, 1186-1195.

Suh, H.C., Leeanansaksiri, W., Ji, M., Klarmann, K.D., Renn, K., Gooya, J., Smith, D., McNiece, I., Lugthart, S., Valk, P.J., *et al.* (2008). Id1 immortalizes hematopoietic progenitors in vitro and promotes a myeloproliferative disease in vivo. Oncogene *27*, 5612-5623.

Sun, X.H., Copeland, N.G., Jenkins, N.A., and Baltimore, D. (1991). Id proteins Id1 and Id2 selectively inhibit DNA binding by one class of helix-loop-helix proteins. Molecular and cellular biology *11*, 5603-5611.

Szlanka, T., Haracska, L., Kiss, I., Deak, P., Kurucz, E., Ando, I., Viragh, E., and Udvardy, A. (2003). Deletion of proteasomal subunit S5a/Rpn10/p54 causes lethality, multiple mitotic defects and overexpression of proteasomal genes in Drosophila melanogaster. Journal of cell science *116*, 1023-1033.

Takai, N., Miyazaki, T., Fujisawa, K., Nasu, K., and Miyakawa, I. (2001). Id1 expression is associated with histological grade and invasive behavior in endometrial carcinoma. Cancer letters *165*, 185-193.

Tam, W.F., Gu, T.L., Chen, J., Lee, B.H., Bullinger, L., Frohling, S., Wang, A., Monti, S., Golub, T.R., and Gilliland, D.G. (2008). Id1 is a common downstream target of oncogenic tyrosine kinases in leukemic cells. Blood *112*, 1981-1992.

Tamura, M., and Noda, M. (1994). Identification of a DNA sequence involved in osteoblast-specific gene expression via interaction with helix-loop-helix (HLH)-type transcription factors. The Journal of cell biology *126*, 773-782.

Tang, J., Gordon, G.M., Muller, M.G., Dahiya, M., and Foreman, K.E. (2003). Kaposi's sarcoma-associated herpesvirus latency-associated nuclear antigen induces expression of the helix-loop-helix protein Id-1 in human endothelial cells. Journal of virology *77*, 5975-5984.

Tang, R., Hirsch, P., Fava, F., Lapusan, S., Marzac, C., Teyssandier, I., Pardo, J., Marie, J.P., and Legrand, O. (2009). High Id1 expression is associated with poor prognosis in 237 patients with acute myeloid leukemia. Blood *114*, 2993-3000.

Tokuzawa, Y., Yagi, K., Yamashita, Y., Nakachi, Y., Nikaido, I., Bono, H., Ninomiya, Y., Kanesaki-Yatsuka, Y., Akita, M., Motegi, H., *et al.* (2010). Id4, a new candidate gene for senile osteoporosis, acts as a molecular switch promoting osteoblast differentiation. PLoS genetics *6*, e1001019.

Vandeputte, D.A., Troost, D., Leenstra, S., Ijlst-Keizers, H., Ramkema, M., Bosch, D.A., Baas, F., Das, N.K., and Aronica, E. (2002). Expression and distribution of id helix-loop-helix proteins in human astrocytic tumors. Glia *38*, 329-338.

Venditti, A., Tamburini, A., Buccisano, F., Scimo, M.T., Del Poeta, G., Maurillo, L., Cox, M.C., Abruzzese, E., Tribalto, M., Masi, M., *et al.* (2000). A phase-II trial of all trans retinoic acid and low-dose cytosine arabinoside for the treatment of high-risk myelodysplastic syndromes. Annals of hematology *79*, 138-142.

Wang, H., Wang, X.Q., Xu, X.P., and Lin, G.W. (2010a). ID4 methylation predicts high risk of leukemic transformation in patients with myelodysplastic syndrome. Leukemia research *34*, 598-604.

Wang, H., Yu, Y., Guo, R.W., Shi, Y.K., Song, M.B., Chen, J.F., Yu, S.Y., Yin, Y.G., Gao, P., and Huang, L. (2010b). Inhibitor of DNA binding-1 promotes the migration and proliferation of endothelial progenitor cells in vitro. Molecular and cellular biochemistry *335*, 19-27.

Wang, X., Xu, K., Ling, M.T., Wong, Y.C., Feng, H.C., Nicholls, J., and Tsao, S.W. (2002). Evidence of increased Id-1 expression and its role in cell proliferation in nasopharyngeal carcinoma cells. Molecular carcinogenesis *35*, 42-49.

Wilson, J.W., Deed, R.W., Inoue, T., Balzi, M., Becciolini, A., Faraoni, P., Potten, C.S., and Norton, J.D. (2001). Expression of Id helix-loop-helix proteins in colorectal adenocarcinoma correlates with p53 expression and mitotic index. Cancer research *61*, 8803-8810.

Wong, Y.C., Wang, X., and Ling, M.T. (2004). Id-1 expression and cell survival. Apoptosis : an international journal on programmed cell death *9*, 279-289.

Wood, A.D., Chen, E., Donaldson, I.J., Hattangadi, S., Burke, K.A., Dawson, M.A., Miranda-Saavedra, D., Lodish, H.F., Green, A.R., and Gottgens, B. (2009). ID1 promotes expansion and survival of primary erythroid cells and is a target of JAK2V617F-STAT5 signaling. Blood *114*, 1820-1830.

Yan, W., Young, A.Z., Soares, V.C., Kelley, R., Benezra, R., and Zhuang, Y. (1997). High incidence of T-cell tumors in E2A-null mice and E2A/Id1 double-knockout mice. Molecular and cellular biology *17*, 7317-7327.

Yates, P.R., Atherton, G.T., Deed, R.W., Norton, J.D., and Sharrocks, A.D. (1999). Id helix-loop-helix proteins inhibit nucleoprotein complex formation by the TCF ETS-domain transcription factors. The EMBO journal *18*, 968-976.

Ying, Q.L., Nichols, J., Chambers, I., and Smith, A. (2003). BMP induction of Id proteins suppresses differentiation and sustains embryonic stem cell self-renewal in collaboration with STAT3. Cell *115*, 281-292.

Yokota, Y., Mansouri, A., Mori, S., Sugawara, S., Adachi, S., Nishikawa, S., and Gruss, P. (1999). Development of peripheral lymphoid organs and natural killer cells depends on the helix-loop-helix inhibitor Id2. Nature *397*, 702-706.

Yu, L., Liu, C., Vandeusen, J., Becknell, B., Dai, Z., Wu, Y.Z., Raval, A., Liu, T.H., Ding, W., Mao, C., *et al.* (2005). Global assessment of promoter methylation in a mouse model of cancer identifies ID4 as a putative tumor-suppressor gene in human leukemia. Nature genetics *37*, 265-274.

Zhang, X., Ling, M.T., Wong, Y.C., and Wang, X. (2007). Evidence of a novel antiapoptotic factor: role of inhibitor of differentiation or DNA binding (Id-1) in anticancer drug-induced apoptosis. Cancer science *98*, 308-314.

Zhang, Y., Hassan, M.Q., Li, Z.Y., Stein, J.L., Lian, J.B., van Wijnen, A.J., and Stein, G.S. (2008). Intricate gene regulatory networks of helix-loop-helix (HLH) proteins support regulation of bone-tissue related genes during osteoblast differentiation. Journal of cellular biochemistry *105*, 487-496.

Zheng, W., Wang, H., Xue, L., Zhang, Z., and Tong, T. (2004). Regulation of cellular senescence and p16(INK4a) expression by Id1 and E47 proteins in human diploid fibroblast. The Journal of biological chemistry *279*, 31524-31532.

13

PU.1, a Versatile Transcription Factor and a Suppressor of Myeloid Leukemia

Shinichiro Takahashi
Division of Hematology, Kitasato University School of Allied Health Sciences, Sagamihara, Kanagawa, Japan

1. Introduction

PU.1 is a member of the Ezb transformation-specific sequence (Ets) family of transcription factors, and is expressed in granulocytic, monocytic and B-lymphoid cells (Chen et al., 1995b; Klemsz et al., 1990). PU.1 expression levels increase during the differentiation of granulocytes (Chen et al., 1995b). PU.1-deficient mice exhibit defects in the development of neutrophils, macrophages and B cells (McKercher et al., 1996; Scott et al., 1994). Therefore, PU.1 is indispensable for myeloid differentiation during normal hematopoiesis. Moreover, mice carrying hypomorphic PU.1 alleles that reduce PU.1 expression to 20% of its normal levels were reported to develop acute myeloid leukemia (AML) (Rosenbauer et al., 2004), suggesting that disruption of the function of this transcription factor plays a pivotal role in myeloid leukemia biology through the control of numerous target genes. Binding sites for PU.1 are found on almost all myeloid-specific promoters. Notable target genes are receptors for the cytokines, *macrophage colony-stimulating factor* (*M-CSF*), *granulocyte colony-stimulating factor* (*G-CSF*) and *granulocyte macrophage colony-stimulating factor* (*GM-CSF*) (Hohaus et al., 1995; Smith et al., 1996; Zhang et al., 1994), the characteristic antigens *CD11b*/*CD18* (Rosmarin et al., 1995), primary granule enzymes (Iwama et al., 1998) and the transcription factors c-Jun and JunB (Steidl et al., 2006). In addition, a transcriptional repressor function of PU.1 toward a certain set of genes has been demonstrated. Although the importance of the PU.1 function as a positive regulator of these myeloid genes has been widely examined and reviewed, studies on the role of PU.1 as a transcriptional repressor are relatively scarce. The author's group and others demonstrated that loss of PU.1 function resulted in upregulation of several drug-resistance or growth-regulating genes, including *metallothionein* (*MT*), *vimentin* (*VIM*), *c-myc* and *Flt3,* through disruption of the transcriptional repressor function (Imoto et al., 2010; Inomata et al., 2006; Iseki et al., 2009). This review summarizes the current understanding of the molecular functions of PU.1. Moreover, this review has a particular focus on the transcriptional function of PU.1 as an activator as well as a repressor. Furthermore, the role of PU.1 in the biology of myeloid leukemia is discussed.

2. PU.1, a member of the ETS transcription factor family

The Ets family of transcription factors is so named because the first gene was identified in the E26 avian retrovirus. Ets factors constitute a relatively large gene family, with 27 members encoded by the human genome (Sharrocks, 2001). As precisely reviewed by Oikawa and Yamada (Oikawa & Yamada, 2003), Ets family proteins can be divided into several subfamilies on the basis of their structural compositions and the similarities in their DNA-binding Ets domains. Most of them have the Ets domains in their C-terminal regions. However, several Ets family proteins, such as the ternary complex factor (TCF) subfamily members, have the Ets domains in their N-terminal regions. In addition, besides the conserved Ets domain, a subset of Ets family proteins (e.g. Ets-1, Ets-2, ERG, TEL) have another evolutionarily conserved domain called the pointed domain at their N-terminal regions, which forms a helix-loop-helix (HLH) structure for protein-protein interactions (Oikawa & Yamada, 2003). PU.1 is the most distantly related member of the Ets family proteins having only about 40% identity with Ets-1 in its DNA-binding domain (Oikawa & Yamada, 2003).

3. Structure of PU.1

Spi-1, the gene name for PU.1, was first identified by Moreau-Gachelin and colleagues as the product of a gene targeted by recurrent insertions of the Spleen Focus Forming Virus (SFFV) in Friend's erythroleukemia. An important and unusual feature of the genomic locus *Spi-1* for SFFV proviral integration is that rearrangements caused by SFFV integration were found in 95% of the erythroid tumors examined (Moreau-Gachelin et al., 1988). They subsequently isolated PU.1 (for purine-rich box 1) as a factor that binds to a purine-rich motif in the MHC class II gene promoter. Basically, monomeric PU.1 binds to the consensus DNA site 5'-AAAG(A/C/G)GGAAG-3' via its C-terminal Ets domain and activates transcription via its N-terminal glutamine-rich and acidic domains (Klemsz et al., 1990) (Figure 1).

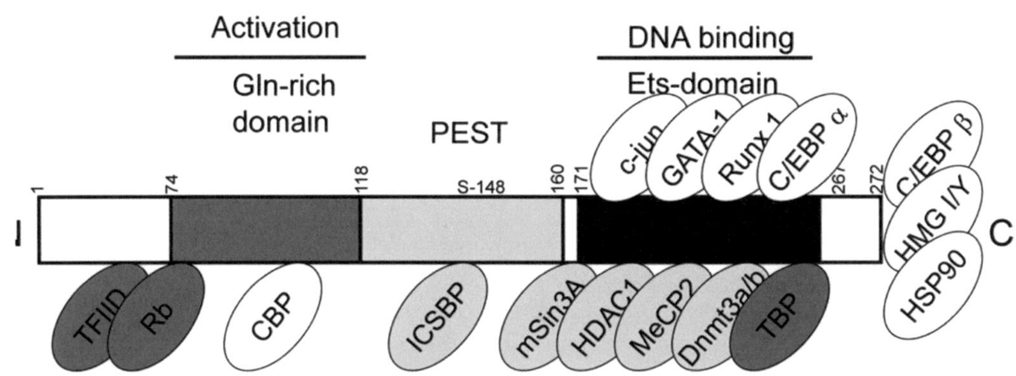

Fig. 1. Schematic presentation of PU.1 and its interacting partners. Proteins involved in transcription are shown in ovals, with transcriptional repressors shown in light gray and basic transcription factors shown in dark gray.

PU.1 is encoded by the *Spi-1 (sfpi1)* gene located on chromosome 11 in humans (chromosome 2 in mice). PU.1 transcripts are 1333 nucleotides long and are produced from the splicing of five exons (Kastner & Chan, 2008). The PU.1 protein is 272 amino acids long (predicted MW: 31 kDa). The structure of PU.1 is shown in Figure 1. The DNA-binding Ets domain shows sequence similarity with other members of the Ets family and is contained within amino acids 171–267 of the C-terminus (Klemsz et al., 1990). The Ets domain corresponds to the DNA-binding domain and recognizes sequences harboring the core GGAA motif. This domain is also involved in the protein-protein interactions between PU.1 and other factors such as GATA-1 (Nerlov et al., 2000), c-Jun (Behre et al., 1999), Runx 1 or C/EBPα (Petrovick et al., 1998).

The activation domain of PU.1 is located within the N-terminus and consists of several regions rich in either acidic amino acids or glutamines (designated the Gln-rich domain) (Klemsz & Maki, 1996). The activation domain at the N-terminal 75 amino acids of PU.1 has been shown to interact *in vitro* with the basal transcription factor IID (TFIID) and the tumor suppressor retinoblastoma (Rb) protein (Hagemeier et al., 1993). Yamamoto *et al.* (Yamamoto et al., 1999) previously found that this transcriptional activation domain of amino acids 74–122 binds to a transcriptional coactivator, cAMP response element-binding protein (CREB)-binding protein (CBP). CBP potentiated PU.1-mediated transcription of a reporter gene driven by multimerized PU.1-binding sites, suggesting that CBP functions as a coactivator for PU.1 (Yamamoto et al., 1999). A region from amino acids 118–160, which has large numbers of prolines, glutamic acids, serines and threonines, is called the PEST domain (Klemsz & Maki, 1996). This domain plays important roles in the protein-protein interactions, particularly those with interferon (IFN) consensus sequence-binding protein (ICSBP, also called IFN regulatory factor-8) (Nakano et al., 2005).

The C-terminal region of PU.1 has been reported to interact with the leucine zipper transcription factor CCAAT/enhancer-binding protein (C/EBP) β, DNA-binding protein HMG I/Y, multifunctional phosphatase MKP-1 and chaperone protein HSP90 (Nagulapalli et al., 1995) as well as the basic transcription factor TATA box-binding protein (TBP) (Kihara-Negishi et al., 2001).

The PU.1 protein is also the target of phosphorylation events, notably on serine 148, which are regulated by various extracellular signals and play critical roles in modifying the activity of this factor (Joo et al., 2004). These aspects will be discussed later in section 7.

4. Role of PU.1 in normal hematopoiesis, especially in the myeloid lineage, through the regulation of its target genes

As described in the introduction, PU.1 is expressed in B-lymphoid, granulocytic and monocytic cells (Chen et al., 1995b; Klemsz et al., 1990). PU.1 expression levels increase during the differentiation of granulocytes (Chen et al., 1995b). PU.1-deficient mice exhibit defects in the development of neutrophils, macrophages and B cells, although the generation of erythroid and megakaryocytic cells is intact (McKercher et al., 1996; Scott et al., 1994).

In the erythroid lineage, the expression of PU.1 is downregulated during terminal differentiation of murine erythroleukemia (MEL) cells by treatment with dimethylsulfoxide (Hensold et al., 1996). Enforced expression of PU.1 in MEL cells inhibits erythroid differentiation (Oikawa et al., 1999; Yamada et al., 2001). In contrast to the lack of PU.1 expression in the myelomonocytic lineage, which results in impairment of the differentiation, overexpression of PU.1 results in erythroid differentiation blockade.

Expression of PU.1 is observed in $CD34^+$ hematopoietic progenitors and differentiation commitment toward the myeloid and lymphoid lineages appears to be determined by the expression levels of PU.1, since high PU.1 levels promote macrophage differentiation and relatively low PU.1 levels induce B-cell differentiation (DeKoter & Singh, 2000).

Collectively, PU.1 functions in multiple hematopoietic lineages including myeloid, lymphoid and erythroid cells. Many reviews describing the roles of PU.1 in hematopoiesis have been published (Gallant & Gilkeson, 2006; Kastner & Chan, 2008; Oikawa et al., 1999; Oikawa & Yamada, 2003). Therefore, this section of the present review particularly focuses on the roles of PU.1 in myeloid lineage development through the regulation of its target genes.

Early myeloid differentiation is controlled by PU.1 and other families of transcription factors, such as C/EBPs, AML1/Runx1, retinoic acid receptor α (RARα), c-Myb and others (Friedman, 2002). C/EBPα and C/EBPε knockout mice also have defects in the development of mature macrophages and neutrophils (Yamanaka et al., 1997; Zhang et al., 1999). Hence, PU.1, as well as the C/EBP family members, is a critical master regulator for the determination of the developmental pathway toward the myeloid lineage in hematopoietic cells.

Gene	Level of regulation	References
M-CSFR	Promoter	(Zhang et al., 1994) (Li et al., 2005)
GM-CSFRα	Promoter	(Hohaus et al., 1995)
G-CSFR	Promoter	(Smith et al., 1996)
CD11b	Promoter	(Chen et al., 1993)
CD18	Promoter	(Rosmarin et al., 1995) (Bottinger et al., 1994)
MPO	Enhancer	(Ford et al., 1996)
NE	Enhancer	(Nuchprayoon et al., 1999)
NE	Promoter	(Oelgeschlager et al., 1996)
PR3	Promoter	(Sturrock et al., 1996)
Lysozyme	Enhancer	(Ahne & Stratling, 1994)
$gp91^{phox}$	Promoter	(Suzuki et al., 1998)
$p47^{phox}$	Promoter	(Li et al., 1997)
c-Jun	Unknown	(Steidl et al., 2006)
JunB	Promoter	(Steidl et al., 2006)
PU.1	Promoter	(Chen et al., 1995a)

Table 1. PU.1 target genes play crucial roles in myeloid lineage development

Binding sites for PU.1 are found on almost all myeloid-specific promoters. A large collection of PU.1-dependent promoters have been identified, which control an array of genes encoding predominantly growth factor receptors, adhesion molecules and characteristic enzymes. Notable target genes are receptors for cytokines, adhesion molecules, primary granule enzymes and transcription factors.

The M-CSF receptor (M-CSFR) (Zhang et al., 1994), GM-CSF receptor α (GM-CSFRα) (Hohaus et al., 1995) and G-CSF receptor (G-CSFR) (Smith et al., 1996) gene promoters were reported to be directly regulated by PU.1. These promoters are regulated by PU.1 in combination with C/EBPα (Hohaus et al., 1995; Li et al., 2005; Smith et al., 1996). By employing sense or antisense PU.1 expression, Celada *et al.* (Celada et al., 1996) showed that PU.1 is necessary for M-CSF-dependent proliferation of macrophages, through the control of M-CSFR expression. Another group demonstrated that PU.1-deficient myeloid progenitors can proliferate *in vitro* in response to the multilineage cytokines interleukin (IL)-3, IL-6 and stem cell factor, but are unresponsive to the myeloid-specific cytokines GM-CSF, G-CSF and M-CSF (DeKoter et al., 1998). Expression of M-CSFR or G-CSFR in PU.1-deficient marrow cells did not rescue myeloid development, indicating that PU.1 is required beyond the induction of these cytokine receptors (DeKoter et al., 1998; Henkel et al., 1999).

The CD11b (or macrophage-1 antigen; MAC-1) leukocyte integrin subunit exists on the surface of human granulocytes and monocytes/macrophages coupled with the CD18 (β) subunit in a heterodimer. This heterodimer mediates multifaceted adherence reactivity of these myeloid cells, including the ability to adhere to endothelial cells (Arnaout, 1990). The CD11b promoter was reported to be positively regulated by both Sp1 and PU.1 (Chen et al., 1993). CD18 promoter activity is also regulated by PU.1 (Bottinger et al., 1994; Rosmarin et al., 1995). Consistently, CD11b/CD18 are undetectable on the surfaces of cells lacking PU.1 (Henkel et al., 1996; Olson et al., 1995). These molecules are from the β2 integrin chain, otherwise known as complement receptor 3 (CR3) (Ehlers, 2000). The CD11b subunit of CR3 promotes phagocytosis and macrophage migration by binding to extracellular matrix proteins, coagulation proteins and a variety of microbial antigens (Ehlers, 2000).

Primary granule enzymes are a group of serine proteases or closely related molecules found in cells of the granulocyte series. PU.1-deficient myeloid promoters lack or exhibit low expression of primary granule enzymes, including myeloperoxidase (MPO), neutrophil elastase (NE), proteinase 3 (PR3) and lysozyme (Iwama et al., 1998). Ford *et al.* (Ford et al., 1996) demonstrated that the MPO upstream enhancer is accessible in multipotent cell chromatin, but functionally incompetent before granulocyte commitment. Multipotent cells contain both PU.1 and C/EBPα as enhancer-binding activities. It was reported that a 220-bp portion of the second intron of the *PR3* gene, which contains an Sp1 consensus site flanked by two Ets family consensus sequences that bind PU.1, functions as an enhancer of NE expression (Nuchprayoon et al., 1999). In addition, PU.1 cooperates with C/EBP α and c-Myb to regulate the NE promoter (Oelgeschlager et al., 1996). PR3 expression has also been shown to be regulated by PU.1 (Sturrock et al., 1996). PU.1-deficient neutrophils do not express secondary granule components, including collagenase, lysozyme and lactoferrin, and have limited ability to ingest and kill bacteria (Anderson et al., 1998; Iwama et al., 1998). The activity of the lysozyme gene enhancer was demonstrated to be controlled by PU.1 in avian macrophages (Ahne & Stratling, 1994). In addition, the expression of $gp91^{phox}$ and $p47^{phox}$, which are both components of nicotinamide adenine dinucleotide phosphate (NADPH) phagocyte oxidase, is positively regulated by PU.1 (Li et al., 1997; Suzuki et al., 1998).

In addition to these myeloid-specific genes, several transcription factors play crucial roles in the phenotype of PU.1-deficient mice. Steidl *et al.* (Steidl et al., 2006) examined the transcriptome of preleukemic hematopoietic stem cells (HSCs) from mice in which PU.1 was knocked down to identify transcriptional changes. They demonstrated that the transcription factors c-Jun and JunB were among the top downregulated targets. They concluded that the decreased levels of c-Jun and especially JunB contribute to the development of PU.1 knockdown-induced AML by blocking differentiation and increasing self-renewal. It was previously reported that PU.1 autoregulates its expression in myeloid cells (Chen et al., 1995a). However, autoregulation by PU.1 remains uncertain, since the expression of GFP reporters driven by the endogenous PU.1 promoter remains high in PU.1-null hematopoietic cells (Back et al., 2005; Dakic et al., 2005).

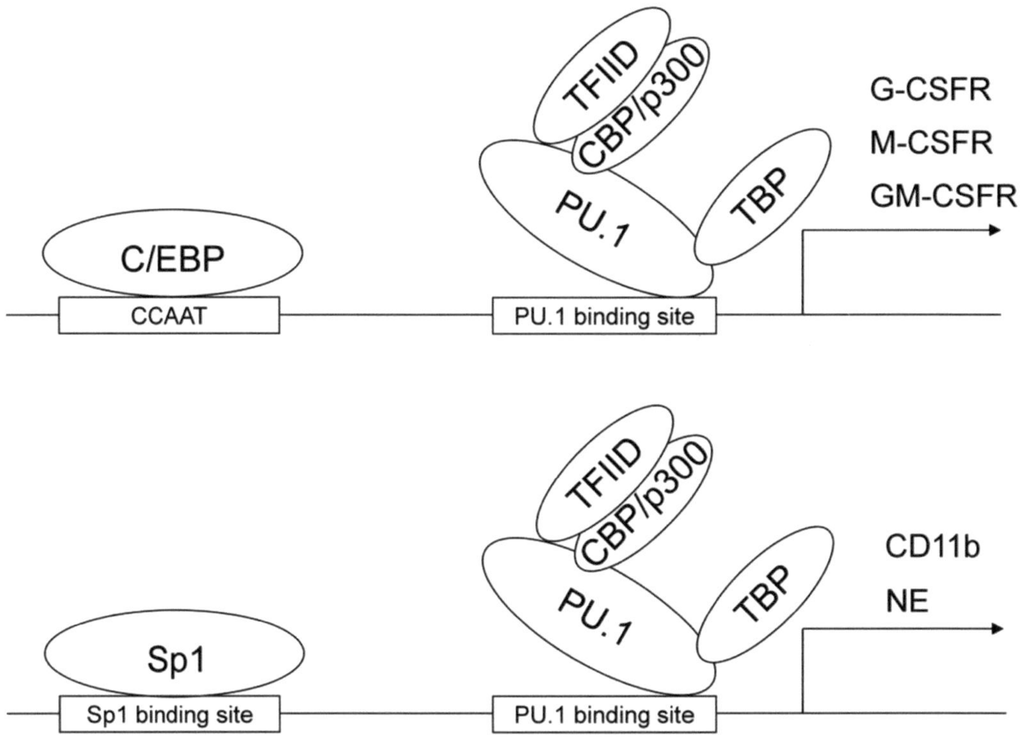

Fig. 2. PU.1 as a transcriptional activator. The known myeloid promoters regulated by a set of transcription factors in combination with PU.1 are depicted.

Table 1 shows a list of myeloid genes that are known to be positively regulated by PU.1. Collectively, PU.1 plays a pivotal role in myeloid development through the regulation of cytokines, receptors, transcription factors and various myeloid specific genes.

The majority of the PU.1-dependent promoters in the myeloid lineage share several structural features, including a PU.1-binding site close to the site(s) of transcriptional initiation, no TATA box and a cluster of binding sites for Sp1 and members of the C/EBP or core-binding factor (CBF) families (Fisher & Scott, 1998; Tenen et al., 1997). A schematic layout of the transcription factors binding to the proximal promoter regions is shown in Figure 2. The G-CSFR, M-CSFR and GM-CSFR promoters are regulated by PU.1 and C/EBPs, whereas the CD11b and NE promoters are regulated by PU.1 in combination with Sp1.

In contrast to PU.1 or C/EBPs, the other transcription factors are widely expressed outside of the hematopoietic system, indicating that myeloid-specific expression may be principally caused by PU.1 or unique combinations of adjoining transcription factors working in concert with PU.1 (Fisher & Scott., 1998). In this group of myeloid promoters, as depicted in Figure 2, binding of PU.1 close to the start point of transcription may facilitate recruitment to the TFIID complex and promote the binding of adjoining transcription factors. TFIID is a protein complex consisting of TBP and a set of TBP-associated factors (TAFs) (Pugh, 1996). Binding of TFIID to the promoter region is the first step in the assembly process that forms the transcription initiation complex. Not only does the N-terminal of PU.1 interact with TFIID, but its C-terminal was reported to interact with TBP (Kihara-Negishi et al., 2001) (Figures 1 and 2). Even though PU.1 may make the initial contact with TFIID, other transcriptional factors (e.g. C/EBPs, Sp1) are likely to help stabilize the TFIID complex through TAF interactions. The PU.1-initiated cooperative stabilization of TFIID may be sufficient to evoke myeloid-specific expression for this group of genes.

5. Regulation of PU.1

As described in the previous section, expression of PU.1 is critical for hematopoiesis. Therefore, the regulatory mechanisms of PU.1 expression have been extensively studied. To date, most aspects of PU.1 regulation have been explained by invoking two regulatory elements, the promoter and an upstream regulatory element (URE) at –14 kb upstream of the transcription start site of the *Spi-1* gene encoding PU.1.

The *Spi-1* promoter contains octamer-binding sites that affect B cell expression (Chen et al., 1996). As described in the previous section, PU.1 was demonstrated to bind to its own promoter to regulate itself in myeloid cells (Chen et al., 1995a). *Spi-1* promoter activity can also be directed in myeloid cells by C/EBPα and AP-1 (Cai et al., 2008) (Figure 3). Although the promoter alone cannot drive reporter expression in a chromatin context, a search for added regulatory function yielded the conserved URE at around –14 kb, reported to be a myeloid-specific enhancer, that enhanced the promoter activity in a myeloid cell line (Li et al., 2001). Huang *et al.* (Huang et al., 2008) demonstrated that AML1/Runx1 binds to functionally important sites within the URE and regulates PU.1 expression at both embryonic and adult stages of development. As described later in section 8, NF-κB was reported to regulate PU.1 through a novel site within the upstream URE (Bonadies et al., 2010). Zarnegar *et al.* (Zarnegar et al., 2010) recently uncovered a set of conserved *cis*-regulatory regions for *Spi-1*. One is a novel enhancer (–10 kb) that can amplify myeloid cell-specific expression of PU.1. The other is a separate pro-T-cell-specific silencer element (–9 kb). The enhancer element at –9 kb functions as a weak silencer in myeloid cells. The schematic layout is presented in Figure 3. Using a combination of transgenic studies, global chromatin assays and detailed molecular analyses, Leddin *et al.* (Leddin et al., 2011) presented evidence that PU.1 is regulated by a novel mechanism involving crosstalk between different *cis*-elements together with lineage-restricted autoregulation. They revealed that myeloid progenitors express C/EBPα, which binds to the URE and induces activation of an enhancer at –12 kb to allow the formation of a second PU.1 autoregulatory loop and binding of additional PU.1 driven-transcription factors, such as early growth response 2 (EGR2). In this model, PU.1 regulates its expression in B cells and macrophages by differently associating with cell type-specific transcription factors at one of its *cis*-regulatory elements to establish differential activity patterns at other elements.

Other mechanisms underlying the regulation of PU.1 expression have been demonstrated. Ebralidze *et al.* (Ebralidze et al., 2008) identified naturally occurring antisense transcripts overlapping the PU.1 coding region. They demonstrated that noncoding antisense RNAs are regulated by shared evolutionarily conserved *cis*-regulatory elements, and further showed that antisense RNAs inhibit PU.1 expression by modulating RNA translation. Vigorito *et al.* (Vigorito et al., 2007) carried out gene expression profiling of activated B cells and validated PU.1 as a direct target of microRNA-155 (miR-155)-mediated inhibition. Using mouse bone marrow (BM) cells, Hu *et al.* (Hu et al., 2010) revealed HOXA9-mediated upregulation, which is frequently observed in AML, of miR-155 in fractionated bone marrow progenitors. Furthermore, they revealed that ectopic expression of miR-155 resulted in a decrease in PU.1 protein (Hu et al., 2010). These findings suggest that the expression of PU.1 is controlled both transcriptionally and post-transcriptionally.

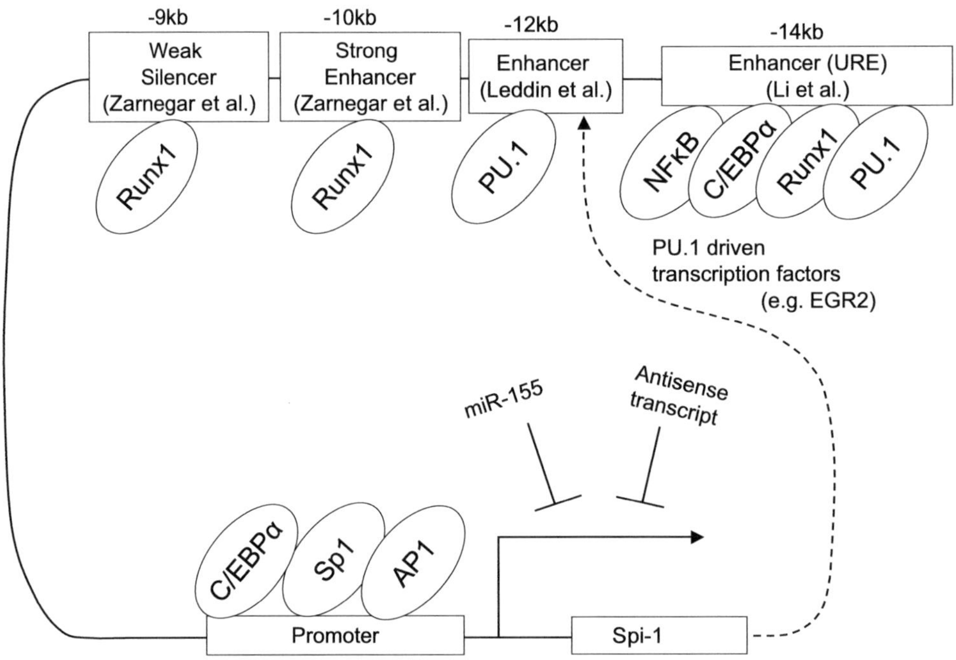

Fig. 3. Regulation of PU.1 expression.

6. PU.1 suppressive targets

Stiedl *et al.* (Steidl et al., 2006) revealed that ~21,500 of 45,000 transcripts were expressed in PU.1-knockdown HSCs, among which 225 transcripts were downregulated and 97 were upregulated in PU.1-knockdown HSCs. These findings indicate that PU.1 not only activates but also represses a substantial number of genes in HSCs. Consistent with this notion, several PU.1 suppressive targets have been identified and reported to date. Table 2 shows a list of the known PU.1 suppressive targets.

Borras *et al.* (Borras et al., 1995) first identified PU.1 as a transcriptional repressor. They examined the ability of PU.1 to regulate the expression of the *major histocompatibility complex I-Ab* gene. Their results indicated that PU.1 represses *I-Ab* expression, possibly by binding to a PU.1 box that is located between the Y-box and the transcription start site (Borras et al., 1995). The *c-myc* promoter (–138 to +517) was found to be a target for downregulation by PU.1 in a dose-dependent manner by luciferase assays (Kihara-Negishi et al., 2001). These authors also found that the *c-fos*, *SV-40*, *β-actin* and *PCNA* promoters are suppressed by expression of PU.1, without binding to a PU.1-binding site. They further showed that the *c-myc* minimal promoter including a TATA box is sufficient to exert PU.1 repression. Using luciferase assays, they demonstrated that a restricted region of PU.1 including the PEST domain is responsible for PU.1-mediated transcriptional repression. They clearly demonstrated that C-terminal amino acids 101–272 of PU.1 formed a complex with mSin3A and HDAC1 *in vivo* (Kihara-Negishi et al., 2001) (Figure 1). By affinity purification assays, Suzuki *et al.* (Suzuki et al., 2003) found that PU.1 bound directly to methyl-CpG-binding protein (MeCP) 2 via the C-terminal Ets domain. They revealed that MeCP2 was integrated into the PU.1–mSin3A–HDAC complex. The same group clearly revealed an interaction between PU.1 and DNA methyltransferase (Dnmt) 3a and Dnmt3b via the Ets domain (Suzuki et al., 2006). They further showed that the CpG sites in the *p16(INK4A)* promoter were methylated by PU.1 overexpression in NIH3T3 cells, accompanied by downregulation of *p16* (*INK4A*) gene expression (Suzuki et al., 2006). Moreover, hematopoietic precursor cells expressing PU.1 showed downregulation of the c-Myb protein levels. Transient expression of PU.1 in cotransfection assays in different cell lines resulted in inhibition of *c-myb* promoter activity through the PU.1-binding site (Bellon et al., 1997).

Gene	Level of regulation	References
Major histocompatibility complex I-Ab	Promoter	(Borras et al., 1995)
c-myc	Promoter	(Kihara-Negishi et al., 2001) (Kihara-Negishi et al., 2005)
c-fos, SV-40, β-actin, PCNA	Promoter	(Kihara-Negishi et al., 2001)
p16 (INK4A)	Promoter	(Suzuki et al., 2006)
c-Myb	Promoter	(Bellon et al., 1997)
CD11c	Promoter	(Lopez-Rodriguez & Corbi, 1997)
MT-1s, VIM	Promoter	(Imoto et al., 2010)
Annexin 1	Unknown	(Iseki et al., 2009)
Flt3	Promoter	(Inomata et al., 2006)

Table 2. Suppressive gene targets regulated by PU.1

It was reported that PU.1 negatively regulates the *CD11c integrin* gene promoter through recognition of the PU.1-binding site at the major transcriptional start site (Lopez-Rodriguez

& Corbi, 1997). The inhibitory action of PU.1 on CD11c is in contrast to its positive regulatory effect on the other integrin-related *CD11b/CD18* gene promoters (Rosmarin et al., 1995), as described in section 4. The opposite changes in CD11b and CD11c expression that take place in extravasating and maturing blood monocytes (Prieto et al., 1994) might be explained by the differential actions of PU.1 on the regulatory regions of the *CD11b* and *CD11c* genes.

The author's group recently revealed that *MT-1* and *VIM* gene expression is directly regulated by PU.1 (Imoto et al., 2010). The MT proteins comprise a group of low molecular weight cysteine-rich intracellular proteins that can be activated by a variety of stimuli, including metal ions, oxidative stress, cytokines, glucocorticoids and growth factors (Cherian et al., 2003). MT was reported to be a potential negative regulator of apoptosis (Shimoda et al., 2003). VIM is a cytoskeletal protein that belongs to the intermediate filament family (Lazarides, 1982). VIM suppresses the apoptotic effect of chemotherapeutic treatment (Belichenko et al., 2001). These findings imply that induced expression of MT, as well as VIM, may function in anti-apoptosis mechanisms in leukemia cells. We demonstrated that MeCP2 and PU.1 bind to the CpG-rich regions in the *MT-1* and *VIM* promoters. Bisulfite sequencing analyses of the PU.1-bound regions of these promoters revealed that the proportions of methylated CpG sites are tightly correlated with the PU.1 expression levels (Imoto et al., 2010). Importantly, the mRNA expression levels of the *MT-1* and *VIM* genes were inversely correlated with PU.1 mRNA expression in 43 primary AML specimens (MT-1G: $R=-0.50$, $p<0.001$; MT-1A: $R=-0.58$, $p<0.0005$; VIM: $R=-0.39$, $p<0.01$) (Imoto et al., 2010).

The author's group also demonstrated an inverse correlation between the mRNA expression of Annexin 1 and PU.1 in AML specimens (Iseki et al., 2009). In addition, the author and colleagues have reported that the *Flt3* gene promoter is suppressed by overexpression of PU.1, and that there is a significant negative correlation between FLT3 and PU.1 ($r=-0.43$, $p<0.05$) (Inomata et al., 2006). Therefore, PU.1 downregulation, which is important in the pathogenesis of AML as described in section 8, may impact on the overexpression of FLT3, which is frequently observed in AML, leading to activation of the FLT3 pathway (Ozeki et al., 2004; Takahashi, 2011).

Together with these findings, PU.1 represses several genes through its epigenetic activity under certain circumstances. The repression of PU.1 is directed in at least two ways. The author's group demonstrated that PU.1 binds to the methylated CpG-rich region with MeCP2, where no consensus PU.1-binding sites were found (Imoto et al., 2010). The other way is direct binding of PU.1 to PU.1-binding sites, as demonstrated in the promoters of the *CD11c, p16 (INK4A), major histocompatibility complex I-Ab, c-myb* and other genes (Borras et al., 1995; Lopez-Rodriguez & Corbi, 1997; Suzuki et al., 2006). In addition, some suppressive target genes of PU.1 may be indirect effects (e.g. Iseki et al., 2009), because direct binding to their promoters has not been demonstrated. A schematic layout of the complex of PU.1 and its corepressors binding to these promoters is shown in Figure 4.

7. Putative regulatory mechanisms for PU.1 as a transcriptional activator or repressor

As mentioned above, Kihara-Negishi *et al.* (Kihara-Negishi et al., 2001) showed a direct interaction of PU.1 with mSin3A. On the other hand, the same group previously demonstrated a direct interaction of PU.1 with the transcriptional coactivator CBP, which

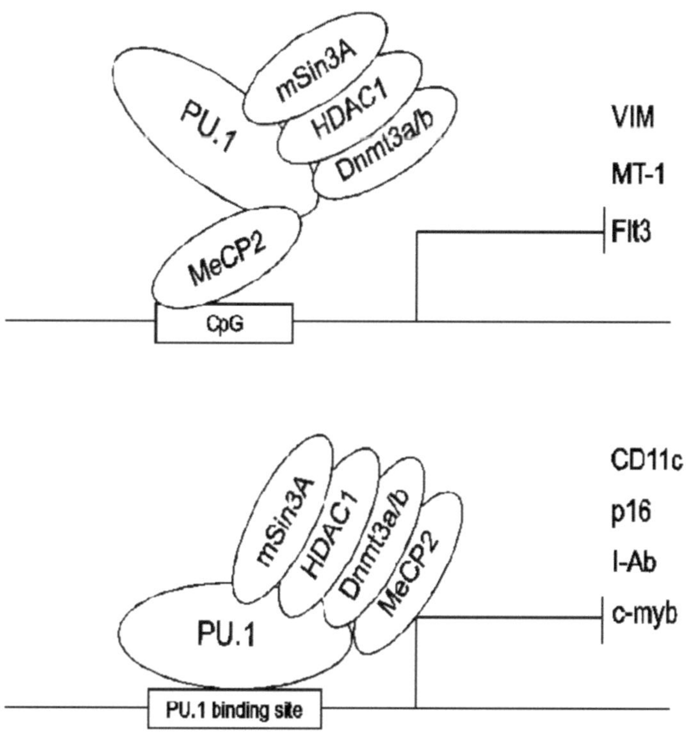

Fig. 4. PU.1 as a transcriptional repressor. This is a schematic picture about the hypothetical formation of the PU.1 repressor complexes, because some of these informations are putative. Since the *Flt3 gene* promoter has a CpG-rich region without a functional PU.1-binding site (Inomata et al., 2006), Flt3 may be classified into the upper group, although direct binding of PU.1 to the *Flt3 gene* promoter has not been examined.

enhances the transcriptional activity of PU.1 (Yamamoto et al., 1999). Of particular interest is the regulatory mechanism of the selection of the interacting partners, CBP and mSin3A-HDAC, which possess opposite functions in the regulation of gene expression. Posttranslational modification of PU.1, such as phosphorylation or acetylation, may be involved in the preferential recruitment of coactivators or corepressors.

In general, the expression of PU.1 is usually unaffected by most stimuli that regulate gene activation and its expression levels remain relatively constant (Yordy & Muise-Helmericks 2000). PU.1 is primarily regulated post-transcriptionally by phosphorylation (Lloberas et al., 1999; Yordy & Muise-Helmericks, 2000). PU.1 is potentially phosphorylated on five separate serine residues (Ser41, Ser45, Ser132, Ser133 and Ser148) and is an *in vitro* substrate for casein kinase II (CKII) (Lodie et al., 1997). Lodie *et al.* (Lodie et al., 1997) revealed that lipopolysaccharide stimulation induces phosphorylation of PU.1 at Ser148 (Figure 1), located within a CKII consensus motif, which increases the transactivation function of PU.1. PU.1 is also phosphorylated at Ser142 by stimulation of IL-3-induced p38 MAPK-mediated pathways (Wang et al., 2003). Mutation of Ser142 to alanine attenuates the IL-3-enhanced transactivation activity of PU.1. In contrast, Breig *et al.* (Breig et al., 2010) recently described that Ser41, but not Ser148, is necessary for Spi-1/PU.1-mediated repression of hemoglobin expression in Friend erythroleukemia cells. Phosphorylation of critical residues in PU.1 may switch the function of this transcription factor from an activator to a repressor. Kihara-Negishi *et al.* (Kihara-Negishi et al., 2005) examined whether acetylation regulates the physical and functional activities of PU.1 in MEL cells. They found that PU.1 is acetylated *in vivo* and that its repressor activity is reduced when the putative acetylation motifs in the Ets domain are mutated. The mutant cooperates with the coactivator CBP, similar to the case for wild-type PU.1, but shows insufficient cooperation with the corepressor mSin3A, which binds to the Ets domain of PU.1. These observations are summarized in Table 3.

The modifications of each functional domain (as depicted in Figure 1), which are required for transcriptional activation or repression, may result in the dissociation of cofactors, leading to changes in the transcriptional ability of PU.1.

However, a question still remains. As described in the previous section, in a same-cell population like HSCs (Steidl et al., 2006), some genes are suppressed while other genes are upregulated by PU.1. How are these genes differently regulated even in the same cells? It is possible that the context of the promoter may be important, and that promoter-specific cofactors may modify PU.1 and regulate the activity of this protein. These mechanisms remain to be elucidated in future studies.

Site	Cells	Responsible Signaling	Effect	Ref.
Ser41, Ser45, Ser132, Ser133 and Ser 148	Raw264.7 (macrophage) cells	Casein Kinase II	Phosphorylation of Ser 148 increases transactivation function.	(Lodie et al., 1997)
Ser 142	Ba/F3 (IL-3 dependent pro B cells)	p38MAP kinase	Phosphorylation of Ser 142 increases transactivation of PU.1, resulted in the stimulation of mcl-1 gene transcription.	(Wang et al., 2003)
Ser 41	Friend erythro-leukemia cells	PI3 kinase /Akt	Ser 41 is responsible for the PU.1 mediated repression, and phosphorylation of this site impairs its repression activity.	(Breig et al., 2010)
Lysine -rich acetylation motifs (a.a.221-223, 244-249)	Zinc inducible PU.1 transgenic MELB8/3 cells, 293T cells	Unknown	The repressor activity of PU.1 was impaired by mutations of both two acetylation motifs	(Kihara -Negishi et al., 2005)

Table 3. List of the post-translational modifications of PU.1

8. Role of PU.1 in the pathogenesis of AML

For many years, it has been known that irradiated mice frequently develop AML after a long latent period, and that nearly all of their tumors contain an interstitial deletion in one copy of chromosome 2 that includes the *PU.1* gene (Hayata et al., 1983; Silver et al., 1999; Trakhtenbrot et al., 1988). Subsequent studies revealed that mice with γ-irradiation-induced myeloid leukemia acquired both a deletion in one copy of chromosome 2 and a point mutation in the ETS domain of PU.1, which impaired DNA binding of the other PU.1 allele (Cook et al., 2004; Suraweera et al., 2005). These single amino acid substitutions were shown to alter the function of PU.1 by reducing its transactivation activity. Grisolano *et al* (Grisolano et al., 1997) previously showed that 10–20% of transgenic mice expressing PML-RARα in their early myeloid cells develop acute promyelocytic leukemia (APL) after a long latent period. The penetrance of APL development increases substantially when RARα-PML is coexpressed in early myeloid cells (Pollock et al., 1999) or when young mice are sublethally irradiated (Walter et al., 2004). In both scenarios, the vast majority of APL tumors contain a large (>20 Mb) interstitial deletion in one copy of chromosome 2 that invariably includes the *PU.1* gene (Walter et al., 2004; Zimonjic et al., 2000). These data strongly suggest that PU.1 acts in a similar manner to a tumor suppressor in myeloid progenitors, and that deletion of one allele, followed by a reduction in the function of the other allele, is relevant for AML pathogenesis. Indeed, PU.1 is expressed at low levels in most cases of human AML (Steidl et al., 2006).

PU.1 expression and/or function appear to be suppressed by several leukemogenic fusion products, such as RUNX1-ETO (Vangala et al., 2003), FLT3-ITD (Mizuki et al., 2003) and PML-RARα (Mueller et al., 2006a). Following these initial reports of suppressed PU.1 function in human AML, the leukemic potential of tumor progenitors with critically reduced PU.1 function has been illustrated by a series of mouse models. The level of PU.1 expression is critical for specifying cell fate and, if perturbed, even modest decreases in PU.1 can lead to leukemias and lymphomas (DeKoter & Singh, 2000a; Rosenbauer et al., 2004). Mice with an engineered deletion of the URE of PU.1 show decreased PU.1 expression and subsequently develop AML, through suppression of the AP-1 transcription factors JunB and c-Jun, by blocking differentiation and increasing self-renewal as described in the previous section. However, while these observations indicate that low but detectable amounts of PU.1 might favor the malignant potential of leukemic cells, this view was challenged by a report suggesting that complete loss of PU.1 can also lead to AML (Metcalf et al., 2006).

As described in section 5, the URE is important for the regulation of PU.1. Several reports have described associations between genetic abnormalities of this region and AML biology. In an analysis of 209 AML patient specimens, Steidl *et al.* (Steidl et al., 2007) revealed that a distal single nucleotide polymorphism (SNP) alters the long-range regulation of the *PU.1* gene in AML. The homozygous SNP within a highly conserved distal enhancer element in humans, which is 2.4-fold more frequent in AML with a complex karyotype (24.3%) than in AML with a normal karyotype (10.0%), leads to decreased enhancer activity and reduces PU.1 expression in myeloid progenitors in a development-dependent manner (Steidl et al., 2007). Bonadies *et al.* (Bonadies et al., 2010a) examined the URE sequence in 120 AML patients. They identified one AML patient with heterozygous loss of the entire URE sequence with markedly reduced PU.1 expression. The link between PU.1 URE mutations and AML pathogenesis might be explained by another model. The same group also identified NF-κB as an activator of PU.1 expression through a novel site within the upstream

URE (Bonadies et al., 2010b). They found sequence variations of this particular NF-κB site in four of 120 AML patients. These variant NF-κB sequences failed to mediate activation of PU.1, and AML patients with such variant sequences had suppressed PU.1 mRNA expression. These findings suggest that the change of a single base pair in a distal element critically affects the regulation of the tumor suppressor gene *PU.1*, thereby contributing to the development of AML.

Mutations of PU.1 have previously been examined by several groups. Mueller *et al.* (Mueller et al., 2002; Mueller et al., 2003) identified 10 mutant alleles of the *PU.1* gene in 9 of 126 AML patients. However, these findings could not be confirmed in two subsequent studies. Vegesna *et al.* (Vegesna et al., 2002) analyzed 381 samples of hematopoietic and solid malignancies, including 60 cases of *de novo* AML and 60 cases of myelodysplastic syndromes (MDS), and were not able to identify *PU.1* coding region mutations. Similarly, Lamandin *et al.* (Lamandin et al., 2002) failed to detect *PU.1* gene mutations in 77 primary AML samples. Collectively, direct genetic inactivation of the *PU.1* gene in myeloid leukemia has only been found in very rare cases. Although there is no doubt that a reduction in PU.1 expression plays a very important role in the pathogenesis of AML, its mutations in human myeloid leukemia biology remain unclear.

9. Perspectives and conclusions

The author has summarized the recent advances in the molecular biology of the PU.1 transcription factor, with a focus on its functions as both a transcriptional activator and repressor. In addition, the role of PU.1 in AML biology has been described.

In 2009, inactivating mutations of the *Ten-Eleven-Translocation oncogene family member 2* (*TET2*) gene were identified in about 15% of patients with various myeloid malignancies, such as MDS (19%), myeloproliferative disorders (12%), secondary AML (24%) and chronic myelomonocytic leukemia (22%) (Delhommeau et al., 2009). TET2 can convert 5-methylcytosine (5-mC) to 5-hydroxymethylcytosine (5-hmC) (Ko et al., 2010), which is hypothesized to be an intermediate in the demethylation of DNA. Ko *et al.* (Ko et al., 2010) demonstrated that disruption of TET2 enzymatic activity favors myeloid tumorigenesis.

Consistent with this observation, it was reported that Dnmt3a mutations were detected in 62 of 281 (22.1%) AML patients (Ley et al., 2010). These mutations were highly enriched in a group of patients with an intermediate-risk cytogenetic profile, as well as in FLT3 receptor mutations (25 of 61 (41.0%) patients; $p<0.003$) (Ley et al., 2010). Walter *et al.* (Walter et al., 2011) also described relatively frequent mutations of Dnmt3a in MDS. They performed sequencing in patients with MDS and identified 13 heterozygous mutations with predicted translational consequences in 12 of 150 (8.0%) patients. Yan *et al.* (Yan et al., 2011) discovered mutations in DNMT3a in 23 of 112 (20.5%) cases with the M5 subtype of AML. The DNMT mutants showed reduced enzymatic activity or aberrant affinity for histone H3 *in vitro*. Notably, there were alterations in the DNA methylation patterns and/or gene expression profiles, such as *HOXB* genes, in samples with DNMT3a mutations compared with those without such mutations (Yan et al., 2011). These recent findings strongly suggest a link between recurrent genetic alterations and aberrant DNA methylation status in myeloid malignancies.

As shown in Figures 1 and 4, PU.1 interacts with DNMT3a and DNMT3b (Suzuki et al., 2006) and suppresses its target genes through Dnmt activity (Imoto et al., 2010; Suzuki et al., 2006). Since the expression of DNMT3s is constant in AML specimens (Ley et al., 2010), it is tempting to speculate that DNMT3a mutations exert their leukemogenic potential, at least in part, by functional impairment of PU.1 epigenetic activities as a transcriptional repressor, mainly through downregulation of its expression. It is possible that this may also play an important role in AML pathogenesis (Figure 5).

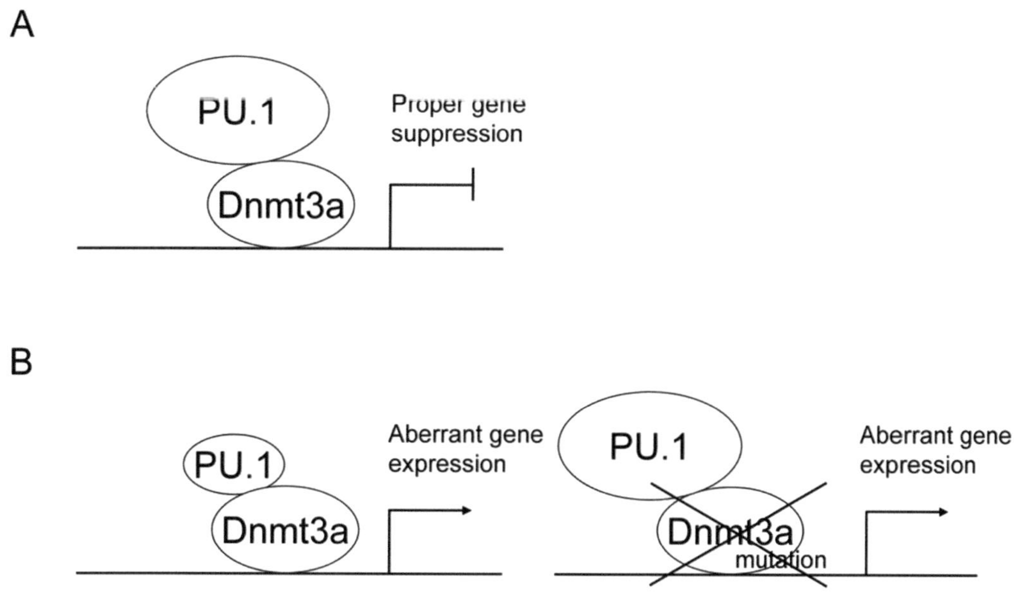

Fig. 5. Putative mechanisms of deregulated PU.1 repressor activity in AML. A, Normal cells. B, AML cells. A reduction in PU.1 expression (left panel), as well as mutations in Dnmt3a (right panel), result in aberrant target gene expression, which plays a role in the pathogenesis of AML.

Collectively, not only deregulation of proper myeloid-specific gene expression by downregulation of PU.1, but also insufficient recruitment of such epigenetic factors may play important roles in leukemia pathogenesis. Further clarification of the functions of this versatile transcription factor, with a particular focus on its function as a transcriptional repressor, may reveal the molecular biology of myeloid leukemia.

10. Acknowledgments

I thank Dr. Alison Sherwin (Edanz Editing) for helpful advice on the English language and editing of this manuscript. This work was supported in part by Grants-in-Aid for Scientific Research (No. 23590687) from the Ministry of Education, Science and Culture, Japan, Mitsubishi Pharma Research Foundation, Nakayama Foundation for Human Science, Takeda Science Foundation, and a foundation from Kitasato University School of Allied Health Sciences (Grant-in-Aid for Research Project, No. 2010-1004, No. 2011-1001).

11. References

Ahne, B. & Stratling, W.H. (1994) Characterization of a myeloid-specific enhancer of the chicken lysozyme gene. Major role for an Ets transcription factor-binding site. *J Biol Chem,* Vol. 269, No.27, (July 1994), pp. 17794-801.

Anderson, K.L.; Smith, K.A.; Pio, F.; Torbett, B.E. & Maki, R.A. (1998) Neutrophils deficient in PU.1 do not terminally differentiate or become functionally competent. *Blood*, Vol. 92, No.5, (September 1998), pp. 1576-85.

Arnaout, M.A. (1990) Structure and function of the leukocyte adhesion molecules CD11/CD18. *Blood*, Vol. 75, No.5, (March 1990), pp. 1037-50.

Back, J.; Allman, D.; Chan, S. & Kastner, P. (2005) Visualizing PU.1 activity during hematopoiesis. *Exp Hematol*, Vol. 33, No.4, (April 2005), pp. 395-402.

Behre, G.; Whitmarsh, A.J.; Coghlan, M.P.; Hoang, T.; Carpenter, C.L.; Zhang, D.E.; Davis, R.J. & Tenen, D.G. (1999) c-Jun is a JNK-independent coactivator of the PU.1 transcription factor. *J Biol Chem*, Vol. 274, No.8, (February 1999), pp. 4939-46.

Belichenko, I.; Morishima, N. & Separovic, D. (2001) Caspase-resistant vimentin suppresses apoptosis after photodynamic treatment with a silicon phthalocyanine in Jurkat cells. *Arch Biochem Biophys*, Vol. 390, No.1, (June 2001), pp. 57-63.

Bellon, T.; Perrotti, D. & Calabretta, B. (1997) Granulocytic differentiation of normal hematopoietic precursor cells induced by transcription factor PU.1 correlates with negative regulation of the c-myb promoter. *Blood*, Vol. 90, No.5, (September 1997), pp. 1828-39.

Bonadies, N.; Pabst, T. & Mueller, B.U. (2010a) Heterozygous deletion of the PU.1 locus in human AML. *Blood*, Vol. 115, No.2, (January 2010), pp 331-4.

Bonadies, N.; Neururer, C.; Steege, A.; Vallabhapurapu, S.; Pabst, T. & Mueller, B.U. (2010b) PU.1 is regulated by NF-kappaB through a novel binding site in a 17 kb upstream enhancer element. *Oncogene*, Vol. 29, No.7, (February 2010), pp. 1062-72.

Borras, F.E.; Lloberas, J.; Maki, R.A. & Celada, A. (1995) Repression of I-A beta gene expression by the transcription factor PU.1. *J Biol Chem*, Vol. 270, No.41, (October 1995), pp. 24385-91.

Bottinger, E.P.; Shelley, C.S.; Farokhzad, O.C. & Arnaout, M.A. (1994) The human beta 2 integrin CD18 promoter consists of two inverted Ets cis elements. *Mol Cell Biol*, Vol. 14, No.4, (April 1994), pp. 2604-15.

Breig, O.; Theoleyre, O.; Douablin, A. & Baklouti, F. (2010) Subtle distinct regulations of late erythroid molecular events by PI3K/AKT-mediated activation of Spi-1/PU.1 oncogene autoregulation loop. *Oncogene*, Vol. 29, No.19, (May 2010), pp. 2807-16.

Cai, D.H.; Wang, D.; Keefer, J.; Yeamans, C.; Hensley, K. & Friedman, A.D. (2008) C/EBP alpha:AP-1 leucine zipper heterodimers bind novel DNA elements, activate the PU.1 promoter and direct monocyte lineage commitment more potently than C/EBP alpha homodimers or AP-1. *Oncogene*, Vol. 27, No.19, (April 2008), pp. 2772-9.

Celada, A.; Borras, F.E.; Soler, C.; Lloberas, J.; Klemsz, M.; van Beveren, C.; McKercher, S. & Maki, R.A. (1996) The transcription factor PU.1 is involved in macrophage proliferation. *J Exp Med*, (July 1996), Vol. 184, No.1, pp. 61-9.

Chen, H.; Ray-Gallet, D.; Zhang, P.; Hetherington, C.J.; Gonzalez, D.A.; Zhang, D.E.; Moreau-Gachelin, F. & Tenen, D.G. (1995a) PU.1 (Spi-1) autoregulates its expression in myeloid cells. *Oncogene*, Vol. 11, No.8, (October 1995), pp. 1549-60.

Chen, H.; Zhang, P.; Radomska, H.S.; Hetherington, C.J.; Zhang, D.E. & Tenen, D.G. (1996) Octamer binding factors and their coactivator can activate the murine PU.1 (spi-1) promoter. *J Biol Chem*, Vol. 271, No.26, (June 1996), pp. 15743-52.

Chen, H.M.; Pahl, H.L.; Scheibe, R.J.; Zhang, D.E. & Tenen, D.G. (1993) The Sp1 transcription factor binds the CD11b promoter specifically in myeloid cells in vivo and is essential for myeloid-specific promoter activity. J Biol Chem, Vol. 268, No.11, (April 1993), pp. 8230-9.

Chen, H.M.; Zhang, P.; Voso, M.T.; Hohaus, S.; Gonzalez, D.A.; Glass, C.K.; Zhang, D.E. & Tenen, D.G. (1995b) Neutrophils and monocytes express high levels of PU.1 (Spi-1) but not Spi-B. *Blood*, Vol. 85, No.10, (May 1995), pp. 2918-28.

Cherian, M.G.; Jayasurya, A. & Bay, B.H. (2003) Metallothioneins in human tumors and potential roles in carcinogenesis. Mutat Res, Vol. 533, No.1-2, (December 2003), pp. 201-9.

Cook, W.D.; McCaw, B.J.; Herring, C.; John, D.L.; Foote, S.J.; Nutt, S.L. & Adams, J.M. (2004) PU.1 is a suppressor of myeloid leukemia, inactivated in mice by gene deletion and mutation of its DNA binding domain. *Blood*, Vol. 104, No.12, (December 2004), pp. 3437-44.

Dakic, A.; Metcalf, D.; Di Rago, L.; Mifsud, S.; Wu, L. & Nutt, S.L. (2005) PU.1 regulates the commitment of adult hematopoietic progenitors and restricts granulopoiesis. *J Exp Med*, Vol. 201, No.9, (May 2005), pp. 1487-502.

DeKoter, R.P. & Singh, H. (2000) Regulation of B lymphocyte and macrophage development by graded expression of PU.1. *Science*, Vol. 288, No.5470, (May 2000), pp. 1439-41.

DeKoter, R.P.; Walsh, J.C. & Singh, H. (1998) PU.1 regulates both cytokine-dependent proliferation and differentiation of granulocyte/macrophage progenitors. *Embo J*, Vol. 17, No.15, (August 1998), pp. 4456-68.

Delhommeau, F.; Dupont, S.; Della Valle, V.; James, C.; Trannoy, S.; Masse, A.; Kosmider, O.; Le Couedic, J.P.; Robert, F.; Alberdi, A.; Lecluse, Y.; Plo, I.; Dreyfus, F.J.; Marzac, C.; Casadevall, N.; Lacombe, C.; Romana, S.P.; Dessen, P.; Soulier, J.; Viguie, F.; Fontenay, M.; Vainchenker, W. & Bernard, O.A. (2009) Mutation in TET2 in myeloid cancers. *N Engl J Med*, Vol. 360, No.22, (May 2009), pp. 2289-301.

Ebralidze, A.K.; Guibal, F.C.; Steidl, U.; Zhang, P.; Lee, S.; Bartholdy, B.; Jorda, M.A.; Petkova, V.; Rosenbauer, F.; Huang, G.; Dayaram, T.; Klupp, J.; O'Brien, K.B.; Will, B.; Hoogenkamp, M.; Borden, K.L.; Bonifer, C. & Tenen, D.G. (2008) PU.1 expression is modulated by the balance of functional sense and antisense RNAs regulated by a shared cis-regulatory element. *Genes Dev*, Vol. 22, No.15, (August 2008), pp. 2085-92.

Ehlers, M.R. (2000) CR3: a general purpose adhesion-recognition receptor essential for innate immunity. *Microbes Infect*, Vol. 2, No.3, (Mar 2000), pp. 289-94.

Fisher, R.C. & Scott, E.W. (1998) Role of PU.1 in hematopoiesis. *Stem Cells*, Vol. 16, No.1, (January 1998), pp. 25-37.

Ford, A.M.; Bennett, C.A.; Healy, L.E.; Towatari, M.; Greaves, M.F. & Enver, T. (1996) Regulation of the myeloperoxidase enhancer binding proteins Pu1, C-EBP alpha, -beta, and -delta during granulocyte-lineage specification. *Proc Natl Acad Sci U S A*, Vol. 93, No.20, (October 1996), pp. 10838-43.

Friedman, A.D. (2002) Transcriptional regulation of granulocyte and monocyte development. *Oncogene*, Vol. 21, No.21, (May 2002), pp. 3377-90.

Gallant, S. & Gilkeson, G. (2006) ETS transcription factors and regulation of immunity. *Arch Immunol Ther Exp (Warsz)*, Vol. 54, No.3, (May-June 2006), pp. 149-63.

Grisolano, J.L.; Wesselschmidt, R.L.; Pelicci, P.G. & Ley, T.J. (1997) Altered myeloid development and acute leukemia in transgenic mice expressing PML-RAR alpha under control of cathepsin G regulatory sequences. *Blood*, Vol. 89, No.2, (January 1997), pp. 376-87.

Hagemeier, C.; Bannister, A.J.; Cook, A. & Kouzarides, T. (1993) The activation domain of transcription factor PU.1 binds the retinoblastoma (RB) protein and the transcription factor TFIID in vitro: RB shows sequence similarity to TFIID and TFIIB. *Proc Natl Acad Sci U S A*, Vol. 90, No.4, (February 1993), pp. 1580-4.

Hayata, I.; Seki, M.; Yoshida, K.; Hirashima, K.; Sado, T.; Yamagiwa, J. & Ishihara, T. (1983) Chromosomal aberrations observed in 52 mouse myeloid leukemias. *Cancer* Res, Vol. 43, No.1, (January 1983), pp. 367-73.

Henkel, G.W.; McKercher, S.R.; Leenen, P.J. & Maki, R.A. (1999) Commitment to the monocytic lineage occurs in the absence of the transcription factor PU.1. *Blood*, Vol. 93, No.9, (May 1999), pp. 2849-58.

Henkel, G.W.; McKercher, S.R.; Yamamoto, H.; Anderson, K.L.; Oshima, R.G. & Maki, R.A. (1996) PU.1 but not ets-2 is essential for macrophage development from embryonic stem cells. *Blood*, Vol. 88, No.8, (October 1996), pp. 2917-26.

Hohaus, S.; Petrovick, M.S.; Voso, M.T.; Sun, Z.; Zhang, D.E. & Tenen, D.G. (1995) PU.1 (Spi-1) and C/EBP alpha regulate expression of the granulocyte-macrophage colony-stimulating factor receptor alpha gene. *Mol Cell Biol*, Vol. 15, No.10, (October 1995), pp. 5830-45.

Hu, Y.L.; Fong, S.; Largman, C. & Shen, W.F. (2010) HOXA9 regulates miR-155 in hematopoietic cells. *Nucleic Acids Res*, Vol. 38, No.16, (September 2010), pp. 5472-8.

Huang, G.; Zhang, P.; Hirai, H.; Elf, S.; Yan, X.; Chen, Z.; Koschmieder, S.; Okuno, Y.; Dayaram, T.; Growney, J.D.; Shivdasani, R.A.; Gilliland, D.G.; Speck, N.A.; Nimer, S.D. & Tenen, D.G. (2008) PU.1 is a major downstream target of AML1 (RUNX1) in adult mouse hematopoiesis. *Nat Genet*, Vol. 40, No.1, (January 2008), pp. 51-60.

Imoto, A.; Okada, M.; Okazaki, T.; Kitasato, H.; Harigae, H. & Takahashi, S. (2010) Metallothionein-1 isoforms and vimentin are direct PU.1 downstream target genes in leukemia cells. *J Biol Chem*, Vol. 285, No.14, (April 2010), pp. 10300-9.

Inomata, M.; Takahashi, S.; Harigae, H.; Kameoka, J.; Kaku, M. & Sasaki, T. (2006) Inverse correlation between Flt3 and PU.1 expression in acute myeloblastic leukemias. *Leuk Res*, Vol. 30, No.6, (June 2006), pp. 659-64.

Iseki, Y.; Imoto, A.; Okazaki, T.; Harigae, H. & Takahashi, S. (2009) Identification of annexin 1 as a PU.1 target gene in leukemia cells. *Leuk Res*, Vol. 33, No.12, (December 2009), pp. 1658-63.

Iwama, A.; Zhang, P.; Darlington, G.J.; McKercher, S.R.; Maki, R. & Tenen, D.G. (1998) Use of RDA analysis of knockout mice to identify myeloid genes regulated in vivo by PU.1 and C/EBPalpha. *Nucleic Acids Res*, Vol. 26, No.12, (June 1998), pp. 3034-43.

Joo, M.; Park, G.Y.; Wright, J.G.; Blackwell, T.S.; Atchison, M.L. & Christman, J.W. (2004) Transcriptional regulation of the cyclooxygenase-2 gene in macrophages by PU.1. *J Biol Chem*, Vol. 279, No.8, (February 2004), pp. 6658-65.

Kastner, P. & Chan, S. (2008) PU.1: a crucial and versatile player in hematopoiesis and leukemia. *Int J Biochem Cell Biol*, Vol. 40, No.1, (January 2008), pp. 22-7.

Kihara-Negishi, F.; Suzuki, M.; Yamada, T.; Sakurai, T. & Oikawa, T. (2005) Impaired repressor activity and biological functions of PU.1 in MEL cells induced by mutations in the acetylation motifs within the ETS domain. *Biochem Biophys Res Commun*, Vol. 335, No.2, (September 2005), pp. 477-84.

Kihara-Negishi, F.; Yamamoto, H.; Suzuki, M.; Yamada, T.; Sakurai, T.; Tamura, T. & Oikawa, T. (2001) In vivo complex formation of PU.1 with HDAC1 associated with PU.1 mediated transcriptional repression. *Oncogene*, Vol. 20, No.42, (September 2001), pp. 6039-47.

Klemsz, M.J. & Maki, R.A. (1996) Activation of transcription by PU.1 requires both acidic and glutamine domains. *Mol Cell Biol*, Vol. 16, No.1, (January 1996), pp. 390-7.

Klemsz, M.J.; McKercher, S.R.; Celada, A.; Van Beveren, C. & Maki, R.A. (1990) The macrophage and B cell-specific transcription factor PU.1 is related to the ets oncogene. *Cell*, Vol. 61, No.1, (April 1990), pp. 113-24.

Ko, M.; Huang, Y.; Jankowska, A.M.; Pape, U.J.; Tahiliani, M.; Bandukwala, H.S.; An, J.; Lamperti, E.D.; Koh, K.P.; Ganetzky, R.; Liu, X.S.; Aravind, L.; Agarwal, S.; Maciejewski, J.P. & Rao, A. (2010) Impaired hydroxylation of 5-methylcytosine in myeloid cancers with mutant TET2. *Nature*, Vol. 468, No.7325, (December 2010), pp. 839-43.

Lamandin, C.; Sagot, C.; Roumier, C.; Lepelley, P.; De Botton, S.; Cosson, A.; Fenaux, P. & Preudhomme, C. (2002) Are PU.1 mutations frequent genetic events in acute myeloid leukemia (AML)? *Blood*, Vol. 100, No.13, (December 2002), pp. 4680-1.

Lazarides, E. (1982) Intermediate filaments: a chemically heterogeneous, developmentally regulated class of proteins. *Annu Rev Biochem*, Vol. 51, (July 1982), pp. 219-50.

Leddin, M.; Perrod, C.; Hoogenkamp, M.; Ghani, S.; Assi, S.; Heinz, S.; Wilson, N.K.; Follows, G.; Schonheit, J.; Vockentanz, L.; Mosammam, A.M.; Chen, W.; Tenen, D.G.; Westhead, D.R.; Gottgens, B.; Bonifer, C. & Rosenbauer, F. (2011) Two distinct auto-regulatory loops operate at the PU.1 locus in B cells and myeloid cells. *Blood*, Vol. 117, No.10, (March 2011), pp. 2827-38.

Ley, T.J.; Ding, L.; Walter, M.J.; McLellan, M.D.; Lamprecht, T.; Larson, D.E.; Kandoth, C.; Payton, J.E.; Baty, J.; Welch, J.; Harris, C.C.; Lichti, C.F.; Townsend, R.R.; Fulton, R.S.; Dooling, D.J.; Koboldt, D.C.; Schmidt, H.; Zhang, Q.; Osborne, J.R.; Lin, L.; O'Laughlin, M.; McMichael, J.F.; Delehaunty, K.D.; McGrath, S.D.; Fulton, L.A.; Magrini, V.J.; Vickery, T.L.; Hundal, J.; Cook, L.L.; Conyers, J.J.; Swift, G.W.; Reed, J.P.; Alldredge, P.A.; Wylie, T.; Walker, J.; Kalicki, J.; Watson, M.A.; Heath, S.; Shannon, W.D.; Varghese, N.; Nagarajan, R.; Westervelt, P.; Tomasson, M.H.; Link, D.C.; Graubert, T.A.; Dipersio, J.F.; Mardis, E.R. & Wilson, R.K. (2010) DNMT3A Mutations in Acute Myeloid Leukemia. *N Engl J Med*, Vol.363, No.25, (November 2010), pp.2424-2433.

Li, S.L.; Valente, A.J.; Zhao, S.J. & Clark, R.A. (1997) PU.1 is essential for p47(phox) promoter activity in myeloid cells. *J Biol Chem*, Vol. 272, No.28, (July 1997), pp. 17802-9.

Li, X.; Vradii, D.; Gutierrez, S.; Lian, J.B.; van Wijnen, A.J.; Stein, J.L.; Stein, G.S. & Javed, A. (2005) Subnuclear targeting of Runx1 is required for synergistic activation of the myeloid specific M-CSF receptor promoter by PU.1. *J Cell Biochem*, Vol. 96, No.4, (November 2005), pp. 795-809.

Li, Y.; Okuno, Y.; Zhang, P.; Radomska, H.S.; Chen, H.; Iwasaki, H.; Akashi, K.; Klemsz, M.J.; McKercher, S.R.; Maki, R.A. & Tenen, D.G. (2001) Regulation of the PU.1 gene by distal elements. *Blood*, Vol. 98, No.10, (November 2001), pp. 2958-65.

Lloberas, J.; Soler, C. & Celada, A. (1999) The key role of PU.1/SPI-1 in B cells, myeloid cells and macrophages. Immunol Today, Vol. 20, No.4, (April 1999), pp. 184-9.

Lodie, T.A.; Savedra, R., Jr.; Golenbock, D.T.; Van Beveren, C.P.; Maki, R.A. & Fenton, M.J. (1997) Stimulation of macrophages by lipopolysaccharide alters the phosphorylation state, conformation, and function of PU.1 via activation of casein kinase II. *J Immunol*, Vol. 158, No.4, (February 1997), pp. 1848-56.

Lopez-Rodriguez, C. & Corbi, A.L. (1997) PU.1 negatively regulates the CD11c integrin gene promoter through recognition of the major transcriptional start site. *Eur J Immunol*, Vol. 27, No.8, (August 1997), pp. 1843-7.

McKercher, S.R.; Torbett, B.E.; Anderson, K.L.; Henkel, G.W.; Vestal, D.J.; Baribault, H.; Klemsz, M.; Feeney, A.J.; Wu, G.E.; Paige, C.J. & Maki, R.A. (1996) Targeted disruption of the PU.1 gene results in multiple hematopoietic abnormalities. *Embo J*, Vol. 15, No.20, (October 1996), pp. 5647-58.

Metcalf, D.; Dakic, A.; Mifsud, S.; Di Rago, L.; Wu, L. & Nutt, S. (2006) Inactivation of PU.1 in adult mice leads to the development of myeloid leukemia. *Proc Natl Acad Sci U S A*, Vol. 103, No.5, (January 2006), pp. 1486-91.

Moreau-Gachelin, F.; Tavitian, A. & Tambourin, P. (1988) Spi-1 is a putative oncogene in virally induced murine erythroleukaemias. *Nature*, Vol. 331, No.6153, (January 1988), pp. 277-80.

Mueller, B.U.; Pabst, T.; Osato, M.; Asou, N.; Johansen, L.M.; Minden, M.D.; Behre, G.; Hiddemann, W.; Ito, Y. & Tenen, D.G. (2002) Heterozygous PU.1 mutations are associated with acute myeloid leukemia. *Blood*, Vol. 100, No.3, (August 2002), pp. 998-1007.

Mueller, B.U.; Pabst, T.; Osato, M.; Asou, N.; Johansen, L.M.; Minden, M.D.; Behre, G.; Hiddemann, W.; Ito, Y. & Tenen, D.G. (2003) Heterozygous PU.1 mutations are associated with acute myeloid leukemia. *Blood*, Vol. 101, No.5, (March 2003), pp. 2074.

Nagulapalli, S.; Pongubala, J.M. & Atchison, M.L. (1995) Multiple proteins physically interact with PU.1. Transcriptional synergy with NF-IL6 beta (C/EBP delta, CRP3). *J Immunol*, Vol. 155, No.9, November 1995, pp. 4330-8.

Nakano, N.; Nishiyama, C.; Masuoka, N.; Nishiyama, M.; Yamane, H.; Okumura, K. & Ogawa, H. (2005) Analysis of PU.1/ICSBP (IRF-8) complex formation with various PU.1 mutants: molecular cloning of rat Icsbp (Irf-8) cDNA. *Immunogenetics*, Vol. 56, No.12, (March 2005), pp. 871-7.

Nerlov, C.; Querfurth, E.; Kulessa, H. & Graf, T. (2000) GATA-1 interacts with the myeloid PU.1 transcription factor and represses PU.1-dependent transcription. *Blood*, Vol. 95, No.8, (April 2000), pp. 2543-51.

Nuchprayoon, I.; Shang, J.; Simkevich, C.P.; Luo, M.; Rosmarin, A.G. & Friedman, A.D. (1999) An enhancer located between the neutrophil elastase and proteinase 3 promoters is activated by Sp1 and an Ets factor. *J Biol Chem*, Vol. 274, No.2, (January 1999), pp. 1085-91.

Oelgeschlager, M.; Nuchprayoon, I.; Luscher, B. & Friedman, A.D. (1996) C/EBP, c-Myb, and PU.1 cooperate to regulate the neutrophil elastase promoter. *Mol Cell Biol*, Vol. 16, No.9, (September 1996), pp. 4717-25.

Oikawa, T. & Yamada, T. (2003) Molecular biology of the Ets family of transcription factors. *Gene*, Vol. 303, (January 2003), pp. 11-34.

Oikawa, T.; Yamada, T.; Kihara-Negishi, F.; Yamamoto, H.; Kondoh, N.; Hitomi, Y. & Hashimoto, Y. (1999) The role of Ets family transcription factor PU.1 in hematopoietic cell differentiation, proliferation and apoptosis. *Cell Death Differ*, Vol. 6, No.7, (July 1999), pp. 599-608.

Olson, M.C.; Scott, E.W.; Hack, A.A.; Su, G.H.; Tenen, D.G.; Singh, H. & Simon, M.C. (1995) PU. 1 is not essential for early myeloid gene expression but is required for terminal myeloid differentiation. *Immunity*, Vol. 3, No.6, (December 1995), pp. 703-14.

Ozeki, K.; Kiyoi, H.; Hirose, Y.; Iwai, M.; Ninomiya, M.; Kodera, Y.; Miyawaki, S.; Kuriyama, K.; Shimazaki, C.; Akiyama, H.; Nishimura, M.; Motoji, T.; Shinagawa, K.; Takeshita, A.; Ueda, R.; Ohno, R.; Emi, N. & Naoe, T. (2004) Biologic and clinical significance of the FLT3 transcript level in acute myeloid leukemia. *Blood*, Vol. 103, No.5, (March 2004), pp. 1901-8.

Petrovick, M.S.; Hiebert, S.W.; Friedman, A.D.; Hetherington, C.J.; Tenen, D.G. & Zhang, D.E. (1998) Multiple functional domains of AML1: PU.1 and C/EBPalpha synergize with different regions of AML1. *Mol Cell Biol*, Vol. 18, No.7, (July 1998), pp. 3915-25.

Pollock, J.L.; Westervelt, P.; Kurichety, A.K.; Pelicci, P.G.; Grisolano, J.L. & Ley, T.J. (1999) A bcr-3 isoform of RARalpha-PML potentiates the development of PML-RARalpha-driven acute promyelocytic leukemia. *Proc Natl Acad Sci U S A*, Vol. 96, No.26, (December 1999), pp. 15103-8.

Prieto, J.; Eklund, A. & Patarroyo, M. (1994) Regulated expression of integrins and other adhesion molecules during differentiation of monocytes into macrophages. *Cell* Immunol, Vol. 156, No.1, (June 1994), pp. 191-211.

Pugh, B.F. (1996) Mechanisms of transcription complex assembly. *Curr Opin Cell Biol*, Vol. 8, No.3, (June 1996), pp. 303-11.

Rosenbauer, F.; Wagner, K.; Kutok, J.L.; Iwasaki, H.; Le Beau, M.M.; Okuno, Y.; Akashi, K.; Fiering, S. & Tenen, D.G. (2004) Acute myeloid leukemia induced by graded reduction of a lineage-specific transcription factor, PU.1. *Nat Genet*, Vol. 36, No.6, (June 2004), pp. 624-30.

Rosmarin, A.G.; Caprio, D.; Levy, R. & Simkevich, C. (1995) CD18 (beta 2 leukocyte integrin) promoter requires PU.1 transcription factor for myeloid activity. *Proc Natl Acad Sci U S A*, Vol. 92, No.3, (January 1995), pp. 801-5.

Scott, E.W.; Simon, M.C.; Anastasi, J. & Singh, H. (1994) Requirement of transcription factor PU.1 in the development of multiple hematopoietic lineages. *Science*, Vol. 265, No.5178, (September 1994), pp. 1573-7.

Sharrocks, A.D. (2001) The ETS-domain transcription factor family. *Nat Rev Mol Cell Biol*, Vol. 2, No.11, (November 2001), pp. 827-37.

Shimoda, R.; Achanzar, W.E.; Qu, W.; Nagamine, T.; Takagi, H.; Mori, M. & Waalkes, M.P. (2003) Metallothionein is a potential negative regulator of apoptosis. *Toxicol Sci*, Vol. 73, No.2, (June 2003), pp. 294-300.

Silver, A.; Moody, J.; Dunford, R.; Clark, D.; Ganz, S.; Bulman, R.; Bouffler, S.; Finnon, P.; Meijne, E.; Huiskamp, R. & Cox, R. (1999) Molecular mapping of chromosome 2 deletions in murine radiation-induced AML localizes a putative tumor suppressor gene to a 1.0 cM region homologous to human chromosome segment 11p11-12. *Genes Chromosomes Cancer*, Vol. 24, No.2, (February 1999), pp. 95-104.

Smith, L.T.; Hohaus, S.; Gonzalez, D.A.; Dziennis, S.E. & Tenen, D.G. (1996) PU.1 (Spi-1) and C/EBP alpha regulate the granulocyte colony-stimulating factor receptor promoter in myeloid cells. *Blood*, Vol. 88, No.4, (August 1996), pp. 1234-47.

Steidl, U.; Rosenbauer, F.; Verhaak, R.G.; Gu, X.; Ebralidze, A.; Otu, H.H.; Klippel, S.; Steidl, C.; Bruns, I.; Costa, D.B.; Wagner, K.; Aivado, M.; Kobbe, G.; Valk, P.J.; Passegue, E.; Libermann, T.A.; Delwel, R. & Tenen, D.G. (2006) Essential role of Jun family transcription factors in PU.1 knockdown-induced leukemic stem cells. *Nat Genet*, Vol. 38, No.11, (November 2006), pp. 1269-77.

Steidl, U.; Steidl, C.; Ebralidze, A.; Chapuy, B.; Han, H.J.; Will, B.; Rosenbauer, F.; Becker, A.; Wagner, K.; Koschmieder, S.; Kobayashi, S.; Costa, D.B.; Schulz, T.; O'Brien, K.B.; Verhaak, R.G.; Delwel, R.; Haase, D.; Trumper, L.; Krauter, J.; Kohwi-Shigematsu, T.; Griesinger, F. & Tenen, D.G. (2007) A distal single nucleotide polymorphism alters long-range regulation of the PU.1 gene in acute myeloid leukemia. *J Clin Invest*, Vol. 117, No.9, (September 2007), pp. 2611-20.

Sturrock, A.; Franklin, K.F. & Hoidal, J.R. (1996) Human proteinase-3 expression is regulated by PU.1 in conjunction with a cytidine-rich element. *J Biol Chem*, Vol. 271, No.50, (December 1996), pp. 32392-402.

Suraweera, N.; Meijne, E.; Moody, J.; Carvajal-Carmona, L.G.; Yoshida, K.; Pollard, P.; Fitzgibbon, J.; Riches, A.; van Laar, T.; Huiskamp, R.; Rowan, A.; Tomlinson, I.P. & Silver, A. (2005) Mutations of the PU.1 Ets domain are specifically associated with murine radiation-induced, but not human therapy-related, acute myeloid leukaemia. *Oncogene*, Vol. 24, No.22, (May 2005), pp. 3678-83.

Suzuki, M.; Yamada, T.; Kihara-Negishi, F.; Sakurai, T.; Hara, E.; Tenen, D.G.; Hozumi, N. & Oikawa, T. (2006) Site-specific DNA methylation by a complex of PU.1 and Dnmt3a/b. *Oncogene*, Vol. 25, No.17, (April 2006), pp. 2477-88.

Suzuki, M.; Yamada, T.; Kihara-Negishi, F.; Sakurai, T. & Oikawa, T. (2003) Direct association between PU.1 and MeCP2 that recruits mSin3A-HDAC complex for PU.1-mediated transcriptional repression. *Oncogene*, Vol. 22, No.54, (November 2003), pp. 8688-98.

Suzuki, S.; Kumatori, A.; Haagen, I.A.; Fujii, Y.; Sadat, M.A.; Jun, H.L.; Tsuji, Y.; Roos, D. & Nakamura, M. (1998) PU.1 as an essential activator for the expression of gp91(phox) gene in human peripheral neutrophils, monocytes, and B lymphocytes. *Proc Natl Acad Sci U S A*, Vol. 95, No.11, (May 1998), pp. 6085-90.

Takahashi, S. (2011) Downstream molecular pathways of FLT3 in the pathogenesis of acute myeloid leukemia: biology and therapeutic implications. *J Hematol Oncol*, Vol. 4, No. 13, (April 2011), pp.1-10.

Tenen, D.G.; Hromas, R.; Licht, J.D. & Zhang, D.E. (1997) Transcription factors, normal myeloid development, and leukemia. *Blood*, Vol. 90, No.2, (July 1997), pp. 489-519.

Trakhtenbrot, L.; Krauthgamer, R.; Resnitzky, P. & Haran-Ghera, N. (1988) Deletion of chromosome 2 is an early event in the development of radiation-induced myeloid leukemia in SJL/J mice. *Leukemia*, Vol. 2, No.8, (August 1988), pp. 545-50.

Vegesna, V.; Takeuchi, S.; Hofmann, W.K.; Ikezoe, T.; Tavor, S.; Krug, U.; Fermin, A.C.; Heaney, A.; Miller, C.W. & Koeffler, H.P. (2002) C/EBP-beta, C/EBP-delta, PU.1, AML1 genes: mutational analysis in 381 samples of hematopoietic and solid malignancies. *Leuk Res*, Vol. 26, No.5, (May 2002), pp. 451-7.

Vigorito, E.; Perks, K.L.; Abreu-Goodger, C.; Bunting, S.; Xiang, Z.; Kohlhaas, S.; Das, P.P.; Miska, E.A.; Rodriguez, A.; Bradley, A.; Smith, K.G.; Rada, C.; Enright, A.J.; Toellner, K.M.; Maclennan, I.C. & Turner, M. (2007) microRNA-155 regulates the generation of immunoglobulin class-switched plasma cells. *Immunity*, Vol. 27, No.6, (December 2007), pp. 847-59.

Walter, M.J.; Ding, L.; Shen, D.; Shao, J.; Grillot, M.; McLellan, M.; Fulton, R.; Schmidt, H.; Kalicki-Veizer, J.; O'Laughlin, M.; Kandoth, C.; Baty, J.; Westervelt, P.; Dipersio, J.F.; Mardis, E.R.; Wilson, R.K.; Ley, T.J. & Graubert, T.A. (2011) Recurrent DNMT3A mutations in patients with myelodysplastic syndromes. *Leukemia*, Mar18 [Epub ahead of print].

Walter, M.J.; Park, J.S.; Lau, S.K.; Li, X.; Lane, A.A.; Nagarajan, R.; Shannon, W.D. & Ley, T.J. (2004) Expression profiling of murine acute promyelocytic leukemia cells reveals multiple model-dependent progression signatures. *Mol Cell Biol*, Vol. 24, No.24, (December 2004), pp. 10882-93.

Wang, J.M.; Lai, M.Z. & Yang-Yen, H.F. (2003) Interleukin-3 stimulation of mcl-1 gene transcription involves activation of the PU.1 transcription factor through a p38 mitogen-activated protein kinase-dependent pathway. *Mol Cell Biol*, Vol. 23, No.6, (March 2003), pp. 1896-909.

Yamamoto, H.; Kihara-Negishi, F.; Yamada, T.; Hashimoto, Y. & Oikawa, T. (1999) Physical and functional interactions between the transcription factor PU.1 and the coactivator CBP. *Oncogene*, Vol. 18, No.7, (February 1999), pp. 1495-501.

Yamanaka, R.; Barlow, C.; Lekstrom-Himes, J.; Castilla, L.H.; Liu, P.P.; Eckhaus, M.; Decker, T.; Wynshaw-Boris, A. & Xanthopoulos, K.G. (1997) Impaired granulopoiesis, myelodysplasia, and early lethality in CCAAT/enhancer binding protein epsilon-deficient mice. *Proc Natl Acad Sci U S A*, Vol. 94, No.24, (November 1997), pp. 13187-92.

Yan, X.J.; Xu, J.; Gu, Z.H.; Pan, C.M.; Lu, G.; Shen, Y.; Shi, J.Y.; Zhu, Y.M.; Tang, L.; Zhang, X.W.; Liang, W.X.; Mi, J.Q.; Song, H.D.; Li, K.Q.; Chen, Z. & Chen, S.J. (2011) Exome sequencing identifies somatic mutations of DNA methyltransferase gene DNMT3A in acute monocytic leukemia. *Nat Genet*, Vol. 43, No.4, (March 2011), pp. 309-15.

Yordy, J.S. & Muise-Helmericks, R.C. (2000) Signal transduction and the Ets family of transcription factors. *Oncogene*, Vol. 19, No.55, (December 2000), pp. 6503-13.

Zarnegar, M.A.; Chen, J. & Rothenberg, E.V. (2010) Cell-type-specific activation and repression of PU.1 by a complex of discrete, functionally specialized cis-regulatory elements. *Mol Cell Biol*, Vol. 30, No.20, (October 2010), pp. 4922-39.

Zhang, D.E.; Hetherington, C.J.; Chen, H.M. & Tenen, D.G. (1994) The macrophage transcription factor PU.1 directs tissue-specific expression of the macrophage colony-stimulating factor receptor. *Mol Cell Biol*, Vol. 14, No.1, (January 1994), pp. 373-81.

Zhang, P.; Behre, G.; Pan, J.; Iwama, A.; Wara-Aswapati, N.; Radomska, H.S.; Auron, P.E.; Tenen, D.G. & Sun, Z. (1999) Negative cross-talk between hematopoietic regulators:

GATA proteins repress PU.1. *Proc Natl Acad Sci U S A*, Vol. 96, No.15, (July 1999), pp. 8705-10.

Zimonjic, D.B.; Pollock, J.L.; Westervelt, P.; Popescu, N.C. & Ley, T.J. (2000) Acquired, nonrandom chromosomal abnormalities associated with the development of acute promyelocytic leukemia in transgenic mice. *Proc Natl Acad Sci U S A*, Vol. 97, No.24, (November 2000), pp. 13306-11.

14

Vav1: A Key Player in Agonist-Induced Differentiation of Promyelocytes from Acute Myeloid Leukemia (APL)

Valeria Bertagnolo, Federica Brugnoli and Silvano Capitani
University of Ferrara, Section of Human Anatomy,
Department of Morphology and Embryology,
Italy

1. Introduction

Acute promyelocytic leukemia (APL) is the M3 subtype of acute myeloid leukemia (AML), characterized by aberrant hyperproliferation of progenitors originally committed to terminal differentiation into granulocytes but blocked at the promyelocytic stage. Although clinical studies have introduced treatments employing arsenic trioxide, anthracyclines and anti-CD33 monoclonal antibodies, all-*trans* retinoic acid (ATRA)-based therapy represents, until today, the standard cure of APL patients (Lo-Coco & Ammatuna, 2006; Tallman, 2007). ATRA treatment of APL constitutes, at present, the only example of successful differentiation therapy of a human cancer, in which tumor cells are induced to complete their maturation to neutrophils. Studies on both APL blasts and APL-derived cell lines have elucidated that ATRA acts throughout a complex network that includes the degradation of the PML/RARα fusion protein and the activation of RARα-mediated gene transcription (Breitman et al., 1980; Lanotte et al., 1991; Yang et al., 2003). In addition, it has been reported that ATRA- and phorbol 12-myristate 13-acetate (PMA)-mediated differentiation of human myeloid leukemia cell lines results in changes of their sensitivity to chemotherapeutic drugs, suggesting that advantages in the cure of APL and other malignancies could be obtained by combining differentiating agents and conventional anticancer drugs (Jasek et al., 2008; Kogan, 2009; Nasr et al., 2008).

Even if the mechanism by which ATRA interacts with its receptor located on specific DNA sequences is well known, the events mediated by the ATRA target genes, able to elicit the integrated signaling networks that promote maturation of tumoral promyelocytes, have not been fully clarified and are currently under study to also identify specific molecular targets for new therapies of APL.

One of the proteins up-regulated by ATRA in APL-derived cells and that resulted chiefly involved in the maturation program of tumoral promyelocytes is Vav1, the sole member of the Vav family of proteins physiologically expressed only in haematopoietic cells, where it works as an important signal transducer in immune response (Katzav, 2009; Tybulewicz, 2005). Relevant insights into the function of Vav1 in hematopoietic cells have been provided by studies with knockout mice, demonstrating that the targeted down-modulation of Vav1 compromises maturation of both lymphoid and myeloid cells (Zhang et al., 1994). In particular, a severe impairment of IL-2 production and calcium mobilization in response to external stimuli has been found in T and B cells (Fujikawa et al., 2003; Haubert & Weckbecker, 2010) and the defective motility observed in the Vav1$^{-/-}$ neutrophils, concomitant with the decrease in migration, has been demonstrated to reduce the capacity for an innate immune response (Phillipson et al., 2009). Vav1 has a critical role also in regulating the acquisition by macrophages of maturation-related competence, as demonstrated by the smaller adhesive area, the reduced motility and the lower migration speed of macrophages from Vav1-deficient mice (Hall et al., 2006; Wells et al., 2005). More recently, Vav1 activity has been demonstrated to be required specifically for SDF1α-dependent perivascular homing and subsequent engraftment of hematopoietic stem cells (Sanchez-Aguilera et al., 2011). In both lymphoid and myeloid cells, Vav1 is involved in the dynamic regulation of the filamentous actin cytoskeleton, critical to numerous physical cellular processes, including adhesion, migration and phagocytosis (Cougoule et al., 2006; Stricker et al., 2010).

Vav1 contains an array of structural motifs that enable it to play a role in several distinct cell functions, like cytoskeletal reorganization and regulation of gene expression during proliferation, maturation, and apoptosis of hematopoietic cells (Clevenger et al., 1995; Fischer et al., 1998; Kong et al., 1998). The Vav1 domains include a DH region which exhibits a GDP/GTP exchange activity for the RhoA, Rac1 and CDC42 small GTPases, a PH domain interacting with phosphoinositides, two SH3 domains and one SH2 domain mediating protein-protein interactions, a CH domain that functions as an actin-binding motif and an AC region that contains 3 regulatory tyrosines. Vav1 also possesses 2 putative nuclear localization signals, indicative for a role of the protein also inside the nuclear compartment (Bustelo, 2001).

In both myeloid and lymphoid cells, the best known function of Vav proteins is the guanosine exchange factor (GEF) for small G proteins which is modulated, at variance with the other exchange factors for Rho/Rac in humans, by phosphorylation on tyrosine residues (Bustelo, 2002). However, some functions of Vav1 in hematopoietic cells are independent of its GEF activity and are attributed to its ability to interact with a number of signalling molecules, in both cytoplasm and nucleus. In particular, inside the nuclear compartment Vav1 seems to play its most intriguing role as part of transcriptionally active complexes (Houlard et al., 2002) and by interacting with components of the DNA-dependent protein kinase complex as well as with hnRNP proteins (Romero et al., 1996, 1998).

In addition to the role played in the acquisition of a mature phenotype by normal hematopoietic cells, Vav1 has been found to promote the agonist-induced completion of the differentiation program of tumoral myeloid precursors. In cell lines derived from APL patiens treated with differentiating agents Vav1 plays indeed multiple roles aimed to regulate different aspects of maturation along the neutrophilic and the monocytic/macrophagic lineages. Since Vav1 may be recruited by various differentiating agents and plays a central role in the completion of the differentiation program of leukemic promyelocytes along diverse hematopoietic lineages, it might be considered a common target for developing new therapeutic strategies for the different subtypes of myeloid leukemias.

2. Vav1 and netrophil-like phenotypical maturation

Promyelocytes derived from APL, which are blocked at different steps of their neutrophil differentiation, contain levels of Vav1 variably lower than those found in mature

neutrophils. Treatments with differentiating doses of ATRA induce a significant increase of Vav1 expression in primary blasts obtained from the bone marrow of APL patients as well as in the APL-derived cell lines HL-60 and NB4. A similar increase of Vav1 is observed when normal CD34+ hematopoietic progenitors are treated with a cytokine cocktail promoting granulocytic differentiation, clearly indicating that an adequate expression of Vav1 has to be achieved along with neutrophil maturation of both normal precursors and poorly differentiated neoplastic cells (Bertagnolo et al., 2005). These evidence, obtained in a variety of normal and neoplastic cells under different experimental conditions, ascribe to Vav1 the potential role of a ubiquitous key player in the path leading myeloid precursors to acquire the mature phenotype of differentiated neutrophils.
The issue of whether the increase of Vav1 observed in differentiation of tumoral promyelocytes is merely designed to the function of the protein in mature cells or, more intriguingly, it is functionally relevant to the maturation mechanism, has been addressed by studies in which the expression of Vav1 was forcedly modulated. The experiments have been performed in ATRA treated HL-60 and NB4 cells, which are blocked at different levels of granulocytic differentiation, and thus constitute models well suited to better understand the role of Vav1 in the maturation process. As a consequence of Vav1 over-expression during ATRA treatment of both cell lines, the expression of the myeloid surface marker CD11b increases, indicating that Vav1 supports the role of ATRA in regulating the maturation process. On the other hand, the sole over-expression of Vav1 is capable to significantly induce the expression of CD11b only in HL-60 cells, that, compared to NB4 cells, are blocked to a less differentiated stage (Bertagnolo et al., 2005). This suggests the existence of a direct and ATRA-independent role of Vav1 in regulating the expression of CD11b, at least in cells that are blocked at early stages of the neutrophilic maturation.
Neutrophils radically change in shape during development and functional life (Sanchez & Wangh, 1999). Accordingly, profound rearrangements of the cell morphology take place throughout differentiation of myeloid precursors along the granulocytic lineage, and the nucleus is the cell compartment that undergoes the biggest architectural changes by a mechanism still largely unknown. Modifications of the nuclear shape constitute one of the markers of neutrophil maturation of tumoral promyelocytes and are particularly evident after treatment with ATRA of HL-60 cells, according to the notion that this cell type is blocked at an early stage of maturation. On the other hand, the sole over-expression of Vav1 is unable to induce nuclear modifications in both HL-60 and NB4 cells, indicating that other ATRA-induced events are required to regulate the maturation-related rearrangements of cell morphology (Bertagnolo et al, 2005).
The use of siRNAs specific for Vav1 unequivocally demonstrates that Vav1 is not dispensable for the progression of tumoral promyelocytes along the granulocytic lineage. In fact, the down-modulation of Vav1 expression during ATRA treatment of both HL-60 and NB4 cells counteracts the agonist-induced increase of CD11b expression and prevents the maturation-related modifications of cell/nucleus morphology, definitely assigning to Vav1 a crucial role in regulating phenotypical maturation of APL-derived cells (Bertagnolo et al, 2005, 2008).

2.1 Tyrosine phosphorylation of Vav1

In parallel with the increase of Vav1 expression, ATRA treatment of HL-60 and NB4 cells also induces Vav1 tyrosine phosphorylation. Since, in the whole cell, the rise of the phosphosphorylation level is almost proportional to the increase in total Vav1 amount, ATRA seems to ensure to differentiating cells the achievement of an adequate amount of tyrosine phosphorylated Vav1, according with the functions of Vav1 in mature neutrophils. On the other hand, the accumulation of tyrosine-phosphorylated Vav1 inside the nuclear compartment seems to be a distinctive feature of the differentiation process induced by ATRA in APL-derived cells (Bertagnolo et al., 2005). In fact, a progressive increase of tyrosine phosphorylated Vav1 inside the nucleus accompanies the agonist-induced maturation (Bertagnolo et al., 1998), indicative of a specific role of tyrosine phosphorylated Vav1 inside the nuclear compartment. The tyrosine phosphorylation level of nuclear Vav1 reaches a maximum in ATRA-treated NB4 cells, which constitute the cell model with the most advanced level of neutrophil maturation among APL-derived precursors (Bertagnolo et al., 2005), clearly correlating tyrosine phosphorylated Vav1 with the maturation-related events that occur inside the nuclear compartment and opening the question of which kinase/s is/are involved in this process.

In both myeloid and lymphoid cells, Vav1 is phosphorylated in tyrosine/s by receptors with intrinsic tyrosine kinase activity or by membrane and/or cytoplasmic tyrosine kinases of the Syk/Zap70, Src and Jak families (Bustelo, 2002). More recently, also the c-Abl kinase has been reported to be specifically involved in regulating the activity of Vav1 in integrin-mediated neutrophil adhesion (Cui et al., 2009). Recruitment and phosphorylation of Vav1 depend on its ability to interact with a number of signalling proteins by means of its various domains. In particular, the interaction between the SH2 domain of Vav1 and phosphorylated proteins is thought to serve for recruitment of activated kinases, which in turn can phosphorylate Vav1 (Bustelo, 2002). The Syk/ZAP-70 family of tyrosine kinases constitutes an example of proteins that contain two SH2 domains, a tandem sequence that might confer high specificity in tyrosine kinase- mediated signalling. In addition, both ZAP-70 and Syk contain a consensus binding sequence for the Vav1 SH2 domain that seems to be critical for antigen receptor-mediated signal transduction (Ottinger et al., 1998).

Experiments performed with HL-60 cells have demonstrated the association of tyrosine phosphorylated Syk with the Vav1-SH2 domain, in both whole cell and nuclear compartment, as a consequence of ATRA treatment (Bertagnolo et al., 2001). These data are in agreement with the notion that activation of Syk occurs in differentiating HL-60 cells (Qin & Yamamura, 1997) and mature neutrophils, in which it regulates migration (Schymeinsky et al., 2006) and the formation of lamellipodia during phagocytosis (Shi et al., 2006). While in whole HL-60 cells the Vav1/Syk association takes place regardless of their phosphorylation level and of ATRA treatment, the formation of Vav1/Syk complexes inside the nuclear compartment strongly increases during the differentiation process, suggesting a specific role for this tyrosine kinase in the nucleus. The role of Syk in phosphorylating Vav1 has been demonstrated by means of *in vitro* assays (Bertagnolo et al., 2001) and confirmed by the use of a pharmacological model of Syk inhibition, in which both HL-60 and NB4 cells were treated with Piceatannol (Bertagnolo et al., 2001, 2008), a tyrosine kinase inhibitor with a reported selectivity for Syk (Law et al, 1999; Seow et al., 2002).

The Syk-dependent tyrosine phosphorylation of Vav1 during the ATRA-induced phenotypical differentiation is not relevant for the expression of the surface marker CD11b, as indicated by the use of Piceatannol in both HL-60 and NB4 cells, but seems to play a crucial role in regulating the reorganization of cell architecture. In fact, when Piceatannol is administered in combination with ATRA, the modifications of nuclear morphology typical of granulocytic differentiation are almost completely abrogated, similarly to what observed when the expression of Vav1 is down-modulated during the differentiation treatment (Bertagnolo et al., 2008). However, since Piceatannol fails to abrogate completely the ATRA-induced tyrosine phosphorylation of Vav1 in both HL-60 and NB4 cells (Bertagnolo et al., 2008), other kinase/s, in addition to Syk, are probably recruited by ATRA in these cell models.

The results from these inhibition studies support the hypothesized action model that requires tyrosine phosphorylated Vav1 in maturation of tumoral myeloid precursors. Nevertheless, the issue needs further investigations, in order to identify the kinase/s involved. In fact, by extending the analysis to other tyrosine kinase inhibitors, it has been found that PP1 and AG490, inhibitors of Src and Jak tyrosine kinase families, respectively, did not affect to any significant extent the tyrosine phosphorylation of Vav1 (Bertagnolo et al., 2004), leaving open the question of which other tyrosine kinases, in addition to Syk, phosphorylate Vav1 during maturation of tumoral promyelocytes.

2.1.1 Participation to protein complexes with signaling molecules

In addition to the obvious interaction with tyrosine kinases, the optimal phosphorylation of Vav1 seems to require the association with adaptor molecules that facilitate the spatial proximity between Vav1 and the upstream kinases. These associations also depend on the tyrosine phosphorylation of the involved proteins and often require the engagement of either the SH3 or the SH2 domains of Vav1 as interacting motifs (Bustelo, 2002). In this context, SLP-76, an adaptor protein predominantly expressed in T cells and myeloid cells and which is a substrate for ZAP-70 and Syk tyrosine kinases, has been reported to associate, via tyrosine-phosphorylated residues in its NH2-terminal domain, with the SH2 domain of Vav1 after ligation of the T-cell antigen receptor (Tuosto et al., 1996; Pauker & Barda-Saad,, 2011). SLP-76 was also described as an important adaptor molecule that is regulated by Syk in C-reactive protein-stimulated platelets (Gross et. al, 1999) and that plays a critical role in FcRI-mediated activation of mast cells *in vivo* and *in vitro* (Pivniouk et al., 1999).

Some of the Vav1-interacting molecules play a role in down modulation of Vav1 signals. A potential negative regulator of Vav1 is Cbl, which down-modulates Syk/ZAP-70 and other protein tyrosine kinases (Lupher et al., 1999). Cbl associates with Vav1 upon T-cell receptor stimulation of primary murine lymphocytes and Jurkat T cells. This interaction appears to require the whole SH3-SH2-SH3 COOH-terminal domain of Vav1 and a proline-rich sequence of Cbl and seems to inhibit the Vav1-dependent signal transduction (Bustelo et al., 1997). Very recently, Chiang & Hodes (2011) have demonstrated a role of Cbl in repressing signaling events that can mediate thymic differentiation in the absence of Vav1, since Cbl inactivation rescued defective T cell development in Vav1-/- mice.

The molecules involved in the recruitment and phosphorylation of Vav1 during the ATRA-dependent granulocytic differentiation of tumoral promyelocytes were investigated in HL-60 cells by using GST-fusion NH2-terminal and COOH-terminal Vav1-SH3 and GST-fusion Vav1-SH3-SH2-SH3 proteins. One of the proteins interacting with Vav1 in HL-60 cells is the adaptor molecule Cbl, present only in the cytoplasm and strongly phosphorylated in response to ATRA treatment. The Vav1/Cbl interaction in HL-60 cells occurs also in control conditions and requires the entire SH3-SH2-SH3 domain of Vav1 (Bertagnolo et al., 2001).

The adaptor protein SLP-76 has been also identified as a phosphorylated protein interacting with the SH3-SH2-SH3 fragment of Vav1 in both cells and nuclei of HL-60 after ATRA treatment. Similarly to Cbl, SLP-76 associates with Vav1 also in control conditions, without quantitative changes due to the differentiation process. Vav1-associated SLP-76 was more abundant in nuclei than in whole cell lysates, indicating a preferential association into the nucleus of these two molecules, in contrast with an exclusive cytoplasmic distribution of Vav1/Cbl complexes (Bertagnolo et al., 2001).

The interaction of Vav1 with Cbl and SLP-76 in HL-60 cells may be correlated to the transmembrane signaling mediated by CD38, an early biomarker of ATRA-induced differentiation in the HL-60 cell line, in which it may play a causal role in myeloid differentiation (Lamkin et al., 2006). A correlation between Vav1 and CD38-activated signaling has been recently demonstrated by experiments in which the expression of a cytosolic deletion mutant of CD38 caused failure to up-regulate ATRA-induced proteins such as CD11b, Vav1 and Fgr, this latter able to phosphorylate Vav1 after ATRA treatment of HL-60 cells (Congleton et al., 2011).

Exclusive of the ATRA treatment of HL-60 seems to be the compartmentalized association between Vav1 and interacting proteins during ATRA treatment, since Cbl/Vav1 complexes are located in the cytoplasm while SLP-76/Vav1 complexes reside in the inner nuclear compartment. This suggests that Vav1 is recruited by one or more signal transduction cascades, starting from cell membrane and directed to the nucleus and involving the two adaptor proteins Cbl and SLP-76, which may then discretely regulate the amount of Vav1 in the cytoplasmic and nuclear compartments (Fig. 1).

The Vav1-associated protein complexes identified in HL-60 cells also contain the tyrosine kinase Syk. In particular, Vav1/Cbl/Syk complexes have been found in cytoplasm whereas Vav1/SLP-76/Syk complexes have been demonstrated inside the nuclear compartment. These associations are present in control conditions and result strongly increased after ATRA treatment (Bertagnolo et al., 2001). This suggests that, during the maturation of APL-derived myeloid precursors, a sequence of signals originated from membrane receptors and directed to the nuclear compartment is ended to regulate the amount of tyrosine phosphorylated Vav1 inside the nucleus (Fig. 1) and that this pathway may involve the negative regulation of Cbl on Vav1 activity.

In both cells and nuclei of HL-60 cells, other signalling molecules associate with Vav1 as a consequence of ATRA treatment. They include the γ1 isoform of PI-PLC and the p85 regulatory subunit of PI3K. In particular, ATRA treatment increases the binding of tyrosine-phosphorylated Vav1 to both N-terminal and C-terminal SH2 domains of p85 (Bertagnolo et al., 1998). Since Vav1 is the only member of the Vav1/PLC-γ1/PI3K complex to possess a nuclear localization sequence (Bustelo, 2001), it is conceivable that Vav1 is directly involved in regulating the amount of PLC-γ1 and PI3K inside the nuclear compartment.

2.1.2 Phosphorylation of Vav1 on Tyr745

Vav1 contains 31 tyrosine residues whose phosphorylation was originally investigated almost exclusively in relation to the function of Vav1 as a GEF. A crucial role in this context seems to be played by Tyr174 in both lymphoid and myeloid cells, even if other mechanisms have emerged in the last few years as regulators of Vav1 GEF activity, and recent data suggest that Tyr174 is coversely involved in roles of Vav1 not mediated by GEF activity (Katzav, 2009). In addition to Tyr174, other conserved residues, Tyr142 and Tyr160, have been described to be phosphorylated in activated Vav1. It has also been suggested that phosphorylation of the tyrosines located inside the acidic region of Vav1 may allow Tyr142, Tyr160, and Tyr174 to become docking sites for kinases, which can then phosphorylate additional tyrosine residues in Vav proteins (Miletic et al., 2006; Yu et al., 2010). Recently, several of the tyrosine residues at the carboxyl terminus of Vav1 have been shown to be phosphorylated in cancer cells, raising the possibility that also these tyrosine residues play an important role in Vav1 function (Lazer et al., 2010).

The residue Tyr174, phosphorylated by members of Syk/Zap70 and Src tyrosine kinase families, plays a central role in regulating GEF activity of Vav1 in mature neutrophils, including β2 integrin-mediated neutrophil migration *in vitro* and neutrophil recruitment during the inflammatory response *in vivo* (Schymeinsky et al., 2006). In APL-derived cells, ATRA induces the phosphorylation of Tyr174 in NB4 but not in HL-60 cells and independently of the activity of Syk (Bertagnolo et al., 2011). Both cytofluorimetrical analysis of CD11b expression and migration assays on NB4 cells over-expressing the Tyr174Phe-mutated Vav1 have ruled out any relevant role for this tyrosine residue in supporting the activity of ATRA in this cell line (Bertagnolo et al., 2010). Since phosphorylation of Tyr174 in neutrophils has been mainly associated to the GEF activity of Vav1 in mature cells, these findings suggest that the ATRA-induced phosphorylation of Tyr174 occurs in parallel with differentiation and may constitute a marker of the acquisition of a mature phenotype. This hypothesis is confirmed by the failure of ATRA in inducing the phosphorylation of Tyr174 in HL-60 cells, that reach indeed only a partially differentiatiated phenotype (Bertagnolo et al., 2011).

Since the phosphorylation of Vav1 on the Tyr174 residue seems unrelated to the path by which tyrosine phosphorylated Vav1 affects the ATRA-induced maturation of APL-derived cells, proteomic studies have been undertaken to identify other tyrosine residues phosphorylated after ATRA treament in both HL-60 and NB4 cells. Mass spectra analysis performed on Vav1 immunoprecipitated from NB4 whole cells identified Tyr745 as an ATRA-induced phosphorylated residue, within a highly conserved Vav1 sequence. The analysis of maturation-related features in differentiating NB4 cells over-expressing the Tyr745Phe-mutated form of Vav1 have clearly shown that phosphorylation of this tyrosine residue is crucial in regulating CD11b expression as well as in promoting the acquisition of migratory capabilities (Bertagnolo et al., 2010). Even if Tyr745 has never been correlated with the known roles of Vav1, multiple sequence alignment analysis of proteins from different species indicates that this is a highly conserved aminoacid, likely involved in physiological roles of Vav1.

Inhibition studies have ruled out the role of Syk in phosphorylating Tyr745 as a consequence of ATRA treatment and, at present, no data are available about the involved tyrosine kinase. This is in part due to the fact that analysis performed with softwares designed to predict cell signaling interactions using short sequence motifs failed to recognize the Tyr745 of Vav1 as a putative phosphorylation site by the known tyrosine kinases. However, some tyrosine residues of Vav1 are not surface exposed and/or may be involved in intramolecular interactions, thereby precluding their tyrosine phosphorylation and impairing their recognition by the data base analysis. Since Tyr745 is located inside a short helix on the SH2 domain of Vav1, its phosphorylation could be an event secondary to phosphorylation of other tyrosine residues, which may induce conformational changes of Vav1 allowing Tyr745 to become accessible to a specific tyrosine kinase.

2.1.3 GEF activity

The best known function of tyrosine phosphorylated Vav1 is a catalytic role as a GEF towards the Rho family of GTPases, in which Tyr174 is crucial. Tyr174 lies within an α-helix and binds directly with the GTPase interaction pocket of the DH domain, blocking access to substrate and inhibiting Vav1 GEF activity. Phosphorylation releases Tyr174 from the binding pocket, relieving the auto-inhibition (Bustelo et al., 2001). The activity of the DH domain is also regulated by the CH domain, as deletion of this domain results in constitutively active GEF activity. It has been suggested that the Vav1 CH domain can bind to the C1 region, occluding the DH domain and blocking access to GTPases. CH–C1 interaction apparently stabilizes the inhibitory Tyr174–DH interaction. In addition, the PH domain regulates Vav1 catalytic activity by interaction with two inositol lipids: phosphatidylinositol 4, 5- bisphosphate (PIP_2) and phosphatidylinositol 3, 4, 5-trisphosphate (PIP_3). Whereas the binding of PIP_3 moderately enhances the in vitro GEF activity of Vav1, binding to PIP_2 has an inhibitory effect. Consistent with this model, Vav1 carrying a single mutation in its PH domain is constitutively active and induces cytoskeleton rearrangements as a consequence of Rac activation. Deletions of C1 domain or mutations that disrupt its structural integrity inhibit Vav1 GEF activity. High resolution X-ray structure of DH–PH–C1 domains suggests that PH and C1 domains contribute to GEF activity by stabilizing the DH domain structure and not through direct contacts with GTPases (Bustelo, 2002).

GEF activity of Vav1 has long been regarded as the key for transferring the signal from activated receptors to the cytoskeleton. Among the molecules constituting the cytoskeleton architecture, actin seems to be a preferred target of the Vav1-dependent GEF activity. Several partners are involved in the pathway by which Vav1 affects actin cytoskeleton. It has been reported that Vav1 is a preferential exchange factor for Rac1, which in turn may activate phosphatidylinositol-4-phosphate (PIP) 5-kinase which phosphorylates PIP to PIP_2. PIP_2 may function as an activator of actin-binding proteins, like talin and vinculin, that attach the cytoskeleton to the cell membrane. Another potential target for the GEF activity of Vav1, Cdc42, may activate the WASP protein, a key mediator of actin polymerization (Hornstein et al., 2004). Finally, Vav1-activated small G proteins play an essential role in regulating actin cytoskeleton dynamics by also interacting with the p21-activated serine-threonine kinase (PAK) family of actin-regulatory enzymes (Daniels & Bokoch, 1999).

In both lymphoid and myeloid cells, like other proteins with a GEF activity, Vav1 mediates a number of cytoskeletal-associated cellular processes, being an essential part of the molecular link connecting activated receptors to the actin cytoskeleton. A consistent number of studies (reviewed in Hornstein et al., 2004) have reported the role of Vav1 in the formation of immunological synapse and in phagocytosis of T cells. In non adherent neutrophils, stimulation of chemoattractant receptors induces a complex sequence of events: actin reorganization, shape changes, development of polarity and reversible adhesion, all culminating in chemotaxis. The complex signaling mechanisms that regulate neutrophil migration are well studied, and Vav1 appears to be a major point of the inhibitory crosstalk between adhesion receptors and cytokine receptors (Gakidis et al., 2004). In particular, the activity of Vav1 as GEF for Rac2 is inhibited in adherent cells, as a possible consequence of the activation by adhesion of one or more tyrosine phosphatases responsible of dephosphorylating Vav1. On the other hand, experiments performed with Vav1-/- mice have demonstrated that motility and mobilization into peripheral blood induced in neutrophils by FMLP are significantly reduced, as well as the generation of filamentous actin (Kim et al., 2003). Studies performed in a rat model have demonstrated that the M-CSF-induced chemotaxis of bone marrow macrophages is initiated by the 3-phosphoinositide-dependent GEF activity of Vav1 on Rac (Vedham et al., 2005).

In APL-derived HL-60 cells, ATRA treatment induces an increase of total GEF activity, not attributable to Vav1, as deduced by *in vitro* assays on Ras/Rac small G proteins performed on Vav1 immunoprecipitated from both whole cells and isolated nuclei (Bertagnolo et al., 2001). This implies that, in this cell model, the Syk-dependent tyrosine phosphorylation of Vav1 is not ended to regulate its GEF activity and that alternative pathways have to be considered to explain the mechanism by which Vav1 affects the organization of cytoskeleton and nucleoskeleton during maturation of tumoral promyelocytes.

2.2 GEF-independent activity of phosphorylated Vav1

2.2.1 Regulation of actin cytoskeleton

In addition to act as a GEF, Vav1 may mediate actin reorganization through other, GEF-independent mechanisms. The presence in its structure of a number of tyrosines and domains potentially involved in protein-protein interactions suggests for Vav1 a role in actin polymerization as an adapter protein that links signaling and cytoskeletal molecules. In T cells, Vav1 binds constitutively Talin and Vinculin, anchoring the actin cytoskeleton to the plasma membrane, and the cytoskeletal protein Zyxin (Hornstein et al., 2004). In the same cell model, a direct link between Vav1 and dynamin 2 (Dyn2), a component of the cytoskeletal regulators, has also been demonstrated (Gomez et al., 2005).

A mechanism by means of which tyrosine-phosphorylated Vav1 regulates cytoskeleton of ATRA-treated tumoral promyelocytes, identified in HL-60 cells, implies the interaction of Vav1 with the p85 regulatory subunit of PI3K. Studies aimed to establish the functional meaning of this interaction have demonstrated that, in maturating myeloid precursors, PI3K activity closely depends on its association with tyrosine phosphorylated Vav1 and that when Vav1/PI3K interaction and/or PI3K activity are abrogated, the phenotypic differentiation of ATRA-treated HL-60 is compromised (Bertagnolo et al., 1999, 2004). These evidence assign to Vav1/PI3K interaction a prominent function in the regulation of cytoskeleton alternative to the described role of 3-phosphoinositides on GEF activity of Vav1 (Han et al., 1998).

Also actin participates in the ATRA-induced protein complexes containing Vav1 and PI3K in HL-60 cells. Remarkably, when the association between Vav1 and PI3K is inhibited, the formation of PI3K/actin complexes is reduced, suggesting that the interaction of PI3K with Vav1 is essential for its association with actin (Bertagnolo et al., 2004). Since the recovery of 3-phosphoinositides is strongly reduced when the Vav1-dependent PI3K/actin interaction is abrogated, it can be concluded that Vav1 regulates the physical contact of PI3K with their cytoskeleton-associated substrates. These observations suggest that in addition to playing a regulatory role in Vav1 activation, PI3K activity may itself be regulated by Vav1.

PI3K is likely to play essential roles in granulocytic differentiation of tumoral myeloid precursors, considering that both down-modulation of its expression and pharmacological inhibition of its activity during ATRA treatment significantly reduce the tendency of HL-60 cells to acquire the differentiated phenotype (Bertagnolo et al., 1999). The response to ATRA and the downstream effects of PI3K observed during the induced differentiation support the notion that PI3K is recruited in the path controling cytoskeleton in mature granulocytes. In fact, PI3K is activated in response to chemotactic factors in murine and human neutrophils (Cicchetti et al., 2002; Niggli & Keller, 1997; Stephens et al., 2002) in which newly produced PIP_3 is involved in determining the localization and possibly the crosslinking/stabilization of actin filaments (Chen et al., 2003; Hannigan et al., 2002; Wang et al., 2002). In vitro experiments have demonstrated that PI3K may affect actin-related modifications of cytoskeleton also by directly affecting PAK kinase activity (Menard & Mattingly, 2004). PI3K has a more general influence on cytoskeleton by determining the amount of the inositol-containing lipids, that have emerged as major players in regulating actin assembly at several levels and with different mechanisms, including the direct interaction with cytoskeletal proteins, such as vinculin and gelsolin (Janmey et al., 1999, Takenawa & Itoh, 2001).

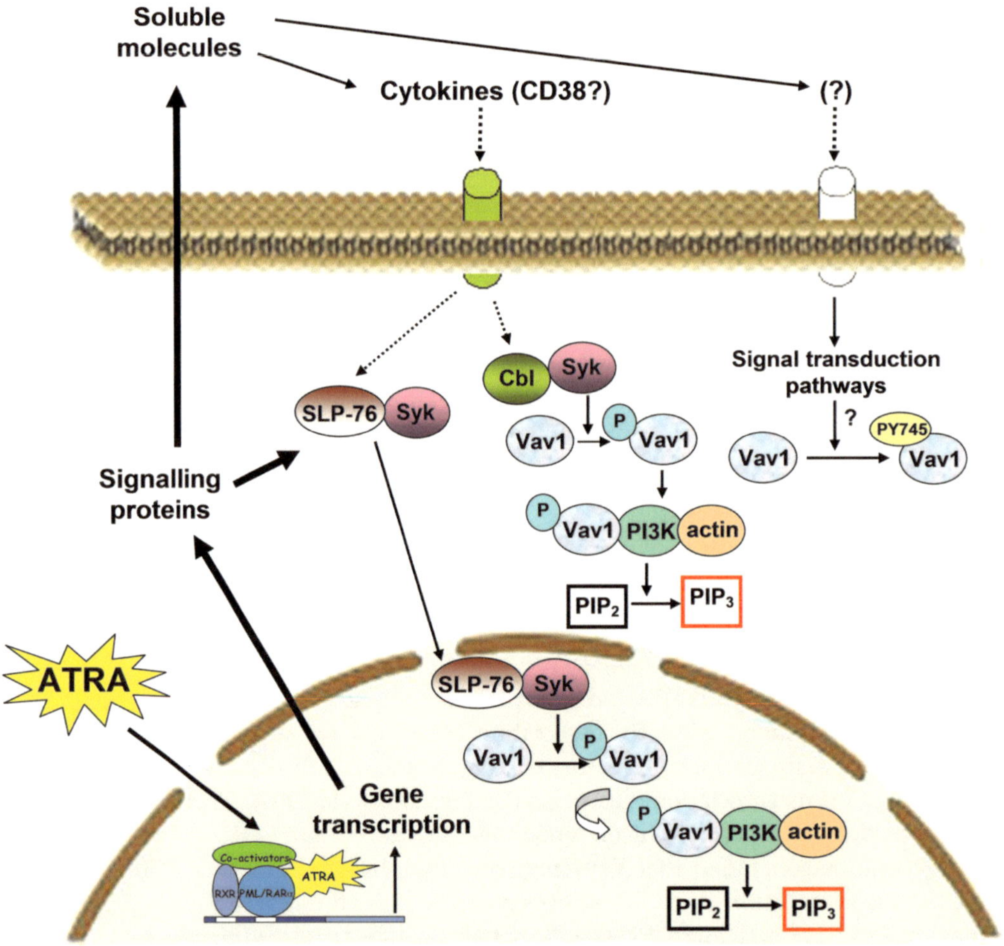

Fig. 1. Schematic representation of the recruitment and phosphorylation of Vav1 in ATRA-treated promyelocytes.

Since, in ATRA-treated promyelocytes, both PI3K activity and the modifications of the nucleus architecture depend on the formation of Vav1/PI3K complexes, Vav1 may be important for targeting PI3K to its nuclear substrates. The association of Vav1 with other lipid modifying enzymes, including specific PI-PLC isoforms (Bertagnolo et al., 1998;), suggests a more general role of Vav1 in determining the composition of the actin-associated phosphoinositide pool and, ultimately, in regulating actin polymerization in differentiating HL-60 cells.

2.2.2 Regulation of gene expression

Microarray analysis performed on APL-derived cell lines has identified several genes whose expression is modified by ATRA treatment, including genes for a number of cytokines, in turn involved in the differentiative program of tumoral promyelocytes (Hsu et al., 1999; Visani et al., 1996). As a consequence of ATRA administration, tyrosine-phosphorylated Vav1 accumulates inside the nuclear compartment of APL-derived cells and becomes involved in the changes of nuclear morphology. Since local reorganization of nuclear architecture is required for both transcription and post-transcriptional events, it is conceivable that Vav1 plays a role in regulating ATRA-related gene expression.
An array analysis performed on HL-60 cells focussed on genes coding for cytokines and cytokine receptors indicates that the inhibition of the Syk-dependent tyrosine-phosphorylation of Vav1 during ATRA treatment prevents the ATRA-induced expression of 8 genes (Bertagnolo et al., 2005). Among them, the thymosin beta-10 (TMSB10) gene has been found, encoding for a small G-actin binding protein that induces depolymerization of intracellular F-actin pools and thus deeply affects actin architecture (Liu et al., 2004; Rho et al., 2004). Tyrosine-phosphorylated Vav1 is also involved in regulating the ATRA-induced expression of the gene for Notch homolog, that codifies for a molecule playing a role in mediating cell fate decisions during hematopoiesis (Ohishi et al., 2003) and whose signaling might be necessary for the proliferation and survival of AML cells, possibly through the maintenance of the expression of c-Myc and Bcl2, as well as the phosphorylation of the Rb protein (Li et al., 2010). The involvement of Vav1 in regulating ATRA-dependent expression of cytokines and/or growth factors has been ascertained by silencing Vav1 during ATRA admistration, further confirming that the increase of Vav1 expression is not an epiphenomenon but constitutes a key event able to actually promote the granulocytic maturation of tumoral myeloid precursors.
The evidence that Vav1 has a role in regulating ATRA-dependent gene expression in APL-derived cells suggests the participation of Vav1 to transcriptional complexes activated by ATRA, also considering that, in both myeloid and lymphoid cells, Vav1 seems to be involved in regulating DNA transcription, by direct interaction with, or as a facilitator of, transcription factors (Katzav, 2004). In particular, Vav1 regulates Nuclear Factor of Activated T-cells (NFAT), Activator Protein-1 (AP-1) and Nuclear Factor κB (NF-κB) in T-cells in response to TCR stimulation, and exerts a specific role in regulating the CREB-dependent gene transcription (Haubert & Weckbecker, 2010; Schneider & Rudd, 2008). Direct evidence for the presence of Vav1 as a component of an active transcriptional complex has been reported by Houlard et al. (2002) demonstrating the participation of Vav1 in complexes with NFAT and NF-kB-like, as facilitator of their transcriptional activity.
In APL-derived cells, nuclear Vav1 associates with PU.1 (Brugnoli et al., 2010), a transcription factor induced by ATRA and able to play a crucial role in the completion of granulocytic differentiation of APL-derived myeloid precursors (Mueller et al., 2006). In particular, the down-modulation of PU.1 by means of specific siRNAs has allowed to establish that, like in other tumoral myeloid precursors (Denkinger et al., 2002), PU.1 regulates the expression of Vav1 induced by ATRA in NB4 cells (Brugnoli et al., 2010).
In AML-derived myeloid precursors, PU.l represents a major determinant of the myeloid expression of CD11b (Kastner & Chan, 2008; Pahl et al., 1993), an integrin receptor whose surface expression increases concurrently with CD11b mRNA levels during myeloid differentiation of APL-derived cell lines (Barber et al., 2008). Chromatin immunoprecipitation (ChIP) experiments performed on NB4 cells treated with ATRA have

demonstrated that PU.1 is recruited to its consensus sequence within the *CD11b* promoter (Brugnoli et al., 2010). Since the over-expression of PU.1 might influence phenotype and restore differentiation of primary myeloid leukemic blasts (Durual et al., 2007), and its silencing counteracts the ATRA ability to induce the expression of the granulocytic marker CD11b (Mueller et al., 2006), PU.1 may be used by ATRA to promote CD11b expression during the late stages of the maturation of APL-derived cells. This is confirmed by *in vitro* experiments demonstrating the formation of PU.1-containing complexes on the *CD11b* promoter (Brugnoli et al., 2010).

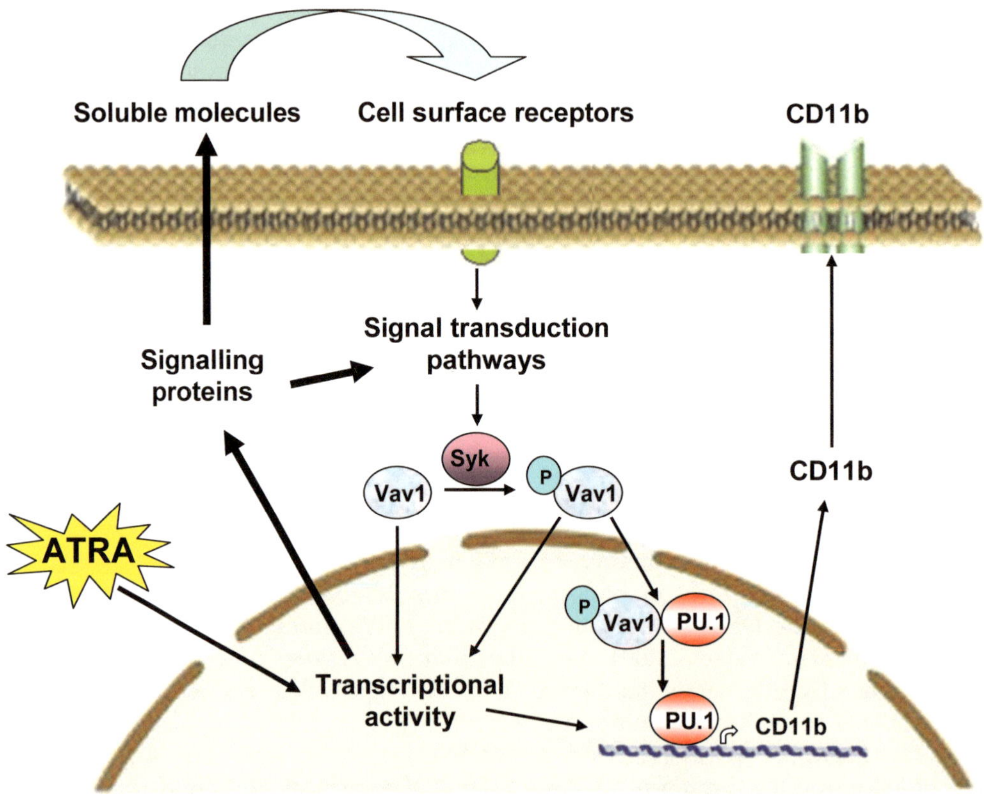

Fig. 2. Schematic representation of the involvement of Vav1 in regulating gene expression in differentiating promyelocytes.

Also Vav1 is recruited to the PU.1 consensus sequence on the *CD11b* promoter in untreated NB4 cells. ATRA treatment, by inducing an increase in Syk-dependent tyrosine phosphorylation of Vav1, displaces this protein from existing molecular complexes on the *CD11b* promoter. Accordingly, the specific inhibition of Syk activity is accompanied by the appearance of a Vav1-containing complex (Brugnoli et al., 2010). The participation of Vav1 to molecular complexes including PU.1 has been ruled out by EMSA experiments. On the other hand, both expression and tyrosine phosphorylation levels of Vav1 seem to play a role in regulating the formation of PU.1-containing complexes. In fact, when the amount of Vav1 is forcedly reduced or its tyrosine phosphorylation is inhibited during the differentiation treatment, the formation of a PU.1-containing complex is negatively affected (Brugnoli et al.,

2010). It is then conceivable that Vav1, and in particular tyrosine-phosphorylated Vav1, regulates the recruitment of PU.1 to its consensus sequence on the *CD11b* promoter region and, possibly, the expression of this surface antigen.

3. Vav1 and protein expression

Proteome analysis currently provides the opportunity to identify global changes in gene expression by directly measuring protein amount. A number of recent studies have used this approach to evaluate protein expression during differentiation/apoptosis induced by different agonists in APL-derived cells. In particular, it has been reported that ATRA modulates the expression level of structural and signal transduction proteins as well as of molecules involved in the different phases of protein synthesis (Dong et al, 2006; Harris et al., 2004; Wan et al., 2001; Wang et al., 2004;).

On the basis of the evidence that inside the nucleus of a number of different cell lines, including APL-derived cells, Vav1 participates to molecular complexes with DNA-related proteins (Brugnoli et al., 2010; Houlard et al., 2002; Romero et al., 1998) a more general role of Vav1 in regulating events ended to control protein expression can be hypothesized. 2D electrophoresis followed by mass spectrometry have established that, in both HL-60 and NB4 cells, the down-modulation of Vav1 abrogates the capacity of ATRA of modulating the expression of proteins associated to cytoskeleton and involved in proliferation and of apoptosis-related proteins, as well as of molecules implicated in metabolism, synthesis, folding and degradation of proteins (Bertagnolo et al., 2008). The majority of the identified proteins are affected by Vav1 down-modulation only in one of the two analyzed cell lines, according to the notion that HL-60 and NB4 cells, even if both derived from patients with APL, show peculiar genotypic and phenotypic profiles (Barber et al., 2008). Interestingly, in NB4 cells, the lack of Vav1 affects the ATRA-dependent expression of the Splicing factor, arg/ser rich 3 (Sfrs3), a member of SR proteins, known as non-snRNP splicing factors, that may affect both constitutive and alternative splicing of mRNA (Sanford et al., 2005). This evidence further supports the role of Vav1 in regulating the ATRA-dependent gene expression.

Some of the identified proteins are differentially expressed, as a consequence of Vav1-down-modulation during ATRA treatment, in both cell lines, suggesting that they may constitute a common part of the signalling activated by ATRA in APL-derived promyelocytes. Notably, this group of proteins includes the ε isoform of the 14-3-3 family of proteins, specifically involved in the caspase networks (Liou et al., 2007). The increased expression of 14-3-3ε in both HL-60 and NB4 cells when Vav1 is down-modulated during ATRA treatment suggests that the amount of Vav1 may be critical in determining the mechanism of caspase activation in APL.

Vav1 also affects the ATRA-dependent expression of α-enolase, a multifunction protein involved in glycolysis and up-regulated in the sera of a number of cancer patients, in which it seems to have a role in tumorigenesis (Zou et al., 2005). α-enolase is expressed at high levels in most AML subtypes in which it might contribute to the adverse evolution of the disease (Lopez-Pedrera et al., 2006). Since down-modulation of Vav1 during ATRA treatment of APL-derived cells reduces the expression of α-enolase (Bertagnolo et al., 2008), it has been suggested that Vav1 promotes the differentiation of tumoral promyelocytes by also targeting metabolic pathways.

The proteasome component "splice isoform 2 subunit α3" is down-modulated as well in HL-60 and NB4 cells under the same experimental conditions (Bertagnolo et al., 2008). Since proteasome is the major cellular proteolytic machinery responsible for degradation of normal and damaged proteins (Von Mikecz, 2006), Vav1 may also be involved in regulating protein degradation during ATRA dependent maturation of tumoral promyelocytes.
Also the component of microtubules α-tubulin is affected by down-modulation of Vav1 during ATRA treatment (Bertagnolo et al., 2008), indicating that Vav1, in addition to regulate cytoskeleton reorganization, takes part to the profound architectural changes of differentiating promyelocytes by regulating the expression of cytoskeleton components.

4. Vav1 and monocytic/macrophagic differentiation

The human promyelocytic leukemia cell lines HL-60 and NB4 can be differentiated either toward neutrophils by ATRA or to monocytes/macrophages by PMA (Murao et al., 1983; Song & Norman, 1998). PMA is a stable analogue of 2, 3-diacylglycerol that induces, even if with dynamics not identical in HL-60 and NB4 cells, morphological and functional changes related to monocyte maturation, accompanied by a loss of proliferative capacity (Jasek et al., 2008). Immunochemical and immunocytochemical analysis demonstrate that the expression of Vav1 increases also during the PMA-induced acquisition of a monocyte-like phenotype of HL-60 and NB4 cells (Bertagnolo et al., 2011). This is consistent with the notion that also mature monocytes express Vav1 and that proper amounts of the protein are necessary for their inflammation related functions (Bhavsar et al., 2009; Hall et al., 2006). In the same cell types, PMA also induces a relevant increase of tyrosine phosphorylation of Vav1. On the other hand, and in constrast to what observed in the ATRA-treatment of the same cell line, no role for Syk was demonstrated in this event (Bertagnolo et al., 2011), consistent with the notion that, at least in HL-60 cells, Syk might exert a narrower role, restricted to directing cells toward granulocyte differentiation (Qin & Yamamura, 1997). In both HL-60 and NB4 cells, PMA induces a relevant increase of tyrosine phosphorylation of Vav1 on the Tyr174 residue (Bertagnolo et al., 2011), according to the GEF role played by Vav1 in myeloid cells. These results are also in agreement with other data indicating that, in macrophage-like differentiated HL-60 cells, the activity of Syk is ended to regulate the roles played by mature cells in immune response, including their complement-mediated phagocytosis, in which the kinase regulates both actin dynamics and the Vav1-RhoA activation pathway (Shi et al., 2006).
Also in differentiation of APL-derived cells to monocytes/macrophages, a crucial role for Vav1 in determining the acquisition of maturation-related features has been demonstrated by silencing the expression of Vav1 induced by PMA (Bertagnolo et al., 2011). Under these conditions, the expression of CD11b, which is induced by PMA and constitutes a marker also for monocyte differentiation, is significantly reduced, similarly to what demonstrated during the treatment with ATRA of HL-60 and NB4 cells (Bertagnolo et al. 2011). This suggests that, in differentiating APL-derived cells, Vav1 plays a role in regulating the expression of the CD11b surface antigen regardless the agonist employed and the maturation lineage. Since in NB4 cells treated with ATRA Vav1 is recuited to protein/DNA complexes on the *CD11b* promoter (Brugnoli et al., 2010), it can be speculated that Vav1 plays a specific role in driving the expression of CD11b as part of the transcriptional machinery also during the differentiation of NB4 cells along the monocytic/macrophagic lineage.

Also cell adhesion is affected by down-modulation of Vav1 during PMA treatment of HL-60 and NB4 cells, in terms of both number of adherent cells and of adhesion area of cells that remain attached to the flask bottom. These results are in agreement with the data obtained with macrophages from Vav1-/- mice, showing a smaller adhesive area or a decreased adhesion efficiency (Wells et al., 2005).

4.1 Regulation of actin

As above reported, the main known functional role of tyrosine phosphorylated Vav1 is to regulate cytoskeleton reorganization, a phenomenon at the basis of both adhesion and migration of monocytes/macrophages. Vav1 regulates cell architecture not only by means of its GEF activity but also by interacting with proteins in turn involved in cytoskeleton reorganization. In addition, in both HL-60 and NB4 cells, Vav1 affects the ATRA-induced expression of the microtubule component α-tubulin.

Contrarily to what observed during granulocytic differentiation, Vav1 down-modulation does not have any effect on expression and architectural organization of α-tubulin during PMA-induced monocytic/macrophagic maturation of NB4 cells (Bertagnolo et al., 2011). This indicates that, during the maturation process of APL-derived cells, Vav1 exerts an agonist- and lineage-specific role in regulating α-tubulin. From a more general point of view, concerning microtubule organization, it can be speculated that the role of Vav1 is restricted to the control of the motility of mature cells, as also suggested by the evidence that changes in microtubule dynamics contribute to the reduced migration speed of Vav1-/- macrophages in response to CSF-1 (Wells et al., 2005).

In living cells, the F-actin cytoskeleton encompasses a variety of different structures that are essential for many different aspects of cell physiology. In particular, dynamic modulation of the filamentous actin cytoskeleton is critical to numerous physical cellular processes, including adhesion, migration and phagocytosis, all requiring precise regulation of cell shape (Stricker et al., 2010). Recent data demonstrate that Vav proteins, including Vav1, are required for actin cytoskeleton reorganization during migration of macrophages, by coupling RhoA and Rac1 activity to adhesion receptors (Bhavsar et al., 2009). Also in ATRA-induced maturation of cells derived from APL Vav1 seems to regulate actin organization.

In HL-60 and NB4 cells treated with PMA, an unprecedented involvement of Vav1 in regulating the increase of actin expression has been shown very recently (Bertagnolo et al., 2011), that constitutes a further confirmation that Vav1, besides being involved in the formation of filaments, takes part to cytoskeleton reorganization as a modulator of protein expression.

The modifications of cell shape in the different cell processes seem to be regulated by the existence of the F-actin cortex, a thin, membrane-bound F-actin network (Stricker et al., 2010). Defective actin-cap formation has been found in lymphocytes from a Vav-deficient mice, clearly correlating Vav1 activity with the regulation of cell shape (Holsinger et al., 1998). Furthermore, a recent work in which adhesive micropatterned surfaces have been used to control the overall shape of fibroblasts, has demonstrated that the shape of the nucleus is tightly regulated through a perinuclear actin cap, which is located above and around the interphase nucleus (Khatau et al., 2009). A wide variety of contractile F-actin networks with different architectures and polarity have also been found near cell adhesion surfaces, correlated with the migratory capability of adherent cells (Stricker et al., 2010). By means of confocal analysis of PMA-treated adherent NB4 cells, it has been demonstrated the existence of an agonist-induced F-actin network, in which F-actin colocalyzes with Vav1, that sharply defines the cytoplasmatic cell border, accumulates inside thin and long cell processes and surrounds the nuclear compartment (Bertagnolo et al., 2011). Since the existence of cytoplasmatic processes in PMA-treated adherent cells are indicative of migratory activity (Stricker et al., 2010), Vav1/F-actin co-localization in cytoplasm protrusions is suggestive of a synergy of the two molecules in controling cell motility. This is in agreement with the role described for Vav proteins in the maintenance of normal morphology and migratory behaviour in macrophages (Bhavsar et al., 2009). The strong Vav1/F-actin co-localization observed at the nuclear periphery and, in particular, in the region above the nucleus, suggests that the two proteins may cooperate in regulating the shape of the nucleus through an actin filament structure similar to the perinuclear actin cap described by Khatau et al. (2009). On the other hand, the role of Vav1 in modulating cell adhesion of PMA-treated cells seems to be related to its ability to regulate expression of integrins, like CD11b, rather than to a direct effect on actin-based cytoskeleton.

5. Conclusion

The present review focuses on the role of the multidomain protein Vav1 in promoting and sustaining the completion of the differentiation program of tumoral promyelocytes. Vav1 is a key protein in the ATRA- and PMA-induced maturation of APL-derived cells, since either its down-modulation or over-expression respectively prevents or potentiates the ability of these agonists to induce the acquisition of a mature phenotype. Alternatively to the best known function of Vav1 as a GEF for small G proteins, ended to regulate cell shape by affecting actin assembly, other mechanisms by which Vav1 affects myeloid differentiation have been described, reflecting the great interactive and regulatory potential of Vav1, which make the full understanding of its functions a very difficult, yet fascinating story.

An example of the complex role played by Vav1 during myeloid differentiation of APL-derived cells is the interaction of Vav1 with various lipid-modifying enzymes ended to regulate the pool of phosphoinositides associated to cytoskeleton. The resulting modifications of actin cytoskeleton contribute to the changes of cellular and nuclear shape occurring in differentiating tumoral promyelocytes (Fig. 3).

The participation of Vav1 to molecular complexes with other adaptor proteins differently distributed in the cytoplasm and in the nucleus suggests the existence of a signal sequence originated from membrane receptors and directed to the nuclear compartment. Inside the nucleus of APL-derived cells, Vav1 seems to play its most intriguing role by regulating the expression of CD11b, a surface marker of both granulocyte and monocyte differentiation, and of a number of ATRA-modulated proteins (Fig. 3). The nuclear issue assumes thus great relevance, confering to Vav1 compartimentalized strategic roles in regulating the maturation process of tumoral promyelocytes.

The bulk of the studies reviewed here are mostly concerned with two cell lines, HL-60 and NB4, derived from APL patients, driven to achieve differentiation by treatment with drugs of the retinoids or phorbol esters families. Even though a better understanding of the functional engagement of Vav1 will be required before converting scientific achievements into clinical advances, Vav1 might be considered a common target for developing new therapeutic strategies for the different subtypes of myeloid leukemias.

In addition, it can be speculated that the identified pathways involving Vav1 are of more general interest and may be potentially extended also outside the haemopoietic/immunological systems.

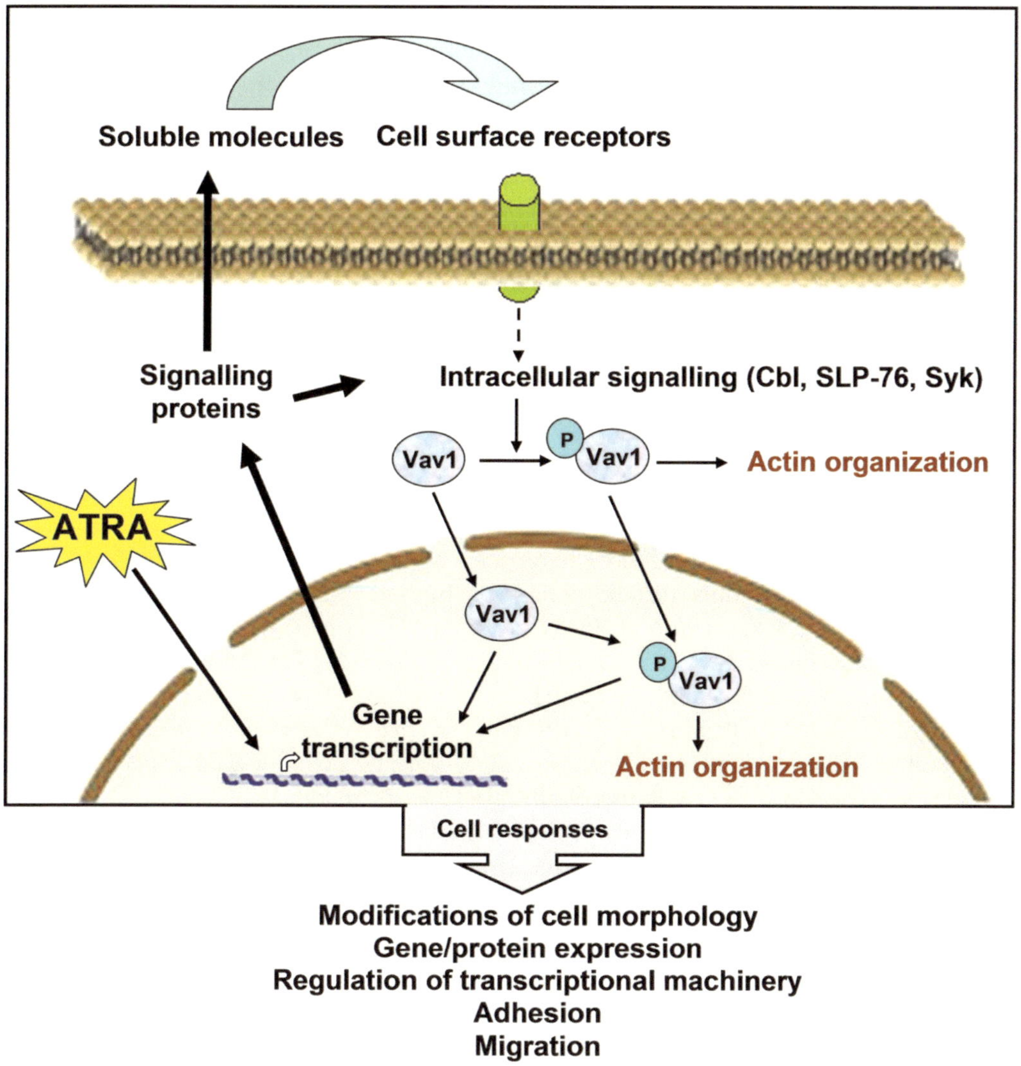

Fig. 3. Overall role of Vav1 in regulating maturation of APL-derived promyelocytes.

6. Acknowledgments

The authors are supported by MIUR (Cofin 2008 and FIRB Accordi di Programma 2010), MAE (Italy-Croatia bilateral project 2009-2011) and by University of Ferrara (Italy).

7. References

Barber, N., Belov, & L., Christopherson, R.I. (2008). All-trans retinoic acid induces different immunophenotypic changes on human HL60 and NB4 myeloid leukaemias. *Leukemia Research*, Vol.32, No.2, (February 2008), pp. 315-322.

Bertagnolo, V., Marchisio, M., Volinia, S., Caramelli, E. & Capitani, S. (1998). Nuclear association of tyrosine-phosphorylated Vav to phospholipase C-gamma1 and phosphoinositide 3-kinase during granulocytic differentiation of HL-60 cells. *FEBS Letters,* Vol.441, No.3, (December 1998), pp. 480-484.

Bertagnolo, V., Neri, L.M., Marchisio, M., Mischiati, C. & Capitani, S. (1999). Phosphoinositide 3-kinase activity is essential for all-trans-retinoic acid-induced granulocytic differentiation of HL-60 cells. *Cancer Research,* Vol. 59, No.3, (February 1999), pp. 542-546.

Bertagnolo, V., Marchisio, M., Brugnoli, F., Bavelloni, A., Boccafogli, L., Colamussi, M.L., & Capitani, S. (2001). Requirement of tyrosine-phosphorylated Vav for morphological differentiation of all-trans-retinoic acid-treated HL-60 cells. *Cell Growth & Differentiation,* Vol.12,No.4, (April 2001), pp. 193-200.

Bertagnolo, V., Brugnoli, F., Marchisio, M., Celeghini, C., Carini, C., & Capitani, S. (2004). Association of PI 3-K with tyrosine phosphorylated Vav is essential for its activity in neutrophil-like maturation of myeloid cells. *Cellullar Signaling,* Vol.16, No.4, (April 2004), pp. 423-433.

Bertagnolo, V., Brugnoli, F., Mischiati, C., Sereni, A., Bavelloni, A., Carini, C., & Capitani, S. (2005). Vav promotes differentiation of human tumoral myeloid precursors. *Experimental Cell Research,* Vol.306, No.1, (May 2005), pp. 56-63.

Bertagnolo, V., Grassilli, S., Bavelloni, A., Brugnoli, F., Piazzi, M., Candiano, G., Petretto, A., Benedusi, M., & Capitani, S. (2008). Vav1 modulates protein expression during ATRA-induced maturation of APL-derived promyelocytes: a proteomic-based analysis. *Journal of Proteome Research,* Vol. 7, No.9, (September 2008), pp. 3729-3736.

Bertagnolo, V., Grassilli, S., D'Aguanno, S., Brugnoli, F., Bavelloni, A., Faenza, I., Nika, E., Urbani, A., Cocco, L., & Capitani, S. (2010). Mass spectrometry-based identification of Y745 of Vav1 as a tyrosine residue crucial in maturation of acute promyelocytic leukemia-derived cells. *Journal of Proteome Research,* Vol.9, No.2, (February 2010), pp. 752-760.

Bertagnolo, V., Nika, E., Brugnoli, F., Bonora, M., Grassilli, S., Pinton, P., & Capitani, S. (2011). Vav1 is a crucial molecule in monocytic/macrophagic differentiation of myeloid leukemia-derived cells. *Cell and Tissue Research,* [Epub ahead of print], (June 2011), DOI: 10.1007/s00441-011-1195-5.

Bhavsar, P.J., Vigorito, E., Turner, M., & Ridley, A.J. (2009). Vav GEFs regulate macrophage morphology and adhesion-induced Rac and Rho activation. *Experimental Cell Research,* Vol.315, No.19, (November 2009), pp. 3345-3358.

Breitman, T.R., Selonick, S.E., & Collins, S.J. (1980). Induction of differentiation of the human promyelocytic leukemia cell line (HL-60) by retinoic acid. *Proceedings of the National Academy of Sciences of the United States of America,* Vol.77, No.5, (May 1980), pp. 2936-2940.

Brugnoli, F., Lambertini, E., Varin-Blank, N., Piva, R., Marchisio, M., Grassilli, S., Miscia, S., Capitani, S., & Bertagnolo, V. (2010). Vav1 and PU.1 are recruited to the CD11b promoter in APL-derived promyelocytes: role of Vav1 in modulating PU.1-containing complexes during ATRA-induced differentiation. *Experimental Cell Research,* Vol.316, No.1, (January 2010), pp. 38-47.

Bustelo, X. R., Crespo, P., Lopez-Barahona, M., Gutkind, J. S., & Barbacid, M. (1997). Cbl-b, a member of the Sli-1/c-Cbl protein family, inhibits Vav-mediated c-Jun N-terminal kinase activation. *Oncogene*, Vol.15, No.21, (November 1997), pp. 2511–2520, 1997.

Bustelo, X.R. (2001). Vav proteins, adaptors and cell signaling. *Oncogene,* Vol.20, No.44, (October 2001), pp. 6372-6381.

Bustelo, X.R. (2002). Regulation of Vav proteins by intramolecular events. *Frontiers in Biosciences,* Vol.7, (January 2002), pp. 24-30.

Chen, L., Janetopoulos, C., Huang, Y.E., Iijima, M., Borleis, J., & Devreotes, P.N. (2003). Two phases of actin polymerization display different dependencies on PI(3,4,5)P3 accumulation and have unique roles during chemotaxis. *Molecular Biology of the Cell,* Vol.14, No.12, (December 2003), pp. 5028-5037.

Chiang, J., & Hodes, R.J. (2011). Cbl Enforces Vav1 Dependence and a Restricted Pathway of T Cell Development. *PLoS ONE,* Vol.6, No.4, (April 2011), e18542.

Cicchetti, G., Allen, P.G., & Glogauer, M. (2002). Chemotactic signaling pathways in neutrophils: From receptor to actin assembly. *Critical Reviews in Oral Biology & Medicine*, Vol.13, No.3, (May 2002), pp. 220–228.

Clevenger, C.V., Ngo, W., Sokol, D.L., Luger, S.M. & Gewirtz, A.M. (1995). Vav is necessary for prolactin-stimulated proliferation and is translocated into the nucleus of T-cell line. *The Journal of Biological Chemistry*, Vol.270, No.22, (June 1995), pp. 13246-13253.

Congleton, J., Jiang, H., Malavasi, F., Lin, H., & Yen, A. (2011). ATRA-induced HL-60 myeloid leukemia cell differentiation depends on the CD38 cytosolic tail needed for membrane localization, but CD38 enzymatic activity is unnecessary. *Experimental Cell Research,* Vol.317, No.7, (April 2011), pp. 910-919.

Cougoule, C., Hoshino, S., Dart, A., Lim, J., & Caron, E. (2006). Dissociation of recruitment and activation of the small G-protein Rac during Fcgamma receptor-mediated phagocytosis. *The Journal of Biological Chemistry,* Vol.281, No.13, (March 2006), pp. 8756-8764.

Cui, L., Chen, C., Xu, T., Zhang, J., Shang, X., Luo, J., Chen, L., Ba, X., & Zeng, X. (2009). c-Abl kinase is required for beta 2 integrin-mediated neutrophil adhesion. *Journal of Immunology,* Vol.182, No.5, (March 2009), pp. 3233–3242.

Daniels, R.H., & Bokoch, G.M. (1999). p21-activated protein kinase: a crucial component of morphological signaling? *Trends in Biochemical Sciences,* Vol.24, No.9, (September 1999), pp. 350-355.

Denkinger, D.J., Lambrecht, T.Q., Cushman-Vokoun, & A.M., Kawahara, R.S. (2002). PU.1 regulates the expression of the vav proto-oncogene. *Journal of Cellular Biochemistry,* Vol.84, No.4, (January 2002), pp. 772-783.

Dong, H., Ying, T., Li, T., Cao, T., Wang, J., Yuan, J., Feng, E., Han, B., Hua, F., Yang, Y., Yuan, J., Wang, H., & Xu, C. (2006). Comparative proteomic analysis of apoptosis induced by sodium selenite in human acute promyelocytic leukemia NB4 cells. *Journal of Cellular Biochemistry,* Vol.98, No.9, (August 2006), pp. 1495-1506.

Durual, S., Rideau, A., Ruault-Jungblut, S., Cossali, D., Beris, P., Piguet, V., & Matthes T. (2007). Lentiviral PU.1 overexpression restores differentiation in myeloid leukemic blasts. *Leukemia,* Vol.21, No.5, (May 2007), pp. 1050-1059.

Fischer, K.D., Kong, Y.Y., Nishina, H., Tedford, K., Marengère, L.E., Kozieradzki, I., Sasaki, T., Starr, M., Chan, G., Gardener, S., Nghiem, M.P., Bouchard, D., Barbacid, M., Bernstein, A., & Penninger, J.M. (1998). Vav is a regulator of cytoskeletal reorganization mediated by the T-cell receptor. *Current Biology,* Vol.8, No.10, (May 1998), pp. 554-562.

Fujikawa, K., Miletic, A.V., Alt, F.W., Faccio, R., Brown, T., Hoog, J., Fredericks, J., Nishi, S., Mildiner, S., Moores, S.L., Brugge, J., Rosen, F.S., & Swat, W. (2003) Vav1/2/3-null mice define an essential role for Vav family proteins in lymphocyte development and activation but a differential requirement in MAPK signaling in T and B cells. *The Journal of Experimental Medicine,* Vol.198, No.10, (November 2003), pp. 1595-1608.

Gakidis, M.A., Cullere, X., Olson, T., Wilsbacher, J.L., Zhang, B., Moores, S.L., Ley, K., Swat, W., Mayadas, T., & Brugge, J.S. (2004). Vav GEFs are required for beta2 integrin-dependent functions of neutrophils. *The Journal of Cell Biology,* Vol.166, No.2, (July 2004), pp. 273-282.

Gomez, T. S., Hamann, M. J., McCarney, S., Savoy, D. N., Lubking, C. M., Heldebrant, M. P., Labno, C. M., McKean, D. J., McNiven, M. A., Burkhardt, J. K. & Billadeau, D. D. (2005). Dynamin 2 regulates T cell activation by controlling actin polymerization at the immunological synapse. *Nature Immunology,* Vol.6, No.3, (March 2005), pp. 261-270.

Gross, B. S., Ran Lee, J., Clements, J. L., Turner, M., Tybulewicz,V. L. J., Findell, P. R., Koretzky, G. A., & Watson, S. P. (1999). Tyrosine phosphorylation of SLP-76 is downstream of Syk following stimulation of the collagen receptor in platelets. *The Journal of Biological Chemistry,* Vol.274, No.9, (February 1999), pp. 5963–5971.

Hall, A.B., Gakidis, M.A., Glogauer, M., Wilsbacher, J.L., Gao, S., Swat, W., & Brugge, J.S. (2006). Requirements for Vav guanine nucleotide exchange factors and Rho GTPases in FcgammaR- and complement-mediated phagocytosis. *Immunity,* Vol.24, No.3, (March 2006), pp. 305-316.

Han, J., Luby-Phelps, K., Das, B., Shu, X., Xia, Y., Mosteller, R.D., Krishna, U.M., Falck, J.R., White, M.A., & Broek, D. (1998). Role of substrates and products of PI 3-kinase in regulating activation of Rac-related guanosine triphosphatases by Vav. *Science,* Vol.279, No.5350, (January 1998), pp. 558-560.

Hannigan, M., Zhan, L., Li, Z., Ai, Y., Wu, D., Huang, C.K. (2002). Neutrophils lacking phosphoinositide 3-kinase gamma show loss of directionality during *N*-formyl-Met-Leu-Phe-induced chemotaxis. *Proceedings of the National Academy of Sciences of the United States of America,* Vol.99, No.6, (March 2002), pp. 3603–3608.

Harris, M.N., Ozpolat, B., Abdi, F., Gu, S., Legler, A., Mawuenyega, K.G., Tirado-Gomez, M., Lopez-Berestein, G., & Chen, X.(2004). Comparative proteomic analysis of all-trans-retinoic acid treatment reveals systematic posttranscriptional control mechanisms in acute promyelocytic leukemia. *Blood,* Vol.*104,* No.5, (September 2004), pp. 1314-1323.

Haubert, D., & Weckbecker, G. (2010). Vav1 couples the T cell receptor to cAMP response element activation via a PKC-dependent pathway. *Cellular Signaling,* Vol.22, No.6, (June 2010), pp. 944-954.

Holsinger, L.J., Graef, I.A., Swat, W., Chi, T., Bautista, D.M., Davidson, L., Lewis, R.S., Alt, F.W., & Crabtree, G.R. (1998). Defects in actin-cap formation in Vav-deficient mice implicate an actin requirement for lymphocyte signal transduction. *Current Bioloogy,* Vol.8, No.10, (May 1998), pp. 563-572.

Hornstein, I., Alcover, A., & Katzav, S. (2004). Vav proteins, masters of the world of cytoskeleton organization. *Cellular Signalling* Vol.16, No.1, (January 2004), pp. 1-11.

Houlard, M., Arudchandran, R., Regnier-Ricard, F., Germani, A., Gisselbrecht, S., Blank, U., Rivera, J., & Varin-Blank, N. (2002). Vav1 is a component of transcriptionally active complexes.*The Journal of Experimental Medicine,* Vol.195, No.9, (May 2002), pp. 1115-1127.

Hsu, H.C., Tsai, W.H., Chen, P.G., Hsu, M.L., Ho, C.K., & Wang, S.Y. (1999). In vitro effect of granulocyte-colony stimulating factor and all-trans retinoic acid on the expression of inflammatory cytokines and adhesion molecules in acute promyelocytic leukemic cells. *European Journal of Haematology,* Vol.63, No.1, (July 1999), pp.11–18.

Janmey, P.A., Xian, W., & Flanagan, L.A. (1999). Controlling cytoskeleton structure by phosphoinositide-protein interactions: phosphoinositide binding protein domains and effects of lipid packing. *Chemistry and Physics of Lipids,* Vol.101, No.1, (August 1999), pp. 93-107.

Jasek, E., Mirecka, J., & Litwin, J.A. (2008). Effect of differentiating agents (all-trans retinoic acid and phorbol 12-myristate 13-acetate) on drug sensitivity of HL60 and NB4 cells in vitro. *Folia Histochemica et Cytobiologica,* Vol.46, No.3, (December 2008), pp.323-330, ISSN, 0239-8508.

Kastner P., & Chan, S. (2008). PU.1: a crucial and versatile player in hematopoiesis and leukemia. *The International Journal of Biochemistry and Cell Biology,* Vol.40, No.1, (n.d.), pp. 22-27.

Katzav, S. (2004). Vav1: an oncogene that regulates specific transcriptional activation of T cells. *Blood,* Vol.103, No.7, (April 2004), pp. 2443-2451.

Katzav, S. (2009). Vav1: a hematopoietic signal transduction molecule involved in human malignancies. *The International Journal of Biochemistry & Cell Biology,* Vol.41, No.6, (June 2009), pp. 1245-1248.

Khatau, S.B., Hale, C.M., Stewart-Hutchinson, P.J., Patel, M.S., Stewart, C.L., Searson, P.C., Hodzic, D., & Wirtz, D. (2009). A perinuclear actin cap regulates nuclear shape. *Proceedings of the National Academy of Sciences of the United States of America,* Vol.106, No.45, (November 2009), pp. 19017-19122.

Kim, C., Marchal, C.C., Penninger, J. & Dinauer M.C. (2003). The hemopoietic Rho/Rac guanine nucleotide exchange factor Vav1 regulates N-formyl-methionyl-leucyl-phenylalanine-activated neutrophil functions. *Journal of Immunology,* Vol.171, No.8, (October 2003), pp. 4425-4430.

Kogan, S.C. (2009). Curing APL: differentiation or destruction? *Cancer Cell,* Vol.15, No.1, (January 2009), pp. 7-8.

Kong, Y.Y., Fischer, K.D., Bachmann, M.F., Mariathasan, S., Kozieradzki, I., Nghiem, M.P., Bouchard, D., Bernstein, A., Ohashi, P.S. & Penninger, J.M. (1998). Vav regulates peptide-specific apoptosis in thymocytes. *The Journal of Experimental Medicine,*Vol.188, No.11, (December 1998), pp. 2099-2111.

Lamkin T.J., Chin, V., Varvayanis, S., Smith, J.L., Sramkoski, R.M., Jacobberger, J.W., & Yen, A. (2006). Retinoic acid-induced CD38 expression in HL-60 myeloblastic leukemia cells regulates cell differentiation or viability depending on expression levels. *Journal of Cellular Biochemistry,* Vol.97, No.6, (April 2006), pp. 1328–1338.

Lanotte M., Martin-Thouvenin, V., Najman, S. Balerini, P., Valensi, F., & Berger, R. (1991). NB4, a maturation inducible cell line with t(15;17) marker isolated from a human acute promyelocytic leukemia (M3). *Blood,* Vol.77, No.5, (March 1991), pp. 1080-1086.

Law, D. A., Nannizzi-Alaimo, L., Ministri, K., Hughes, P. E., Forsyth, J.,Turner, M., Shattil, S. J., Ginsberg, M. H., Tybulewicz, V. L. J., & Phillips,D. R. (1999). Genetic and pharmacological analyses of Syk function in aII-b3 signaling in platelets. *Blood,* Vol.93, No.8, (April 1999), pp. 2645–2652.

Lazer, G., Pe'er, L., Farago, M., Machida, K., Mayer, B.J., & Katzav, S. (2010). Tyrosine residues at the carboxyl terminus of Vav1 play an important role in regulation of its biological activity. *The Journal of Biological Chemistry,* Vol.285, No.30, (July 2010), pp. 23075-23085.

Li, G.H., Fan, Y.Z., Liu, X.W., Zhang, B.F., Yin, D.D., He, F., Huang, S.Y., Kang, Z.J., Xu, H., Liu, Q., Wu, Y.L., Niu, X.L., Zhang, L., Liu, L., Hao, M.W., Han, H., & Liang, Y.M. (2010). Notch signaling maintains proliferation and survival of the HL60 human promyelocytic leukemia cell line and promotes the phosphorylation of the Rb protein. *Molecular and Cellular Biochemistry,* Vol.340, No. 1-2, (July 2010), pp. 7–14.

Liou, J.Y., Ghelani, D., Yeh, S., & Wu, K.K. (2007). Nonsteroidal anti-inflammatory drugs induce colorectal cancer cell apoptosis by suppressing 14-3-3epsilon. *Cancer Research,* Vol.67, No.7, (April 2007), pp. 3185-3191.

Liu, C.R., Ma, C.S., Ning, J.Y., You, J.F., Liao, S.L., & Zheng, J. (2004). Differential thymosin beta 10 expression levels and actin filament organization in tumor cell lines with different metastatic potential. *Chinese Medical Journal,* Vol.117, No.2, (February 2004), pp. 213– 218.

Lo-Coco F., & Ammatuna, E. (2006). The biology of acute promyelocytic leukemia and its impact on diagnosis and treatment. *Hematology,* (January 2006), pp. 156-161.

López-Pedrera, C., Villalba, J.M., Siendones, E., Barbarroja, N. Gómez-Díaz, C., Rodríguez-Ariza, A., Buendía, P., Torres, A., & Velasco, F. (2006). Proteomic analysis of acute myeloid leukemia: Identification of potential early biomarkers and therapeutic targets. *Proteomics,* Vol.6, No.S1, (April 2006), pp. 293-299.

Lupher, M.L., Jr., Rao, N., Eck, M.J., & Band, H. The Cbl protooncoprotein: a negative regulator of immune receptor signal transduction. *Immunology Today,* Vol.20, No.8, (August 1999), pp. 375–382.

Menard, R.E., & Mattingly, R.R. (2004). Gbetagamma subunits stimulate p21-activated kinase 1 (PAK1) through activation of PI3-kinase and Akt but act independently of Rac1/Cdc42. *FEBS Letters,* Vol.556, No.1-3, (January 2004), pp. 187-192.

Miletic, A.V., Sakata-Sogawa, K., Hiroshima, M., Hamann, M.J., Gomez, T. S., Ota, N., Kloeppel, T., Kanagawa, O., Tokunaga, M., Billadeau, D.D., & Swat, W. (2006). Vav1 acidic region tyrosine 174 is required for the formation of T cell receptor-induced microclusters and is essential in T cell development and activation. *The Journal of Biological Chemistry,* Vol.281, No.50, (December 2006), pp. 38257–38265.

Mueller, B.U., Pabst, T., Fos, J., Petkovic, V., Fey, M.F., Asou, N., Buergi, U., & Tenen, D.G. (2006). ATRA resolves the differentiation block in t(15;17) acute myeloid leukemia by restoring PU.1 expression. *Blood,* Vol.107, No.8, (April 2006), pp. 3330-3338.

Murao, S., Gemmell, M.A., Callaham, M.F., Anderson, N.L., & Huberman, E. (1983). Control of macrophage cell differentiation in human promyelocytic HL-60 leukemia cells by 1,25-dihydroxyvitamin D3 and phorbol-12-myristate-13-acetate. *Cancer Research,* Vol.43, No.10, (October 1983), pp. 4989-4996.

Nasr, R., Guillemin, M.C., Ferhi, O., Soilihi, H., Peres, L., Berthier, C., Rousselot, P., Robledo-Sarmiento, M., Lallemand-Breitenbach, V., Gourmel, B., Vitoux, D., Pandolfi, P.P., Rochette-Egly, C., Zhu, J., & de Thé, H. (2008). Eradication of acute promyelocytic leukemia-initiating cells through PML-RARA degradation. *Nature Medicine,* Vol.14, No.12, (December 2008), pp. 1333-1342.

Niggli, V., & Keller, H. (1997). The phosphatidylinositol 3-kinase inhibitor wortmannin markedly reduces chemotactic peptide-induced locomotion and increases in cytoskeletal actin in human neutrophils. *European Journal of Pharmacology,* Vol.335, No.1, (September 1997), pp. 43–52.

Ohishi, K., Katayama, N., Shiku, H., Varnum-Finney, B., & Bernstein, I.D. (2003). Notch signalling in hematopoiesis. *Seminars in Cell & Developmental Biology,* Vol.14, No.2, (April 2003), pp. 143– 150.

Ottinger, E., Botfield, M.C., & Shoelson, S.E. (1998). Tandem SH2 domains confer high specificity in tyrosine kinase signaling. *The Journal of Biological Chemistry,* Vol.273, No.2, (January 1998), pp. 729–735.

Pahl H.L., Scheibe, R.J., Zhang, D.E., Chen, H.M., Galson, D.L., Maki, R.A., & Tenen, D.G. (1993). The proto-oncogene PU.1 regulates expression of the myeloid-specific CD11b promoter. *The Journal of Biological Chemistry,* Vol.268, No.7, (March 1993), pp. 5014-5020.

Pauker, M.H., & Barda-Saad, M. (2011). Studies of novel interactions between Nck and VAV SH3 domains. *Communicative & Integrative Biology,* Vol.4, No.2, (March/April 2011), pp. 175-177.

Phillipson, M., Heit, B., Parsons, S.A., Petri, B., Mullaly, S.C., Colarusso, P., Gower, R.M., Neely, G., Simon, S.I., & Kubes, P. (2009). Vav1 is essential for mechanotactic crawling and migration of neutrophils out of the inflamed microvasculature. *Journal of Immunology,* Vol.182, No.11, (June 2009), pp. 6870-6878.

Pivniouk, V.I., Martin, T.R., Lu-Kuo, J.M., Katz, H.R., Oettgen, H.C., & Geha, R.S. (1999). SLP-76 deficiency impairs signaling via the high-affinity IgE receptor in mast cells. *The Journal of Clinical Investigation,* Vol.103, No.12, (June 1999), pp. 1737–1743.

Qin, S., & Yamamura, H. (1997). Up-regulation of Syk activity during HL60 cell differentiation into granulocyte but not into monocyte/macrophage-lineage. *Biochemical and Biophysical Ressearch Communications,* Vol.236, No.3, (July 1997), pp. 697-701.

Rho, S.B., Chun, T., Lee, S.H., Park, K., & Lee, J.H. (2004). The interaction between E-tropomodulin and thymosin beta-10 rescues tumor cells from thymosin beta-10 mediated apoptosis by restoring actin architecture. *FEBS Letters,* Vol.557, No.1-3, (January 2004), pp. 57–63.

Romero, F., Dargemont, C., Pozo, F., Reeves, W.H., Camonis, J., Gisselbrecht, S., & Fischer S. (1996). p95vav associates with the nuclear protein Ku-70. *Molecular and Cellular Biology,* Vol.16, No.1, (January 1996), pp. 37-44.

Romero, F., Germani, A., Puvion, E., Camonis, J., Varin-Blank, N., Gisselbrecht, S., & Fischer, S. (1998). Vav binding to heterogeneous nuclear ribonucleoprotein (hnRNP) C. Evidence for Vav-hnRNP interactions in an RNA-dependent manner. *The Journal of Biological Chemistry,* Vol.273, No.10, (March 1998), pp. 5923-5931.

Sanchez, J.A., & Wangh, L.J. (1999). New insights into the mechanisms of nuclear segmentation in human neutrophils. *Journal of Cellular Biochemistry,* Vol.73, No.1, (April 1999), pp. 1-10.

Sanchez-Aguilera, A., Lee, Y.J., Lo Celso, C., Ferraro, F., Brumme, K., Mondal, S., Kim, C., Dorrance, A., Luo, H.R., Scadden, D.T, & Williams D.A. (2011). Guanine nucleotide exchange factor Vav1 regulates perivascular homing and bone marrow retention of hematopoietic stem and progenitor cells. *Proceedings of the National Academy of Sciences of the United States of America,* Vol.108, No.23, (June 2011), pp. 9607-9612.

Sanford, J.R., Ellis, J., & Cáceres, J.F. (2005). Multiple roles of arginine/serine-rich splicing factors in RNA processing. *Biochemical Society Transactions,* Vol.33, No.3, (June 2005), pp. 443-446.

Schneider H., &. Rudd, C.E. (2008). CD28 and Grb-2, relative to Gads or Grap, preferentially co-operate with Vav1 in the activation of NFAT/AP-1 transcription. *Biochemical and Biophysical Ressearch Communications,* Vol.369, No.2, (May 2008), pp. 616-621.

Schymeinsky, J., Sindrilaru, A., Frommhold, D., Sperandio, M., Gerstl, R., Then, C., Mócsai, A., Scharffetter-Kochanek, K., & Walzog, B. (2006). The Vav binding site of the non-receptor tyrosine kinase Syk at Tyr 348 is critical for beta2 integrin (CD11/CD18)-mediated neutrophil migration. *Blood,* Vol.108, No.12, (December 2006), pp. 3919-3927.

Seow C.J., Chue, S.C., & Wong, W.S. (2002). Piceatannol, a Syk-selective tyrosine kinase inhibitor, attenuated antigen challenge of guinea pig airways in vitro. *European Journal of Pharmacology,* Vol.443, No.1-3, (May 2002), pp. 189-196.

Shi, Y., Tohyama, Y., Kadono, T., He, J., Miah, S.M., Hazama, R., Tanaka, C., Tohyama, K., & Yamamura, H. (2006). Protein-tyrosine kinase Syk is required for pathogen engulfment in complement-mediated phagocytosis. *Blood,* Vol.107, No.11, (June 2006), pp. 4554-4562.

Song, X., & Norman, A.W. (1998). 1Alpha,25-dihydroxyvitamin D3 and phorbol ester mediate the expression of alkaline phosphatase in NB4 acute promyelocytic leukemia cells. *Leukemia Research,* Vol.22, No.1, (January 1998), pp. 69-76.

Stephens, L., Ellson, C., & Hawkins, P. (2002). Roles of PI3Ks in leukocyte chemotaxis and phagocytosis. *Current Opinion in Cell Biology,* Vol.14, No.2, (April 2002), pp. 203–213.

Stricker, J., Falzone, T., & Gardel, M.L. (2010). Mechanics of the F-actin cytoskeleton. *Journal of Biomechanics,* Vol.43, No.1, (January 2010), pp. 9-14.

Takenawa, T., & Itoh, T. (2001). Phosphoinositides, key molecules for regulation of actin cytoskeletal organization and membrane traffic from the plasma membrane. *Biochimica et Biophysica Acta,* Vol.1533, No.3, (October 2001), pp. 190-106.

Tallman, M. (2007). Treatment of relapsed or refractory acute promyelocytic leukemia. *Best Practice & Research Clinical Haematology,* Vol.20, No.1, (March 2007), pp. 57-65.

Tuosto, L., Michel, F., & Acuto, O. (1996). p95vav associates with tyrosine-phosphorylated SLP-76 in antigen-stimulated T cells. *The Journal of Experimental Medicine,* Vol.184, No.3, (September 1996), pp. 1161–1166.

Tybulewicz, V.L. (2005). Vav-family proteins in T-cell signalling. *Current Opinion in Immunology,* Vol.17, No.3, (June 2005), 267-274.

Vedham, V., Phee, H., & Coggeshall, K.M. (2005). Vav activation and function as a rac guanine nucleotide exchange factor in macrophage colony-stimulating factor-induced macrophage chemotaxis. *Molecular and Cellular Biology,* Vol.25, No.10, (May 2005), pp. 4211-4220.

Visani, G., Tosi, P., Ottaviani, E., Zaccaria, A., Baccini, C., Manfroi, S., Pastano, R., Remiddi, C., Morelli, A., Molinari, A.L., Zanchini, R., & Tura, S. (1996). All-trans retinoic acid and in vitro cytokine production by acute promyelocytic leukemia cells. *European Journal of Haematology,* Vol.57, No.4, (October 1996), pp. 301–306.

Von Mikecz, A. (2006). The nuclear ubiquitin-proteasome system. *Journal of Cell Science,* Vol.119, No.10, (May 2006), pp. 1977-1984.

Wan, J., Wang, J., Cheng, H., Yu, Y. Xing, G., Oiu, Z., Qian, X., & He, F.(2001). Proteomic analysis of apoptosis initiation induced by all-trans retinoic acid in human acute promyelocytic leukemia cells. *Electrophoresis,* Vol.22, No.14, (August 2001), pp. 3026-3037.

Wang, D., Jensen, R., Gendeh, G., Williams, K. & Pallavicini, M.G. (2004). Proteome and transcriptome analysis of retinoic acid-induced differentiation of human acute promyelocytic leukemia cells, NB4. *Journal of Proteome Research,* Vol.3, No.3, (May-June 2004), pp. 627-635.

Wang, F., Herzmark, P., Weiner, O.D., Srinivasan, S., Servant, G., & Bourne, H.R. (2002). Lipid products of PI3Ks maintain persistent cell polarity and directed motility in neutrophils. *Nature Cell Biology,* Vol.4, No.7, (July 2002), pp. 513–518.

Wells, C.M., Bhavsar, P.J., Evans, I.R., Vigorito, E., Turner, M., Tybulewicz, V., & Ridley A.J. (2005). Vav1 and Vav2 play different roles in macrophage migration and cytoskeletal organization. *Experimental Cell Research,* Vol.1, No.2, (November 2005), pp. 303-310.

Yang, L., Zhao, H., Li, S.W., Ahrens, K., Collins, C., Eckenrode, S., Ruan, Q.G., McIndoe, R.A., & She, J.X. (2003). Gene expression profiling during all-trans retinoic acid-induced cell differentiation of acute promyelocytic leukemia cells. *The Journal of Molecular Diagnostics,* Vol.5, No.4, (November 2003), pp. 212-221.

Yu, B., Martins, R.S., Li, P., Amarasinghe, G.K., Umetani, J., Fernandez-Zapico, M.E., Billadeau,D.D., Machius, M., Tomchick, D.R., Rosen, M.K. (2010). Structural and Energetic Mechanisms of Cooperative Autoinhibition and Activation of Vav1. *Cell,* Vol.140, (January 22), pp. 246–256.

Zhang, R., Tsai, F.Y., & Orkin, S.H. (1994). Hematopoietic development of vav-/- mouse embryonic stem cells. *Proceedings of the National Academy of Sciences of the United States of America* Vol.91, No.26, (December 1994), pp. 12755-12759.

Zou, L., Wu, Y., Pei, L., Zhong, D., Gen, M., Zhao, T., Wu, J., Ni, B., Mou, Z., Han, J., Chen, Y., Zhi, Y. (2005). Identification of leukemia-associated antigens in chronic myeloid leukemia by proteomic analysis. *Leukemia Research,* Vol.29, No.12, (December 2005), pp. 1387-1391.

15

p15INK4b, a Tumor Suppressor in Acute Myeloid Leukemia

Joanna Fares[1,2], Linda Wolff[1] and Juraj Bies[1]
[1]*Laboratory of Cellular Oncology, National Cancer Institute, NIH, Bethesda, Maryland,*
[2]*Georgetown University, Department of Biochemistry and Molecular Biology, Washington DC, USA*

1. Introduction

p15INK4b expression is lost in a striking 80% of all patients suffering from acute myeloid leukemia (AML). Specific inactivation of the gene by aberrant promoter hypermethylation is also detected in about 50% of patients diagnosed with myelodysplastic syndromes (MDS) and almost 60% of patients with myeloproliferative disorders (MPD). More importantly, a strong correlation between the methylation levels of *p15INK4b* and poor prognosis is now well established in these patients. Hypermethylation levels also provide a marker for subsequent transformation and progression of the disease to a more aggressive phenotype. These clinical observations establish the repression of *p15INK4b* expression by promoter hypermethylation as the most prevalent genetic abnormality in myeloid leukemia. The *p15INK4b* gene (also referred to as *CDKN2B* and *MTS2*) encodes a 15kDa cyclin dependent kinase inhibitor (CDKI). Specific and preferential epigenetic targeting of *p15INK4b* for silencing over other CDKIs such as *p16INK4a* and *p21WAF/CIP* in AML, MDS and MPD patients strongly supports a role for this protein as a tumor suppressor in hematological malignancies of the myeloid lineage.

This chapter provides a review of the literature outlining the high prevalence of *p15INK4b* loss of expression in human myeloid malignancies, as well as the latest research carried out in mice which supports a role for p15Ink4b as a tumor suppressor. It also focuses on the well established function of p15INK4b in the control of the cell cycle, as well as its role during early and late myeloid cells development. Finally, this chapter discusses the multiple mechanisms by which *p15INK4b* is silenced and presents a few examples of clinical studies of drugs that target *p15INK4b* for re-expression. These include treatments for reversing aberrant DNA methylation, and are currently being tested and used for the therapy of MDS and AML.

2. Role of p15INK4b in myeloid malignancies

2.1 Inactivation in human AML and MDS

p15INK4b silencing by promoter hypermethylation occurs almost exclusively in cancers of the hematopoietic system, and is observed in acute leukemias of myeloid (AML) and lymphoid (ALL) origins (Drexler, 1998). Aberrant hypermethylation occurs at the gene's

CpG islands which extend throughout the promoter region, exon 1 and part of intron 1 (Herman et al., 1996). DNA methylation is the addition of methyl groups on cytosine bases on the DNA molecules of mammalian cells which affects gene expression (Deaton et al., 2011). Methylation is carried out by the enzymes DNA methyltransferases (DNMT) which catalyze the reaction converting cytosine to 5-methylcytosine (Bird et al., 2002). In the earlier studies DNA methylation was assessed by southern blotting and methylation-specific PCR technique and more recently by more sensitive assays including bisulfate pyrosequencing and genome-wide sequencing methods (Deaton et al., 2011).

Despite the broad clinical diversity of AML, with more than a hundred cytogenetic alterations described (Vardiman et al., 2002; Trost et al., 2006), aberrant methylation of *p15INK4b* has been reported in up to 80% of patients with primary and secondary AML. Hypermethylation levels have been shown to correlate with a reduction in the mRNA and the protein expression levels of p15INK4b (Cameron et al., 1999; Matsuno et al., 2005). Furthermore, density of the methylation has been shown to vary greatly between and within AML patients and its levels closely correlate with the degree of transcriptional repression (Aggerholm et al., 1999, Cameron et al., 1999). AML classification into ten different subtypes was originally defined by the French-American-British (FAB) cooperative group (Bennett et al., 1976, 1985). Numerous studies have been conducted to assess the methylation levels of *p15INK4b* on samples of patients with AML across the different FAB subtypes (Herman et al., 1996, 1997; Aggerholm et al., 1999; Guo et al., 2000; Chim et al., 2001a, 2001b; Christiansen et al., 2003; Garcia-Manero et al., 2003; Teofili et al., 2003; Shimamoto et al., 2005). In patients with adult and childhood AML, hypermethylation of *p15INK4b* in cells isolated from bone marrow and peripheral blood is observed in nearly all morphological FAB subtypes. Higher frequencies are generally observed in the M1, M2, M3 and M4 subtypes than in the M5, M6 or M7 subtypes and are found to occur in the vast majority of the patients' leukemic cells (Aggerholm et al., 1999; Wong et al., 2000; Shimamoto et al., 2005; Tsellou et al., 2005). In patients with therapy-induced AML (t-AML), aberrant methylation of *p15INK4b* (in over 90% of patients) is found to be independent from the patient's type of previous therapy which ranges from alkylating agents, topoisomerase II inhibitors to radiotherapy (Christiansen et al., 2003).

A similar pattern of aberrant methylation is also well documented in patients with MDS (Uchida et al., 1997; Quesnel et al., 1998; Aoki et al., 2000; Tien et al., 2001; Christiansen et al., 2003; Teofili et al., 2003). The FAB classification system for MDS is mainly based on the percentage of blast cells in the bone marrow and the peripheral blood and the degree of cytopenia (Bennet et al., 1982). Methylation levels have also been shown to increase during follow-up and in conversion to overt AML (Tien et al., 2001, Christiansen et al., 2003). Importantly, aberrant DNA methylation of *p15INK4b* was found to be one of the most dominant molecular events in MDS progression to AML (Jiang et al., 2009). Similar to AML, cytogenetics of MDS is also a crucial factor in the prognosis and development of the disease (Haase et al., 2007). The World Health Organization (WHO) classification system for myeloid neoplasms was developed and takes into consideration both morphology and cytogenetic abnormalities (Harris et al., 2000). In MDS patients, methylation of *p15INK4b* is associated with an increased percentage of immature myeloblasts in the bone marrow (Christiansen et al., 2003). The presence of DNA hypermethylation at the *p15INK4b* promoter is found predominantly in high risk MDS patients with increased levels being reported in the subtypes characterized by advanced stages of the disease such as refractory anemia with excess blasts (RAEB). Reduced levels are reported in patients with the early stages of MDS such as refractory anemia (RA) and refractory anemia with ringed sideroblasts (RARS) (Uchida et al., 1997; Christiansen et al., 2003). However, more recently, it was found that even in patients with the RARS subtype, which falls within the lower risk of MDS, *p15INK4b* was found to be the most frequently methylated gene (>20% of cases) of 25 known tumor suppressors that were evaluated in the study (Valencia et al., 2011). Although most studies have been conducted in MDS in adults, comparable levels of aberrant methylation patterns have been observed in pediatric MDS patients as well (Hasegawa et al., 2005), and a similar correlation with the disease subtypes has been established (Rodrigues et al., 2010).

In chronic myelomonocytic leukemia (CMML), aberrant methylation of *p15INK4b* is found in about 60% of cases and is associated with a high proportion of blastic transformation (Tessema et al., 2003). CMML is a disease that was originally categorized under myelodysplastic disorders, but is now classified by the WHO as a disorder that bridges MDS with myeloproliferative features (Harris et al., 1999). In these patients, genomic sequencing techniques have revealed that hypermethylation spans a wide area in the 5′ region of the gene and is correlated with reduced expression of the mRNA levels. High variability between and within individual patients, consistent with observations in AML patients, were also reported (Tessema et al., 2003, Aggerholm et al., 1999, Cameron et al., 1999). In the pediatric form of the disease, juvenile myelomonocytic leukemia (JMML), *p15INK4b* hypermethylation is found to be a less frequent, however, still significant event (17% of cases) (Hasegawa et al., 2005).

With regards to cytogenetic abnormalities, *p15INK4b* methylation levels have been found to occur at higher frequencies in AML/MDS patients with an unfavorable karyotype (Wong et al., 2000; Galm et al., 2005; Shimamoto et al., 2005; Markus et al., 2007). Cases with unmethylated or low levels of hypermethylated *p15INK4b* were associated with normal karyotype or with those karyotypic abnormalities that are associated with a favorable prognosis (Wong et al., 2000; Markus et al., 2007). Studies have consistently reported an increased tendency for *p15INK4b* hypermethylation in unfavorable cytogenetics (Shimamoto et al., 2005). These results suggest interplay between *p15INK4b* loss of expression and the frequent chromosomal translocations, inversions and deletions observed in AML and MDS. The mechanisms underlying *p15INK4b* hypermethylation are not completely understood, but a few theories involving maintaining and de-novo DNA methylation through action of DNA methyltransferases (DNMT), as well as histone modification pathways have been suggested to play a role (Paul et al., 2010). Specifically in t-AML and therapy-induced MDS (t-MDS), deletion or loss of chromosome arm 7q, which is the most common cytogenetic abnormality in those categories, has been found to be closely associated with hypermethylation of *p15INK4b* (Christiansen et al., 2003).

p15INK4b is now used as an independent prognosticator in AML and MDS (Chim et al., 2001b; Teofili et al., 2003; Christiansen et al., 2003; Shimamoto et al., 2005; Chim et al., 2006). In the many categories of the diseases, aberrant *p15INK4b* methylation levels have been associated with a generally poor prognosis. In studies that monitor patients across all AML FAB subtypes, patients without *p15INK4b* hypermethylation at diagnosis had increased complete remission rates which also correlated with increased survival times (Shimamoto et al., 2005; Deneberg et al., 2010). Consistent with these observations, in APL patients, abnormal *p15INK4b* methylation was associated with a shorter disease-free survival (DFS) period and a higher incidence of relapse during the 5-year follow up period (Teofili et al.,

2003). In the relapsed patients, the *p15INK4b* hypermethylation levels remained persistent following treatment. In contrast, the patients without detectable hypermethylation displayed prolonged survival (Chim et al., 2001b). Additionally, as previously stated, patients with MDS with high methylation levels at diagnosis had a significantly higher chance of the disease progressing to AML (Tien et al., 2001; Jiang et al., 2009). It was also reported that in early stage of MDS, the *p15INK4b* hypermethylation is a negative risk factor for patients, closely correlating with leukemic transformation (Aggerholm et al., 2006). The same correlation has been shown in patients with t-MDS, in which methylation resulted in significantly shorter survival (Christiansen et al., 2003). A recent study showed that the high levels of methylation in lower risk MDS categories suggest a poor prognosis in those patients as well (Valencia et al, 2011). In JMML p15INK4b hypermethylation was associated with reduced overall survival rates and higher relapse of the disease following hematopoietic stem cell transplantation (Olk-Batz et al., 2011). All these results suggest that lack of *p15INK4b* expression, mediated by promoter hypermethylation, not only affects the prognosis in patients with AML and MDS, but can be used to predict the outcome of the diseases.

The studies described above confirm that aberrant hypermethylation levels of *p15INK4b* have important prognostic implications for clinical monitoring in MDS and assessment of risk of progression into AML. However, its potential use as a biomarker in leukemia excluded estimation of minimal residual disease in patients who have achieved clinical remission, and its implications in terms of subsequent relapse. A study aiming at addressing this issue, evaluated *p15INK4b* methylation levels in AML patients in complete clinical remission (Agrawal et al., 2007). The study reported that even in remission, leukemia patients that harbored a significant amount of methylation in the bone marrow cells had a higher risk for leukemia relapse. Moreover, the time of disease-free survival was found to be significantly reduced in correlation with the amount of residual hypermethylation of the *p15Ink4b* gene. Concurrently, low levels of *p15INK4b* methylation during complete remission were associated with reduced relapse rates during the 12 month follow-up. It was suggested that analysis of *p15INK4b* methylation levels during clinical remission can be potentially used as a prognosticator for the occurrence of relapse (Agrawal et al., 2007).

In recent years, it has been suggested in a number of studies that DNA methylation of *p15INK4b* could also help predict response to therapy (Grovdal et al., 2007; Shen et al., 2009). Grövdal et al. (2007) studied DNA methylation patterns in older patients with high risk MDS and AML following MDS. Patients were treated with conventional induction therapy. Methylation levels of *p15INK4b*, *E-cadherin*, and *HIC1* (hypermethylated in cancer 1), were assessed prior to initiation of treatment. Abnormal levels of methylation of *p15INK4b* alone did not correlate with decreased complete remission (CR), but all patients with all three genes methylated did not achieve CR. Another study, in which patients with MDS and AML were treated with the DNA methyltransferase inhibitor 5-azacytidine (5-aza-C), reported consistent results with these observations (Raj et al., 2007; Tran et al., 2011). Patients with levels exceeding 24% methylation in the *p15Ink4b* promoter region did not respond to treatment (Raj et al., 2007). The possibility of using methylation of *p15INK4b* as an indicator for treatment outcome is still under investigation. However, results suggest that studying *p15INK4b* methylation density in conjunction with other altered genes at diagnosis and monitoring its levels following treatment might have predictive information with respect to the patient's response to treatment.

Although hypermethylation is the most common mode of inactivation of *p15INK4b* in myeloid neoplasms, other silencing mechanisms have also been described. In AML with chromosome 16 inversion (*inv16*), the overall *p15INK4b* methylation levels are found to be very low and almost comparable to levels in normal patients. However, expression of the gene is severely suppressed. In this type of AML, the inversion (16) results in a fusion protein between the core binding factor (CBFβ) and the smooth myosin heavy chain gene (SMMHC). This chimeric transcription factor CBFβ-SMMHC binds directly to the promoter of *p15INK4b* and represses its expression (Markus et al., 2007). These results further emphasize an important role of *p15INK4b* silencing in leukemogenesis of the myeloid lineage, and suggest, that in the absence of a repressive epigenetic event, other mechanisms may result in inhibition of *p15INK4b* expression (Markus et al., 2007).

2.2 Inactivation in other types of human leukemias

In B and T cell acute lymphoblastic leukemias (B-ALL, T-ALL), *p15INK4b* hypermethylation as well as deletion of the entire 9p21 locus which includes *p15INK4b*, *p16INK4a* and *ARF* genes has been reported (Roussel, 1999; Ruas et al., 1998). Homozygous deletions of *p16INK4a* and *p15INK4b* are found in approximately 30% of childhood acute lymphoblastic leukemia at first presentation, with striking rates in T-ALL (60 to 80%), and lower rates in B-cell precursor ALL (5 to 20%) (Drexler HG, 1998; Chim et al., 2001a). Further studies have analyzed methylation levels of the two genes in these disease categories specifically in terms of overall survival and absence of relapse at 6 years of follow-up. *p15INK4b* and *p16INK4a* methylation levels were found to occur at similar rates (35%) in adults and children with mature B-ALL (Graf-Einsiedel et al., 2002). Deletion of the entire locus was observed in 12% and 30% of children and adults, respectively. Interestingly, results show that deletion is associated with poor overall survival (OS) in adults only, but not in children (Van Zutven et al., 2005; Mirebeau et al., 2006; Kim et al., 2009). Furthermore, it did not affect the type of relapse or DFS time in children. In untreated adult patients with precursor B-ALL, high methylation levels of *p15INK4b* (found in 43% of patients) were significantly associated with decreased DFS at 4 years (Hoshino et al., 2002). Recent methylation profiles in 95 children with ALL supported older studies showing that methylation of *p15INK4b* occurred predominantly in T-ALL as opposed to B-ALL, and *p15INK4b* is one of the most commonly methylated genes among the 14 genes analyzed (Takeuchi et al., 2011). A clear correlation between increased methylation and prognoses in T-ALL has not been established.

2.3 p15Ink4b as a tumor suppressor in mice

To define the role of p15INK4b as a tumor suppressor in AML, mouse models have been developed and characterized (Latres et al., 2000; Wolff et al., 2003a, 2004; Bies et al., 2010). These have provided strong experimental evidence to support the hypothesis that loss of p15INK4b function plays an important role in the development of myeloid leukemia.

A p15Ink4b$^{-/-}$ mouse model was first described by Latres et al. (2000). Mice were generated by genetic targeting with elimination of the second coding exon of the p15Ink4b gene. Knockout mice were viable, fertile, and did not exhibit any behavioral abnormalities. Mouse embryonic fibroblasts were found to have a higher proliferation rate and plating efficiency when compared to their wild type counterparts. More importantly, they were more susceptible to transformation with *c-myc* and *ras* oncogenes, confirming the reported results that p15Ink4b participates in the tumor suppressor activity triggered after inappropriate oncogenic *ras* activation of the Raf-Mek-Erk pathway (Malumbres et al., 2000). However, with respect to AML, deleting p15Ink4b did not result in leukemogenesis in these mice. Of note, extramedullary hematopoiesis and lymphoid hyperplasia in the spleen were observed in mice aged less than 9 months and resulted in death of over 75% of the mice at an older age. Taken together, these experimental results were the first to suggest that p15Ink4b might be playing a tumor suppressor role in AML (Latres et al., 2000).

A role for p15Ink4b in myeloid neoplasia in mice was first supported by the finding that retrovirus-induced AML had hypermethylation of the CpG promoter region of the *p15Ink4b* gene. Based upon this, further mouse models were developed to determine if loss of p15Ink4b increases susceptibility to myeloid leukemia when additional oncogenic events were provided by retroviral insertional mutagenesis. For these studies, a specific retrovirus with a broad tropism and the capability of inducing a high incidence of myeloid leukemia was constructed (Wolff et al., 2003b and 2004). It consists of a recombinant virus incorporating Moloney murine leukemia virus (Mo-MuLV) sequences, and regulatory LTR sequences of retrovirus 4070A. The recombinant virus, named MOL4070LTR, combines the capacity of 4070A to accelerate myeloid disease with the wide tropism of Mo-MuLV, and successfully produced myeloid disease when inoculated intraperitoneally into wild-type FVB and BALB/c mice as neonates (Wolff et al., 2003b). The *p15Ink4b* knockout mice were developed using the same targeting vector as described by Latres et al. (2000), and MOL4070LTR was inoculated into neonates. While there was no incidence of disease in control wild-type mice (p15Ink4b$^{+/+}$), a significant percentage of heterozygous mice (p15Ink4b$^{+/-}$) developed myeloid leukemia within a year. Surprisingly, a smaller percentage of homozygous knockout mice (p15Ink4b$^{-/-}$) developed myeloid tumors (Wolff et al., 2003a). Further experiments demonstrated that in heterozygous p15Ink4b$^{+/-}$ mice, the second remaining *p15Ink4b* allele was actually hypermethylated, with a reduction of its mRNA expression. This data supported the fact that p15Ink4b functions as a tumor suppressor for myeloid leukemia, however, it was difficult to explain why mice heterozygous for the null allele were more susceptible than homozygous null mice. One explanation might be that in the homozygous null mice, *p15Ink4b* is lost in all the tissues and loss of expression in one tissue may have compensating effects on loss in another tissue.

A new mouse system in which deletion of the gene is restricted to the myeloid lineage was developed to mimic more closely myeloid lineage disease in man (Bies et al., 2010). The mouse strain utilizes a Cre-loxP system for conditional deletion of the *p15Ink4b* gene through action of Cre recombinase exclusively expressed in blood cells of the myeloid lineage (Clausen et al., 1999). In this model, Cre recombinase specifically recognizes loxP sites to mediate efficient excision of exon 2 of the *p15Ink4b* gene in myeloid cells. In order to monitor disease development in mice with targeted *p15Ink4b* deletion (p15Ink4b$^{fl/fl}$ LysMcre), white cell counts were performed in circulating blood from targeted and wild-type animals from different age groups. Interestingly, p15Ink4b$^{fl/fl}$LysMcre mice showed a significant increase in the number of circulating monocytes compared to control mice (p15Ink4b$^{wt/wt}$LysMcre), whereas neutrophils, lymphocytes, platelets and red blood cell counts were not affected. Monocytosis remained in targeted mice beyond 8 months of age, while wild-type mice showed a marked decrease in monocytes resulting in an even greater significance in the statistical comparisons (Figure 3A). Expansion of myelomonocytic cells in the bone marrow (BM) of p15Ink4b$^{fl/fl}$LysMcre mice was also observed. Analysis of BM cells for the cell surface markers Gr-1, Mac-1 and c-Kit revealed that BM cells from p15Ink4b$^{fl/fl}$LysMcre mice had a significant increase in both mature myeloid (Gr-1$^+$/Mac-1$^+$) and monocytic (Gr-1$^{-/lo}$/Mac-1$^+$) cells. This increase correlated with a significantly higher proportion of immature myeloid (Mac-1$^{+/lo}$/c-Kit$^+$) cells in the BM. Inactivation of *p15Ink4b* in myeloid cells promoted a mild preleukemic myeloproliferative-like disease (Bies et al., 2010). A small percentage of the targeted mice spontaneously progressed to a form of leukemia featuring an increased number of mature circulating myeloid cells in the peripheral blood, as well as an increase in the number of progenitors in the BM. The disease observed in mice most closely resembled an advanced form of CMML (Bies et al., 2010). However, the disease did not progress to an acute form of leukemia over the period of 15 months in any of the mice. These results were in agreement with studies carried on in the embryonal p15Ink4b$^{-/-}$ mice, and suggested that inactivation of the *p15Ink4b* gene without an additional genetic/epigenetic hit is not sufficient to cause acute leukemia. Retrovirus-induced mutagenesis in p15Ink4b$^{fl/fl}$LysMcre mice was used to identify genetic changes that

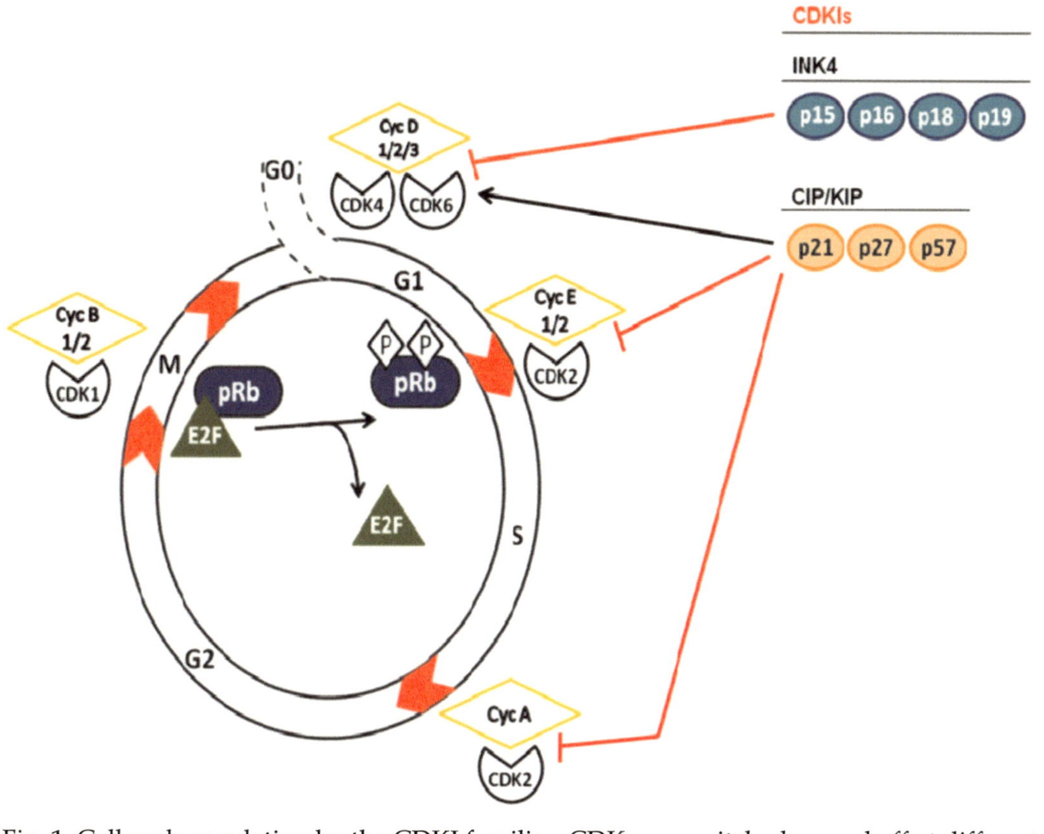

Fig. 1. Cell cycle regulation by the CDKI families. CDKs are switched on and off at different times during the cell cycle; the cyclins Ds-dependent kinases 4 and 6, and CDK2/cyclin E, CDK2/cyclin A regulate G1 progression and entry into the S phase. CDK1/cyclin B regulates entry and exit from mitosis. The CDK/cyclin complexes phosphorylate pRb to allow for the transcription of genes under the control of E2Fs which include factors necessary for cell cycle progression. CIP/KIP family members of CDKI can be either activators or inhibitors of cyclin/CDK assembly (Sherr & Roberts, 1999).

could cooperate with the loss of p15Ink4b in leukemia development. Mice inoculated with the MOL4070LTR retrovirus were monitored for 15 months for signs of disease. Control mice developed leukemia with low penetrance, whereas the incidence of retrovirus-induced leukemia was statistically highly significant for the p15Ink4b$^{fl/fl}$LysMcre animals. Additionally, phenotypic analyses of tumor cells demonstrated a strong bias towards the development of AML in the knockout animals. Myeloid-specific inactivation of *p15Ink4b* results in retrovirus-induced development of tumors mostly monocytic (F4/80$^+$, F4/80$^+$/Mac1$^+$) and myelomonocytic (F4/80$^+$/Mac1$^+$/Gr-1$^+$), whereas there was an equal distribution of lymphoid and monocytic tumors in the control mice (Figure 3B). Results generated using this model complement the embryonal *p15nk4b*$^{-/-}$ studies and demonstrate an active role for *p15Ink4b* silencing in promoting the establishment of preleukemic conditions. These results also provided strong experimental evidence that p15Ink4b functions as a tumor suppressor for myeloid leukemia development (Bies et al., 2010).

3. Conventional and novel functions of p15INK4b

3.1 p15INK4B as a regulator of the cell cycle

p15INK4b belongs to the INK4 family of cyclin-dependent kinases inhibitors (CDKIs). The family comprises three other members - p16INK4a, p18INK4c and p19INK4d and is one of two families of CDKIs that have been identified and defined based on their structure and CDK specificities. INK4 proteins all show a high and exclusive specificity towards the activity of cyclin-dependent kinase 4 (CDK 4) and cyclin-dependent kinase 6 (CDK6) during the early and mid-G1 phase of the cell cycle (Sherr & Roberts, 1999). The cell cycle is comprised of 4 phases, G1, S, G2 (also referred to as interphase), and M phase (mitosis). Entrance of cells from the quiescent G0/G1 phase into cycle is governed by the actions of kinases CDK4/CDK6 and CDK2 that are activated by cyclins Ds and Es, respectively (Figure 1).

During the transition to S phase, CDKs hyperphosphorylate pRb causing its dissociation from the nuclear transcription factors E2Fs. E2Fs regulate the transcription of genes which are required for the completion of the cell cycle and include cyclins A and E, thymidine synthetase and PCNA (Korenjak & Brehm, 2005). Throughout the S, G2 and M phases, pRb is kept in a hyperphosphorylated state by an orchestrated mechanism that involves sequential activities of multiple cyclins/CDKs (Sherr & Roberts, 1999). INK4 proteins inhibit CDKs/cyclin Ds complexes and, therefore, function in G1-S checkpoint control. When INK4 proteins block formation of these complexes, the pRb is in a hypophosphorylated, active state and interacts with E2F to inhibit its function (Korenjak & Brehm, 2005). Structural studies have demonstrated that INK4 proteins perform their inhibitory activity by allosteric competition with cyclins Ds to bind CDK4 and CDK6. CDK4/6-INK4s protein complexes have reduced affinity toward the D-type cyclins (Jeffrey et al., 2000; Yuan et al 2000).

p15INK4b and *p16INK4a* are tandemly linked on human chromosome 9p21 within a 40kb DNA region, whereas *p18INK4c* and *p19INK4d* are located in the chromosomal regions 1p32.3 and 19p13.2, respectively. The 9p21 chromosomal locus is referred to as the *INK4/ARF* locus has been tightly linked to the formation of many types of tumors (Nobori et al., 1994). In addition to *p15INK4b* and *p16INK4a*, it also encodes a third gene called *p14ARF*, originally identified as an alternative transcript of *p16INK4a* (Figure 2). *p14ARF* is transcribed from exon 1β and exons 2 and 3 of *p16INK4a*, but using a different reading frame (Figure 2). The p14ARF protein (p19Arf in mouse) is immunologically and functionally unrelated to the p16INK4a protein; they are not considered to be isoforms and do not share sequence homology or overlapping roles in the cell (Ozenne et al., 2010; Sherr CJ, 2006). Furthermore, p14ARF bears little or no structural similarities with the INK4 family members, and is unable to bind or inhibit CDKs. It is not considered to be part of the INK4 family of inhibitors, but it still participates in the negative regulation of the cell cycle by antagonizing the effects of MDM2, a ubiquitin ligase that targets the tumor suppressor protein p53 for degradation by the 26S proteasome (Ruas et al., 1998).

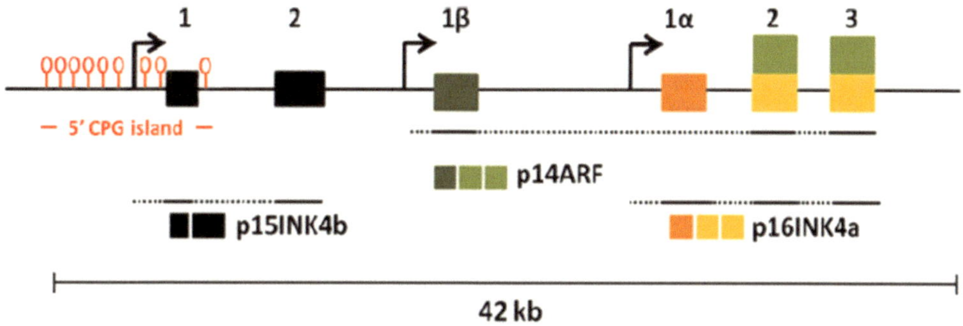

Fig. 2. 9p21 chromosomal locus showing the promoters and exons that are involved in the transcription of *p15INK4b*, *p14ARF* and *p16INK4a* genes. The CpG island is depicted for the *p15INK4b* gene only and extends throughout the promoter region, exon 1 and part of intron 1 (Herman et al., 1996).

INK4 family members are highly conserved among species, with over 90% identity between the human and the corresponding mouse proteins. In human, the four proteins share roughly 40% sequence homology with each other and have a very closely related structure, characterized by the presence of ankyrin motif tandem repeats. Four ankyrin repeats are found in p15INK4b and p16INK4a, and five repeats in p18INK4c and p19INK4d (Yuan et al., 2000). Ankyrin motif repeats consist of a helix-loop-helix structure that promotes protein-protein interaction (Li et al., 1999). Structural studies involving programmed mutations and generation of chimeric proteins have revealed that the third ankyrin repeat is necessary for the interaction with CDK4 and CDK6, and is responsible for the inhibitory activity of these CDKIs. Crystallography work on the CDK6 bound p16INK4a, p18INK4c and p19INK4d suggested that the INK4 proteins bind to one side of the catalytic cleft, opposite to the cyclin binding site, and that binding and recognition are mediated mostly via hydrogen bonds (Brotherton et al., 1998; Noh et al., 1999; Russo et al., 1998). INK4 proteins were found not to interfere with the cyclin binding site which is consistent with the presence of INK4s/cyclin Ds/CDK4 or CDK6 ternary complexes. When bound in the absence of cyclin D, they cause a conformation switch in CDK4 and CDK6 which distorts the cyclin and the ATP-binding sites leading to rapid recycling of unbound D-type cyclins by the ubiquitin-dependent 26S proteasome. The specificity towards CDK 4 and CDK6 was found to be due primarily to the critical residues involved in the hydrogen bonds with INK4 proteins which are conserved exclusively in CDK4 and CDK6, but not in the other CDKs (Russo et al., 1998). Interestingly, several of the residues necessary for recognition and binding have been reported to be mutated in cancer (Li et al., 1999).

The structural similarities observed between the INK4 proteins are consistent with the shared biological and biochemical properties of these molecules. However, the expression pattern of each of the human INK4 proteins appears to be highly specific to the cell type and tissue localization, as well as the differentiation stage of the cells (Shwaller et al., 1997; Thullberg et al., 2000). For instance, in normal hematopoietic cells, the expression of p15INK4b is shown to be lineage restricted, and is mainly detected in monocytes and lymphocytes, but not in any of the erythroid precursors (Teofili et al., 1998). Myeloid-restricted expression of *p15INK4b* is observed in peripheral blood and bone marrow and its levels are reported to be increased during megakaryocyte and monocyte/macrophage differentiation (Furukawa et al., 2000; Teofili et al., 2001; Haviernik et al., 2003).

p15INK4b, in particular, is an important downstream effector of anti-proliferative signaling by the transforming growth factor- β1 (TGF-β1) (Hannon & Beach, 1994). In different human and mouse cell lines, treatment with this negative growth factor, as well as interleukin 6 (IL-6) or Interferon β (IFN- β) leads to G0/G1 cell cycle arrest (Schmidt et al., 2004; Haviernik et al., 2003). Treatment with TGF-β1 induces a significant increase in the transcription levels of *p15INK4b*, but also induces a major increase in p15INK4b protein stability (Sandhu et al., 1997). Following treatment with TGF-β1, p15INK4b-CDK4/6 complexes are more abundant compared to the Cyclin D-Cdk4 complexes indicating strong inhibitor activity (Sandhu et al., 1997). In contrast to *p15INK4b*, whose expression is absent in hematopoietic stem cells, but increases as the cells mature along the myeloid lineage, *p16INK4a* is highly expressed in hematopoietic stem cells, and down-regulated with differentiation of all lineages (Furukawa et al., 2000). *p18INK4c* is found to be the most homogeneously and abundantly expressed member of the family, whereas *p19INK4d* is the most restricted, and its expression is limited to lymphoid cell, epithelial cells, seminiferous tubes and adrenal gland cells (Thullberg et al., 2000). The differential expression patterns of the INK4 proteins, suggest non-overlapping physiological functions.

Despite their common function in regulation of the cell cycle, the four members are found to be differentially involved in tumorigenesis. Mouse knock-out models along with genetic screenings of human tumors and gene expression profiling of cell lines have been used to help elucidate the role of these cell cycle inhibitors in the establishment and progression of cancer (Cánepa et al., 2007). In concordance with the molecular analysis of human tumor tissues, mice deficient in different Ink4 proteins display an increased susceptibility to the development of various types of tumors with variable penetrance. *p16INK4a* is a family member that has a prominent role in carcinomas of the pancreas and the bladder, glioblastomas, leukemias and melanomas among others. Its expression is lost by several mechanisms including point mutations, small deletion and epigenetic modifications which have been reported in thousands of human cancers (Serrano et al., 1996; Krimpenfort et al., 2001). On the other hand, as previously described, *p15INK4b* is noted to be silenced primarily by an epigenetic mechanism in human cancers, and loss of its expression through hypermethylation of its promoter region is well documented in hematologic neoplasms in particular (Drexler HG, 1998; Roussel, 1999). In these types of cancers, inactivation of *p15INK4b* has been reported in the absence of aberrant modification or deletion of *p16INK4a*. In contrast with p15INK4b and p16INK4a, p18INK4c was originally found to play a more limited role as a human tumor suppressor, and p19INK4d is not thought to be involved in the pathogenesis of cancer (Thullberg et al., 2000). *p18Ink4c*-null mice are viable but display an unusual phenotype with pronounced gigantism, lymphomas and more importantly pituitary hyperplasia (Franklin et al., 1998). Later examination of these mice revealed that p18Ink4c is a haploinsufficient tumor suppressor for spontaneous and carcinogen-induced pituitary tumors and lymphomas (Bai et al., 2003). Loss of p16Ink4a expression was shown to be a necessary event in conjunction with loss of p18Ink4c for the mice to develop aggressive advanced stages of pituitary carcinoma (Morishita et al., 2004). Furthermore, it is now clear that p18INK4c is a tumor suppressor in human glioblastoma multiform and hepatocellular carcinoma (Solomon, 2008a and 2008b). Interestingly, studies in mice deficient for p19Ink4d have not revealed increased susceptibility to any cancer or other proliferative diseases, suggesting a limited or nonexistent role in carcinogenesis (Buchold et al. 2007, Zindy et al, 2000).

Although these cell cycle regulators exhibit overlapping and surely compensatory activities mainly due to their structural similarities (Krimpenfort et al., 2007), their temporal and tissue-restricted expression patterns as well as their differential involvement in the pathogenesis of human cancers clearly suggest that they can harbor specific and distinct functions during development.

3.2 Function as a regulator of cell fate during early myelopoiesis

The strikingly high prevalence of *p15INK4b* loss of expression during the development of myeloid disease in human patients has triggered scientists to explore alternate functions for this CDKI. As a cell cycle regulator, p15INK4b was suggested to be one of the players determining the fine balances in differentiation and proliferation of myeloid cells. To test this hypothesis, the previously described p15Ink4b germline knockout mice as well as murine transplant models were used. Results revealed a novel role for the protein during early and late stages of myeloid cells development (Rosu-Myles et al., 2007, 2008).

Myelopoiesis is the process by which an undifferentiated progenitor cell gives rise to mature differentiated functional myeloid cells. The process takes place in the bone marrow and is driven by a pool of hematopoietic cytokines that have different binding specificities to cell surface markers in a stage and lineage dependent manner. Committed progenitors with a restricted myeloid lineage fate arise from earlier common myeloid progenitor cells (CMP), who themselves originate from hematopoietic stem cells (HSC) (Akashi et al. 2000).

In p15Ink4b knockout mice (p15Ink4b$^{-/-}$), loss of p15Ink4b was found to favor the differentiation of CMPs into granulocyte macrophage progenitors (GMP) which results in an imbalance between the erythroid and myeloid compartments (Rosu-Myles et al 2007). This defect was in the bipotent differentiation capacity of the CMP, and did not affect the frequency of early long-term HSCs, or their ability to self-renew and proliferate. Therefore, this finding differs from the traditional role of p15Ink4b in regulating the cell cycle. As shown in Figure 3A, the increased number of myeloid progenitors was found to occur at the expense of differentiation of CMPs towards the erythroid progenitors .Furthermore, competitive repopulating assays have shown that the defect is intrinsic to the cells. Loss of p15Ink4b provided a competitive advantage over the wild-type cells within the myeloid compartment (Rosu-Myles et al., 2007).

Interestingly, an earlier study carried out in p18Ink4c$^{-/-}$ mice, had shown that this CDKI also impacts cell fate but targets a different cell type. Deletion of p18Ink4c was found to result in a long-term engraftment advantage in HSCs. The observed effects were not due to increased proliferation capacity of the cells, but rather to an enhanced potential of self-renewal of these cells as opposed to differentiation. This lead to an efficient expansion of HSCs as well as hematopoietic progenitor pools, which fully retained their multi-lineage differentiation potential (Yuan et al., 2004).

3.3 Function in cell cycle arrest in late myeloid cell development

In addition to its hypothesized role in cell fate decision of early myeloid progenitors, p15Ink4b is implicated during the late stages of myelopoiesis. In this case its role appears to be the induction of cell-cycle arrest. p15Ink4b expression has been shown to increase specifically during myeloid differentiation in vivo both in human bone marrow and peripheral blood cells (Teofili et al. 2000); and in vitro, in murine M1 myeloblastic cells which undergo monocytic differentiation following treatment with IL-6 (Schmidt et al 2004).

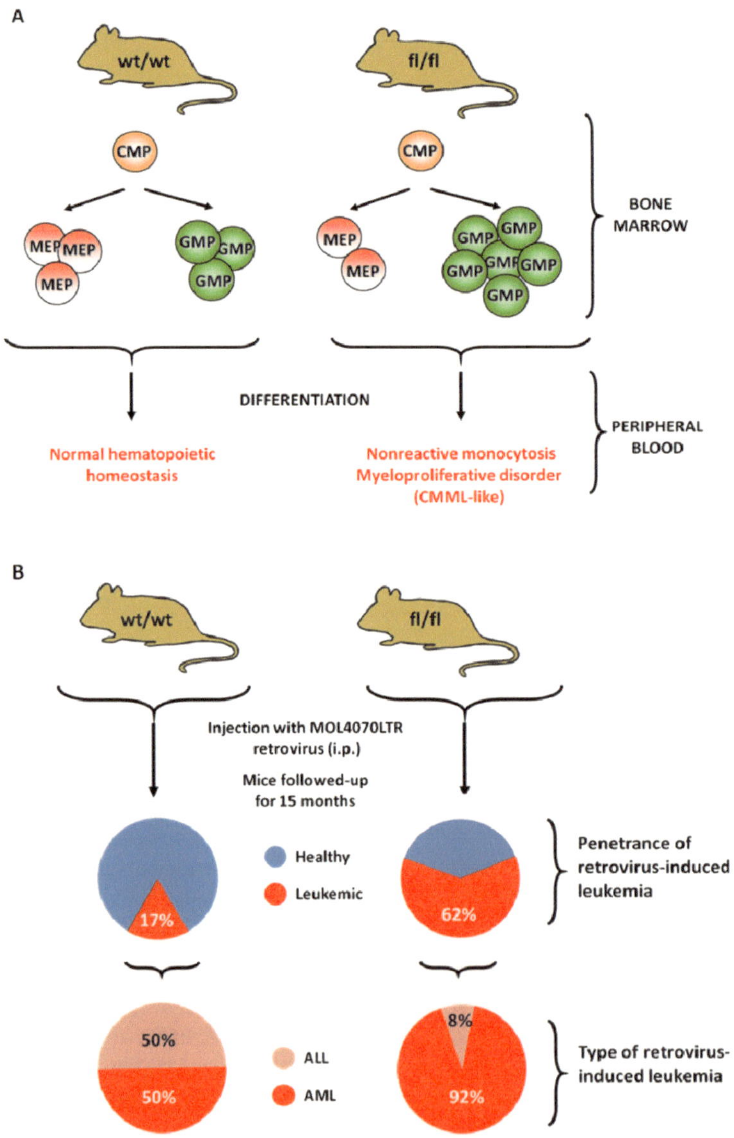

Fig. 3. The loss of p15Ink4b in myeloid lineage results in: A. Imbalance in the myeloid progenitor pools and nonreactive monocytosis; B. Increased incidence of the retrovirus-induced leukemia with preference toward the myeloid phenotype.

The M1 leukemia cell line, does not express p53, proliferates autonomously and is often used as a model for monocytic differentiation. When terminal differentiation is induced in these cells, upregulation of p15Ink4b expression is accompanied by inhibition of Cdk4 kinase activity as well as by a decrease in levels of phosphorylated Rb (Bergh et al., 1999). Furthermore, over-expression of p15Ink4b in M1 cells causes cell cycle arrest in the G1 phase, providing additional evidence for the implication of the protein in maturation and cell cycle inhibition of late stage progenitors (Haviernik et al., 2003). This function is further supported by studies in human CD34+ hematopoietic progenitor cells. When expression of p15INK4b is triggered, higher levels of the protein are associated with transcriptional upregulation of genes known to induce myeloid differentiation, such as the colony stimulating factor 1 receptor gene (c-fms), the myeloperoxidase gene (mpo) and lactoferrin (lf), among others (Furukawa et al 2000). Overexpression of p15INK4b is also linked with a dramatic decrease in early blast progenitor populations and an increase in the numbers of cells that adopt a myeloid morphology (Teofili et al., 2000).

This data suggests that p15INK4b has functions during both the early and late stages of myelopoiesis; in early progenitors, p15Ink4b influences cell fate by altering the balance between myeloid and erythroid progenitors, whereas during late myelopoiesis, p15INK4b appears to be causing withdrawal from the cell-cycle in response to cytokines.

4. Targeting p15INK4b for re-expression in AML and MDS

The reversible nature of epigenetic alterations makes them very attractive therapeutic targets for AML and MDS. In the case of *p15INK4b*, these epigenetic alterations consist of DNA methylation as well as chromatin remodeling by post-transcriptional histone modifications. Studying the association of *p15INK4b* promoter DNA methylation with histone modifications revealed important insight into the interplay of these two types of epigenetic mechanisms (Paul et al., 2010). Histones undergo post-transcriptional modifications that target primarily the N-terminal tail regions, and involve the attachment of phospho, acetyl, methyl, ribosyl, and small ubiquitin-like modifier or ubiquitin groups on the side chains of the different amino acids residues of histone molecules (Biancotto et al., 2010). Acetylation and de-acetylation of lysine residues are catalyzed by two groups of enzymes with opposing actions: histone acetyltransferases (HAT) and histone deacetylases (HDAC) (Jenuwein & Allis, 2001), whereas histone methyltransferases (HMT), and histone demethylases (HDM) control the balance of histone methylations. Similar to DNA methylation, histone modifications are fully biochemically reversible, result in changes in the protein structure and affect the affinity of histone tails to DNA molecules (Varier & Timmers, 2011). Paul et al. (2010) found that in AML cell lines with aberrant *p15INK4b* DNA hypermethylation, the histone 3 trimethylated at lysine 4 (H3K4me3), which is a transcriptional activation mark, was at lower levels than in AML cell lines without hypermethylation. Interestingly, irrespective of the methylation status of *p15INK4b*, this study also reported the presence of the repressive mark H3K27me3 (histone 3 trimethylated at lysine 27) at the 9p21 locus. Human AML blasts with hypermethylation of *p15INK4b* were similarly found to have H3K27me3, but lacked H3K4me3 at the gene.

The tight collaboration of the different epigenetic alterations in silencing the *p15INK4b* gene makes combinatorial therapeutics a promising approach for its reexpression. Importantly, removal of methyl groups from hypermethylated CpG clusters associated with the gene promoter reverses the inhibitory effects and restores normal gene expression (Jones &

Baylin, 2002). The DNMT inhibitor 5-azacytidine (5-aza-C) and its analogue 5-aza-deoxycytidine (5-aza-dC, Decitabine) are powerful hypomethylating agents that are used in the therapy of high-risk MDS and AML. It has been demonstrated that they can lead to the reversal of hypermethylation and subsequent reexpression of the *p15INK4b* gene in patients with MDS (Daskalakis et al., 2002; Farinha et al., 2004; Gore et al., 2006; Santos et al., 2010). It was shown that treatment of patient blasts with hypomethylating agent Decitabine also affects histone modifications. Paul et al. (2010) provided evidence that the levels of H3K4me3 increased with retention of H3K27me3, thus inducing a state of bivalency. The use of other HMT inhibitors such as 3-Deazaneplanocin A (DZNep) have been reported to successfully decrease global DNA methylation levels, but not to induce re-expression of specific genes including *p15INK4b* (Flotho et al., 2009; Miranda et al., 2009).
HDAC inhibitors such as Trichostatin A (TSA) have been used for targeting of histone acetylations. In the case of AML samples with *p15INK4b* hypermethylation, it was shown that TSA treatment alone is insufficient to increase p15INK4b expression levels (Scott et al., 2007; Paul et al., 2010). However, studies that incorporated the use of both HDAC and DNMT inhibitors have proven successful at inducing higher levels of p15INK4b expression (Cameron et al., 1999; Scott et al., 2007; Paul et al., 2010).

5. Conclusion

p15INK4b is a CDK inhibitor whose expression is lost in a very high proportion of patients with MDS and AML. This implicates an important role for the loss of the protein expression in the development of myeloid disease in humans. Its role in myeloid leukemogenesis as a tumor suppressor is now confirmed by research carried out in several mouse models. In addition to its role in inhibiting CDKs to arrest the cell cycle during late myeloid development, it is now known to affect cell fate decisions during early myelopoiesis. In myeloid progenitors, loss of p15Ink4b results in an imbalance in the progenitor pools, and favors the expansion of GMPs at the expense of MEPs. Importantly, when deleted in the cells of the myeloid lineage only, mice develop nonreactive monocytosis and are strongly predisposed to succumb to retrovirus-induced leukemia, especially of myeloid origin. These results validate a tight link between loss of p15INK4b and human myeloid neoplasia. Clinical observations that associate *p15INK4b* demethylation and re-expression with improved prognosis and survival, further stress the importance of this gene in AML and MDS treatment.

6. References

Aggerholm A, Guldberg P, Hokland M & Hokland P (1999). Extensive intra- and inter-individual heterogeneity of p15INK4B methylation in acute myeloid leukemia. *Cancer Research*, Vol.59, No.2, (January 2009), pp. 436-441, ISSN 0008-5472

Aggerholm A, Holm MS, Guldberg P, Olesen LH & Hokland P (2006). Promoter hypermethylation of p15INK4B, HIC1, CDH1, and ER is frequent in myelodysplastic syndrome and predicts poor prognosis in early-stage patients. *European Journal of Hematology*, Vol.76, No.1, (January 2006), pp. 23-32, ISSN 0902-4441

Agrawal S, Unterberg M, Koschmieder S, zur Stadt U, Verbeek W, Büchner T, Berdel WE, Serve H & Müller-Tidow C (2007). DNA methylation of tumor suppressor genes in clinical remission predicts the relapse risk in acute myeloid leukemia. *Cancer Research,* Vol.67, No.3, (February 2007), pp. 1370-1377, ISSN 0008-5472

Akashi K, Traver D, Miyamoto T & Weissman IL (2000). A clonogenic common myeloid progenitor that gives rise to all myeloid lineages. *Nature,* Vol.404, No.6774, (March 2000), pp. 193-197, ISSN 0028-0836

Aoki E, Uchida T, Ohashi H, Nagai H, Murase T, Ichikawa A, Yamao K, Hotta T, Kinoshita T, Saito H & Murate T(2000). Methylation status of the p15INK4B gene in hematopoietic progenitors and peripheral blood cells in myelodysplastic syndromes. *Leukemia,* Vol.14, No.4, pp. 586-593, ISSN 0887-6924

Bai F, Pei XH, Godfrey VL & Xiong Y. (2003) Haploinsufficiency of p18(INK4c) sensitizes mice to carcinogen-induced tumorigenesis. *Molecular and Cellular Biology,* Vol.23, No.4, (February 2003), pp. 1269–1277, ISSN 0270-7306

Bennett JM, Catovsky D, Daniel MT, Flandrin G, Galton DA, Gralnick HR & Sultan C (1976). Proposals for the classification of the acute leukaemias, French-American-British (FAB) co-operative group. *British Journal of Haematology* Vol.33, No.4, (August 1976), pp. 451-458, ISSN 0007-1048

Bennett JM, Catovsky D, Daniel MT, Flandrin G, Galton DA, Gralnick HR & Sultan C (1982). Proposals for the classification of the myelodysplastic syndromes. *British Journal of Haematology,* Vol.51, No.2, (June 1982), pp. 189-199, ISSN 0007-1048

Bennett JM, Catovsky D, Daniel MT, Flandrin G, Galton DA, Gralnick HR & Sultan C (1985). Proposed revised criteria for the classification of acute myeloid leukemia. A report of the French-American-British Cooperative Group. *Annals of Internal Medicine,* Vol. 103, No.4, (October 1985), pp. 620-625, ISSN 0003-4819

Bergh G, Ehinger M, Olsson I, Jacobsen SE & Gullberg U (1999). Involvement of the retinoblastoma protein in monocytic and neutrophilic lineage commitment of human bone marrow progenitor cells. *Blood,* Vol.94, No.6, (September 1999), pp. 1971-1978, ISSN 0006-4971

Biancotto C, Frigè G & Minucci S (2010). Histone modification therapy of cancer. *Advances in Genetics,* Vol.70, pp. 341-386, ISSN 0065-2660

Bies J, Sramko M, Fares J, Rosu-Myles M, Zhang S, Koller R & Wolff L (2010). Myeloid-specific inactivation of p15Ink4b results in monocytosis and predisposition to myeloid leukemia. *Blood,* Vol.116, No.6, (August 2010), pp. 979-987, ISSN 0006-4971

Bird A (2002). DNA methylation patterns and epigenetic memory. *Genes and Development,* Vol.16, No.1, (January 2002), pp. 6-21, ISSN 0890-9369

Brotherton DH, Dhanaraj V, Wick S, Brizuela L, Domaille PJ, Volyanik E, Xu X, Parisini E, Smith BO, Archer SJ, Serrano M, Brenner SL, Blundell TL & Laue ED (1998). Crystal structure of the complex of the cyclin D-dependent kinase Cdk6 bound to the cell cycle inhibitor $p19^{INK4d}$. *Nature,* Vol.395, No.6699, (September 1998), pp. 244–250, ISSN 0028-0836

Buchold GM, Magyar PL & O'Brien DA (2007). Mice lacking cyclin-dependent kinase inhibitor p19Ink4d show strain-specific effects on male reproduction. *Molecular Reproduction and Development,* Vol.74, No.8, (August 2007), pp. 1008-1020, ISSN 1040-452X

Cameron EE, Baylin SB & Herman JG (1999). p15(INK4B) CpG island methylation in primary acute leukemia is heterogeneous and suggests density as a critical factor for transcriptional silencing. *Blood,* Vol.94, No.7, (October 1999), pp. 2445-2451, ISSN 0006-4971

Cánepa ET, Scassa ME, Ceruti JM, Marazita MC, Carcagno AL, Sirkin PF & Ogara MF (2007). INK4 proteins, a family of mammalian CDK inhibitors with novel biological functions. *IUBMB Life,* Vol.59, No.7, (July 2007), pp. 419-426, ISSN 1521-6543

Chim CS, Liang R, Tam CY & Kwong YL (2001). Methylation of p15 and p16 genes in acute promyelocytic leukemia: potential diagnostic and prognostic significance. *Journal of Clinical Oncology,* Vol.19, No.7, (April 2001), pp. 2033-2040, ISSN 0732-183X

Chim CS, Tam CY, Liang R & Kwong YL (2001). Methylation of p15 and p16 genes in adult acute leukemia: lack of prognostic significance. *Cancer,* Vol.91, No.12, (June 2001), pp. 2222-2229, ISSN 0008-543X

Chim CS & Kwong YL (2006). Adverse prognostic impact of CDKN2B hyper-methylation in acute promyelocytic leukemia. *Leukemia and Lymphoma,* Vol.47, No.5, (May 2006), pp. 815-825, ISSN 1042-8194

Christiansen DH, Andersen MK & Pedersen-Bjergaard J (2003). Methylation of p15INK4B is common, is associated with deletion of genes on chromosome arm 7q and predicts a poor prognosis in therapy-related myelodysplasia and acute myeloid leukemia. *Leukemia,* Vol.17, No.9, (September 2003), pp. 1813-1819, ISSN 0887-6924

Clausen BE, Burkhardt C, Reith W, Renkawitz R & Forster I (1999). Conditional gene targeting in macrophages and granulocytes using LysMcre mice. *Transgenic Research,* Vol.8, No.4, (August 1999), pp. 265-277, ISSN 0962-8819

Daskalakis M, Nguyen TT, Nguyen C, Guldberg P, Köhler G, Wijermans P, Jones PA & Lübbert M (2002). Demethylation of a hypermethylated P15/INK4B gene in patients with myelodysplastic syndrome by 5-Aza-2'-deoxycytidine (decitabine) treatment. *Blood,* Vol.100, No.8, (October 2002), pp. 2957-2964. ISSN 0006-4971

Deaton AM & Bird A (2011). CpG islands and the regulation of transcription. *Genes and Development,* Vol.25, No.10, (May 2011), pp. 1010-1022, ISSN 0890-9369

Deneberg S, Grövdal M, Karimi M, Jansson M, Nahi H, Corbacioglu A, Gaidzik V, Döhner K, Paul C, Ekström TJ, Hellström-Lindberg E & Lehmann S (2010). Gene-specific and global methylation patterns predict outcome in patients with acute myeloid leukemia. *Leukemia,* Vol.24, No.5, (May 2010), pp. 932-941, ISSN 0887-6924

Drexler HG (1998). Review of alterations of the cyclin-dependent kinase inhibitor INK4 family genes p15, p16, p18 and p19 in human leukemia-lymphoma cells. *Leukemia,* Vol.12, No.6, (June 1998), pp. 845-859, ISSN 0887-6924

Farinha NJ, Shaker S, Lemaire M, Momparler L, Bernstein M & Momparler RL (2004). Activation of expression of p15, p73 and E-cadherin in leukemic cells by different concentrations of 5-aza-2'-deoxycytidine (Decitabine). *Anticancer Research,* Vol.24, No.1, (January 2004), pp. 75-78, ISSN 0250-7005

Flotho C, Claus R, Batz C, Schneider M, Sandrock I, Ihde S, Plass C, Niemeyer CM & Lübbert M (2009). The DNA methyltransferase inhibitors azacitidine, decitabine and zebularine exert differential effects on cancer gene expression in acute myeloid leukemia cells. *Leukemia,* Vol.23, No.6, (June 2009), pp. 1019-1028, ISSN 0887-6924

Franklin, D.S., Godfrey, V.L., Lee, H., Kovalev, G.I., Schoonhoven, R., Chen-Kiang, S., Su, L. & Xiong, Y (1998). CDK inhibitors p18(INK4c) and p27(Kip1) mediate two separate pathways to collaboratively suppress pituitary tumorigenesis. *Genes and Development,* Vol.12, No.18, (September 1998), pp. 2899–2911, ISSN 0890-9369

Furukawa Y, Kikuchi J, Nakamura M, Iwase S, Yamada H & Matsuda M (2000) Lineage-specific regulation of cell cycle control gene expression during haematopoietic cell differentiation. *British Journal of Haematology,* Vol.110, No.3, (September 2000), pp. 663-673, ISSN 0007-1048

Galm O, Wilop S, Lüders C, Jost E, Gehbauer G, Herman JG & Osieka R (2005). Clinical implications of aberrant DNA methylation patterns in acute myelogenous leukemia. *Annals of Hematology,* Vol.84, No.1, (December 2005), pp. 39-46, ISSN 0939-5555

Garcia-Manero G (2003). Prognostic implications of epigenetic silencing of p15INK4B in acute promyelocytic leukemia. *Leukemia,* Vol.17, No.5, (May 2003), pp. 839-840, ISSN 0887-6924

Gore SD, Baylin S, Sugar E, Carraway H, Miller CB, Carducci M, Grever M, Galm O, Dauses T, Karp JE, Rudek MA, Zhao M, Smith BD, Manning J, Jiemjit A, Dover G, Mays A, Zwiebel J, Murgo A, Weng LJ & Herman JG (2006). Combined DNA methyltransferase and histone deacetylase inhibition in the treatment of myeloid neoplasms. *Cancer Research,* Vol.66, No.12, (June 2006), pp. 6361-6369, ISSN 0008-5472

Guo SX, Taki T, Ohnishi H, Piao HY, Tabuchi K, Bessho F, Hanada R, Yanagisawa M & Hayashi Y (2000). Hypermethylation of p16 and p15 genes and RB protein expression in acute leukemia. *Leukemia Research,* Vol.24, No.1, (January 2000), pp. 39-46, ISSN 0145-2126

Graf Einsiedel H, Taube T, Hartmann R, Wellmann S, Seifert G, Henze G & Seeger K. (2002). Deletion analysis of p16(INKa) and p15(INKb) in relapsed childhood acute lymphoblastic leukemia. *Blood,* Vol.99, No.12 (June 2002), pp. 4629-4631, ISSN 0006-4971

Grövdal M, Khan R, Aggerholm A, Antunovic P, Astermark J, Bernell P, Engström LM, Kjeldsen L, Linder O, Nilsson L, Olsson A, Wallvik J, Tangen JM, Oberg G, Jacobsen SE, Hokland P, Porwit A & Hellström-Lindberg E (2007). Negative effect of DNA hypermethylation on the outcome of intensive chemotherapy in older patients with high-risk myelodysplastic syndromes and acute myeloid leukemia following myelodysplastic syndrome. *Clinical Cancer Research,* Vol.13, No.23, (December 2007), pp. 7107-7112, ISSN 1078-0432

Haase D, Germing U, Schanz J, Pfeilstöcker M, Nösslinger T, Hildebrandt B, Kundgen A, Lübbert M, Kunzmann R, Giagounidis AA, Aul C, Trümper L, Krieger O, Stauder R, Müller TH, Wimazal F, Valent P, Fonatsch C & Steidl C (2007). New insights into the prognostic impact of the karyotype in MDS and correlation with subtypes: evidence from a core dataset of 2124 patients. *Blood,* Vol.110, No.13, (December 2007), pp. 4385-4395, ISSN 0006-4971

Hannon GJ & Beach D (1994). p15INK4B is a potential effector of TGF-beta-induced cell cycle arrest. *Nature,* Vol.371, No.6494, (September 1994), pp. 257-261, ISSN 0028-0836

Harris NL, Jaffe ES, Diebold J, Flandrin G, Muller-Hermelink HK, Vardiman J, Lister TA & Bloomfield CD (1999). World Health Organization classification of neoplastic diseases of the hematopoietic and lymphoid tissues: report of the Clinical Advisory Committee meeting-Airlie House, Virginia, November 1997. *Journal of Clinical Oncology,* Vol.17, No.12, (December 1999), pp. 3835-3849, ISSN 0732-183X

Harris NL, Jaffe ES, Diebold J, Flandrin G, Muller-Hermelink HK, Vardiman J, Lister TA & Bloomfield CD (2000). The World Health Organization classification of hematological malignancies report of the Clinical Advisory Committee Meeting, Airlie House, Virginia, November 1997. *Modern Pathology,* Vol.13, No.2, (February 2000), pp.193-207, ISSN 0893-3952

Hasegawa D, Manabe A, Kubota T, Kawasaki H, Hirose I, Ohtsuka Y, Tsuruta T, Ebihara Y, Goto Y, Zhao XY, Sakashita K, Koike K, Isomura M, Kojima S, Hoshika A, Tsuji K & Nakahata T (2005). Methylation status of the p15 and p16 genes in paediatric myelodysplastic syndrome and juvenile myelomonocytic leukaemia. *British Journal of Haematology,* Vol.128, No.6, (March 2005), pp.805-812, ISSN 0007-1048

Haviernik P, Schmidt M, Hu X & Wolff L (2003).Consistent inactivation of p19(Arf) but not p15(Ink4b) in murine myeloid cells transformed in vivo by deregulated c-Myc. *Oncogene,* Vol.22, No.11, (March 2003), pp. 1600-1610, ISSN 0950-9232

Herman JG, Jen J, Merlo A & Baylin SB (1996). Hypermethylation-associated inactivation indicates a tumor suppressor role for p15INK4B. *Cancer Research,* Vol.56, No.4, (February 1996), pp. 722-727, ISSN 0008-5472

Herman JG, Civin CI, Issa JP, Collector MI, Sharkis SJ & Baylin SB (1997). Distinct patterns of inactivation of p15INK4B and p16INK4A characterize the major types of hematological malignancies. *Cancer Research,* Vol.57, No.5, (March 1997), pp. 837-841, ISSN 0008-5472

Hoshino K, Asou N, Okubo T, Suzushima H, Kiyokawa T, Kawano F & Mitsuya H (2002). The absence of the p15INK4B gene alterations in adult patients with precursor B-cell acute lymphoblastic leukaemia is a favourable prognostic factor. *British Journal of Haematology,* Vol.117, No.3, (June 2002), pp. 531-540, ISSN 0007-1048

Jeffrey PD, Tong L & Pavletich NP (2000). Structural basis of inhibition of CDK-cyclin complexes by INK4 inhibitors. *Genes and Development*, Vol.14, No.24, (December 2000), pp. 3115-3125, ISSN 0890-9369

Jenuwein T & Allis CD (2001). Translating the histone code. *Science,* Vol.293, No.5532, (August 2001), pp. 1074-1080, ISSN 0036-8075

Jiang Y, Dunbar A, Gondek LP, Mohan S, Rataul M, O'Keefe C, Sekeres M, Saunthararajah Y & Maciejewski JP (2009). Aberrant DNA methylation is a dominant mechanism in MDS progression to AML. *Blood,* Vol.113, No.6, (February 2009), pp.1315-1325, ISSN 0006-4971

Jones PA & Baylin SB. (2002). The fundamental role of epigenetic events in cancer. *Nature Reviews Genetics,* Vol.3, No.6, (June 2002), pp. 415-428 ISSN 1471-0056

Kim M, Yim SH, Cho NS, Kang SH, Ko DH, Oh B, Kim TY, Min HJ, She CJ, Kang HJ, Shin HY, Ahn HS, Yoon SS, Kim BK, Shin HR, Han KS, Cho HI & Lee DS (2009). Homozygous deletion of CDKN2A (p16, p14) and CDKN2B (p15) genes is a poor prognostic factor in adult but not in childhood B-lineage acute lymphoblastic leukemia: a comparative deletion and hypermethylation study. *Cancer Genetics and Cytogenetics,* Vol.195, No.1, (November 2009), pp. 59-65, ISSN 0165-4608

Korenjak M & Brehm A (2005). E2F-Rb complexes regulating transcription of genes important for differentiation and development. *Current Opinion in Genetics and Development,* Vol.15, No.5, (October 2005), pp. 520-527, ISSN 0959-437X

Krimpenfort P, Quon KC, Mooi WJ, Loonstra A & Berns A (2001). Loss of p16INK4A confers susceptibility to metastatic melanoma in mice. *Nature,* Vol.413, No.6851, (September 2001), pp. 83-86, ISSN 0028-0836

Krimpenfort P, Ijpenberg A, Song JY, van der Valk M, Nawijn M, Zevenhoven J & Berns A (2007). p15Ink4b is a critical tumor suppressor in the absence of p16INK4A. *Nature,* Vol.448, No.7156, (August 2007), pp.943-946, ISSN 0028-0836

Latres E, Malumbres M, Sotillo R, Martín J, Ortega S, Martín-Caballero J, Flores JM, Cordón-Cardo C & Barbacid M (2000). Limited overlapping roles of p15(INK4b) and p18(INK4c) cell cycle inhibitors in proliferation and tumorigenesis. *EMBO Journal,* Vol.19, No.13, (July 2000), pp. 3496-3506, ISSN 0261-4189

Li J, Byeon IJ, Ericson K, Poi MJ, O'Maille P, Selby T & Tsai MD (1999). Tumor suppressor INK4: determination of the solution structure of p18INK4c and demonstration of the functional significance of loops in p18INK4c and p16INK4A. *Biochemistry,* Vol.38, No.10, (March 1999), pp.2930-2940, ISSN 0006-2960

Malumbres M, Pérez De Castro I, Hernández MI, Jiménez M, Corral T & Pellicer A (2000). Cellular response to oncogenic ras involves induction of the Cdk4 and Cdk6 inhibitor p15(INK4b). *Molecular and Cellular Biology,* Vol.20, No.8, (April 2000), pp. 2915-2925, ISSN 0270-7306

Markus J, Garin MT, Bies J, Galili N, Raza A, Thirman MJ, Le Beau MM, Rowley JD, Liu PP & Wolff L (2007). Methylation-independent silencing of the tumor suppressor INK4b (p15) by CBFbeta-SMMHC in acute myelogenous leukemia with inv(16). *Cancer Research,* Vol.67, No.3, (February 2007), pp. 992-1000, ISSN 0008-5472

Matsuno N, Hoshino K, Nanri T, Kawakita T, Suzushima H, Kawano F, Mitsuya H & Asou N (2005). p15 mRNA expression detected by real-time quantitative reverse transcriptase-polymerase chain reaction correlates with the methylation density of the gene in adult acute leukemia. *Leukemia Research,* Vol.29, No.5, (May 2005), pp. 557-564, ISSN 0145-2126

Mirebeau D, Acquaviva C, Suciu S, Bertin R, Dastugue N, Robert A, Boutard P, Méchinaud F, Plouvier E, Otten J, Vilmer E & Cavé H (2006). The prognostic significance of CDKN2A, CDKN2B and MTAP inactivation in B-lineage acute lymphoblastic leukemia of childhood. Results of the EORTC studies 58881 and 58951. *Haematologica,* Vol.91, No.7, (July 2006), pp. 881-885, ISSN 0390-6078

Miranda TB, Cortez CC, Yoo CB, Liang G, Abe M, Kelly TK, Marquez VE & Jones PA (2009). DZNep is a global histone methylation inhibitor that reactivates developmental genes not silenced by DNA methylation. *Molecular Cancer Therapeutics,* Vol.8, No.6, (June 2009), pp. 1579-1588, ISSN 1535-7163

Morishita A, Masaki T, Yoshiji H, Nakai S, Ogi T, Miyauchi Y, Yoshida S, Funaki T, Uchida N, Kita Y, Funakoshi F, Usuki H, Okada S, Izuishi K, Watanabe S, Kurokohchi K & Kuriyama S (2004). Reduced expression of cell cycle regulator p18(INK4C) in human hepatocellular carcinoma. *Hepatology,* Vol.40, No.3, (September 2004), pp. 677-686, ISSN 0270-9139

Nobori T, Miura K, Wu DJ, Lois A, Takabayashi K & Carson DA (1994). Deletions of the cyclin-dependent kinase-4 inhibitor gene in multiple human cancers. *Nature,* Vol.368, No.6473, (April 1994), pp. 753-756, ISSN 0028-0836

Noh SJ, Li Y, Xiong Y & Guan KL (1999). Identification of functional elements of p18INK4C essential for binding and inhibition of cyclin-dependent kinase (CDK) 4 and CDK6. *Cancer Research,* Vol.59, No.3, (February 1999), pp. 558-564, ISSN 0008-5472

Olk-Batz C, Poetsch AR, Nöllke P, Claus R, Zucknick M, Sandrock I, Witte T, Strahm B, Hasle H, Zecca M, Stary J, Bergstraesser E, De Moerloose B, Trebo M, van den Heuvel-Eibrink MM, Wojcik D, Locatelli F, Plass C, Niemeyer CM, Flotho C & the European Working Group of Myelodysplastic Syndromes in Childhood (EWOG-MDS) (2011). Aberrant DNA methylation characterizes juvenile myelomonocytic leukemia with poor outcome. *Blood,* Vol.117, No.18, (May 2011), pp. 4871-4880, ISSN 0006-4971

Ozenne P, Eymin B, Brambilla E & Gazzeri S (2010). The ARF tumor suppressor: structure, functions and status in cancer. *International Journal of Cancer,* Vol.127, No.10, (November 2010), pp. 2239-2947, ISSN 0020-7136

Paul TA, Bies J, Small D & Wolff L (2010). Signatures of polycomb repression and reduced H3K4 trimethylation are associated with p15INK4b DNA methylation in AML. *Blood,* Vol.115, No.15, (April 2010), pp. 3098-3108, ISSN 0006-4971

Quesnel B, Guillerm G, Vereecque R, Wattel E, Preudhomme C, Bauters F, Vanrumbeke M & Fenaux P (1998) Methylation of the p15(INK4b) gene in myelodysplastic syndromes is frequent and acquired during disease progression. *Blood,* Vol.91, No.8, (April 1998), pp. 2985–2990, ISSN 0006-4971

Raj K, John A, Ho A, Chronis C, Khan S, Samuel J, Pomplun S, Thomas NS & Mufti GJ (2007). CDKN2B methylation status and isolated chromosome 7 abnormalities predict responses to treatment with 5-azacytidine. *Leukemia,* Vol.21, No.9, (September 2007), pp. 1937-1944, ISSN 0887-6924

Rodrigues EF, Santos-Rebouças CB, Gonçalves Pimentel MM, Mencalha AL, Dobbin J, Da Costa ES, Fernandez Cde S, Bouzas LF, Abdelhay E & De Souza Fernandez T (2010). Epigenetic alterations of p15(INK4B) and p16(INK4A) genes in pediatric primary myelodysplastic syndrome. *Leukemia and Lymphoma,* Vol.51, No.10, (October 2010), pp. 1887-1894, ISSN 1042-8194

Rosu-Myles M, Taylor BJ & Wolff L (2007). Loss of the tumor suppressor p15Ink4b enhances myeloid progenitor formation from common myeloid progenitors. *Experimental Hematology,* Vol.35, No.3, (March 2007), pp. 394-406, ISSN 0301-472X

Rosu-Myles M & Wolff L (2008). p15Ink4b: dual function in myelopoiesis and inactivation in myeloid disease. *Blood Cells, Molecules and Diseases,* Vol.40, No.3, (May 2008), pp. 406-409, ISSN 1079-9796

Roussel, M.F (1999). The INK4 family of cell cycle inhibitors in cancer. *Oncogene,* Vol.18, No.38, (September 1999), pp. 5311–5317, ISSN 0950-9232

Ruas M & Peters G. (1998). The p16INK4A/CDKN2A tumor suppressor and its relatives. *Biochimica et Biophysica Acta (BBA) - Reviews on Cancer,* Vol.1378, No.2, (October 1998), pp. 115-77, ISSN 0304-419X

Russo AA, Tong L, Lee JO, Jeffrey PD & Pavletich NP (1998). Structural basis for inhibition of the cyclin-dependent kinase Cdk6 by the tumour suppressor p16INK4A. *Nature,* Vol.395, No.6699, (September 1998), pp. 237-243, ISSN 0028-0836

Sandhu C, Garbe J, Bhattacharya N, Daksis J, Pan CH, Yaswen P, Koh J, Slingerland JM & Stampfer MR (1997).Transforming growth factor beta stabilizes p15INK4B protein, increases p15INK4B-cdk4 complexes, and inhibits cyclin D1-cdk4 association in human mammary epithelial cells. *Molecular and Cellular Biology,* Vol.17, No.5, (May 1997), pp. 2458-2467, ISSN 0270-7306

Santos FP, Kantarjian H, Garcia-Manero G, Issa JP & Ravandi F (2010).Decitabine in the treatment of myelodysplastic syndromes. *Expert Review of Anticancer Therapy,* Vol.10, No.1, (January 2010), pp. 9-22, ISSN 1473-7140

Schmidt M, Bies J, Tamura T, Ozato K & Wolff L (2004). The interferon regulatory factor ICSBP/IRF-8 in combination with PU.1 up-regulates expression of tumor suppressor p15(Ink4b) in murine myeloid cells. *Blood,* Vol.103, No.11, (June 2004), pp. 4142-4149, ISSN 0006-4971

Schwaller J, Pabst T, Koeffler HP, Niklaus G, Loetscher P, Fey MF & Tobler A (1997). Expression and regulation of G1 cell-cycle inhibitors (p16INK4A, p15INK4B, p18INK4C, p19INK4D) in human acute myeloid leukemia and normal myeloid cells. *Leukemia,* Vol.11, No.1, (January 1997), pp. 54-63, ISSN 0887-6924

Scott SA, Lakshimikuttysamma A, Sheridan DP, Sanche SE, Geyer CR & DeCoteau JF (2007). Zebularine inhibits human acute myeloid leukemia cell growth in vitro in association with p15INK4B demethylation and reexpression. *Experimental Hematology,* Vol.35, No.2, (February 2007), pp. 263-273, ISSN 0301-472X

Serrano, M., Lee, H., Chin, L., Cordon-Cardo, C., Beach, D. & DePinho, R.A (1996). Role of the INK4A locus in tumor suppression and cell mortality. *Cell,* Vol.85, No.1, (April 1996), pp. 27–37, ISSN 0092-8674

Shen L, Kantarjian H, Guo Y, Lin E, Shan J, Huang X, Berry D, Ahmed S, Zhu W, Pierce S, Kondo Y, Oki Y, Jelinek J, Saba H, Estey E & Issa JP (2009). DNA methylation predicts survival and response to therapy in patients with myelodysplastic syndromes. *Journal of Clinical Oncology,* Vol.28, No.4, (February 2009), pp. 605-613, ISSN 0732-183X

Sherr CJ & Roberts JM. (1999). CDK inhibitors: positive and negative regulators of G1-phase progression. *Genes and Development,* Vol.13, No.12, (June 1999), pp. 1501-1512, ISSN 0890-9369

Sherr CJ (2006). Divorcing ARF and p53: an unsettled case. *Nature Reviews Cancer,* Vol.6, No.9, (September 2006), pp. 663-673, ISSN 1474-175X

Shimamoto T, Ohyashiki JH & Ohyashiki K (2005). Methylation of p15(INK4b) and E-cadherin genes is independently correlated with poor prognosis in acute myeloid leukemia. *Leukemia Research,* Vol.29, No.6, (June 2005), pp. 653-659, ISSN 0145-2126

Solomon DA, Kim JS, Jean W & Waldman T (2008). Conspirators in a capital crime: co-deletion of p18INK4c and p16INK4A/p14ARF/p15INK4b in glioblastoma multiforme. *Cancer Research,* Vol.68, No.21, (November 2008), pp. 8657-8560, ISSN 0008-5472

Solomon DA, Kim JS, Jenkins S, Ressom H, Huang M, Coppa N, Mabanta L, Bigner D, Yan H, Jean W & Waldman T. (2008). Identification of p18 INK4c as a tumor suppressor gene in glioblastoma multiforme. *Cancer Research,* Vol.68, No.8, (April 2008), pp. 2564-2569, ISSN 0008-5472

Takeuchi S, Matsushita M, Zimmermann M, Ikezoe T, Komatsu N, Seriu T, Schrappe M, Bartram CR & Koeffler HP (2011). Clinical significance of aberrant DNA methylation in childhood acute lymphoblastic leukemia. *Leukemia Research,* n.d. ISSN 0145-2126

Teofili L, Rutella S, Chiusolo P, La Barbera EO, Rumi C, Ranelletti FO, Maggiano N, Leone G & Larocca LM (1998). Expression of p15INK4B in normal hematopoiesis. *Experimental Hematology,* Vol.26, No.12, (November 1998), pp. 1133-1139, ISSN 0301-472X

Teofili L, Morosetti R, Martini M, Urbano R, Putzulu R, Rutella S, Pierelli L, Leone G & Larocca LM (2000). Expression of cyclin-dependent kinase inhibitor p15INK4B during normal and leukemic myeloid differentiation. *Experimental Hematology,* Vol.28, No.5, (May 2000), pp. 519-526, ISSN 0301-472X

Teofili L, Martini M, Di Mario A, Rutella S, Urbano R, Luongo M, Leone G & Larocca LM (2001). Expression of p15(ink4b) gene during megakaryocytic differentiation of normal and myelodysplastic hematopoietic progenitors. *Blood,* Vol.98, No.2, (July 2001), pp. 495-497, ISSN 0006-4971

Teofili L, Martini M, Luongo M, Diverio D, Capelli G, Breccia M, Lo Coco F, Leone G & Larocca LM (2003). Hypermethylation of GpG islands in the promoter region of p15(INK4b) in acute promyelocytic leukemia represses p15(INK4b) expression and correlates with poor prognosis. *Leukemia,* Vol.17, No.5, (May 2003), pp. 919–924, ISSN 0887-6924

Tessema M, Länger F, Dingemann J, Ganser A, Kreipe H & Lehmann U (2003). Aberrant methylation and impaired expression of the p15(INK4b) cell cycle regulatory gene in chronic myelomonocytic leukemia (CMML). *Leukemia,* Vol.17, No.5, (May 2003), pp. 910-918, ISSN 0887-6924

Thullberg M, Bartkova J, Khan S, Hansen K, Rönnstrand L, Lukas J, Strauss M & Bartek J (2000). Distinct versus redundant properties among members of the INK4 family of cyclin-dependent kinase inhibitors. *FEBS Letters,* Vol.470, No.2, (March 2000), pp. 161-166, ISSN 0014-5793

Tien HF, Tang JH, Tsay W, Liu MC, Lee FY, Wang CH, Chen YC & Shen MC (2001). Methylation of the p15(INK4B) gene in myelodysplastic syndrome: It can be detected early at diagnosis or during disease progression and is highly associated with leukaemic transformation. *British Journal of Hematology,* Vol.112, No.1, (January 2001), pp. 148–154, ISSN 0007-1048

Tran HT, Kim HN, Lee IK, Kim YK, Ahn JS, Yang DH, Lee JJ & Kim HJ (2011). DNA methylation changes following 5-azacitidine treatment in patients with myelodysplastic syndrome. *Journal of Korean Medical Science,* Vol.26, No.2, (February 2011), pp. 207-213, ISSN 1011-8934

Trost D, Hildebrandt B, Beier M, Müller N, Germing U & Royer-Pokora B (2006). Molecular cytogenetic profiling of complex karyotypes in primary myelodysplastic syndromes and acute myeloid leukemia. *Cancer Genetics and Cytogenetics,* Vol.165, No.1, (February 2006), pp. 51-63, ISSN 0165-4608

Tsellou E, Troungos C, Moschovi M, Athanasiadou-Piperopoulou F, Polychronopoulou S, Kosmidis H, Kalmanti M, Hatzakis A, Dessypris N, Kalofoutis A & Petridou E (2005). Hypermethylation of CpG islands in the promoter region of the p15INK4B gene in childhood acute leukaemia. *European Journal of Cancer,* Vol.41, No.4, (March 2005), pp. 584-589, ISSN 0959-8049

Uchida T, Kinoshita T, Nagai H, Nakahara Y, Saito H, Hotta T & Murate T (1997). Hypermethylation of the p15INK4B gene in myelodysplastic syndromes. *Blood,* Vol.90, No.4, (August 1997), pp. 1403-1409, ISSN 0006-4971

Valencia A, Cervera J, Such E, Ibañez M, Gómez I, Luna I, Senent L, Oltra S, Sanz MA & Sanz GF (2011). Aberrant methylation of tumor suppressor genes in patients with refractory anemia with ring sideroblasts. *Leukemia Research,* Vol.35, No.4, (April 2011), pp. 479-483, ISSN 0145-2126

Van Zutven LJ, van Drunen E, de Bont JM, Wattel MM, Den Boer ML, Pieters R, Hagemeijer A, Slater RM & Beverloo HB (2005). CDKN2 deletions have no prognostic value in childhood precursor-B acute lymphoblastic leukaemia. *Leukemia,* Vol.19, No.7, (July 2005), pp. 1281-1284, ISSN 0887-6924

Vardiman JW, Harris NL & Brunning RD (2002). The World Health Organization (WHO) classification of the myeloid neoplasms. *Blood,* Vol.100, No.7, (October 2002), pp. 2292-2302, ISSN 0006-4971

Varier RA & Timmers HT (2011). Histone lysine methylation and demethylation pathways in cancer. *Biochimica et Biophysica Acta (BBA) - Reviews on Cancer,* Vol.1815, No.1, (January 2011), pp. 75-89, ISSN 0304-419X

Wolff L, Garin MT, Koller R, Bies J, Liao W, Malumbres M, Tessarollo L, Powell D & Perella C (2003) Hypermethylation of the Ink4b locus in murine myeloid leukemia and increased susceptibility to leukemia in p15(Ink4b)-deficient mice. *Oncogene,* Vol.22, No.58, (December 2003), pp. 9265-9274, ISSN 0950-9232

Wolff L, Koller R, Hu X & Anver MR (2003). A Moloney murine leukemia virus-based retrovirus with 4070A long terminal repeat sequences induces a high incidence of myeloid as well as lymphoid neoplasms. *Journal of Virology,* Vol.7, No.8, (April 2003), pp. 4965-4971, ISSN 0022-538X

Wolff L, Garin MT, Koller R, Bies J, Tessarollo L, Anver MR, Powell D & Perella C (2004) A novel retrovirus provides the cooperating oncogenic event(s) required to demonstrate the tumor suppressor activity of p15Ink4b in myeloid cells in vivo. *Blood Cells, Molecules and Diseases,* Vol.32, No.1, (January 2004), pp. 226-231, ISSN 1079-9796

Wong IH, Ng MH, Huang DP & Lee JC (2000). Aberrant p15 promoter methylation in adult and childhood acute leukemias of nearly all morphologic subtypes: potential prognostic implications. *Blood,* Vol.95, No.6, (March 2000), pp. 1942–1949, ISSN 0006-4971

Yuan C, Selby TL, Li J, Byeon IJ & Tsai MD (2000). Tumor suppressor INK4: refinement of p16INK4A structure and determination of p15INK4b structure by comparative modeling and NMR data. *Protein Science,* Vol.9, No.6, (June 2000), pp. 1120-1128, ISSN 0961-8368

Yuan Y, Shen H, Franklin DS, Scadden DT & Cheng T (2004). In vivo self-renewing divisions of haematopoietic stem cells are increased in the absence of the early G1-phase inhibitor, p18INK4C. *Nature Cell Biology,* Vol.6, No.5, (May 2004), pp. 436-442, ISSN 1465-7392

Zindy F, Quelle DE, Roussel MF & Sherr CJ (1997). Expression of the p16INK4A tumor suppressor versus other INK4 family members during mouse development and aging. *Oncogene,* Vol.15, No.2, (July 1997) pp. 203-211, ISSN 0950-9232

Zindy F., van Deursen J., Grosveld G., Sherr C.J. & Roussel M.F (2000). INK4d-deficient mice are fertile despite testicular atrophy. *Molecular and Cellular Biology,* Vol.20, No.1, (January 2000), pp. 372–378, ISSN 0270-7306

16

New Molecular Markers in Acute Myeloid Leukemia

Silvia de la Iglesia Iñigo[1], María Teresa Gómez Casares[1], Carmen Elsa López Jorge[1,2], Jezabel López Brito[1] and Pedro Martin Cabrera[3]

[1]*Servicio de Hematología, Hospital de Gran Canaria Doctor Negrín, Las Palmas de GranCanaria*

[2]*Unit Research, Hospital de Gran Canaria Doctor Negrín, Las Palmas de GranCanaria*

[3]*Secció de Citologia Hematològica, Servei d'Anatomia Patològica Hospital Universitari de Bellvitge, Barcelona, Spain*

1. Introduction

Acute leukemia is characterized by abnormal proliferation, inhibition of differentiation and expansion of leukemic cells blocked at the early stage of hematopoiesis. Acute myeloid leukemia (AML) is a malignant hematological disease of hematopoietic precursor cells of non-lymphoid lineage. Recent insights into the molecular mechanisms of AML are challenging the traditional diagnostic classification, prognostic significance and clinical practice of this hematological disorder.

1.1 Concept and classification

AML is a clinically heterogeneous disorder with distinct clinical and biological features. Until the 1970s, diagnosis was based on morphological examination of bone marrow and peripheral blood samples. In 1976, French, American, and British hematologists (the FAB group) defined six subgroups of AML morphological variants (Bennett et al., French-American-British Cooperative Group [FAB], 1976). This classification allowed us to identify several types of AML: M1-M6. Blastic populations were identified using standard staining techniques and consequently classified depending on reactivity to certain cytochemicals, namely, myeloperoxidase and Sudan black B (markers of myeloid differentiation) and nonspecific esterase reactions such as alpha-naphthyl acetate esterase and alpha-naphthyl butyrate esterase (for monocytic lineage). Later on, this group identified two new types of AML (M0 and M7) according to cytochemical and inmunophenotypical features (Bennett et al., FAB, 1985). Over the past decade, refinement in the diagnosis of subtypes of AML and advances in therapeutic approaches have improved the outlook for patients with AML (Döhner et al., 2010).

FAB classification
M0: AML minimally differentiated
M1: AML without maturation
M2: AML with maturation
M3: Acute promyelocytic leukemia
M4: Acute myelomonocytic leukemia
M5: Acute monoblastic leukemia
M6: Acute erythroleukemia
M7: Acute megakaryoblastic leukemia

Table 1. FAB classification of acute myeloid leukemia (AML).

Since several specific cytogenetic and genetic abnormalities in AML are associated with a characteristic morphology and have distinctive clinical behavior (Harris et al., World Health Organization [WHO], 1999). The World Health Organization (WHO), classification of myeloid neoplasms and acute leukemias integrates genetic, clinical data, and morphological features.

Three prognostic groups have been described classically according to cytogenetic findings. The favorable prognostic group includes the following chromosomal abnormalities: t(15;17), t(8;21) and inv(16). Normal karyotype and cytogenetic abnormalities not classified as favorable or adverse comprise the intermediate group. The adverse prognosis group includes patients with complex karyotype, del (5q), 5 or 7 monosomy, 3q abnormalities and t(6;9) (Dohner et al., 2010).

Recently the WHO published a revised and updated edition of the 1998 WHO classification where the importance of gene mutations as diagnostic and prognostic markers in myeloid neoplasms was acknowledged. This group recommended that fluorescence in situ hybridization (FISH), reverse transcriptase–polymerase chain reaction (RT-PCR) and mutational status studies should be guided through clinical, laboratory, and morphologic information. Mutational studies for mutated *NPM1*, *CEBPA*, *FLT3*, *KIT*, *WT1*, and *MLL* are recommended in all cytogenetically normal AML. Table 2 lists the major subgroups of AML in the WHO classification (WHO, 2009).

The genes involved in the pathogenesis of leukemia are normal genes (proto-oncogenes) with either structural alterations or deregulated expression patterns, which generates in turn a novel gene (an oncogene) whose protein product acts on the host cell to enhance malignancy-related characteristics. Oncogene activation and the loss of tumor-suppressor genes are consistently associated with some types of leukemia (Cline, 1994). Some of the molecular alterations involved in the pathogenesis of AML are: translocations, mutations and overexpression of normal genes, which often characterizes a particular subtype of AML. Therefore, there are also activating mutations which lead to increased proliferation or survival, or both, of haematopoietic progenitor cells through the stimulation of tyrosine kinases such as FLT3 or RAS family members. These are considered class I mutations (Haferlach et al., 2007; Schlenk et al., 2008). Class II mutations interfere with transcription and lead to a maturation arrest either through a direct alteration of transcription factors due to gene fusions (CBF-leukemias or PML-RARA positive leukemia) or by indirect interference with transcription (MLL-rearrangements). Cytogenetic and molecular analysis of leukemic blasts, provide critical diagnostic, therapeutic and prognostic information.

Acute myeloid leukemia with recurrent genetic abnormalities
AML with t(8;21)(q22;q22); *RUNX1-RUNX1T1*
AML with inv(16)(p13.1q22) or t(16;16)(p13.1;q22); *CBFB-MYH11*
APL with t(15;17)(q22;q12); *PML-RARA*
AML with t(9;11)(p22;q23); *MLLT3-MLL*
AML with t(6;9)(p23;q34); *DEK-NUP214*
AML with inv(3)(q21q26.2) or t(3;3)(q21;q26.2); *RPN1-EVI1*
AML (megakaryoblastic) with t(1;22)(p13;q13); *RBM15-MKL1*
Provisional entity: AML with mutated NPM1
Provisional entity: AML with mutated CEBPA
Acute myeloid leukemia with myelodysplasia-related changes
Therapy-related myeloid neoplasms
Acute myeloid leukemia, not otherwise specified
AML with minimal differentiation
AML without maturation
AML with maturation
Acute myelomonocytic leukemia
Acute monoblastic/monocytic leukemia
Acute erythroid leukemia
Pure erythroid leukemia
Erythroleukemia, erythroid/myeloid
Acute megakaryoblastic leukemia
Acute basophilic leukemia
Acute panmyelosis with myelofibrosis
Myeloid sarcoma
Myeloid proliferations related to Down syndrome
Transient abnormal myelopoiesis
Myeloid leukemia associated with Down syndrome
Blastic plasmacytoid dendritic cell neoplasm

Table 2. WHO classification of acute myeloid leukemia and related neoplasms.

1.2 Molecular markers

1.2.1 Useful at diagnosis and to evaluate Minimal Residual Disease (MRD)

Molecular techniques allow us to diagnose and classify AML, establishing groups of patients with different disease behaviour and prognosis. In the same way, the development of more specific therapies and the application of risk-adjusted therapeutic approaches have been made possible. Disease relapse can be favored by persistent low numbers of leukemic cells undetectable by conventional techniques. Monitoring of AML patients has given rise to a higher insight into the effectiveness of treatment. At diagnosis, some types of myeloid leukemias display a molecular change that might be useful as a marker of neoplastic disease and MRD (Hilden et al., 1995; Nakao et al., 1996; Foroni et al., 1999; Lo Coco et al., 1999a). Specific molecular alterations of certain hematologic malignancies are useful in the detection of MRD. Translocations are the most widely involved chromosomal abnormalities in AML. These can give rise to an altered function or activity of oncogenes located at or near the translocated breakpoint. The first molecular cytogenetic marker described in AML was t(15;17), which originates a single morphologic phenotype (hyper- or micro-granular French-American-British [FAB] AML-M3 acute myeloid leukemia) (Bernstein et al., 1980). This rearrangement disappears with complete remission and is able to predict a relapse very accurately. The presence of this translocation or its fusion gene (PML/ RARα) is thus a detectable tumor marker in leukemic cells, which allows assessment of the molecular response to therapy in AML-M3 patients (Lo Coco et al., 1999b). *RUNX1-RUNX1T1* and CBFβ-MYH11 are other genetic alterations less likely to predict relapse, since they may persist even when complete remission (CR) has been achieved. However, the applicability of this strategy has been limited to those leukemia subsets characterized by genetic markers. Recent interest has focused on identifying new molecular markers that might prove significant in the diagnosis and follow-up of MRD in AML patients. In recent years, a variety ot potential molecular markers have been identified (see table 2 and table 3) (Radich & Thomson, 1997; Inoue et al., 1994; Kreuzer et al., 2001; Alberta et al., 2003; Lin et al., 2005; Gilliland & Griffin, 2002; Morishita et al., 1992).

Involvement of transcription				
	Prevalence	**Prognostic value**	**Associated mutations**	**Utility in MRD**
CBF-leukemias: Inv 16/t(16;16) CBFB/MYH11 t(8;21);*RUNX1-RUNX1T1*	15%	Favorable (Poor with KIT in normal karyotype leukemia)	FLT3 NRAS KIT	Possible
PML-RARA	10-15%	Favorable	FLT3 (40%)	Yes
MLL mutation	10-30%	Poor	-	Yes
CEBPA mutation	15-20%	Favorable if biallelic	-	Yes
AML1 mutation	1-20%	Poor	FLT3 (in 20% M0)	Yes
Activating mutations				
FLT3-ITD mutation	28-34%	Poor		Possible
FLT3-TKD mutation	20-30%	Controversial	CBF, NPM1	
c-KIT mutation	6-48%	Poor	CBF-leukemias	Yes
RAS mutation	NRAS 11% KRAS 5%	Not influence	FLT3-ITD (24-26%)	-
Other genes alterations				
NPM1 mutation	35%	Favorable (without FLT3)	FLT3	Yes
BAALC overexpression	65%	Poor	-	Possible
EVI-1 overexpression	10-22%	Poor	-	Possible
WT1 overexpression	10-15%	Poor	-	Yes
DNMT3A mutation	20%	Poor	FLT3-ITD	-
IDH1/2 mutation	15%	Controversial	NPM1, FLT3-ITD	-

Table 3. Molecular markers in AML: prevalence, prognostic, associated mutations, genetic alterations and utility in MDR.

1.2.2 Genetic alterations with prognosis value

In recent years, the availability of new genetic and molecular prognostic markers in AML has grown considerably. This is particularly important in the case of patients with normal cytogenetics who comprise the largest subgroup of AML patients (approximately 45%) where many new prognostic factors have been identified. These include gene mutations in FLT3 (Fms-like tyrosine kinase 3; generally FLT3-ITD has been associated with significantly worse survival (Sheikhha et al, 2003)), NPM1 (nucleophosmin 1) and CEBPA (CCAAT enhancer-binding protein-α; generally favorable in cases of biallelic mutations) and gene overexpression as BAALC, WT1, EVI1 and MN1 (Foran, 2010).

Identifying alterations in these genes might provide independent prognostic value in predicting the outcome of acute leukemia, as in the case of the NPM1 mutation gene, which is a relatively frequent abnormality in AML patients and is useful in detecting MRD (Falini et al., 2007).

2. Detailed description of molecular markers

Next, we will describe the most common molecular markers in AML.

2.1 Core Binding Factor (CBF)

Leukemias affecting CBF are characterized by rearrangements of genes that code for components of the heterodimeric transcription factor CBF, which plays an essential role in haematopoiesis (Gabert et al., 2006). CBF complex is a heterodimer composed of RUNX1 (also called AML1) and CBFβ and is the target of at least three common transloctions in AML: t(8;21)/RUNX1-RUNX1T1, t(3;21)/RUNX1-EVI1 and inv(16) or t(16;16) resulting in CBFβ-MYH11. Rearrangements of *AML1* and *CBFB* with other genes lead to chimeric proteins that disrupt the CBF complex, suppressing the activation of transcription.

2.1.1 AML1 (RUNX1) rearrangements

AML1, also called, RUNX1, is normally expressed in all hematopoietic lineages and regulates the expression of several genes specifically linked to hematopoiesis, including the granulocyte colony-stimulating factor receptor, interleukin 3, T-cell receptor, and myeloperoxidase (MPO) genes. The *AML1* gene (on 21q22) is one of the genes most frequently deregulated in leukemias, generally through translocations that produce chimeric messenger RNA. Chimeric protein AML1-ETO (*RUNX1-RUNX1T1)* results from the t(8;21)(q22;q22) involving the AMLI gene on chromosome 21 and the ETO gene on chromosome 8. This rearrangement is detected in approximately 8% of AML cases in children and young adults. *RUNX1-RUNX1T1* is a marker for favourable outcome and an important PCR target for MRD detection. Most patients achieve a CR after induction therapy and those patients benefit most from a postremission therapy with high-dose cytarabin (Bloomfield et al., 1998; Perea et al., 2006). Hence, this marker permits to single out a relatively small subgroup of patients who are more likely to relapse (Gabert et al., 2003). *RUNX1-RUNX1T1* is also frequently associated with c-kit mutations which determine an adverse outcome within this group of patients with favorable prognosis. In addition, the loss of Y chromosome in male patients with t(8;21) leukemia is a negative prognostic factor for the overall survival (Schlenk et al., 2004). While the molecular diagnosis is performed by qualitative and quantitative Real Time RT-PCR (QRT-PCR), MRD monitoring is performed by quantitative QRT-PCR. The rare balanced t(3;21)(q26;q22) was described in AML, mainly after treatment with topoisomerase II inhibitors. This translocation fuses the AML1 gene on 21q22 and the EVI-1 gene on 3q26 resulting in t(3;21)(q26;q22). This translocation is associated with higher WBC and platelets counts but is not, however, predictive for relapse-free or overall survival (Preudhomme et al., 2000; Meyers et al., 1993; Lutghart et al., 2010).

2.1.2 AML1 mutations

AML1 mutations can be found in *de novo* leukemia, particularly subtypes FAB M0 and M7, as well as in patients with trisomy 21 and myelodysplastic syndromes. Testing for mutations can be performed By real time PCR or PCR-single stranded conformational polymorphism (SSCP). A multivariate analysis carried out by Schnittger et al., showed an independent unfavourable prognostic significance of AML1 (or RUNX1) mutations for overall survival (Schnittger et al., 2011).

2.1.3 CBFb-MYH11

Inv(16)(p13;q22) or t(16;16)(p13;q22) are among the most frequent recurring chromosomal rearrangements detected in AML, generally observed in cases showing myelomonocytic differentiation and having abnormal bone marrow eosinophils (M4 Eo AML in the French American British (FAB) classification). Inv(16)(p13;q22) is found in approximately 10-12% of cases of AML. It can occur in all age groups but is predominantly seen in younger patients. This rearrangement results in the disruption of the myosin heavy chain (MYH) gene at 16p13 and the core binding factor β(CBFβ) gene at 16q22 (FAB, 1976). Ten different CBFβ-MYH11 transcripts have been reported, but the frequency of each transcript is variable. CBFB-MYH11 positive patients are considered to have a favourable prognosis. This rearrangement is frequently associated with c-kit and FLT3 mutations which worsen the prognosis. Quantitative QRT-PCR allows monitoring of CR (Gabert et al., 2003; Perea et al., 2005).

2.1.4 CEBPA

The CCAAT/enhancer binding alpha protein (C/EBPα) is the founding member of a family of related leucine zipper transcription factors. Mutations in CEBPA are found in 5-14% of AML and have been associated with a relatively favourable outcome only in biallelic mutations of this gene. There are two main classes of mutation situated at the N- terminal or

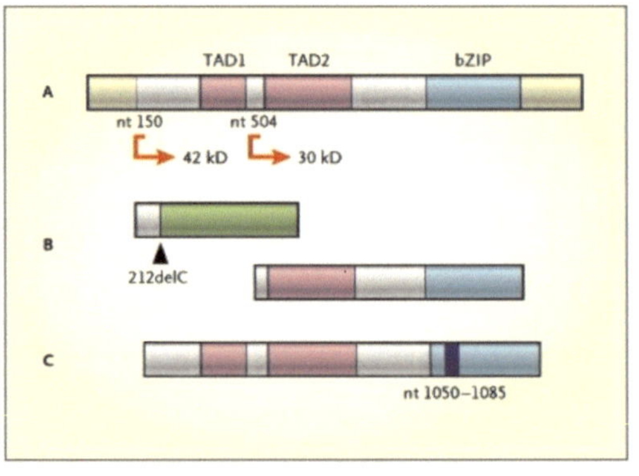

Fig. 1. Schematic representation of CEBPA (by Smith, 2004).

C-terminal basic leucine zipper (bZIP) regions (Figure 1). The latter affect both DNA binding and homo and heterodimerization with other CEBP-proteins. The former introduce a premature stoppage of the translation of the p42 CEBPA protein, preserving a p30 isoform, which was shown to inhibit DNA binding and transactivation by C/EBPα p42. CEBPA mutations are exclusively related to the intermediate risk group karyotype AML. CEBPA insertion, deletions and point mutations are detected usually by DNA sequencing (Wouters et al., 2009; Pabst et al., 2001; Fuchs et al., 2008).

2.2 PML-RARα

Acute promyelocytic leukemia is a distinct subtype of AML (AML-M3) according to the FAB classification. AML-M3 is characterized by t(15;17) that involves the retinoic acid receptor a (RARα) gene on chromosome 17 and the promyelocytic leukemia gene (PML) on chromosome 15. At the molecular level, t(15;17) results in a hybrid PML/ RARα gene, which is easily identified by reverse transcriptase-polymerase chain reaction (RT-PCR). This test provides a rapid and refined diagnosis. The usefulness of minimal residual disease monitoring during follow up (Lo Coco et al., 1992; Lo Coco et al., 1999a) has been well established. The different breakpoints within the PML gene cluster can be located in three regions: bcr1, 2 and 3.

The assessment of remission status at the molecular level by RT-PCR of PML-RARα represents a significant clinical advance with respect to other poorly sensitive methods (morphology, karyotype). The treatment of this disease (arsenicals, liposomal ATRA, other retinoid derivatives, etc) needs to be assessed taking into account the response at the RT-PCR level. The detection of residual PML-RARα transcripts during clinical remission predicts subsequent hematologic relapse. This determines the need for additional treatment given the benefits of anticipating salvage therapy in AML-M3. Figure 3 shows the statistically significant difference between patients treated for molecular relapse and the historical series treated for hematologic relapse (Lo Coco et al., 1999b).

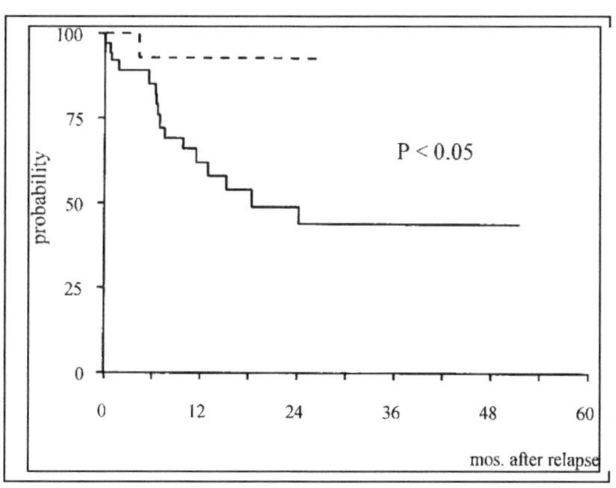

Fig. 2. Kaplan-Meier estimates of overall survival from relapse in patients treated at the time of molecular relapse (dotted line) and in the historical series of patients treated for hematologic relapse (continuous line).

Around 40% of all cases of PML-RARα-positive AML show FLT3 mutations. FLT3-ITD mutations, but not *FLT3-D835*, are associated with characteristic diagnostic hematological features of acute promyelocytic leukemia, in particular with high WBC counts. Also, FLT3 mutations, especially ITD, can adversely affect overall survival and disease-free survival in PML-RARα-positive AML (Beitinjaneh et al., 2010). However, in a large series of 739 patients with acute promyelocytic leukemia treated with ATRA and anthracycline-based chemotherapy, we were unable to demonstrate an independent prognostic value of *FLT3* mutations (Barragan et al., 2011).

2.3 DEK-CAN

AML defined by t(6;9) is a relatively rare disease, associated with specific clinical and morphological features (Garcon et al., 2005). Especially in young adults, the leukemic phase can be preceded by dysplastic features, conferring a bad prognosis. Morphological findings usually correlate with FAB M2 (60%), M4 (30%), or Ml (von Lindern et al., 1990). A chimeric protein is generated, resulting from the fusion between DEK and the 30- terminus of the CAN gene, also known as NUP214 (von Lindern et al., 1990). DEK is a component of metazoan chromatin capable of modifying the structure of DNA by introducing supercoils. CAN is a nuclear pore complex protein implicated in nucleocytoplasmic trafficking. The CAN gene is also involved in several fusion transcripts described in acute leukemia other than DEK in t(6;9)(p23;q34) AML, such as the SET gene and recently with ABL in T-cell acute lymphoblastic leukaemia (ALL). The DEK-CAN transcript can be used as a marker of t(6;9) AML which can be sensitively monitored by the polymerase chain reaction. This offers a great advantage in the diagnosis, monitoring of response to chemotherapy, and detection of minimal residual disease after bone marrow transplantation (von Lindern et al., 1992). DEK-CAN is related with an adverse prognosis (Dohner et al., 2010).

2.4 NPM1

NPM1 gene is located in 5q35 and encodes a phosphoprotein, nucleophosmin, which moves between the nucleus and the cytoplasm. The gene product is thought to be involved in several processes including regulation of the ARF/p53 pathway. Mutations in exon 12 in this gene are associated with AML with normal karyotype (50%) and especially correlate with monocytic leukemias. Patients with *NPM1* mutations have a significantly higher rate of complete remissions (CRs) after standard induction chemotherapy except for cases associated with internal tandem duplications mutations of FLT3 (Falini et al., 2007; Gale et al., 2008). Gale et al. (2008) identified 3 prognostic groups among the NPM1+ AML patients: good in those with only a NPM1 mutation and absence of a FLT3-ITD; intermediate in those with either absence of FLT3-ITD or NPM1 mutations or mutations in both genes; and poor in those with only FLT3-ITD. Monitoring can be performed by quantitative PCR (Schnittger et al., 2009). In our group, the incidence of NPM1 mutation was 30% (17 of 55 patients with AML), being this prevalence similar to that found for FLT3-ITD in the same population (29 %). The 17 NPM1+ AML patients were distributed as follows: eight M1-M2 (47.1 %), four M4-M5 (23.5%), and five not labelled (29.4 %) because cytogenetic studies were not informative due to several reasons. 64.7% of the NPM1+ patients had a normal karyotype, while 5.8% of them had cytogenetic anomalies. FLT3-ITD mutations were found in 41.2 % of the NPM1+ AML cases. In contrast to what has been described in the literature our group did not find a higher incidence of M4 or M5 subtypes (Thiede et al., 2002). In our case, a higher incidence of M1 and M2 subtypes was detected (Table 4). However the differences are most likely attributable to the small sample size of our cohort as compared to the Thiede cohort. The global mortality was analyzed disregarding risk factors, with a mortality of 67 % in the NPM1+/FLT3-ITD- group standing in clear contrast to a 100% death rate in the NPM1+/FLT3-ITD+ group (Lopez Jorge et al., 2006). This was confirmed in another study where we analysed the incidence and prognostic relevance of CD34/CD7/DR surface markers in a group of forty two NPM1positive patients and related it to FLT3-ITD mutations. We found that 84% of the NPM1 positive patients had normal karyotypes. Mutations in FLT3-ITD were detected in 23.8% of the NPM1+ patients. The screening for this mutation could be very useful in the future as patients with normal karyotype and expression of this molecular marker is included in a better prognostic subgroup (Gomez Casares et al., 2009; Dohner et al., 2010).

	N° patients	NPM1+	NPM1-
Patients (%)	55	17 (30.9)	38(69)
Median (range age) (years)	60 (18-95)	58 (18-82)	60 (19-95)
Age, r**FAB subtype**			
M0	5	0	5
M1/M2	8/10	4/4	4/6
M4/M5	12/4	3/1	9/3
M6	1	0	1
Not labeled	15	5	10
Cytogenetic:			
Normal karyotype	24	11	13
del(5)	2	0	2
del(7)	5	0	5
trisomy 8	1	1	0
t(4;11)	1	0	1
t(8;21)	2	0	2
t(10;11)	1	0	1
t(9;11)	1	0	1
t(12;13)	1	0	1
t(3;10)	1	0	1
+11	2	0	2
-Y	2	0	2
Complex: >3 abnormalities	2	0	2
Non determinated	14	5	9
FLT3-ITD+ (%)	16 (29)	7(41.2)	9(23.6)

Table 4. Cytogenetics and demographic characteristics in a group of 55 AML patients (Lopez Jorge et al., 2006).

2.5 c-KIT

KIT is a proto-oncogene located on chromosome band 4q11-12 and encodes a 145-kDa transmembrane glycoprotein member of the type III receptor tyrosine kinase family. Ligand independent activation of KIT results from mutations in the extracellular portion of the receptor (exon 8), transmembrane and juxtamembrane domains (exons 10 and 11, respectively), and activation loop of the tyrosine kinase domain (exon 17). *c-KIT* mutations have been found in a variable but relatively high frequency (up to 50%) in patients with CBF

AML, including both t(8;21) and the other major type of CBF AML inv(16)(p13q22) or t(16;16)(p13;q22). This appears to confer a quite unfavourable prognosis with higher relapse risk (associated to inv(16) or t(8;21)). An adverse effect on OS in AML with inv(16) has been described, particularly those that occur in exon 17 (Paschka et al., 2006). Such patients may warrant more aggressive or alternative therapy. The presence of the *c-KIT* mutation would be also important because it provides a target for novel tyrosine kinase inhibitor (TKI) therapy (Pollard et al., *2010).*

2.6 FLT3

Flt3 is a member of the class III tyrosine kinase receptor family that includes the c-kit, c-fms, and PDGF receptors. The Flt3 receptor is preferentially expressed on hematopoietic stem cells and mediates stem cell differentiation and proliferation. Interaction of the Flt3 receptor with Flt3 ligand causes receptor dimerization, leading to the activation of the receptor tyrosine kinase and receptor autophosphorylation. The phosphorylated Flt3 transduces activation signals through associations with various cytoplasmic proteins, including ras GTPase-activating protein, phospholipase C, and Src family tyrosine kinases. Activation of the Flt3 receptor by ligand-dependent phosphorylation induces cellular proliferation via activation of cytoplasmic mediators. Thus, constitutive activation of the Flt3 pathway may lead to disease proliferation and may block cellular apoptotic response to conventional chemotherapy. An internal tandem duplication of the juxtamembrane (JM) domain-coding sequence of the *FLT3 (FLT3-IT)* gene on chromosome 13 has been identified in a group of patients with AML. Constitutive activation of the Flt3 receptor tyrosine kinase, either by internal tandem duplication (ITD) mutations of the juxtamembrane domain or point mutations clustering in the second tyrosine kinase domain (TKD mutations as D835), has been found in 20% to 30% of patients with AML and in 30% to 45% of patients with normal karyotype (reviewed by Stirewalt and Radich (2003)). ITD mutations have been associated with an increased risk of treatment failure after conventional chemotherapy (overall survival and disease-free survival were worse for ITD positive patients versus *FLT3* wildtype patients), whereas the prognostic relevance of *FLT3* point mutations is less evident (D835 mutants did not appear to have a worse median overal suvival or disease-free survival compared with the wildtype group) (Sheikhha et al., 2003). Recently, Spassov et al analyzed for *WT1* and *FLT3*-internal tandem duplication (*FLT3-ITD*) expression in 30 samples of AML patients and determined that high *WT1* expression correlated with the presence of *FLT3-ITD* ($P = 0{\cdot}014$) and with a lower rate of complete remissions ($P = 0{\cdot}023$) (Spassov et al., 2011). The detection of both molecular markers (*WT1* and *FLT3-ITD*) may be helpful in defining high risk AML patients that need special therapeutic strategies.

Several studies described that a higher mutational load as determined by calculation of *FLT3-ITD/FLT3* wildtype ratio indicates a worse prognosis in mutation carriers. Therefore, it was suggested that not the FLT3-ITD per se, but more likely loss of heterozygosity is associated with the unfavorable outcome in FLT3-ITD mutated AML (Meshinchi et al., 2001; Yanada et al., 2005; Thiede et al., 2002; Schnittger et al., 2011).

2.7 EVI1 overexpression

The ectopic viral integration site 1 (EVI1), located in chromosome 3q26, has been recognized in the last years as one of the most aggressive oncogenes associated to human leukemia (Gröschel et al., 2010). The inappropriate expression of EVI1 in hematopoietic cells has been

implicated in the development or progress of myeloid disorders (Lugthart et al., 2008). Previous studies, applying microarray technology, indicate that high levels of EVI1 expression are detected in 10% -22% of patients with AML (Barjesteh et al., 2003). Although the higher expression of EVI1 gene was clearly associated with myeloid malignancies, is not restricted to this group. It is noteworthy that overexpression of EVI1 was also observed in 13.8% of patients with acute lymphoid leukemia. The correlation between overexpression of EVI1 in bone marrow and poor outcome in AML is a frequent issue of discussion in the literature (Lugthart et al., 2008; Luzardo et al., 2007).
We analyzed the incidence of EVI1 overexpression in haematological malignancies and its value as a prognostic factor. EVI1 overexpression (EVI1+) was examined by RT-PCR in bone marrow and/or peripheral blood samples of 113 AML patients at diagnosis and during follow-up. We found that 23.8% of AML overexpressed EVI1, as established by our previously determined cut-off point. Correlation with FAB subtypes stands as follows: 2M0, 1 M1,3 M2, 6 M4, 7 M5, 1 M6, 4 secondary AML and 3 not labeled. Survival curves in the AML group didn´t show any significant differences in overall survival and disease free survival when comparing EVI1+ to EVI1- populations. In AML samples a greater than expected incidence of EVI1 expression was observed (22.8% vs 11% previously described). When survival curves were analyzed in the AML group with ages ranging from 14 to 60 years, all of them treated with similar chemotherapy schemes, no significant difference was observed. However, a recent collaboration with other groups, showed that *EVI1* overexpression is a poor prognostic marker in patients <65 years in an independent large cohort, and showed that the total absence of *EVI1* expression has a prognostic impact in the outcome of acute myeloid leukemia patients (Vazquez et al.,2011).

2.8 BAALC AND MN1

The Brain and Acute Leukemia Cytoplasmic *(BAALC)*, human gene located on chromosome 8q22.3, has also been found to be an important adverse prognostic factor if overexpressed in normal karyotype AML, suggesting a role for BAALC overexpression in acute leukemia. This gene is highly conserved in mammals. Normally, BAALC is almost exclusively expressed in neuroectoderm-derived tissues. Though little is known about the biological function of BAALC, it is highly expressed in hematopoietic precursor cells as well as leukemic blasts and is down-regulated during differentiation. BAALC has been postulated to play its role in the cytoskeleton network due to its cellular location. BAALC expression is an independent adverse prognostic factor and is associated with a specific gene-expression profile. Recent studies revealed the prognostic impact of BAALC expression in AML and also as a marker in minimal residual disease. Currently, determination of BAALC expression is performed by qualitative and quantitative real-time PCR, although the lack of validation or standardization studies limits its utility (Tanner et al., 2001; Gregory et al., 2009; Baldus et al., 2003; Najima et al., 2010).
The meningioma 1 *(MN1)* gene is localized on human chromosome 22. *MN1* overexpression is a prognostic marker in patients with AML with normal karyotype characterized by an intermediate prognosis. Patients with high *MN1* expression had a significantly worse prognosis (the overall survival was shorter and relapse rate was higher in this group compared to low *MN1* expression group). High *MN1* expression has as well been associated with other AML characteristics like inv(16) or overexpression of *EVI-1* (Heuser et al, 2007). In addition, MN1 is able to induce myeloid leukemias in a murine model (Heuser et al, 2011). This suggested that MN1 may play a functional role in the pathogenesis of AML.

We performed a retrospective analysis of MN1 expression in a group of 49 AML patients with a mean age of 52 years (43 de novo AML and 6 secondary AML). In order to analyze response to chemotherapy, overall survival and correlation to other molecular markers (NPM1, FLT3-ITD, EVI1 and BAALC), patients were further classified into three groups depending on prognosis (favourable with 11 patients, intermediate with 25 and poor with 12). We analysed by real-time PCR the expression of MN1 in patients samples. We used as positive control of expression RNA of KG1 cell line that overexpress MN1. The incidence of MN1 overespression was 65.3%. The study showed that MN1 overexpression correlated to BAALC expression. We did not find relation with other markers, such as EVI-1, NPM-1 and FLT3. MN1 and BAALC overexpression have been associated to induction treatment refractoriness. However, due to the limited sample size in our series, determining whether MN1 or BAALC were actually involved with refractoriness was not possible. The 2-year overall survival was 52% and 53% for MN1 overexpressed and MN1 not overexpressed patients respectively. The 5-year overall survival was 52% and 42% respectively, showing no significant differences. Survival analysis for the intermediate risk AML group did not show significant differences either. MN1 overexpression was not associated with a worse prognosis in any of the studied patients, probably due to a small sample size (Rodriguez et al., 2010).

2.9 WT1

The Wilms' tumor locus was identified as a tumor suppressor gene, which is inactivated in Wilms' tumor, a pediatric kidney cancer. This protein, displaying characteristic features of a transcription factor, and with an expression restricted to kidney and haematopoetic cells, was called Wilms' tumor gene 1 (*WT1*). This gene is located on chromosome 11p13 and encodes a zinc-finger transcription factor influencing the expression of several growth factors and their corresponding receptors. It is also known to be involved in the early stage of hematological cell differentiation. Aberrant expression may be one mechanism by which the normal function of *WT1* is disrupted. However, the exact role of *WT1* in hematopoiesis and leukemogenesis still remains unclear. The abundant overexpression of *WT1* in leukemia creates a very attractive target for quantitative MRD studies in AML, especially in those samples with no specific fusion gene available. The method used to determine the expression of *WT1* gene is the RT-PCR, which will reveal its value as a marker to detect minimal residual disease (Keilholz et al., 2005; Weisser et al., 2005; Inoue et al., 1994; Garg et al., 2003).
Mutations of the coding region (most frequenly in 7 and 9 exons) of the *WT1* gene have also been described and occur in 10–15% of AML (figure 3). Gaidzik et al. concluded that *WT1* mutation as a single molecular marker did not have an impact on outcome. On the other hand, Hou et al. demostrated that *WT1* mutations disappeared in *WT1*-mutated studied patients who achieved complete remission, suggesting its potential use as MRD marker (Gaidzik et al., 2009; Hou et al., 2010).

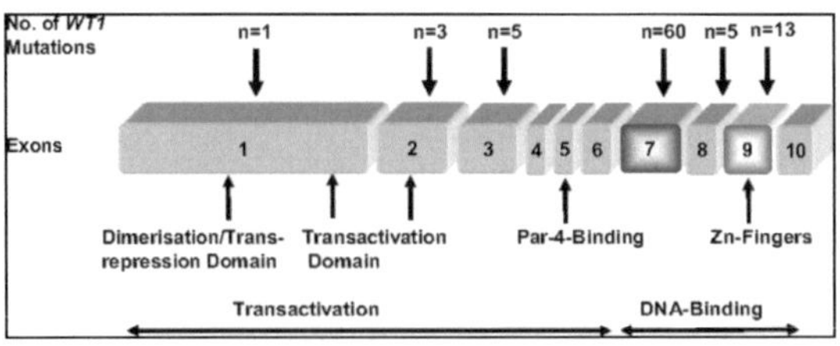

Fig. 3. Structure of the *WT1* gene and localization of the 87 mutations identified by Gaidzik et al.

2.10 MLL rearrangement and MLL-PTD

The *MLL* (mixed lineage leukemia) gene located at 11q23, is fused to a variety of partner genes through chromosomal translocations in acute leukemias. Up to now, more than 40 different *MLL* partner genes have been identified. *MLL* gene contains 100 kb of DNA, but nearly all breakpoints are clustered within a 8.3 kb region. Molecular analysis shows that fusion of the amino terminus of *MLL* to the carboxy terminus of partner genes generates the critical leukemogenic fusion proteins. Abnormalities of the mixed-lineage leukemia (*MLL*) gene can be detected in *de novo* acute myeloid leukemia (AML) and acute lymphoblastic leukemia (ALL) as well as in therapy-related AML, particularly after treatment with DNA topoisomerase II inhibitors (generally less than 5-10% of patients carried this rearrangements).The most common translocation involving 11q23 in acute myeloid leukemia (AML) is t(9;11)(p22;q23), which results in the generation of a fusion transcript of *MLL-AF.* The other common translocations involving 11q23 in AML are t(6;11)(q27;q23), t(10;11)(p12;q23), t(11;19)(q23;p13.1) and t(11;19)(q23;p13.3); these translocations result in the generation of fusion transcripts *MLL-AF6, MLL-AF10, MLL-ELL* or *MLL-ENL,* respectively. In AML, *MLL-AF9* has generally been associated with a more favourable outcome although this finding is controversial. This rearrangement is related to a superior event-free and overall survival as compared to patients with other chromosomal abnormalities or with no detectable rearrangements (Dimartino et al., 1999; Balgobind et al., 2005). In contrast, the other traslocation involving Cr 11q23 are asociated with poor prognostic in more cases (Dimartino et al., 1999; Balgobind et al., 2005). t(9;11)(p22;q23) is classified as intermediate and t(v;11)(v;q23) as adverse prognostic group (Döhner et al., 2010). Therefore, detection and identification of the different types of *MLL* rearrangements is of clinical importance. A recent study indicated that quantification by RQ-PCR of the fusion gene transcript levels at diagnosis may be of prognostic relevance (Shih et al., 2006; Jansen et al., 2005). One type of *MLL* rearrangement not detectable by classic cytogenetic is the partial tandem duplication of *MLL* (*MLL*-PTD). This rearrangement results most commonly from a duplication of a genomic region encompassing either *MLL* exons 5 through 11 or *MLL* exons 5 through 12 that is inserted into intron 4 of a full-length *MLL* gene, thus fusing introns 11 or 12 with intron 4. At a transcriptional level, this results in a unique in-frame fusion of exons 11 or 12 upstream of exon 5. In adult de novo AML with a normal karyotype, the presence of the *MLL*-PTD has been associated with a worse prognosis (ie, shorter duration of remission) when compared with normal karyotype AML without the *MLL*-PTD (Whitman et al., 2005).

2.11 Other molecular markers in research: Renin expression

There have been reports of experimental findings that relate the renin-angiotensin system (RAS) with hematopoiesis. Some studies have identified RAS components located in the bone marrow (Haznedaroglu & Buyukasik, 1997) that might functionally affect cellular proliferation and differentiation in physiological or pathological states (Huckle & Earp, 1994; Comte et al., 1997). It has been demonstrated that the RAS component renin is expressed in the bone marrow microenvironment as well as in hematopoietic cells (Abali et al., 2002). Bone marrow blast cells of some types of AML (M4 and M5 FAB types) express renin (Wulf et al., 1998), however no expression has been detected in normal bone marrow from healthy donors (Gómez Casares et al., 2002). Our group also detected renin expression in AML patients, but it did not relate to monocytic dififerentiation or to the existence of other cytogenetic risk markers (Gómez Casares et al., 2002). Moreover, renin expression has been found to be related to disease activity, disappearing with AML remission and returning with relapse (De la Iglesia et al., 2006).

We did not found statistically significant differences in the outcome between renin-positive and renin-negative patients (De la Iglesia et al., 2006).

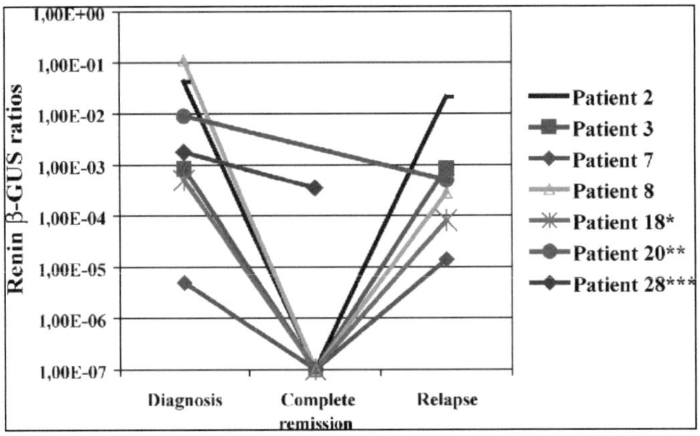

Fig. 4. Renin:βglucuronidase ratios vs clinical state of the quantified patients. *This data belong to third relapse, CR and fourth relapse, respectively. **This patient did not reach CR, continuing the positivity of the renin gene expression. ***Patient 28 in morphological CR was presented with 1% blasts in BM that later disappeared (De la Iglesia et al., 2006).

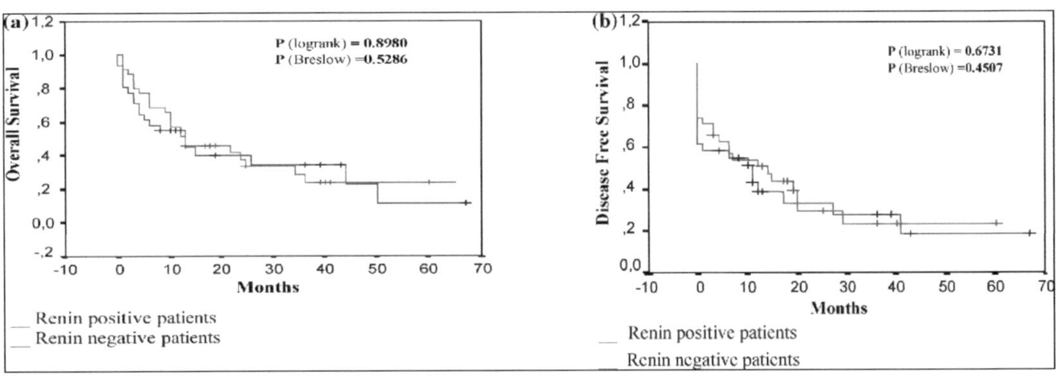

Fig. 5. (a) Overall survival of renin-positive and renin-negative patients with AML. Kaplan-Meier plot showing the correlation between overall survival and renin expression in AML patients. (b)Disease-free survival of renin-positive and renin-negative patients with AML. Kaplan-Meier plot showing the correlation between disease-free survival and renin expression in AML patients. (De la Iglesia et al., 2006).

Renin expression is related to undifferentiated phenotypic cell lines (K562, KU812), since no expression of the renin gene was found in cellular lines that showed a highly differentiated phenotype like HL60 and U937 (Gómez Casares et al., 2002). ACE inhibitors (captopril and trandolapril) and AT1 receptor blocker (losartan) produce a stop in proliferation in K562 cells with captopril (C) 10 mM and trandolapril (T) 2 mM (figure 6a) as well as an increase in the apoptotic rate in renin positive leukemia cell lines (K562) after the treatment with captopril (data not shown) and trandolapril (figure 6b) (De la Iglesia et al., 2009).

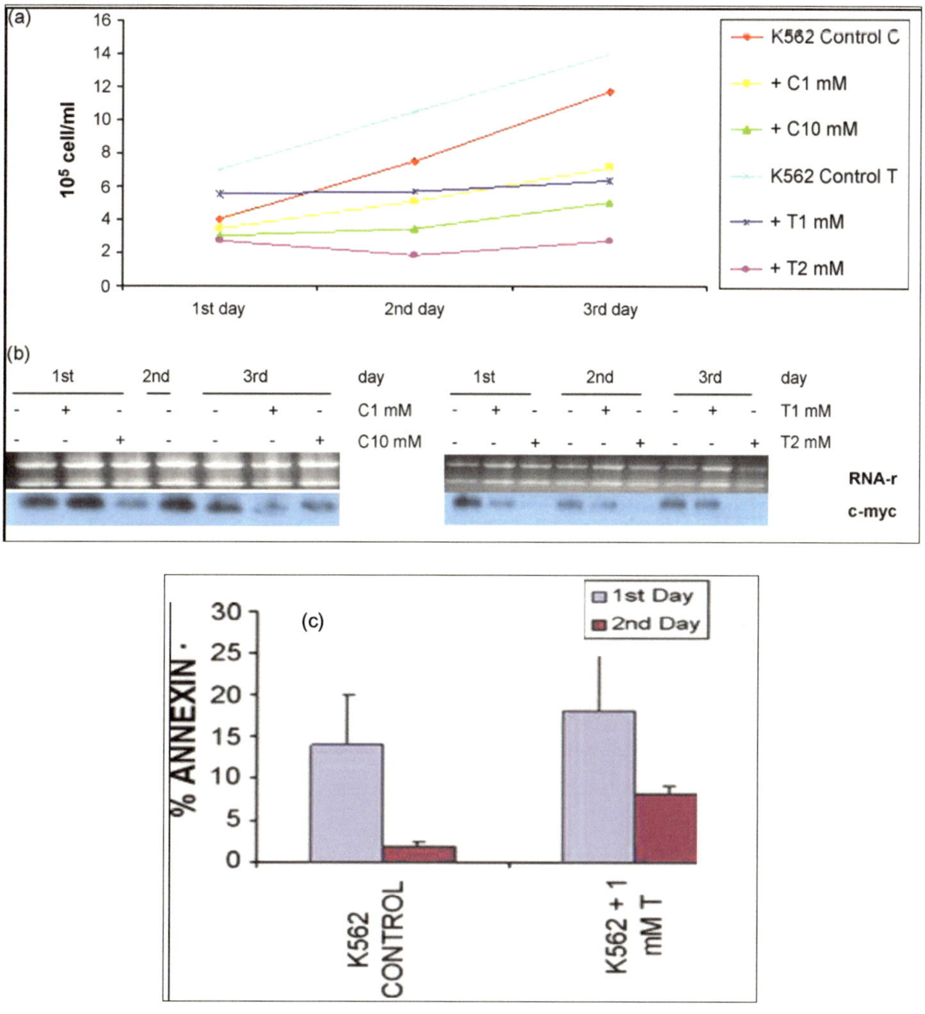

Fig. 6. **(a)** Proliferation in K562 after the treatment with captopril (C) and trandolapril (T). **(b)** C-myc gene expression in K562 after the treatment with the same drugs. **(c)** Apoptosis determined by annexin V binding in K562 and K562 transfected with bcl-2 and bcl-x (Kbcl2 and Kbclx) cells treated with 1mM trandolapril (T) (De la Iglesia et al., 2009). All experiments were performed in triplicate.

The leukaemogenic role of renin gene expression and the implicated molecular pathways have not yet been elucidated but it may offer novel therapeutic approaches in pathological or neoplastic conditions (Haznedaroglu & Öztürk, 2003).

3. Conclusion

The AML embraces very heterogeneous entities with different clinical behaviours. Some of these leukemias have certain chromosomal alterations that are related to specific morphological and clinical subtypes. Their identification has had great impact on different management aspects of these diseases, either from the standpoint of diagnosis, prognosis or development of a treatment plan tailored to the risk of relapse. This has been largely possible thanks to the application of molecular biology studies, which have provided a better and deeper understanding of the pathogenesis of leukemia.

The genetic alterations that occur at different stages fall into two broad groups: those that activate signal transduction as c-KIT and FLT3 (type I) and those which alter transcription factors such as CBF, RAR-α, CEBPA and NPM1 (type II). These two groups work together in leukemogenesis, being very frequent the coexistence of alterations of the two groups in the same patient.

The knowledge of these molecular markers helps us to classify patients within certain prognostic groups. In this way, in patients with normal cytogenetics, it is very important to know if there is a mutation of the FLT3 gene as well as its kind (ITD or TKD), because this information is of great relevance in order to select the appropriate treatment scheme. Moreover, the overexpression of the genes BAALC (under OS, DFS), MN1 (induction failure in patients with normal karyotype) or EVI1 (adverse impact) has been shown to have prognostic significance in AML.

In a laboratory setting there are different ways to classify leukemias. One of them is the rationale showed in the figure 5. According to the cytogenetic or molecular biology at diagnosis, it is possible to perform different determinations which will allow us to classify the patients within a favourable or unfavourable prognostic group. AML patients are classified at the time of diagnosis into three different prognostic groups based on their cytogenetic profiles.

There are plenty of algorithms which allow us to classify patients into different prognostic groups. They are undergoing continuous changes with the enrichment of new data. If we are in the presence of a CBF leukemia (by showing RUNX1-RUNXT1 or inv (16)), mutational analysis of c-kit should be performed, as this mutation translates into a higher risk of relapse. In patients with AML with normal karyotype, we recommend to analyze for FLT3-ITD first, as FLT-ITD3 is a well-known adverse prognostic factor. We then recommend screening for NPM1 mutations as a next step, because it is another mutation with clinical relevance of this subgroup of patients in the absence of FLT3-ITD. Then, given the favourable prognosis of NK-AML with biallelic CEBPA mutation, we recommend a CEBPA mutational analysis in those patients non-carriers of FLT3-ITD or NPM1. Also, FLT3-TKD an others mutations can be analyze in a context of clinical trials, even though there is no prognostic relevance.

There after, it is possible to perform other studies such as the detection of mutations in MLL/AF9 or BAALC, MN1 and EVI1 gene overexpression in order to make a better stratification of the prognosis. Besides working with prognostic and follow up markers with a recognized utility, we are also carrying out experimental work with new, not yet validated markers which will probably help us in the follow up, prognosis, classification and monitoring of AML patients. Renin, EVI1 and WT1 would be markers applicable to AML patients, especially in those with normal karyotype where they will facilitate the monitoring of minimal residual disease.

GENETIC GROUP	SUBSET
Favorable	t(8;21)(q22;q22); *RUNX1-RUNX1T1* inv(16)(p13.1q22) or t(16;16)(p13.1;q22); *CBFB-MYH11* Mutated *NPM1* without *FLT3*-ITD (normal karyotype) Mutated *CEBPA* (normal karyotype)
Intermediate-1	Mutated *NPM1* and *FLT3*-ITD (normal karyotype) Wild-type *NPM1* and *FLT3*-ITD (normal karyotype) Wild-type *NPM1* without *FLT3*-ITD (normal karyotype)
Intermediate-2	t(9;11)(p22;q23); *MLLT3-MLL* Cytogenetic abnormalities not classified as favorable or adverse
Adverse	inv(3)(q21q26.2) or t(3;3)(q21;q26.2); *RPN1-EVI1* t(6;9)(p23;q34); *DEK-NUP214* t(v;11)(v;q23); *MLL* rearranged -5 or del(5q); -7; abnl(17p); complex karyotype

Table 5. Standardized reporting for correlation of cytogenetic and molecular genetic data in AML with clinical data (Döhner. European LeukemiaNet , 2010)

In recent past, treatments had an empirical basis, lack of specificity and, therefore, limited effectiveness combined with high toxicity. The treatment of AML pioneered the search for specific therapies with the use of ATRA in APL. Currently, the ultimate goal of the understanding and classification of molecular aberrations in every AML subtype is to design a targeted therapy, which will reduce the risk of relapse and treatment side effects. That is because the future of AML therapy should be in the search and development of drugs that are directed against specific molecular or fusion proteins aberrations. On the other hand, due to the interaction between different molecular aberrations that arise in AML, the design of these new drugs has to be focused on the combined inhibition of several signalling pathways to achieve maximum clinical benefit.

4. References

Abali H, Haznedaroglu IC, Goker H, Celik I, Ozatli D, Koray Z & Caglar M. (2002). Circulating and Local Bone Marrow Renin-angiotensin System in Leukemic Hematopoiesis: Preliminary Evidences. Hematology, Vol. 7, No.75-82.

Alberta, J. A., Springett, G. M., Rayburn, H., Natoli, T. A., Loring, J., Kreidberg, J. A., & Housman, D. (2003). Role of the WT1 tumor suppressor in murine hematopoiesis. Blood, Vol. 101, No.7, 2570-2574.

Baldus, C. D., Tanner, S. M., Kusewitt, D. F., Liyanarachchi, S., Choi, C., Caligiuri, M. A., Bloomfield, C. D., & Chapelle, A. d. l. (2003). BAALC, a novel marker of human hematopoietic progenitor cells. Experimental Hematology, Vol. 31, No.11, 1051-1056, 0301-472X.

Balgobind, B.V., Raimondi, S.C., Harbott, J., Zimmermann, M., Alonzo, T.A., Auvrignon, A., Beverloo, H.B., Chang, M., Creutzig, U., Dworzak, M.N., Forestier, E., Gibson, B., Hasle, H., Harrison, C.J., Heerema, N.A., Kaspers, G.J., Leszl, A., Litvinko, N., Nigro, L.L., Morimoto, A., Perot, C., Pieters, R., Reinhardt, D., Rubnitz, J.E., Smith, F.O., Stary, J., Stasevich, I., Strehl, S., Taga, T., Tomizawa, D., Webb, D., Zemanova, Z., Zwaan, C.M. & van den Heuvel-Eibrink, M.M. (2009). Novel prognostic subgroups in childhood 11q23/MLL-rearranged acute myeloid leukemia: results of an international retrospective study. Blood, Vol. 114, No. 12, 2489-96.

Barjesteh van Waalwijk van Doorn-Khosrovani, S., Erpelinck, C., van Putten, W. L. J., Valk, P. J. M., van der Poel-van de Luytgaarde, S., Hack, R., Slater, R., Smit, E. M. E., Beverloo, H. B., Verhoef, G., Verdonck, L. F., Ossenkoppele, G. J., Sonneveld, P., de Greef, G. E., Löwenberg, B., & Delwel, R. (2003). High EVI1 expression predicts poor survival in acute myeloid leukemia: a study of 319 de novo AML patients. Blood, Vol. 101, No.3, 837-845.

Barragan, E., Montesinos, P., Camos, M., Gonzalez, M., Calasanz, M. J., Roman-Gomez, J., Gomez-Casares, M. T., Ayala, R., Lopez, J., Fuster, O., Colomer, D., Chillon, C., Larrayoz, M. J., Sanchez-Godoy, P., Gonzalez-Campos, J., Manso, F., Amador, M. L., Vellenga, E., Lowenberg, B., & Sanz, M. A. (2011). Prognostic value of FLT3 mutations in patients with acute promyelocytic leukemia treated with all-trans retinoic acid and anthracycline Haematologica, Vol. 96, No. 10, 1470-1477.

Beitinjaneh, A., Jang, S., Roukoz, H. & Majhail, N.S (2010). Prognostic significance of FLT3 internal tandem duplication and tyrosine kinase domain mutations in acute promyelocytic leukemia: a systematic review. Leuk Res. Vol. 34, No.7:831-6.

Bennett, J. M., Catovsky, D., Daniel, M. T., Flandrin, G., Galton, D. A. G., Gralnick, H. R., & Sultan, C. (1976). Proposals for the Classification of the Acute Leukaemias French-American-British (FAB) Cooperative Group. British Journal of Haematology, Vol. 33, No.4, 451-458, 1365-2141.

Bennett J.M.; Catovsky D.A.N.I.; Daniel,Marie T.; Flandrin G.E.O.R.; Galton D.; Gralnick R.& Sultan C.L.A.U. (1985). Proposed Revised Criteria for the Classification of Acute Myeloid Leukemia. Annals of Internal Medicine, Vol. 103, No.4, 620-625.

Bernstein, R., Mendelow, B., Pinto, M. R., Morcom, G., & Bezwoda, W. (1980). Complex translocations involving chromosomes 15 and 17 in acute promyelocityc leukaemia. British Journal of Haematology, Vol. 46, No.2, 311-314, 1365-2141.

Bloomfield, C.D., Lawrence, D., Byrd, J.C., Carroll, A., Pettenati, M.J., Tantravahi, R., Patil, S.R., Davey, F.R., Berg, D.T., Schiffer, C.A., Arthur, D.C. & Mayer, R.J. (1998). Frequency of prolonged remission duration after high-dose cytarabine intensification in acute myeloid leukemia varies by cytogenetic subtype. Cancer Res, Vol. 58, No.18, 4173-9.

Chellappan, S. P., Hiebert, S., Mudryj, M., Horowitz, J. M., & Nevins, J. R. (1991). The E2F transcription factor is a cellular target for the RB protein. Cell, Vol. 65, No.6, 1053-1061, 0092-8674.

Cline M.J. (1994). The Molecular Basis of Leukemia. New England Journal of Medicine, Vol. 330, No.5, 328-336, 0028-4793.

Comte, L., Lorgeot, V., Volkov, L., Roullet, B., Tubiana, N., & Praloran, V. (1997). AcSDKP plasma concentrations in patients with solid tumors: comparison of two chemotherapeutic regimens. Cancer Letters, Vol. 112, No.1, 1-4, 0304-3835.

De la Iglesia Iñigo, S., Lopez-Jorge, C. E., Gomez-Casares, M. T., Lemes Castellano, A., Martin Cabrera, P., Lopez Brito, J., Suarez Cabrera, A., & Molero Labarta, T. (2009). Induction of apoptosis in leukemic cell lines treated with captopril, trandolapril and losartan: A new role in the treatment of leukaemia for these agents. Leukemia Research, Vol. 33, No.6, 810-816, 0145-2126.

De la Iglesia, S., Gomez-Casares, M.T., Lopez-Jorge, C. E., Gonzalez-Leiza, S.M., Santana, G., Jimenez, S., Gonzalez-San Miguel, J.D., Caballero, A., Perera, M., Lemes, A., Luzardo, H., & Molero,T. (2006). Relevance of renin expression by real-time PCR in acute myeloid leukemia. Leukemia & Lymphoma, Vol. 47, No.3, 409-416, 1042-8194.

Dimartino, J.F., & Cleary, M.L. (1999). Mll rearrangements in haematological malignancies: lessons from clinical and biological studies. Br J Haematol, Vol. 106, No.3, 614-26.

Döhner, H., Estey, E.H., Amadori, S., Appelbaum, F.R., Büchner, T., Burnett, A.K., Dombret, H., Fenaux, P., Grimwade, D., Larson, R.A., Lo-Coco, F., Naoe, T., Niederwieser, D., Ossenkoppele, G.J., Sanz, M.A., Sierra, J., Tallman, M.S., Löwenberg, B. & Bloomfield, C.D.European LeukemiaNet (2010). Diagnosis and management of acute myeloid leukemia in adults: recommendations from an international expert panel, on behalf of the European LeukemiaNet. Blood, Vol 115, No 3, 453-74.

Falini, B., Nicoletti, I., Martelli, M. F., & Mecucci, C. (2007). Acute myeloid leukemia carrying cytoplasmic/mutated nucleophosmin (NPMc+ AML): biologic and clinical features. Blood, Vol. 109, No.3, 874-885.

Foran, J. M. (2010). New Prognostic Markers in Acute Myeloid Leukemia: Perspective from the Clinic. Hematology, Vol. 2010, No.1, 47-55.

Foroni, L., Harrison, C. J., Hoffbrand, A. V., & Potter, M. N. (1999). Investigation of minimal residual disease in childhood and adult acute lymphoblastic leukaemia by molecular analysis. British Journal of Haematology, Vol. 105, No.1, 7-24, 1365-2141.

Fuchs, O., Provaznikova, D., Kocova, M., Kostecka, A., Cvekova, P., Neuwirtova, R., Kobylka, P., Cermak, J., Brezinova, J., Schwarz, J., Markova, J., Salaj, P., Klamova, H., Maaloufova, J., Lemez, P., Novakova, L., & Benesova, K. (2008). CEBPA polymorphisms and mutations in patients with acute myeloid leukemia, myelodysplastic syndrome, multiple myeloma and non-Hodgkin's lymphoma. Blood Cells, Molecules, and Diseases, Vol. 40, No.3, 401-405, 1079-9796.

Gabert, J., Beillard, E., van der Velden, V. H. J., Bi, W., Grimwade, D., Pallisgaard, N., Barbany, G., Cazzaniga, G., Cayuela, J. M., Cave, H., Pane, F., Aerts, J. L. E., De Micheli, D., Thirion, X., Pradel, V., Gonzalez, M., Viehmann, S., Malec, M., Saglio, G., & van Dongen, J. J. M. (2003). Standardization and quality control studies of /`real-time/' quantitative reverse transcriptase polymerase chain reaction of fusion gene transcripts for residual disease detection in leukemia - A Europe Against

Cancer Program. Leukemia : official journal of the Leukemia Society of America, Leukemia Research Fund, U.K, Vol. 17, No.12, 2318-2357, 0887-6924.

Gaidzik, V. I., Schlenk, R. F., Moschny, S., Becker, A., Bullinger, L., Corbacioglu, A., Krauter, J., chlegelberger, B., anser, A., öhner, H., & öhner, K. (2009). Prognostic impact of WT1 mutations in cytogenetically normal acute myeloid leukemia: a study of the German-Austrian AML Study Group. Blood, Vol. 113, No.19, 4505-4511.

Gale, R. E., Green, C., Allen, C., Mead, A. J., Burnett, A. K., Hills, R. K., & Linch, D. C. (2008). The impact of FLT3 internal tandem duplication mutant level, number, size, and interaction with NPM1 mutations in a large cohort of young adult patients with acute myeloid leukemia. Blood, Vol. 111, No.5, 2776-2784.

Garcon, L., Libura, M., Delabesse, E., Valensi, F., Asnafi, V., Berger, C., Schmitt, C., Leblanc, T., Buzyn, A., & Macintyre, E. (2005). DEK-CAN molecular monitoring of myeloid malignancies could aid therapeutic stratification. Leukemia : official journal of the Leukemia Society of America, Leukemia Research Fund, U.K, Vol. 19, No.8, 1338-1344, 0887-6924.

Garg, M., Moore, H., Tobal, K., & Liu Yin, J. A. (2003). Prognostic significance of quantitative analysis of WT1 gene transcripts by competitive reverse transcription polymerase chain reaction in acute leukaemia. British Journal of Haematology, Vol. 123, No.1, 49-59, 1365-2141.

Gomez Casares, M.T., Lemes, A.,Navarro, N., González-San Miguel, J.D., Fumero, S., Bosch, J.M., Martín, P., Fiuza, M.D., López-Jorge, C.E., Luzardo, H., De la Iglesia, S. & Molero T. (2009). Prognostic value of inmunophenotype in AML patients with NPM1 mutation. Poster 0296.14th Congress of EHA.

Gomez Casares, M. T., de la Iglesia, S., Perera, M., Lemes, A., Campo, C., Gonzalez San Miguel, J. D., Bosch, J. M., Suarez, A., Guerra, L., Rodriguez-Perez, J. C., & Molero, T. (2002). Renin Expression in Hematological Malignancies and its Role in the Regulation of Hematopoiesis. Leukemia & Lymphoma, Vol. 43, No.12, 2377-2381, 1042-8194.

Gregory, T., Wald, D., Chen, Y., Vermaat, J., Xiong, Y., & Tse, W. (2009). Molecular prognostic markers for adult acute myeloid leukemia with normal cytogenetics. Journal of Hematology & Oncology, Vol. 2, No.1, 1756-8722.

Gröschel, S., Lugthart, S., Schlenk, R. F., Valk, P. J. M., Eiwen, K., Goudswaard, C., van Putten, W. J. L., Kayser, S., Verdonck, L. F., Lübbert, M., Ossenkoppele, G. J., Germing, U., Schmidt-Wolf, I., Schlegelberger, B., Krauter, J., Ganser, A., Döhner, H., Löwenberg, B., Döhner, K., & Delwel, R. (2010). High EVI1 Expression Predicts Outcome in Younger Adult Patients With Acute Myeloid Leukemia and Is Associated With Distinct Cytogenetic Abnormalities. Journal of Clinical Oncology, Vol. 28, No.12, 2101-2107.

Haferlach, T., Bacher, U., Haferlach, C., Kern, W., & Schnittger, S. (2007). Insight into the molecular pathogenesis of myeloid malignancies. Current Opinion in Hematology, Vol. 14, No.2, 1065-6251.

Harris, N. L., Jaffe, E. S., Diebold, J., Flandrin, G., Muller-Hermelink, H. K., Vardiman, J., Lister, T. A., & Bloomfield, C. D. (1999). World Health Organization Classification of Neoplastic Diseases of the Hematopoietic and Lymphoid Tissues: Report of the Clinical Advisory Committee Meeting-ùAirlie House, Virginia, November 1997. Journal of Clinical Oncology, Vol. 17, No.12, 3835-3849.

Haznedaroglu IC, B. Y. (1997). Current evidence for the existence of a local renin-angiotensin system affecting physiological and pathological haemopoiesis in the bone marrow. British Journal of Haematology, Vol. 99, No.2, 471-471, 1365-2141.

Haznedaroglu, I. C. , Oztürk M.A. (2003). Towards the understanding of the local hematopoietic bone marrow renin-angiotensin system. The International Journal of Biochemistry & Cell Biology, Vol. 35, No.6, 867-880, 1357-2725.

Heuser, M., Argiropoulos, B., Kuchenbauer, F., Yung, E., Piper, J., Fung, S., Schlenk, R. F., Döhner, K., Hinrichsen, T., Rudolph, C., Schambach, A., Baum, C., Schlegelberger, B., Dohner, H., Ganser, A., & Humphries, R. K. (2007). MN1 overexpression induces acute myeloid leukemia in mice and predicts ATRA resistance in patients with AML. Blood, Vol. 110, No.5, 1639-1647.

Heuser, M., Yun, H., Berg, T., Yung, E., Argiropoulos, B., Kuchenbauer, F., Park, G., Hamwi, I., Palmqvist, L., Lai, C.K., Leung, M., Lin, G., Chaturvedi, A., Thakur, B.K., Iwasaki, M., Bilenky, M., Thiessen, N., Robertson, G., Hirst, M., Kent, D., Wilson, N.K., Göttgens, B., Eaves, C., Cleary, M.L., Marra, M., Ganser ,A. & Humphries, R.K.(2011). Cell of origin in AML: susceptibility to MN1-induced transformation is regulated by the MEIS1/AbdB-like HOX protein complex. Cancer Cell. Vol. 20, No.1, 39-52.

Hilden, J. M., Frestedt, J. L., Moore, R. O., Heerema, N. A., Arthur, D. C., Reaman, G. H., & Kersey, J. H. (1995). Molecular analysis of infant acute lymphoblastic leukemia: MLL gene rearrangement and reverse transcriptase-polymerase chain reaction for t(4; 11)(q21; q23). Blood, Vol. 86, No.10, 3876-3882.

Hou, H. A., Huang, T. C., Lin, L. I., Liu, C. Y., Chen, C. Y., Chou, W. C., Tang, J. L., Tseng, M. H., Huang, C. F., Chiang, Y. C., Lee, F. Y., Liu, M. C., Yao, M., Huang, S. Y., Ko, B. S., Hsu, S. C., Wu, S. J., Tsay, W., Chen, Y. C., & Tien, H. F. (2010). WT1 mutation in 470 adult patients with acute myeloid leukemia: stability during disease evolution and implication of its incorporation into a survival scoring system. Blood, Vol. 115, No.25, 5222-5231.

Huckle, W. R. , Earp, H. S. (1994). Regulation of cell proliferation and growth by angiotensin II. Progress in Growth Factor Research, Vol. 5, No.2, 177-194, 0955-2235.

Inoue, K., Sugiyama, H., Ogawa, H., Nakagawa, M., Yamagami, T., Miwa, H., Kita, K., Hiraoka, A., Masaoka, T., & Nasu, K. (1994). WT1 as a new prognostic factor and a new marker for the detection of minimal residual disease in acute leukemia. Blood, Vol. 84, No.9, 3071-3079.

Jansen, M. W. J. C., van der Velden, V. H. J., & van Dongen, J. J. M. (2005). Efficient and easy detection of MLL-AF4, MLL-AF9 and MLL-ENL fusion gene transcripts by multiplex real-time quantitative RT-PCR in TaqMan and LightCycler. Leukemia : official journal of the Leukemia Society of America, Leukemia Research Fund, U.K, Vol. 19, No.11, 2016-2018, 0887-6924.

Keilholz, U., Menssen, H. D., Gaiger, A., Menke, A., Oji, Y., Oka, Y., Scheibenbogen, C., Stauss, H., Thiel, E., & Sugiyama, H. (2005). Wilms' tumor gene 1 (WT1) in human neoplasia. Leukemia : official journal of the Leukemia Society of America, Leukemia Research Fund, U.K, Vol. 19, No.8, 1318-1323, 0887-6924.

Kreuzer, K. A., Saborowski, A., Lupberger, J., Appelt, C., Na, I. K., Le Coutre, P., & Schmidt, C. A. (2001). Fluorescent 5'-exonuclease assay for the absolute quantification of

Wilms' tumor gene (WT1) mRNA: implications for monitoring human leukaemias. British Journal of Haematology, Vol. 114, No.2, 313-318, 1365-2141.

Lin, L. I., Chen, C. Y., Lin, D. T., Tsay, W., Tang, J. L., Yeh, Y. C., Shen, H. L., Su, F. H., Yao, M., Huang, S. Y., & Tien, H. F. (2005). Characterization of CEBPA Mutations in Acute Myeloid Leukemia: Most Patients with CEBPA Mutations Have Biallelic Mutations and Show a Distinct Immunophenotype of the Leukemic Cells. Clinical Cancer Research, Vol. 11, No.4, 1372-1379.

Lo Coco , F., Diverio, D., Falini, B., Biondi, A., Nervi, C., & Pelicci, P. G. (1999). Genetic Diagnosis and Molecular Monitoring in the Management of Acute Promyelocytic Leukemia. Blood, Vol. 94, No.1, 12-22.

Lo Coco, F., Diverio, D., Avvisati, G., Arcese, W., Petti, M. C., Meloni, G., Mandelli, F., Pandolfi, P. P., Grignani, F., Pelicci, P. G., Biondi, A., Rossi, V., Masera, G., Barbui, T., & Rambaldi, A. (1992). Molecular evaluation of residual disease as a predictor of relapse in acute promyelocytic leukaemia. The Lancet, Vol. 340, No.8833, 1437-1438, 0140-6736.

Lo Coco, F., Diverio, D., Avvisati, G., Petti, M. C., Meloni, G., Pogliani, E. M., Biondi, A., Rossi, G., Carlo-Stella, C., Selleri, C., Martino, B., Specchia, G., & Mandelli, F. (1999). Therapy of Molecular Relapse in Acute Promyelocytic Leukemia. Blood, Vol. 94, No.7, 2225-2229.

Lopez-Jorge, C.E., Martin, P.,Lopez Brito, J., Gomez Casares, M.T., Gonzalez San Miguel, J.D., Lemes, A., Ramirez, T., Santana, G., Mataix, R., De La Iglesia, S., Luzardo, H.& Molero, T. (2006). Prevalence of NPM1 mutation in AML and MDR. Póster 0695.11th Congress of the EHA.

Lugthart, S., van Drunen, E., van Norden, Y., van Hoven, A., Erpelinck, C. A. J., Valk, P. J. M., Beverloo, H. B., Löwenberg, B., & Delwel, R. (2008). High EVI1 levels predict adverse outcome in acute myeloid leukemia: prevalence of EVI1 overexpression and chromosome 3q26 abnormalities underestimated. Blood, Vol. 111, No.8, 4329-4337.

Lugthart, S., Groschel, S., Beverloo, H.B., Kayser, S., Valk, P.J., van Zelderen-Bhola, S.L., Jan Ossenkoppele, G., Vellenga, E., van den Berg-de Ruiter, E., Schanz, U., Verhoef, G., Vandenberghe, P., Ferrant, A., Kohne, C.H., Pfreundschuh, M., Horst, H.A., Koller, E., von Lilienfeld-Toal, M., Bentz, M., Ganser, A., Schlegelberger, B., Jotterand, M., Krauter, J., Pabst, T., Theobald, M., Schlenk, RF., Delwel, R., Döhner, K., Löwenberg, B. & Döhner, H. (2010). Clinical, molecular, and prognostic significance of WHO type inv(3)(q21q26.2)/t(3;3)(q21;q26.2) and various other 3q abnormalities in acute myeloid leukemia. J Clin Oncol, Vol.28, No.24, 3890-8.

Luzardo, H., Gómez-Casares, M.T., Gonzalez-San Miguel, J.D., Lopez-Brito, J., Calvo-Villas, J.M., Molines, A., De la Iglesia, S, Caballero, A., López-Jorge, C.E., Santana, G., Suarez, A.& Molero, T. (2007). EVI1 overexpression in a serie of 212 hematological malignancies. Poster 0171.12th Congress of EHA.

Meshinchi, S., Woods, W. G., Stirewalt, D. L., Sweetser, D. A., Buckley, J. D., Tjoa, T. K., Bernstein, I. D., & Radich, J. P. (2001). Prevalence and prognostic significance of Flt3 internal tandem duplication in pediatric acute myeloid leukemia. Blood, Vol. 97, No.1, 89-94.

Meyers, S., Downing, J. R., & Hiebert, S. W. (1993). Identification of AML-1 and the (8;21) translocation protein (AML-1/ETO) as sequence-specific DNA-binding proteins:

the runt homology domain is required for DNA binding and protein-protein interactions. Molecular and Cellular Biology, Vol. 13, No.10, 6336-6345.

Morishita, K., Parganas, E., William, C. L., Whittaker, M. H., Drabkin, H., Oval, J., Taetle, R., Valentine, M. B., & Ihle, J. N. (1992). Activation of EVI1 gene expression in human acute myelogenous leukemias by translocations spanning 300-400 kilobases on chromosome band 3q26. Proceedings of the National Academy of Sciences, Vol. 89, No.9, 3937-3941.

Najima, Y., Ohashi, K., Kawamura, M., Onozuka, Y., Yamaguchi, T., Akiyama, H., & Sakamaki, H. (2010). Molecular monitoring of BAALC expression in patients with CD34-positive acute leukemia. International Journal of Hematology, Vol. 91, No.4, 636-645, 0925-5710.

Nakao, M., Yokota, S., Horiike, S., Taniwaki, M., Kashima, K., Sonoda, Y., Koizumi, S., Takaue, Y., Matsushita, T., Fujimoto, T., & Misawa, S. (1996). Detection and quantification of TEL/AML1 fusion transcripts by polymerase chain reaction in childhood acute lymphoblastic leukemia. Leukemia : official journal of the Leukemia Society of America, Leukemia Research Fund, U.K, Vol. 10, No.9, 1463-1470.

Pabst, T., Mueller, B. U., Zhang, P., Radomska, H. S., Narravula, S., Schnittger, S., Behre, G., Hiddemann, W., & Tenen, D. G. (2001). Dominant-negative mutations of CEBPA, encoding CCAAT/enhancer binding protein-[alpha] (C/EBP[alpha]), in acute myeloid leukemia. Nat Genet, Vol. 27, No.3, 263-270, 1061-4036.

Paschka, P., Marcucci, G., Ruppert, A.S., Mrozek, K., Chen, H., Kittles, R.A., Vukosavljevic, T., Perrotti, D., Vardiman, J.W., Carroll, A.J., Kolitz, J.E., Larson, R.A. & Bloomfield, C.D.; Cancer and Leukemia Group B. (2006). Adverse prognostic significance of KIT mutations in adult acute myeloid leukemia with inv(16) and t(8;21): a Cancer and Leukemia Group B Study. J Clin Oncol, Vol.24, No.24, 3904-11.

Perea, G., Lasa, A., Aventin, A., Domingo, A., Villamor, N., Paz Queipo de Llano, M., Llorente, A., Junca, J., Palacios, C., Fernandez, C., Gallart, M., Font, L., Tormo, M., Florensa, L., Bargay, J., Marti, J. M., Vivancos, P., Torres, P., Berlanga, J. J., Badell, I., Brunet, S., Sierra, J., & Nomdedeu, J. F. (2005). Prognostic value of minimal residual disease (MRD) in acute myeloid leukemia (AML) with favorable cytogenetics t(8;21) and inv(16). Leukemia : official journal of the Leukemia Society of America, Leukemia Research Fund, U.K, Vol. 20, No.1, 87-94, 0887-6924.

Pollard, J. A., Alonzo, T. A., Gerbing, R. B., Ho, P. A., Zeng, R., Ravindranath, Y., Dahl, G., Lacayo, N. J., Becton, D., Chang, M., Weinstein, H. J., Hirsch, B., Raimondi, S. C., Heerema, N. A., Woods, W. G., Lange, B. J., Hurwitz, C., Arceci, R. J., Radich, J. P., Bernstein, I. D., Heinrich, M. C., & Meshinchi, S. (2010). Prevalence and prognostic significance of KIT mutations in pediatric patients with core binding factor AML enrolled on serial pediatric cooperative trials for de novo AML. Blood, Vol. 115, No.12, 2372-2379.

Preudhomme, C., Warot-Loze, D., Roumier, C., Grardel-Duflos, N., Garand, R., Lai, J. L., Dastugue, N., Macintyre, E., Denis, C., Bauters, F., Kerckaert, J. P., Cosson, A., & Fenaux, P. (2000). High incidence of biallelic point mutations in the Runt domain of the AML1/PEBP2αB gene in Mo acute myeloid leukemia and in myeloid malignancies with acquired trisomy 21. Blood, Vol. 96, No.8, 2862-2869.

Radich, J. & Thomson, B. (1997). Advances in the detection of minimal residual disease. Current Opinion in Hematology, Vol. 4, No.4, 1065-6251.

Rodríguez ,C., Gómez Casares, MT., Santana, G., Guedes, S.,Calvo-Villas, JM, López Jorge, CE.,García Bello, MA.,González San Miguel JD., Jiménez, S.,Quiroz, K., Fumero, S., Ramos, Y., Navarro, N. & Molero, T. (2010). Sobreexpresión de MN1 en leucemias agudas de estirpe mieloide. Correlación con otros marcadores moleculares y relación con respuesta al tratamiento y supervivencia global. Poster 0154.LII Reunión Nacional de la SEHH y XXVI Congreso Nacional de la SETH.

Stirewalt, D.L. & Radich, J.P. (2003). The role of FLT3 in haematopoietic malignancies. Nat Rev Cancer. Vol. 3, No.9,:650-65.

Sasaki, O., Meguro, K., Tohmiya, Y., Funato, T., Shibahara, S., & Sasaki, T. (2002). Altered expression of retinoblastoma protein-interacting zinc finger gene, RIZ, in human leukaemia. British Journal of Haematology, Vol. 119, No.4, 940-948, 1365-2141.

Schlenk, RF., Benner, A., Krauter, J., Büchner, T., Sauerland, C., Ehninger, G., Schaich, M., Mohr, B., Niederwieser, D., Krahl, R., Pasold, R., Döhner, K., Ganser, A., Döhner, H. & Heil, G. (2004). Individual Patient Data–Based Meta-Analysis of Patients Aged 16 to 60 Years With Core Binding Factor Acute Myeloid Leukemia: A Survey of the German Acute Myeloid Leukemia Intergroup. J Clin Oncol, Vol. 22, No.18, 3741-50.

Schlenk, RF., Döhner, K., Krauter, J., Fröhling, S., Corbacioglu, A., Bullinger, L., Habdank, M., Späth, D., Morgan, M., Benner, A., Schlegelberger, B., Heil, G., Ganser, A.& Döhner, H.; German-Austrian Acute Myeloid Leukemia Study Group. (2008). Mutations and treatment outcome in cytogenetically normal acute myeloid leukemia. N Engl J Med; Vol. 358, No.18, 1909-18.

Schnittger, S., Kern, W., Tschulik, C., Weiss, T., Dicker, F., Falini, B., Haferlach, C. & Haferlach, T. (2009). Minimal residual disease levels assessed by NPM1 mutation-specific RQ-PCR provide important prognostic information in AML. Blood, Vol. 114, No.11, 2220-31.

Schnittger, S., Bacher, U., Kern, W., Alpermann, T., Haferlach, C., & Haferlach, T. (2011). Prognostic impact of FLT3-ITD load in NPM1 mutated acute myeloid leukemia. Leukemia : official journal of the Leukemia Society of America, Leukemia Research Fund, U.K, 1476-5551.

Schnittger, S., Dicker, F., Kern, W., Wendland, N., Sundermann, J., Alpermann, T., Haferlach, C., & Haferlach, T. (2011). RUNX1 mutations are frequent in de novo AML with noncomplex karyotype and confer an unfavorable prognosis. Blood, Vol. 117, No.8, 2348-2357.

Sheikhha, M.H., Awan, A., Tobal, K. & Liu Yin, J.A. (2003). Prognostic significance of FLT3 ITD and D835 mutations in AML patients. Hematol J, Vol. 4, No.1,41-6.

Shih, L., Liang, D., Fu, J., Wu, J., Wang, P., Lin, T., Dunn, P., Kuo, M., Tang, T., Lin, T., & Lai, C. (2006). Characterization of fusion partner genes in 114 patients with de novo acute myeloid leukemia and MLL rearrangement. Leukemia : official journal of the Leukemia Society of America, Leukemia Research Fund, U.K, Vol. 20, No.2, 218-223, 0887-6924.

Spassov, BV., Stoimenov, AS., Balatzenko, GN., Genova, ML., Peichev, DB. & Konstantinov, SM. (2011). Wilms' tumor protein and FLT3-internal tandem

duplication expression in patients with de novo acute myeloid leukemia. Hematology. Vol.16, No.1, 37-42.
Tanner, S. M., Austin, J. L., Leone, G., Rush, L. J., Plass, C., Heinonen, K., Mrózek, K., Sill, H., Knuutila, S., Kolitz, J. E., Archer, K. J., Caligiuri, M. A., Bloomfield, C. D., & de la Chapelle, A. (2001). BAALC, the human member of a novel mammalian neuroectoderm gene lineage, is implicated in hematopoiesis and acute leukemia. Proceedings of the National Academy of Sciences, Vol. 98, No.24, 13901-13906.
Thiede, C., Steudel, C., Mohr, B., Schaich, M., Schäkel, U., Platzbecker, U., Wermke, M., Bornhäuser, M., Ritter, M., Neubauer, A., Ehninger, G., & Illmer, T. (2002). Analysis of FLT3-activating mutations in 979 patients with acute myelogenous leukemia: association with FAB subtypes and identification of subgroups with poor prognosis. Blood, Vol. 99, No.12, 4326-4335.
Vardiman, J. W., Thiele, J., Arber, D.A., Brunning, R.D., Borowitz, M. J., Porwit, A., Harris, N. L., Le Beau, M. M., Hellström-Lindberg, E., Tefferi, A., & Bloomfield, C. D. (2009). The 2008 revision of the World Health Organization (WHO) classification of myeloid neoplasms and acute leukemia: rationale and important changes. Blood, Vol. 114, No.5, 937-951.
Vazquez, I., Maicas, M., Cervera, J., Agirre, X., Marin-Bejar, O., Marcotegui, N., Vicente, C., Lahortiga, I., Gomez-Benito, M., Carranza, C., Valencia, A., Brunet, S., Lumbreras, E., Prosper, F., Gomez-Casares, M.T., Hernandez-Rivas, J.M., Calasanz, M.J., Sanz, M.A., Sierra, J. & Odero, M.D. (2011). Downregulation of EVI1 is associated with epigenetic alterations and good prognosis in patients with acute myeloid leukemia. Haematologica; Vol. 96, No.10, 448-56.
von Lindern, M., Poustka, A., Lerach, H., & Grosveld, G. (1990). The (6;9) chromosome translocation, associated with a specific subtype of acute nonlymphocytic leukemia, leads to aberrant transcription of a target gene on 9q34. Molecular and Cellular Biology, Vol. 10, No.8, 4016-4026.
von Lindern, M., Fornerod, M., van Baal, S., Jaegle, M., de Wit, T., Buijs, A., & Grosveld, G. (1992). The translocation (6;9), associated with a specific subtype of acute myeloid leukemia, results in the fusion of two genes, dek and can, and the expression of a chimeric, leukemia-specific dek-can mRNA. Molecular and Cellular Biology, Vol. 12, No.4, 1687-1697.
Weisser, M., Kern, W., Rauhut, S., Schoch, C., Hiddemann, W., Haferlach, T., & Schnittger, S. (2005). Prognostic impact of RT-PCR-based quantification of WT1 gene expression during MRD monitoring of acute myeloid leukemia. Leukemia : official journal of the Leukemia Society of America, Leukemia Research Fund, U.K, Vol. 19, No.8, 1416-1423, 0887-6924.
Whitman, S. P., Liu, S., Vukosavljevic, T., Rush, L. J., Yu, L., Liu, C., Klisovic, M. I., Maharry, K., Guimond, M., Strout, M. P., Becknell, B., Dorrance, A., Klisovic, R. B., Plass, C., Bloomfield, C. D., Marcucci, G., & Caligiuri, M. A. (2005). The MLL partial tandem duplication: evidence for recessive gain-of-function in acute myeloid leukemia identifies a novel patient subgroup for molecular-targeted therapy. Blood, Vol. 106, No.1, 345-352.
Wouters, B. J., Löwenberg, B., Erpelinck-Verschueren, C. A. J., van Putten, W. L. J., Valk, P. J. M., & Delwel, R. (2009). Double CEBPA mutations, but not single CEBPA mutations, define a subgroup of acute myeloid leukemia with a distinctive gene

expression profile that is uniquely associated with a favorable outcome. Blood, Vol. 113, No.13, 3088-3091.

Wulf, G. G., Jahns-Streubel, G., Nobiling, R., Strutz, F., Hemmerlein, B., Hiddemann, W., & Wörmann, B. (1998). Renin in acute myeloid leukaemia blasts. British Journal of Haematology, Vol. 100, No.2, 335-337, 1365-2141.

Yanada, M., Matsuo, K., Suzuki, T., Kiyoi, H., & Naoe, T. (2005). Prognostic significance of FLT3 internal tandem duplication and tyrosine kinase domain mutations for acute myeloid leukemia: a meta-analysis. Leukemia: official journal of the Leukemia Society of America, Leukemia Research Fund, U.K, Vol. 19, No.8, 1345-1349, 0887-6924.

17

Analysis of Leukemogenic Gene Products in Hematopoietic Progenitor Cells

Julia Schanda[1], Reinhard Henschler[2], Manuel Grez[1] and Christian Wichmann[1]
[1]*Georg-Speyer-Haus, Institute for Biomedical Research, Frankfurt am Main*
[2]*Institute of Transfusion Medicine, German Red Cross Blood Center, Frankfurt am Main*
Germany

1. Introduction

One major limitation in the development of effective and targeted cancer therapies is the incomplete understanding of the molecular mechanisms driving malignant cell growth and the resistance of residual 'cancer stem cells' to standard therapies, such as chemotherapy and radiation. Consequently, numerous attempts have been made to elucidate the molecular circuits initiating and perpetuating malignant cell transformation.

Among the different cancer entities, leukemias harbor only a few mutations and therefore represent a good model system for the study of oncogenesis. The cloning and subsequent analysis of leukemia-associated gene products have strongly facilitated the understanding of their biological function and the development of appropriate model systems. In early experiments, leukemia-associated oncogenes were ectopically expressed in fibroblasts, a cell type which is not optimal for modeling leukemia initiation and progression. Later, the development of cell separation methods for murine and human hematopoietic precursor cells allowed for the isolation of specific target cells, in large quantities and with high cell population purity (Belvedere et al., 1999). Together with the utilization of retroviral expression vectors, which enable stable integration and expression of a transgene of choice, these cell isolation procedures represent a significant methodological improvement for leukemia modeling approaches in the hematopoietic tissue. With these technologies in hand, the genetic lesions of leukemia can be better modeled in the appropriate cell compartment. By performing cell biology experiments and tumor sample deep sequencing it became clear that both solid tumors and hematological malignancies depend on multiple oncogenic alterations to ultimately result in cellular transformation (Hanahan & Weinberg, 2000, 2011; Kinzler & Vogelstein, 1996). Additionally, the overall number of mutated genes in solid tumors was found to be higher than in leukemias. These observations resulted in the formulation of the multi-hit model of tumorigenesis. Initiating mutations induce stem cell expansion and survival, thereby allowing for the occurrence of additional genetic alterations that result in the progression of malignant transformation. The later stages of this process are characterized by uncontrolled proliferation with overgrowth of the ´healthy´ cell compartment and metastasis, in the case of solid tumors. This multi-hit cancer model has been well described for colon cancer by Kenneth W. Kinzler and Bert Vogelstein (Kinzler &

Vogelstein, 1996). Similarly, it has been suggested for hematopoietic malignancies, that only a concerted signaling network resulting from the activity of several activated oncogenes leads to full transformation of preleukemic cell clones. However, the exact chronological order of these genetic events and the causality of their mutual cooperation are hardly understood (Schuringa et al., 2010).

Myeloid leukemia represents a well-depicted tumor entity in terms of molecular pathogenesis. It is characterized by an uncontrolled proliferation behavior based on the aberrant self-renewal capacity of the myeloid progenitor cell compartment including the erythroid, monocytic and granulocytic lineages. Depending on the morphology and genetics of the cells and its clinical progression, myeloid leukemia is classified as either acute myeloid leukemia (AML) or chronic myeloid leukemia (CML). AML is distinguished by the rapid proliferation of immature myeloid progenitor cells, which overgrow the normal hematopoietic cells. AML is the most common acute leukemia, which predominantly affects adults. Its incidence strongly increases with age, with a median age at diagnosis of 65 years, suggesting that several oncogenic events are required for the onset and progression of the disease (Estey & Dohner, 2006). If left untreated, the disease proceeds rapidly and is typically fatal within weeks or months. To date, numerous AML-specific fusion genes and mutations have been described (Look, 1997). Chromosomal translocations and mutations involving the AML1 gene are amongst the most common alterations found in AML (Schnittger et al., 2011). AML1 is an essential transcription factor that controls the myeloid cell differentiation of progenitor cells into mature blood cells. Both point mutations and chromosomal translocations, such as t(8;21) and t(3;21), disrupt the physiological function of AML1 and hinder the normal maturation process of the progenitor cells (Niebuhr et al., 2008). IIn addition, mutations of the receptor tyrosine kinase, c-kit, are frequently detected in these cells and seem to be associated with poor prognosis due to their correlation with higher relapse rates after chemotherapy (Boissel et al., 2006; Paschka et al., 2006). Mutations of the nucleophosmin (NPM1) gene are also frequently observed in AML. This gene is involved in multiple cellular processes including protein shuttling between the nucleus and cytoplasm, RNA biogenesis, cell cycle control and transcriptional regulation. It is also described as a cellular stress sensor associated with the p53-dependent apoptosis pathway (Grisendi et al., 2006). Commonly identified NPM1 mutations render this protein mislocalized to the cytoplasm. The oncogenic mechanisms behind this phenomenon are currently under intense investigation (Falini et al., 2010; Falini et al., 2007). Among the mutated kinases in AML, mutations of the FLT3 cytokine receptor gene are common and are associated with poor prognosis (Gilliland & Griffin, 2002; Meshinchi et al., 2001). Hyperactive FLT3 induces a strong intracellular signal transduction response, mainly by activating STAT5, a latent transcription factor important for self-renewal and proliferation of hematopoietic progenitors. For this leukemia entity, FLT3-inhibitors blocking its kinase activity are currently being tested in clinical trials (Wiernik, 2010). Isocitrate dehydrogenases, IDH1 and IDH2, represent genes that were recently identified to be frequently mutated in AML with adverse prognosis in cytogenetically normal leukemias (Mardis et al., 2009; Paschka et al., 2010). Mutations in IDH genes have also been found in human brain tumors, including gliomas. Interestingly, the accumulation of an intracellular metabolite, 2-hydroxyglutarate, was discovered in these tumor cells (Dang et al., 2009). This so-called 'oncometabolite' alters the genome-wide histone and DNA methylation patterns, thereby exerting oncogenic activity (Xu et al., 2011).

Chronic myeloid leukemia is characterized by the increased proliferation rate of mature granulocytes and their precursors. The course of disease can be divided into three phases:

the chronic phase, the accelerated phase and the acute phase with typical features of AML (Sawyers, 1999). The t(9;22) chromosomal translocation, also called the Philadelphia chromosome, which generates the fusion protein BCR/ABL, is frequently observed in CML patient samples. The BCR-portion of the fusion protein triggers multimerization of the ABL portion, thereby locking the ABL kinase into a hyperactive state. BCR/ABL multimers induce constitutive intracellular proliferation and survival signaling, thereby triggering the development of leukemia (Hoelbl et al., 2010; Melo & Barnes, 2007). Over the last years, a breakthrough in the treatment of CML was achieved with the development of the ABL-kinase inhibitor, imatinib (Sawyers et al., 2002). BCR/ABL positive CML patients are now treated with one of several targeted, first-line therapies, including imatinib, dasatinib, and nilotinib, which have dramatically increased patient survival rates to nearly 90% since the advent of these therapies. These kinase inhibitors specifically inhibit the oncogenic tyrosine kinase activity of BCR/ABL. For the first time, an inhibitor has been developed that targets a driving oncogene with high efficiency, which is currently used in many clinical trials (Garcia-Manero et al., 2003). Later, it was found that imatinib also targets c-kit, a receptor tyrosine kinase frequently mutated in gastrointestinal stromal tumors (GIST), thereby widening the application spectrum of imatinib to include solid tumors (Demetri, 2002). Currently, large efforts are being made in the development of specific inhibitors for other oncoproteins. The elucidation of the molecular mechanisms controlling the process of leukemic transformation represents a prerequisite for the development of targeted oncogene inhibitors designed to improve current therapeutic strategies for myeloid leukemias.

For both acute and chronic myeloid leukemia, 'leukemia stem cells' are most likely the origin of disease and are probably responsible for recurrence after chemotherapy (Trumpp & Wiestler, 2008). These leukemia stem cells share common features with normal stem cells. They are described as dormant or slowly cycling cells with an increased self-renewal capacity and a resistance to chemotherapeutic drugs. It has been proposed that they reside in the bone marrow niches and can fully regenerate the leukemia after standard chemotherapy. Perturbed self-renewal programs of leukemia stem cells represent a major problem for leukemia therapy. Even in BCR/ABL positive CML, for which a specific oncogene inhibitor is available, CML stem cells are resistant to imatinib treatment (Holyoake et al., 1999). Therefore, lifelong treatment of CML patients with tyrosine kinase inhibitors is necessary (Corbin et al., 2011; Diamond & Melo, 2011).

Most of the current understandings of leukemogenic fusion genes and mutations have resulted from overexpression experiments using either cell line models or primary murine and human hematopoietic stem cells, both *in vitro* and *in vivo*. In these studies, leukemic gene products were usually expressed with the help of retroviral expression vectors resulting in ectopic and stable expression. This represents a convenient experimental strategy to model leukemia in mammalian hematopoietic stem and progenitor cells. The following sections will recapitulate the different retroviral expression vector systems used for modeling leukemia development and will summarize exemplary results acquired from studies of both the murine and human progenitor cell systems.

2. Retroviral vector systems and expression cassettes

When modeling leukemia in the mammalian hematopoietic system, there are two major strategies used to express a leukemia-associated gene product. The creation of knock-in or transgenic mice enables robust transgene expression *in vivo*. However, transgene expression is usually not restricted to a certain tissue and permanent oncogene expression often causes delirious side effects, e.g. embryonic lethality, thereby impeding accurate analysis. Alternatively, genes can be delivered by retroviral vectors directly into the hematopoietic system via bone marrow transplantation of hematopoietic progenitors, transduced with the gene of interest (GOI). Gene marking of few cells also more precisely resembles leukemia development from a single cell clone. In addition, this method provides the advantage of rapid testing of numerous gene expression constructs in contrast to the time-consuming gene-manipulation of mice. Therefore, gamma-retroviral and lentiviral expression vector systems represent attractive and efficient techniques for the stable expression of a gene of interest in hematopoietic progenitor cells. Retroviruses are enveloped RNA viruses. Viral RNA is linear, single-stranded and approximately 7-12 kb in size. The common characteristic of retroviruses is their strategy of replication: the viral RNA is reverse transcribed into linear double-stranded DNA followed by its integration into the genome of the cell (Coffin et al., 2007). The most commonly used delivery system is the gamma-retroviral vector system. These vectors are derived from the Moloney murine leukemia virus (Mo-MLV) genome (Kohn et al., 1987). The murine stem cell virus (MSCV) expression vector is one of the most frequently employed vector systems, as it enables stable and high transgene expression in virtually all cell types (Hawley et al., 1994). This vector is available with several marker genes, such as the enhanced green fluorescent protein (eGFP) and derivatives thereof, which are co-expressed via the internal ribosomal entry site (IRES) elements. One of the disadvantages of gamma-retroviral vectors is their inability to target non-dividing cells. Successful cell transduction is completely dependent on the breakdown of the nuclear membrane during mitosis (Roe et al., 1993). In contrast, lentiviral vectors, which are mostly derived from the HIV-1 genome, are able to integrate into both dividing and non-dividing cells (Lewis et al., 1992; Lewis & Emerman, 1994). Compared with gamma-retroviral vectors, lentiviral vectors have the capacity to incorporate larger transgenes, up to 10 kilobases, although vector titers decrease when using larger inserts (Matrai et al., 2010). The integration of retroviral vectors into the cell genome results in the stable and permanent expression of the transgene, which is transferred to all daughter cells during cell division. Therefore, retrovirally transduced oncogene expressing cells resemble cancer cells in that they pass their oncogenic alterations down to all progeny. However, during integration into the genome there is a risk of insertional mutagenesis (Baum, 2007). This must be kept in mind while analyzing the potential oncogenic effects of a transgene delivered by retroviral vectors. In general, gamma-retro as well as lentiviral vectors integrate into transcriptional units. Gamma-retroviruses tend to integrate either upstream or downstream of the start of transcriptional units (Wu et al., 2003), while lentiviral vectors integrate randomly within a transcriptional unit (Naldini et al., 2006). During retroviral integration into the genome of a cell, there is a risk of proto-oncogene activation close to the integration site of the vector driven by either the enhancer element or the promoter sequences present in the U3 region of the viral long terminal repeats (LTRs). Deletion of the U3 region within the LTRs and the insertion of an internal enhancer/promoter result in the formation of self-inactivating (SIN) vectors with the reduced risk of cellular oncogene activation (Yu et al., 1986). Retroviral particle production and transduction procedures represent convenient routine methods, which can be carried out in any laboratory with the appropriate laboratory biosafety level. For safety reasons, genes required for the assembly of the viral particles, *gag, pol* and *env,* are expressed from separate, so-called 'helper plasmids'. In contrast to the expression vector, which codes for the gene of interest, the helper plasmids do not contain coding sequences for the packaging signal. Therefore, transcribed RNAs from the helper plasmids are not incorporated into the virus particle. With these replication defective retroviral particles, only a single round of transduction is possible. Thus, the risk of generating replication competent virus particles during production is greatly reduced. Retroviral transduction efficacy can be improved by concentrating the viral particles via ultracentrifugation (Kanbe & Zhang, 2004; Naldini et al., 1996). Gamma-retroviral particles can be preloaded onto RetroNectin-coated surfaces. RetroNectin, a recombinant peptide consisting of a mixture of fragments of the fibronectin molecule, co-localizes the viral particles and target cells into close proximity, thereby strongly increasing the efficiency of transduction (Hanenberg et al., 1996). A standard protocol for routine gamma-retroviral particle production and transduction of suspension cells is provided in Table 1. Expression of the gene of interest is usually coupled to the expression of a marker gene. This allows for immediate determination of the viral transduction efficacy as well as for the identification of transduced cells for the measurement of proliferation, differentiation and cell death. EGFP is the most commonly used marker protein, which exhibits a bright green fluorescence after laser excitation at 488 nm. Enrichment of vector-transduced fluorescent-labeled cells can be performed by fluorescence activated cell sorting (FACS). The usage of drug-selectable marker genes, such as neomycin and puromycin, represents another method used to obtain pure populations of transduced cells. Cellular expression of more than one transgene by retroviral vectors can be accomplished by a variety of strategies (Figure 1).

The inclusion of an internal promoter allows for the expression of a second transgene when one transgene is expressed from the vector 5´-LTR. However, this approach also carries the risk of promoter interference with the vector LTR during retroviral particle production, thereby reducing vector titers and expression levels of the GOI (de Felipe et al., 1999). Another commonly employed strategy is the expression of two separate genes from one single transcript using the IRES element derived from the picornavirus (Gallardo et al., 1997). The IRES element allows for the initiation of mRNA translation in a 5′ cap-independent manner (Mountford & Smith, 1995). However, expression levels of the two genes usually differ significantly. Typically, the gene located downstream is expressed at a level ten times lower than that of the other gene (Mizuguchi et al., 2000). The gene of interest and the marker gene can be fused to increase their stability and to allow for expression from one promoter. However, fusing two transgenes can result in functional restriction of the proteins caused by the fusion. Therefore, a short, flexible linker should be used to connect the proteins (Robinson & Sauer, 1998). Repeats of small side chain amino acids, such as glycine, serine and alanine, are well suited for the creation of linker sequences. The expression of two separate transgenes in equimolar amounts can be accomplished using 'self-cleaving' 2A peptides, originating from the foot-and-mouth disease virus (Ryan et al., 1991). The 2A peptide sequence disrupts the peptide bond formation via a ribosomal skip mechanism, which releases the polypeptide from the translational complex and allows the production of the downstream translation product (Donnelly et al., 2001).

Step 1: Retroviral vector production	• For retroviral vector particle production subconfluent (80%) adherent cell lines (e.g. HEK293T, HeLA) are co-transfected with the retroviral expression construct and the appropriate helper plasmids • 6 hours (or overnight) after transfection, exchange the appropriate medium for the target cells • 24 hours later, harvest the viral supernatant: centrifuge the viral supernatant at 1.500 rpm to pellet cell debris and filtrate the supernatant (0.22 μm filter) • Virus supernatant is ready for transduction or can be stored at –80°C for several months
Step 2: Preparation of RetroNectin-coated plates	• One day before transduction (at least 6 hours), add 500 μl RetroNectin (RN) solution (50 μg/ml) to each well of a 24-well plate (non-tissue culture treated) and incubate overnight at room temperature • The next day, discard the RN solution (reusable up to 8 times), add 1 ml stop solution (1xPBS+2% BSA) and incubate for 30 minutes at room temperature • Discard the stop solution, rinse 1x with HBSS solution and 1x with 1xPBS • Coated plates are ready for virus preload (RN coated plates can be stored in 4°C with PBS)
Step 3: Preload of viral particles	• Quickly defrost the virus supernatant and dilute as necessary • Discard the 1xPBS and add the viral supernatant with the appropriate multiplicities of infection (MOI) • Centrifuge at 3000 rpm at 4°C for 20-25 minutes • Discard the viral supernatant and repeat the preload *at least* 3 times, each with the appropriate volume (minimum: 500 μl)
Step 4: Transduction of target cells	• Remove the remaining viral supernatant before adding the cells • Count the cells and dilute the cells to a concentration of 7.5×10^5 cells/ml in the appropriate culture medium • Add 500 μl (minimum) cell suspension to each well and incubate at 37°C and 5% CO_2 for at least 8 hours (or overnight) • Optional: The addition of protamine sulfate (4 μg/ml) might increase the transduction efficiency • Prepare a second RN coated 24-well plate and repeat the preload and transduction procedure for a second, third or fourth transduction (max. 2 transductions per day) • 8 hours after the final transduction, exchange the medium and transfer the transduced cells into a fresh tissue-coated 24-well plate without RN • Optional: Wash the plate 3x with 1x PBS to collect the remaining cells from the plate

Table 1. Vector particle production and transduction standard protocol for suspension cells with gamma-retroviral vectors.

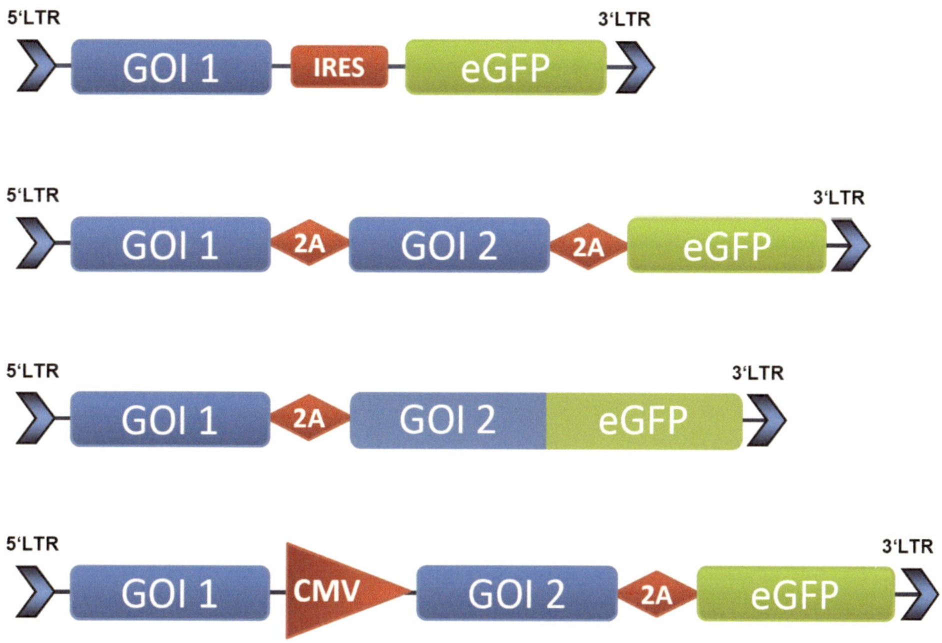

Fig. 1. Retroviral co-expression vector constructs, including eGFP as a marker gene. The depicted co-expression vectors are based on a standard 5'-LTR driven retroviral expression vector (top). 2A elements allow for co-expression of several GOI at equimolar levels. For intracellular stabilization, the GOI can be fused to eGFP. An internal promoter, e.g. the CMV promoter, drives GOI 2 expression independently of GOI 1. LTR, long terminal repeats; GOI, gene of interest; IRES, internal ribosomal entry site; 2A, 2A peptide sequence; eGFP, enhanced green fluorescent protein; CMV, cytomegalovirus.

In the context of the MSCV-based retroviral vectors, it has been shown that coupling four transgenes via three different 2A peptide cleavage sequences can generate four separate proteins both *in vitro* and *in vivo*. One restriction with this system is that the small remaining 2A-tag at the N-terminal end of the protein may potentially affect protein function (Szymczak et al., 2004). Therefore, proper cleavage and function of the individual proteins should be carefully verified. Table 2 summarizes the advantages and disadvantages of the different expression cassettes used for the co-expression of two genes of interest.

The 'lentiviral gene ontology' (LeGO) vectors represent a useful collection of state-of-the-art expression vectors for functional gene analysis. These vectors contain the retroviral enhancer/promoter of the spleen focus-forming virus, which has a broad and high expression pattern. LeGO expression vectors are available with a wide spectrum of different fluorescent markers, e.g. Cerulean, eGFP, tdTomato and mCherry, which are expressed in combination with the gene of interest via IRES elements. LeGO vectors that contain fluorescent marker genes linked via 2A peptides to different drug-selectable genes, e.g. blasticidin, hygromycin, neomycin, puromycin or zeocin, are also available. Furthermore, the expression cassettes of these LeGO vectors are flanked by loxP sites, which allows for displacement of the transgene after introduction of the CRE recombinase (Weber, 2007; Weber et al., 2008; Weber et al., 2010).

	IRES	2A	2nd promoter (internal)	Co-transduction
Advantage	Expression of 2 separate transgenes	Equal expression levels of the 2 genes	Expression of 2 separate transgenes	Independent expression; results in single and double transduced cells
Disadvantage	10x lower expression of the downstream gene	Remaining 2A tag at the end of the N-terminal protein	Low titer of viral particles	Low rate of double transduced cells; increases risk of insertional mutagenesis
Literature	*Gallardo et al., 1997 Mizuguchi et al., 2000*	*Szymczak et al., 2004*	*Felipe et al., 1999*	*Rizo et al., 2010*

Table 2. Overview of expression cassette elements for co-expression of two genes of interest.

To accurately characterize oncogene activity it is important to have the ability to selectively induce and terminate oncogene expression. This is particularly important if the delivered gene product is toxic at high concentrations. The regulation of gene expression can be achieved by using the tetracycline-controlled transactivator (tTA)-responsive promoter (Tet-system), a prokaryotic inducible promoter system that is also applicable to mammalian cells (Gossen & Bujard, 1992). The Tet system comprises two components: one component that drives expression of the transactivator (tTA) and a second component that contains the (tTA)-responsive promoter element for transgene expression. In the first developed 'tet-off' system, the transactivator binds to the promoter in the absence of tetracycline. The addition of tetracycline inhibits its binding, thereby resulting in inhibition of transgene expression (Gossen et al., 1995). To avoid constant tetracycline supplementation, a reverse system ('tet-on' system) allows for transgene expression only in the presence of doxycycline, a tetracycline derivate (Gossen et al., 1995). Traditionally, transactivator and promoter components had to be introduced by two separate transduction steps to obtain inducible gene expression. The development of an 'all-in-one' vector system circumvents this complication. In this system, all components required for tet-regulated transgene expression have been inserted as a bidirectional expression cassette (Heinz et al., 2011). Another means of intracellular oncogene dosage control is the regulation at the protein level. With this type of expression control, the gene of interest can be fused to a small destabilizing domain, thereby mediating the intracellular destruction of the protein by targeting it for proteasomal degradation. Degradation of the fusion protein can be specifically blocked by cell membrane-permeable small molecules, which bind to and inhibit the destabilizing domain mediated degradation, thereby resulting in the accumulation of the expressed transgene (Banaszynski et al., 2006).

3. Murine progenitor cells

Murine hematopoietic stem and progenitor cells have been well characterized. To study these cell types, progenitor cells can be simply isolated from the bone marrow. After femora and tibia preparation, bone marrow cells can be harvested by flushing the bones. Further purification of hematopoietic progenitor cells is typically carried out by 'lineage depletion'. Using this method, differentiated 'lineage positive' cells, such as monocytes and macrophages, T- and B- cells, erythrocytes and granulocytes, are separated from their committed precursors, the 'lineage negative' fraction. Freshly isolated, complete bone marrow suspension cells are incubated with a mixture of magnetically labeled antibodies against cell surface markers for mature blood cells, typically B220, CD4, CD8, Gr-1, Mac-1 and Ter-119. Separation of the lineage negative progenitor cell fraction is performed by passing the labeled and non-labeled cells through magnetic columns (Challen et al., 2009).

Amongst all vertebrates, the murine hematopoietic system is the best characterized. For the subdivision of stem and progenitor cell populations, the LSK- and SLAM-markers have become widely accepted. LSK (lin^-, $Sca1^+$, $c\text{-}kit^+$) cells lack the markers of mature blood cells and simultaneously express high levels of the stem cell markers, Sca1 and c-kit. As little as one hundred LSK cells have been shown to be sufficient for the long-term multilineage repopulation of lethally irradiated recipient mice (Okada et al., 1992). The LSK cell compartment can be further separated into hematopoietic stem cells (HSCs) and multipotent progenitors (MPPs) depending on their diverse expression pattern of the family of 'signaling lymphocyte activation molecule' (SLAM) receptors (Kiel et al., 2005). The SLAM cell surface marker, CD150, is exclusively expressed on HSCs, whereas CD244 is expressed by transiently reconstituting MPPs. CD34 and Flt3 expression patterns further allow for the discrimination between long term-HSC (LT-HSCs; $CD34^-/Flt3^-$) and short term HSCs (ST-HSCs; $CD34^+/Flt3^+$) (Adolfsson et al., 2001; Osawa et al., 1996). ST-HSCs have a reduced self-renewal capacity for a restricted time compared with the life-long self-renewal capacity of LT-HSCs (Adolfsson et al., 2001; Morrison & Weissman, 1994; Yang et al., 2005). Because the murine hematopoietic system has been well characterized, with precisely classified and characterized stem and progenitor cell compartments, and simple precursor cell purification procedures have been established and optimized, murine hematopoietic progenitor cells are well suited for the functional analysis of oncogenic fusion genes and mutations associated with leukemia development.

The cell transforming activity of a given leukemia-associated oncogene can be measured by performing an *in vitro* colony forming unit (CFU) assay. This assay allows for the quantification of colony forming progenitors and their iterative replating capacity. Hematopoietic progenitor cells expressing the gene of interest are plated in methylcellulose at low density. In general, normal progenitor cells only form colonies in the first round of plating. However, oncogene-expressing cells are able to confer serial replating capacity for several rounds of plating. For example, cells expressing the t(8;21) translocation product, AML1/ETO, are able to confer serial replating for up to 13 rounds of plating (Rhoades et al., 2000). Transgene expressing murine progenitor cells can also be cultivated in liquid suspension cultures. Here, cytokines such as IL3, IL6 and SCF must be supplemented continuously. Under these *ex vivo* cultivation parameters specific for cell differentiation, proliferation and apoptosis can be measured under various cell culture conditions, such as serum or cytokine deprivation and hypoxic conditions, which imitate the hypoxic niches of the bone marrow.

Gene modified precursor cells can be further examined *in vivo* in a mouse transplantation model. In this case, immediately after retroviral gene transfer, lineage depleted bone marrow cells stably expressing the oncogene of interest are transplanted into lethally irradiated syngeneic recipient mice. The transplantation is performed by injection of gene-modified cells into the tail vein or the retro-orbital sinus of recipient mice (Larochelle et al., 1995). For successful hematopoietic rescue, transplanted cells must reach the appropriate milieu in the bone marrow niches, which supports their proliferation and differentiation; this cell migration process is referred to as 'homing' (Szilvassy et al., 1999). To analyze disease progression in mice following the transplantation of progenitor cells body weight and blood profile values must be documented carefully over time. If transplanted mice develop any symptoms of leukemia, e.g. sudden body weight reduction, increasing peripheral leukocyte counts or poor general health conditions, they should be sacrificed and analyzed. Blood cells isolated from the periphery, spleen and bone marrow compartment can be studied separately. Flow cytometric analysis conveniently allows for the detection of oncogene expressing blood cells by discerning the expression of the fluorescence marker proteins. Gene marked cells can be examined for cellular differentiation (CD differentiation marker), the proliferation/cell cycle profile and apoptosis by AnnexinV-staining, for example. FACS based methods allow for the parallel analysis of transduced and non-transduced cells, using the latter as the internal experimental control. Transgene expression of leukemic cells must be analyzed by RT-PCR and western immunoblotting, which assesses mRNA and protein levels, respectively. There are highly specific antibodies that can detect epitope-tagged oncoproteins, e.g. Ha- or Flag-tagged proteins, even at very low expression levels (Terpe, 2003). To exclude the potential oncogenic effects of vector-mediated insertional mutagenesis, clonality and integration site analysis must be performed carefully. The oncogene activity of the expressed transgene can be accurately validated by analyzing the downstream signal transduction pathways of the cell. For example, phosphorylated STAT5 and CRKL are regarded as downstream indicators of oncogenic BCR/ABL signaling. Bone marrow and spleen, which are the target organs of leukemic origin, and peripheral blood must be analyzed for the presence of immature blast cells. This can be carried out by conventional blood smear and flow cytometric analysis. For organ histology, samples of each organ, including the spleen, liver, lymph nodes and thymus, are transferred into paraffin, sectioned and examined. Hematoxylin and eosin are the most commonly used staining solutions in histology for light microscopical analysis. A final validation of the leukemia must be demonstrated by re-transplantating the leukemic blood cells into secondary lethally irradiated recipient mice. In these secondary transplanted mice, leukemia onset should appear much earlier than in primary recipients. In 2002, Kogan et al published the 'Bethesda proposals for the classification of hematopoietic neoplasms in mice' (Kogan et al., 2002). As with the World Health Organization (WHO) classification of human disorders, theses proposals utilize morphologic, immunophenotypic, clinical, biological and genetic characteristics to classify neoplasms.

Both methods, the colony-forming assay and the mouse transplantation model are commonly used techniques for the investigation of the transforming potential of oncogenes in leukemia (Figure 2).

The following examples illustrate both the genetic and biochemical approaches utilizing murine hematopoietic progenitor cells for leukemia modeling.

The acute promyelocytic leukemia (APL) associated t(15;17) translocation product, PML/RARα, is one of the most studied fusion proteins associated with AML (Puccetti & Ruthardt, 2004). In the clinical setting, APL patients not only respond well to 'all trans retinoic acid' (ATRA) therapy, which has been well documented (Huang et al., 1988), but also benefit from treatment with arsenic trioxide (Chen et al., 1997), which exerts a profound anti-cancer effect by inducing the degradation of the PML/RARα oncoprotein. Retroviral expression of PML/RARα in murine progenitor cells efficiently induces leukemia development in transplanted lethally irradiated recipient mice (Minucci et al., 2002). The efficacy of arsenic trioxide and ATRA has been recapitulated in PML/RARα mouse models displaying the impressive anti-leukemia effects of both substances (Rego et al., 2000). Furthermore, in transplantation models based on ATRA-resistant APL cell lines, treatment with arsenic trioxide significantly decreases tumor formation (Kinjo et al., 2000). Zhang et al have further showed that arsenic trioxide functions by directly binding to PML/RARα. The researchers identified cysteine residues within the PML portion that are directly bound by arsenic trioxide, which triggered SUMOylation and subsequent degradation of the oncoprotein (Zhang et al., 2010).

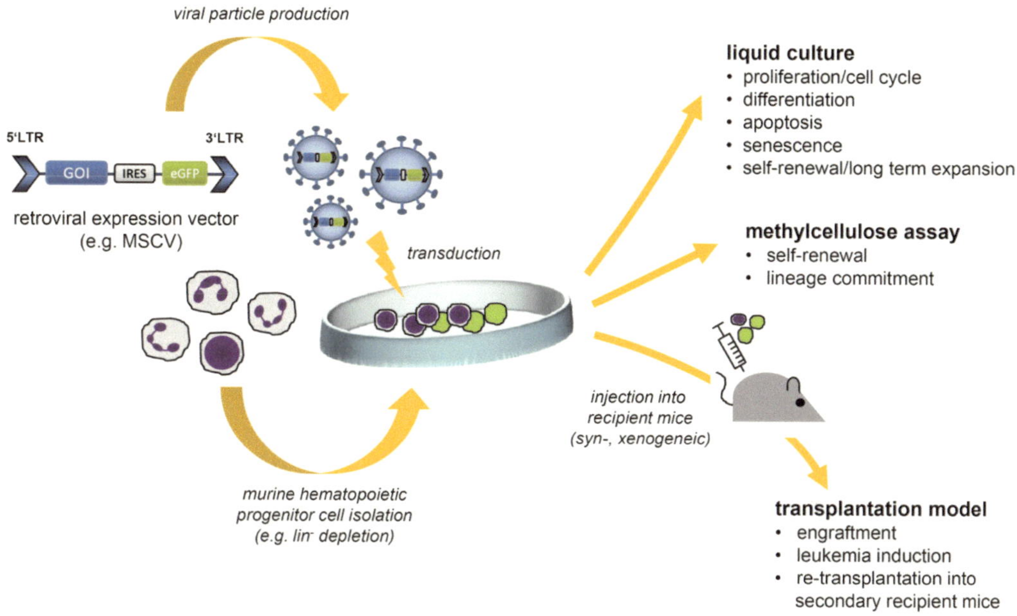

Fig. 2. Functional analysis of gene-modified murine/human hematopoietic progenitor cells. Experimental procedures include cloning of the retroviral expression vector, viral particle production, hematopoietic progenitor cell isolation, transduction and functional analysis in methylcellulose assays, liquid cultures and murine syngeneic or xenogeneic mouse transplantation models. GOI, gene of interest; MSCV, murine stem cell virus; LTR, long terminal repeats; lin-, lineage negative.

Other reports have described that oncogene expression experiments involving murine progenitor cells supported the clinical finding reporting a highly leukemogenic splice variant of the familiar AML1/ETO fusion gene resulting from the translocation t(8;21). Several groups have shown that the full length AML1/ETO protein does not lead to the development of leukemia when transplanting LSK bone marrow cells expressing AML1/ETO into syngeneic mice (de Guzman et al., 2002). However, in similar transplantation experiments performed by Yan and colleagues, one mouse developed leukemia 14 weeks after bone marrow transplantation. Further analysis showed that a C-terminal truncated AML1/ETO protein was expressed in this mouse due to a one-base pair insertion into the full length AML1/ETO gene. Subsequently, the cloning and creation of mice expressing the truncated protein by transplantation of transduced progenitor cells again revealed a rapid leukemia development (Yan et al., 2004). Consequently, these results led to the investigation and identification of a naturally occurring splice variant of AML1/ETO in t(8;21) patients by sophisticated gene expression analysis of patient material. This splice variant, termed AML1/ETO9A, is almost structurally identical to the truncated form expressed in the leukemic mouse. Expression of this newly discovered splice isoform in mice also induced rapid leukemia development (Yan et al., 2006). In conclusion, these oncogene expression experiments using murine progenitor cells led to the clinical identification of a potent oncogenic AML1/ETO splice variant. Further experiments must be performed to understand whether the AML1/ETO splice isoform is the driving oncogene in human t(8;21) leukemia cells.

The usage of oncogene expressing vectors has also facilitated the understanding of the protein domain structure-function relationship. Biophysical and biochemical experiments have been used to identify highly conserved domains within several oncoproteins, which might represent valuable target structures for molecular intervention. This has been demonstrated with the AML1/ETO fusion protein. Here, a central region, the *nervy* homology region 2 (NHR2), was found to play an essential role in the leukemogenic activity of the fusion protein. Analysis of the crystal structure revealed a tetrameric formation that is essential for the serial colony formation capacity of murine progenitor cells in methylcellulose assays (Liu et al., 2006). By performing additional bioinformatic molecular modeling analyses, five amino acids were identified within the large NHR2 tetramer-interface that are important for oligomer formation. Substitution of these critical residues led to the conversion of tetramers into dimers with the complete loss of the transforming abilities of AML1/ETO. Transplantation of retroviral infected murine bone marrow cells expressing the AML1/ETO protein harboring these five substitutions showed that these amino acids play a critical role in transformation, as the mice failed to develop leukemia. Interestingly, the identified amino acids are clustered in one region at the top of the NHR2 dimer surface, thereby representing a potential target site for molecular intervention (Wichmann et al., 2010). These findings, which reveal the molecular determinants of oncogene activity, are the result of a productive combination of bioinformatics, biochemical and cell-biological analyses. Furthermore, proof of concept of oncogene targeting was demonstrated using a synthetic oligomerization domain. This domain was integrated into the AML1/ETO fusion gene, thereby replacing the NHR2 tetramer domain. Specific inhibitors that disrupt the oligomerization of this synthetic domain within AML1/ETO completely blocked the replating capacity of retrovirally transduced AML1/ETO expressing murine progenitor cells (Kwok et al., 2009).

By expressing leukemia fusion genes in murine cells, one can assess exactly which gene product from a balanced translocation, which often generates two different reciprocal fusion genes, is responsible for driving the leukemic activity. Bursen and colleagues have reported interesting findings regarding the function of the reciprocal fusion proteins, AF4/MLL and MLL/AF4, which are generated by the chromosomal translocation t(4;11) in high-risk infant acute mixed lineage leukemia. They analyzed the leukemia-inducing capacity of these two fusion genes in mice by transplantation of retrovirally transduced $Lin^{-}/Sca1^{+}$ cells expressing either one or both of the reciprocal fusion genes. They could show that expression of AF4/MLL alone was sufficient to promote leukemia development, while the reciprocal translocation, MLL/AF4, completely lacked leukemogenic potential (Bursen et al., 2010).

4. The human CD34+ progenitor cell system

Human blood progenitor cells are characterized by the high expression levels of the cell surface marker CD34 and the absence of CD38 expression ($CD34^+/CD38^-$). CD34 is a member of the single-pass transmembrane sialomucin protein family, which is expressed in early hematopoietic and vascular-associated tissues; however, little is known about its exact biological function (Furness & McNagny, 2006). There are a variety of ways to obtain hematopoietic CD34+ cells from the human body. The cells can be isolated from the peripheral blood by leukapheresis after stimulation and mobilization of the bone marrow precursors with G-CSF (granulocytic colony stimulating factor). Bone marrow aspiration represents the classical but invasive isolation method, which also allows for the isolation of large numbers of CD34+ cells. A third option involves the usage of placental derived cord blood cells of which the quality/stemness and engraftment potential are superior to that of adult CD34+ stem cells (Hao et al., 1995). The efficient enrichment of human hematopoietic CD34+ cells can be achieved by immunomagnetic cell sorting, which represents a standard and convenient method in laboratory work (Clarke & Davies, 2001). Magnetic labeled CD34-antibodies are used to recover high-purity populations of CD34+ cells by passing cells through magnetic columns. Isolated CD34+ cells can then be used for clinical and experimental purposes. For transgene expression studies, the cells can be manipulated by retroviral transduction immediately after recovery or after a short pre-cultivation in a cytokine cocktail, which usually contains IL-3, IL6 and SCF for cell cycle activation. Like the murine system, transduced human CD34+ cells can be propagated *in vitro* in methylcellulose assays for colony formation as well as in long-term liquid cultures used to assess self-renewal and proliferation/expansion capacities (Figure 1). Furthermore, human CD34+ cells expressing leukemic gene products can be transplanted into severe combined immunodeficient (NOD/SCID) mice (xenotransplants). Additionally, the NOG (NOD/Shi-scid/IL-$2R\gamma^{null}$) mice accept heterologous transplanted cells more easily than any other type of immunodeficient nude or NOD/SCID mice. Therefore, the NOG mouse system is a highly efficient recipient model for the engraftment, proliferation and differentiation of human cells (Ito et al., 2002).

The transformation of human cells requires additional genetic alterations when compared with their murine counterparts (Hahn et al., 1999; Rangarajan & Weinberg, 2003). This is reflected by the observation that singular expression of several oncogenes induces leukemia in the murine system but fails to transform human CD34+ cells in the NOD/SCID humanized leukemia mouse model. Further evidence of this concept has been demonstrated by gene expression analysis of healthy individuals. Here, oncogenes such as BCR/ABL and AML1/ETO have been frequently detected in individuals completely lacking any sign of disease (Song et al., 2011). As CD34+ cells represent the human hematopoietic stem/progenitor cell population, these cells can be regarded as appropriate target cells used to study the biological effects of oncogenes in human leukemia development.

The following passages provide an overview of recent experiments addressing the leukemogenic activity of several myeloid leukemia associated oncogenes expressed alone or in combination in human hematopoietic CD34+ progenitor cells. In all cases, genes were delivered using gamma-retroviral vectors co-expressing the marker genes eGFP or dNGFR (truncated nerve growth factor receptor), which allowed for the convenient detection of gene-modified cells by FACS analysis.

Grignani et al have reported that ectopic expression of PML/RARα in human CD34+ *ex vivo* cultures rapidly induced the cellular differentiation of progenitor cells towards the promyelocytic stage, followed by a block in further terminal differentiation into granulocytes, which resembled typical features of primary human acute promyelocytic leukemia (Grignani et al., 2000). In cytokine deprived liquid cultures, PML/RARα expressing cells survived and continued to expand, whereas control cells stopped proliferation and died by apoptosis. The terminal differentiation block induced by PML/RARα could be overcome by treatment with ATRA, a drug that has dramatically improved the overall survival of APL patients. They further demonstrated that a mutation of the N-CoR repressor binding interface within the PML portion of the fusion protein completely disrupted the observed biological effects, thereby suggesting that N-CoR triggered transcriptional repression is an essential prerequisite for PML/RARα oncogene activity in human hematopoietic progenitor cells.

Among the AML oncogenes, hyperactive tyrosine kinases play a major role in disease development and have gathered much attention since the kinase inhibitor imatinib has been proven to be highly beneficial for BCR/ABL positive CML patients (Druker et al., 1996; Sawyers et al., 2002; Brandts et al., 2007). Chung and colleagues retrovirally expressed a related constitutive active tyrosine kinase, FLT3-ITD, which is frequently found in AML patient samples associated with poor prognosis (Gilliland & Griffin, 2002). Stable expression of FLT3-ITD conferred a strong short-term proliferative signal in human CD34+ cells with enhanced erythropoiesis for two weeks after transduction *ex vivo*. The cells were blocked in terminal differentiation and colony formation was enhanced when compared with control cells. These effects could be partially substituted by expression of a constitutive active STAT5 mutant, a major downstream target of the hyperactive FLT3-ITD kinase. Moreover, FLT3-ITD triggered effects that could be blocked via inhibition with the FLT3-inhibitor tyrphostin (Chung et al., 2005). Despite these significant effects, FLT3-ITD transgene-expressing CD34+ cells are neither able to expand further in *ex vivo* cultures nor able to induce leukemia in the NOD/SCID mouse transplantation model.

Stable ectopic expression of several leukemogenic fusion genes resulting from chromosomal translocations leads to enhanced *ex vivo* CD34+ cell expansion for up to several months (Abdul-Nabi et al., 2010). This has previously been shown for the t(8;21) associated fusion protein AML1/ETO, which is capable of expanding human CD34+ cells *ex vivo* for several months with a cumulative cell expansion of more than 10^{15}-fold. Retroviral expression of AML1/ETO resulted in a sustained proliferation potential using a cytokine cocktail that included IL3, IL6, SCF, FLT3, GM-CSF, TPO and EPO, all at low concentrations. The cells display the typical differentiation block as observed in myeloid blast cells and grow out from a mixed culture of transduced and non-transduced cells. Even after several weeks in *ex vivo* culture, the cells are capable of colony formation in methylcellulose assays and, more importantly, of engraftment into immunodeficient NOD/SCID mice (Mulloy et al., 2003; Mulloy et al., 2002). Phenotypically, a subpopulation of the cells continues to express CD34, while the majority of the cells express the myeloid specific markers CD13 and CD33, in the absence of erythroid markers. Continuous expansion of the cells completely depends on the CD34+ subgroup. Erythroid differentiation was shown to be blocked by the AML1/ETO fusion protein via direct inhibition of GATA1 transcription factor activity (Choi et al., 2006). However, expression of AML1/ETO does not lead to leukemia development in transplanted immunodeficient NOD/SCID mice, suggesting that additional genetic hits must occur for full-blown AML development. Similar results were obtained from analysis of the inv(16) fusion protein CBFB/MYH11. Expression of this fusion gene also caused enhanced proliferation and expansion of CD34+ cells over several months with retention of the engraftment potential in NOD/SCID mice. However, as also observed with AML1/ETO, transplanted mice do not develop leukemia (Wunderlich et al., 2006). Therefore, both oncogenes confer a preleukemic status and subsequent alterations are required for the transition to overt leukemia.

To decipher the genetic signature of AML, Abdul-Nabi and colleagues have assessed various AML-associated fusion proteins for their ability to enhance CD34+ cell expansion *ex vivo* and subsequently analyzed their gene expression profiles (Abdul-Nabi et al., 2010). In this study, experiments were also performed with gamma-retroviral vectors expressing the fusion genes AML1/ETO, PML/RARα, MLL/AF9 and NUP98/HOXA9 together with eGFP. To identify key target genes responsible for the expansion of CD34+ cells the authors performed gene array analysis of FACS-sorted eGFP+ cells expressing the indicated oncogenes, which identifies the induced and repressed target genes during the *ex vivo* selection process. One interesting candidate gene that was shown to be specifically upregulated due to both AML1/ETO and PML/RARα expression was the p53-inhibiting molecule MDM2. The authors could further show that activation of the gatekeeper protein p53, by blocking the MDM2-p53 protein-protein interaction with the small molecule compound Nutlin-3, was sufficient to completely block AML1/ETO induced selection and expansion of CD34+ progenitor cells. Therefore, Nutlin-3 is proposed to function as an inhibitor for AML1/ETO positive leukemias by reactivating p53 and consecutively eliminating the leukemic cells via the induction of apoptosis. Two independent groups have shown that retroviral expression of the NUP98/HOXA9 fusion gene, which is found in myelodysplastic syndrome (MDS) and AML patients, resulted in a similar outgrowth of transgene expressing cells with maintenance of self-renewal potential *ex vivo* and increased engraftment capacity in NOD/SCID mice (Chung et al., 2006; Takeda et al., 2006). This outgrowth was accompanied by high levels of HOX gene expression, a typical feature for this leukemia entity.

Regardless of their remarkable *ex vivo* cell expansion properties, the AML associated gene products described above, PML/RARα, FLT3-ITD, NUP98/HOXA9 and AML1/ETO, were not able to independently induce leukemia in transplanted NOD/SCID mice. Therefore, it is likely that additional genetic alterations are required for full cellular transformation in AML. In this regard it was shown that oncogenic RAS signaling, triggered by N-Ras^{G12D} overexpression, does increase AML1/ETO engraftment capacity in NOD/SCID mice but is still not sufficient to overcome the leukemia onset defect in the NOD/SCID mouse model (Chou et al., 2011).

Interestingly, MLL rearrangements are typically found in aggressive infant or therapy related leukemias (Aplan, 2006). In contrast to AML derived gene products, ectopic expression of either MLL/AF9 or MLL/ENL mixed-lineage leukemia fusion genes, as a single genetic event, results in the development of myeloid or lymphoid leukemias in the NOD/SCID mouse model approximately 100 days after transplantation (Barabe et al., 2007; Wei et al., 2008). Morphological analysis has revealed that AML and B-ALL leukemias are associated with both MLL rearrangements. Remarkably, *ex vivo* expanded cells gave rise to leukemia in NOD/SCID mice, even after 70 days of *in vitro* culture prior to transplantation in sublethally irradiated mice. The reasons for the striking differences between AML and

MLL fusion genes in their ability to induce leukemia onset in NOD/SCID mice are completely unknown. A direct comparison of deregulated genes may reveal which additional pathways are activated in MLL leukemic human CD34+ cells.

Recently, a report was published describing a true oncogenic cooperativeness in human CD34+ cell expansion and leukemia induction in NOD/SCID mice (Rizo et al., 2010). The authors convincingly have shown that retroviral co-expression of the CML associated oncogene, BCR/ABL, and the polycomb ring finger oncogene, BMI1, leads to leukemia induction within 4-5 months after transplantation. The isolated human leukemia cells were re-transplantable into secondary recipient mice, which induced leukemia with a shortened latency. *In vitro,* the co-expression of both oncogenes in human CD34+ cells allowed for the establishment of myeloid and lymphoid long-term cultures with self-renewing properties. This report also describes a series of valuable cell culture methods for *in vitro* analysis of CD34+ cell proliferation and self-renewal. Finally, the authors have demonstrated that retroviral introduction of BMI1 into primary leukemia cells from CML chronic-phase patients elevated the proliferative capacity and self-renewal properties of the leukemia cells, while shRNA knockdown of BMI1 in blast crisis CML cells completely blocked their proliferation potential. These results highlight BMI1 as an attractive molecular target for blast crisis CML cells, which is especially important given the rates of BCR/ABL positive leukemic stem cell resistance to kinase inhibitors such as imatinib (Corbin et al., 2011). However, the exact molecular mechanisms of BCR/ABL and BMI1 oncogenic co-operation have to be addressed in further studies.

In conclusion, human CD34+ blood progenitor cells represent a powerful cell biology tool used for the analysis of leukemogenic gene product activity. Methods of isolation and purification of CD34+ cells have significantly improved and are broadly available for researchers. The cells can be propagated *ex vivo* and oncogene activity can be analyzed for a wide range of biological parameters, including differentiation, proliferation, self-renewal, senescence and apoptosis, using standard cell biology methods. CD34+ suspension cells can be cultured *ex vivo* as liquid cultures or on stromal layer cells. With the possibility to transplant these cells into sublethally irradiated NOD/SCID mice this is an ideal model system to study the function of human leukemia-associated oncogenes.

5. Conclusions

Powerful retroviral expression vectors and standardized enrichment technologies, which are used for the isolation of hematopoietic precursor cells from the murine and human bone marrow compartment, efficiently enabled the accurate modeling of leukemia initiation and progression in the appropriate cell compartment. Currently available expression vectors allow for the simultaneous expression of several genes, including oncogenes, marker genes for detection and selection genes used to isolate modified cells, which represent practical tools for modeling leukemia progression in hematopoietic cells. Among the introduced strategies, the humanized mouse model based on human CD34+ precursor cell transplantation into NOD/SCID mice represents a credible model system to study human leukemia. As described here, the expression of single oncogenes such as BCR/ABL and AML1/ETO, which are primarily found in older patients, does not lead to leukemia development, implying that disease develops as a result of secondary mutations. In contrast, the expression of several MLL fusion proteins, which are typically found in younger patients, was found to be sufficient to trigger leukemia development with high penetrance.

In total, these approaches will lead to a better understanding of the genetic alterations that are required for the onset of cellular transformation. Furthermore, these studies have the potential to propel the development of effective drugs designed to eradicate leukemia cells.

6. Acknowledgement

The authors are supported by research grants from the NGFN Cancer Network (grant 01GS0450, TP-10), the Deutsche Krebshilfe (grant 102362, TP-7), the LEOWE OSF (TP-C3) and the LOEWE CGT (startup grant CW). The Georg-Speyer-Haus is supported by the Bundesministerium für Gesundheit and the Hessisches Ministerium für Wissenschaft und Kunst.

7. References

Abdul-Nabi, A.M.; Yassin, E.R.; Varghese, N.; Deshmukh, H. & Yaseen, N.R. (2010). In vitro transformation of primary human CD34+ cells by AML fusion oncogenes: early gene expression profiling reveals possible drug target in AML. *PLoS One*, Vol. 5, No. 8, pp. e12464

Adolfsson, J.; Borge, O.J.; Bryder, D.; Theilgaard-Monch, K.; Astrand-Grundstrom, I.; Sitnicka, E.; Sasaki, Y. & Jacobsen, S.E.W. (2001). Upregulation of flt3 expression within the bone marrow Lin(-)Sca1(+)c-kit(+) stem cell compartment is accompanied by loss of self-renewal capacity. *Immunity*, Vol. 15, No. 4, pp. 659-669

Aplan, P.D. (2006). Chromosomal translocations involving the MLL gene: molecular mechanisms. *DNA Repair (Amst)*, Vol. 5, No. 9-10, pp. 1265-1272

Banaszynski, L.A.; Chen, L.C.; Maynard-Smith, L.A.; Ooi, A.G.L. & Wandless, T.J. (2006). A rapid, reversible, and tunable method to regulate protein function in living cells using synthetic small molecules. *Cell*, Vol. 126, No. 5, pp. 995-1004

Barabe, F.; Kennedy, J.A.; Hope, K.J. & Dick, J.E. (2007). Modeling the initiation and progression of human acute leukemia in mice. *Science*, Vol. 316, No. 5824, pp. 600-604

Baum, C. (2007). Insertional mutagenesis in gene therapy and stem cell biology. *Current Opinion in Hematology*, Vol. 14, No. 4, pp. 337-342

Belvedere, O.; Feruglio, C.; Malangone, W.; Bonora, M.L.; Donini, A.; Dorotea, L.; Tonutti, E.; Rinaldi, C.; Pittino, M.; Baccarani, M.; Del Frate, G.; Biffoni, F.; Sala, P.; Hilbert, D.M. & Degrassi, A. (1999). Phenotypic characterization of immunomagnetically purified umbilical cord blood CD34+ cells. *Blood Cells Mol Dis*, Vol. 25, No. 3-4, pp. 141-146

Boissel, N.; Leroy, H.; Brethon, B.; Philippe, N.; de Botton, S.; Auvrignon, A.; Raffoux, E.; Leblanc, T.; Thomas, X.; Hermine, O.; Quesnel, B.; Baruchel, A.; Leverger, G.; Dombret, H. & Preudhomme, C. (2006). Incidence and prognostic impact of c-Kit, FLT3, and Ras gene mutations in core binding factor acute myeloid leukemia (CBF-AML). *Leukemia*, Vol. 20, No. 6, pp. 965-970

Brandts, C.H.; Berdel, W.E. & Serve, H. (2007). Oncogenic signaling in acute myeloid leukemia. *Curr Drug Targets*, Vol. 8, No. 2, pp. 237-246

Bursen, A.; Schwabe, K.; Ruster, B.; Henschler, R.; Ruthardt, M.; Dingermann, T. & Marschalek, R. (2010). The AF4.MLL fusion protein is capable of inducing ALL in mice without requirement of MLL.AF4. *Blood*, Vol. 115, No. 17, pp. 3570-3579

Challen, G.A.; Boles, N.; Lin, K.K.Y. & Goodell, M.A. (2009). Mouse Hematopoietic Stem Cell Identification and Analysis. *Cytometry Part A*, Vol. 75A, No. 1, pp. 14-24

Chen, G.Q.; Shi, X.G.; Tang, W.; Xiong, S.M.; Zhu, J.; Cai, X.; Han, Z.G.; Ni, J.H.; Shi, G.Y.; Jia, P.M.; Liu, M.M.; He, K.L.; Niu, C.; Ma, J.; Zhang, P.; Zhang, T.D.; Paul, P.; Naoe, T.; Kitamura, K.; Miller, W.; Waxman, S.; Wang, Z.Y.; de The, H.; Chen, S.J. & Chen, Z. (1997). Use of arsenic trioxide (As2O3) in the treatment of acute promyelocytic leukemia (APL): I. As2O3 exerts dose-dependent dual effects on APL cells. Blood, Vol. 89, No. 9, pp. 3345-3353

Choi, Y.; Elagib, K.E.; Delehanty, L.L. & Goldfarb, A.N. (2006). Erythroid inhibition by the leukemic fusion AML1-ETO is associated with impaired acetylation of the major erythroid transcription factor GATA-1. *Cancer Res*, Vol. 66, No. 6, pp. 2990-2996

Chou, F.S.; Wunderlich, M.; Griesinger, A. & Mulloy, J.C. (2011). N-Ras(G12D) induces features of stepwise transformation in preleukemic human umbilical cord blood cultures expressing the AML1-ETO fusion gene. *Blood*, Vol. 117, No. 7, pp. 2237-2240

Chung, K.Y.; Morrone, G.; Schuringa, J.J.; Plasilova, M.; Shieh, J.H.; Zhang, Y.; Zhou, P. & Moore, M.A. (2006). Enforced expression of NUP98-HOXA9 in human CD34(+) cells enhances stem cell proliferation. *Cancer Res*, Vol. 66, No. 24, pp. 11781-11791

Chung, K.Y.; Morrone, G.; Schuringa, J.J.; Wong, B.; Dorn, D.C. & Moore, M.A. (2005). Enforced expression of an Flt3 internal tandem duplication in human CD34+ cells confers properties of self-renewal and enhanced erythropoiesis. *Blood*, Vol. 105, No. 1, pp. 77-84

Clarke, C. & Davies, S. (2001). Immunomagnetic cell separation. *Methods Mol Med*, Vol. 58, No. pp. 17-23

Coffin, J.M.; Hughes, S.H. & Varmus, H.E. (2007). *Retroviruses*, Cold Spring Harbor Laboratory Press, ISBN-10: 0-87969-571-4, New York, USA

Corbin, A.S.; Agarwal, A.; Loriaux, M.; Cortes, J.; Deininger, M.W. & Druker, B.J. (2011). Human chronic myeloid leukemia stem cells are insensitive to imatinib despite inhibition of BCR-ABL activity. *J Clin Invest*, Vol. 121, No. 1, pp. 396-409

Dang, L.; White, D.W.; Gross, S.; Bennett, B.D.; Bittinger, M.A.; Driggers, E.M.; Fantin, V.R.; Jang, H.G.; Jin, S.; Keenan, M.C.; Marks, K.M.; Prins, R.M.; Ward, P.S.; Yen, K.E.; Liau, L.M.; Rabinowitz, J.D.; Cantley, L.C.; Thompson, C.B.; Vander Heiden, M.G. & Su, S.M. (2009). Cancer-associated IDH1 mutations produce 2-hydroxyglutarate. *Nature*, Vol. 462, No. 7274, pp. 739-744

de Felipe, P.; Martin, V.; Cortes, M.L.; Ryan, M. & Izquierdo, M. (1999). Use of the 2A sequence from foot-and-mouth disease virus in the generation of retroviral vectors for gene therapy. *Gene Therapy*, Vol. 6, No. 2, pp. 198-208

de Guzman, C.G.; Warren, A.J.; Zhang, Z.; Gartland, L.; Erickson, P.; Drabkin, H.; Hiebert, S.W. & Klug, C.A. (2002). Hematopoietic stem cell expansion and distinct myeloid developmental abnormalities in a murine model of the AML1-ETO translocation. *Molecular and Cellular Biology*, Vol. 22, No. 15, pp. 5506-5517

Demetri, G.D. (2002). Targeting the molecular pathophysiology of gastrointestinal stromal tumors with imatinib. Mechanisms, successes, and challenges to rational drug development. *Hematol Oncol Clin North Am*, Vol. 16, No. 5, pp. 1115-1124

Diamond, J.M. & Melo, J.V. (2011). Mechanisms of resistance to BCR-ABL kinase inhibitors. *Leuk Lymphoma*, Vol. 52 Suppl 1, No. pp. 12-22

Donnelly, M.L.; Luke, G.; Mehrotra, A.; Li, X.; Hughes, L.E.; Gani, D. & Ryan, M.D. (2001). Analysis of the aphthovirus 2A/2B polyprotein 'cleavage' mechanism indicates not a proteolytic reaction, but a novel translational effect: a putative ribosomal 'skip'. *Journal of General Virology*, Vol. 82, No. Pt 5, pp. 1013-1025

Druker, B.J.; Tamura, S.; Buchdunger, E.; Ohno, S.; Segal, G.M.; Fanning, S.; Zimmermann, J. & Lydon, N.B. (1996). Effects of a selective inhibitor of the Abl tyrosine kinase on the growth of Bcr-Abl positive cells. *Nat Med,* Vol. 2, No. 5, pp. 561-566

Estey, E. & Dohner, H. (2006). Acute myeloid leukaemia. *Lancet,* Vol. 368, No. 9550, pp. 1894-1907

Falini, B.; Martelli, M.P.; Bolli, N.; Sportoletti, P.; Liso, A.; Tiacci, E. & Haferlach, T. (2010). Acute myeloid leukemia with mutated nucleophosmin (NPM1): is it a distinct entity? *Blood,* Vol. 117, No. 4, pp. 1109-1120

Falini, B.; Nicoletti, I.; Martelli, M.F. & Mecucci, C. (2007). Acute myeloid leukemia carrying cytoplasmic/mutated nucleophosmin (NPMc+ AML): biologic and clinical features. *Blood,* Vol. 109, No. 3, pp. 874-885

Furness, S.G. & McNagny, K. (2006). Beyond mere markers: functions for CD34 family of sialomucins in hematopoiesis. *Immunol Res,* Vol. 34, No. 1, pp. 13-32

Gallardo, H.F.; Tan, C. & Sadelain, M. (1997). The internal ribosomal entry site of the encephalomyocarditis virus enables reliable coexpression of two transgenes in human primary T lymphocytes. *Gene Therapy,* Vol. 4, No. 10, pp. 1115-1119

Garcia-Manero, G.; Faderl, S.; O'Brien, S.; Cortes, J.; Talpaz, M. & Kantarjian, H.M. (2003). Chronic myelogenous leukemia: a review and update of therapeutic strategies. *Cancer,* Vol. 98, No. 3, pp. 437-457

Gilliland, D.G. & Griffin, J.D. (2002). Role of FLT3 in leukemia. *Curr Opin Hematol,* Vol. 9, No. 4, pp. 274-281

Gossen, M. & Bujard, H. (1992). Tight Control of Gene-Expression in Mammalian-Cells by Tetracycline-Responsive Promoters. *Proceedings of the National Academy of Sciences of the United States of America,* Vol. 89, No. 12, pp. 5547-5551

Gossen, M.; Freundlieb, S.; Bender, G.; Muller, G.; Hillen, W. & Bujard, H. (1995). Transcriptional Activation by Tetracyclines in Mammalian-Cells. *Science,* Vol. 268, No. 5218, pp. 1766-1769

Grignani, F.; Valtieri, M.; Gabbianelli, M.; Gelmetti, V.; Botta, R.; Luchetti, L.; Masella, B.; Morsilli, O.; Pelosi, E.; Samoggia, P.; Pelicci, P.G. & Peschle, C. (2000). PML/RAR alpha fusion protein expression in normal human hematopoietic progenitors dictates myeloid commitment and the promyelocytic phenotype. *Blood,* Vol. 96, No. 4, pp. 1531-1537

Grisendi, S.; Mecucci, C.; Falini, B. & Pandolfi, P.P. (2006). Nucleophosmin and cancer. *Nat Rev Cancer,* Vol. 6, No. 7, pp. 493-505

Hahn, W.C.; Counter, C.M.; Lundberg, A.S.; Beijersbergen, R.L.; Brooks, M.W. & Weinberg, R.A. (1999). Creation of human tumour cells with defined genetic elements. *Nature,* Vol. 400, No. 6743, pp. 464-468

Hanahan, D. & Weinberg, R.A. (2000). The hallmarks of cancer. *Cell,* Vol. 100, No. 1, pp. 57-70

Hanahan, D. & Weinberg, R.A. (2011). Hallmarks of cancer: the next generation. *Cell,* Vol. 144, No. 5, pp. 646-674

Hanenberg, H.; Xiao, X.L.; Dilloo, D.; Hashino, K.; Kato, I. & Williams, D.A. (1996). Colocalization of retrovirus and target cells on specific fibronectin fragments increases genetic transduction of mammalian cells. *Nature Medicine,* Vol. 2, No. 8, pp. 876-882

Hao, Q.L.; Shah, A.J.; Thiemann, F.T.; Smogorzewska, E.M. & Crooks, G.M. (1995). A functional comparison of CD34 + CD38- cells in cord blood and bone marrow. *Blood,* Vol. 86, No. 10, pp. 3745-3753

Hawley, R.G.; Lieu, F.H.L.; Fong, A.Z.C. & Hawley, T.S. (1994). Versatile Retroviral Vectors for Potential Use in Gene-Therapy. *Gene Therapy*, Vol. 1, No. 2, pp. 136-138

Heinz, N.; Schambach, A.; Galla, M.; Maetzig, T.; Baum, C.; Loew, R. & Schiedlmeier, B. (2011). Retroviral and Transposon-Based Tet-Regulated All-In-One Vectors with Reduced Background Expression and Improved Dynamic Range. *Human Gene Therapy*, Vol. 22, No. 2, pp. 166-176

Hoelbl, A.; Schuster, C.; Kovacic, B.; Zhu, B.; Wickre, M.; Hoelzl, M.A.; Fajmann, S.; Grebien, F.; Warsch, W.; Stengl, G.; Hennighausen, L.; Poli, V.; Beug, H.; Moriggl, R. & Sexl, V. (2010). Stat5 is indispensable for the maintenance of bcr/abl-positive leukaemia. *EMBO Mol Med*, Vol. 2, No. 3, pp. 98-110

Holyoake, T.; Jiang, X.; Eaves, C. & Eaves, A. (1999). Isolation of a highly quiescent subpopulation of primitive leukemic cells in chronic myeloid leukemia. *Blood*,Vol. 94, No. 6, pp. 2056-2064

Huang, M.E.; Ye, Y.C.; Chen, S.R.; Chai, J.R.; Lu, J.X.; Zhoa, L.; Gu, L.J. & Wang, Z.Y. (1988). Use of all-trans retinoic acid in the treatment of acute promyelocytic leukemia. *Blood*, Vol. 72, No. 2, pp. 567-572

Ito, M.; Hiramatsu, H.; Kobayashi, K.; Suzue, K.; Kawahata, M.; Hioki, K.; Ueyama, Y.; Koyanagi, Y.; Sugamura, K.; Tsuji, K.; Heike, T. & Nakahata, T. (2002). NOD/SCID/gamma(c)(null) mouse: an excellent recipient mouse model for engraftment of human cells. *Blood*, Vol. 100, No. 9, pp. 3175-3182

Kanbe, E. & Zhang, D.E. (2004). A simple and quick method to concentrate MSCV retrovirus. *Blood Cells Molecules and Diseases*, Vol. 33, No. 1, pp. 64-67

Kiel, M.J.; Yilmaz, O.H.; Iwashita, T.; Terhorst, C. & Morrison, S.J. (2005). SLAM family receptors distinguish hematopoietic stem and progenitor cells and reveal endothelial niches for stem cells. *Cell*, Vol. 121, No. 7, pp. 1109-1121

Kinjo, K.; Kizaki, M.; Muto, A.; Fukuchi, Y.; Umezawa, A.; Yamato, K.; Nishihara, T.; Hata, J.; Ito, M.; Ueyama, Y. & Ikeda, Y. (2000). Arsenic trioxide (As2O3)-induced apoptosis and differentiation in retinoic acid-resistant acute promyelocytic leukemia model in hGM-CSF-producing transgenic SCID mice. *Leukemia*, Vol. 14, No. 3, pp. 431-438

Kinzler, K.W. & Vogelstein, B. (1996). Lessons from hereditary colorectal cancer. *Cell*, Vol. 87, No. 2, pp. 159-170

Kogan, S.C.; Ward, J.M.; Anver, M.R.; Berman, J.J.; Brayton, C.; Cardiff, R.D.; Carter, J.S.; de Coronado, S.; Downing, J.R.; Fredrickson, T.N.; Haines, D.C.; Harris, A.W.; Harris, N.L.; Hiai, H.; Jaffe, E.S.; MacLennan, I.C.; Pandolfi, P.P.; Pattengale, P.K.; Perkins, A.S.; Simpson, R.M.; Tuttle, M.S.; Wong, J.F. & Morse, H.C., 3rd. (2002). Bethesda proposals for classification of nonlymphoid hematopoietic neoplasms in mice. *Blood*, Vol. 100, No. 1, pp. 238-245

Kohn, D.B.; Kantoff, P.W.; Eglitis, M.A.; McLachlin, J.R.; Moen, R.C.; Karson, E.; Zwiebel, J.A.; Nienhuis, A.; Karlsson, S.; O'Reilly, R. & et al. (1987). Retroviral-mediated gene transfer into mammalian cells. *Blood Cells*, Vol. 13, No. 1-2, pp. 285-298

Kwok, C.; Zeisig, B.B.; Qiu, J.H.; Dong, S.O. & So, C.W.E. (2009). Transforming activity of AML1-ETO is independent of CBF beta and ETO interaction but requires formation of homo-oligomeric complexes. *Proceedings of the National Academy of Sciences of the United States of America*, Vol. 106, No. 8, pp. 2853-2858

Larochelle, A.; Vormoor, J.; Lapidot, T.; Sher, G.; Furukawa, T.; Li, Q.; Shultz, L.D.; Olivieri, N.F.; Stamatoyannopoulos, G. & Dick, J.E. (1995). Engraftment of immune-deficient mice with primitive hematopoietic cells from beta-thalassemia and sickle cell anemia patients: implications for evaluating human gene therapy protocols. *Hum Mol Genet*, Vol. 4, No. 2, pp. 163-172

Lewis, P.; Hensel, M. & Emerman, M. (1992). Human-Immunodeficiency-Virus Infection of Cells Arrested in the Cell-Cycle. *Embo Journal*, Vol. 11, No. 8, pp. 3053-3058

Lewis, P.F. & Emerman, M. (1994). Passage through Mitosis Is Required for Oncoretroviruses but Not for the Human-Immunodeficiency-Virus. *Journal of Virology*, Vol. 68, No. 1, pp. 510-516

Liu, Y.; Cheney, M.D.; Gaudet, J.J.; Chruszcz, M.; Lukasik, S.M.; Sugiyama, D.; Lary, J.; Cole, J.; Dauter, Z.; Minor, W.; Speck, N.A. & Bushweller, J.H. (2006). The tetramer structure of the Nervy homology two domain, NHR2, is critical for AML1/ETO's activity. *Cancer Cell*, Vol. 9, No. 4, pp. 249-260

Look, A.T. (1997). Oncogenic transcription factors in the human acute leukemias. *Science*, Vol. 278, No. 5340, pp. 1059-1064

Mardis, E.R.; Ding, L.; Dooling, D.J.; Larson, D.E.; McLellan, M.D.; Chen, K.; Koboldt, D.C.; Fulton, R.S.; Delehaunty, K.D.; McGrath, S.D.; Fulton, L.A.; Locke, D.P.; Magrini, V.J.; Abbott, R.M.; Vickery, T.L.; Reed, J.S.; Robinson, J.S.; Wylie, T.; Smith, S.M.; Carmichael, L.; Eldred, J.M.; Harris, C.C.; Walker, J.; Peck, J.B.; Du, F.; Dukes, A.F.; Sanderson, G.E.; Brummett, A.M.; Clark, E.; McMichael, J.F.; Meyer, R.J.; Schindler, J.K.; Pohl, C.S.; Wallis, J.W.; Shi, X.; Lin, L.; Schmidt, H.; Tang, Y.; Haipek, C.; Wiechert, M.E.; Ivy, J.V.; Kalicki, J.; Elliott, G.; Ries, R.E.; Payton, J.E.; Westervelt, P.; Tomasson, M.H.; Watson, M.A.; Baty, J.; Heath, S.; Shannon, W.D.; Nagarajan, R.; Link, D.C.; Walter, M.J.; Graubert, T.A.; DiPersio, J.F.; Wilson, R.K. & Ley, T.J.(2009). Recurring mutations found by sequencing an acute myeloid leukemia genome. *N Engl J Med*, Vol. 361, No. 11, pp. 1058-1066

Matrai, J.; Chuah, M.K.L. & VandenDriessche, T. (2010). Recent Advances in Lentiviral Vector Development and Applications (vol 18, pg 477, 2010). *Molecular Therapy*, Vol. 18, No. 5, pp. 1055-1055

Melo, J.V. & Barnes, D.J. (2007). Chronic myeloid leukaemia as a model of disease evolution in human cancer. *Nat Rev Cancer*, Vol. 7, No. 6, pp. 441-453

Meshinchi, S.; Woods, W.G.; Stirewalt, D.L.; Sweetser, D.A.; Buckley, J.D.; Tjoa, T.K.; Bernstein, I.D. & Radich, J.P. (2001). Prevalence and prognostic significance of Flt3 internal tandem duplication in pediatric acute myeloid leukemia. *Blood*, Vol. 97, No. 1, pp. 89-94

Minucci, S.; Monestiroli, S.; Giavara, S.; Ronzoni, S.; Marchesi, F.; Insinga, A.; Diverio, D.; Gasparini, P.; Capillo, M.; Colombo, E.; Matteucci, C.; Contegno, F.; Lo-Coco, F.; Scanziani, E.; Gobbi, A. & Pelicci, P.G. (2002). PML-RAR induces promyelocytic leukemias with high efficiency following retroviral gene transfer into purified murine hematopoietic progenitors. *Blood*, Vol. 100, No. 8, pp. 2989-2995

Mizuguchi, H.; Xu, Z.L.; Ishii-Watabe, A.; Uchida, E. & Hayakawa, T. (2000). IRES-dependent second gene expression is significantly lower than cap-dependent first gene expression in a bicistronic vector. *Molecular Therapy*, Vol. 1, No. 4, pp. 376-382

Morrison, S.J. & Weissman, I.L. (1994). The Long-Term Repopulating Subset of Hematopoietic Stem-Cells Is Deterministic and Isolatable by Phenotype. *Immunity*, Vol. 1, No. 8, pp. 661-673

Mountford, P.S. & Smith, A.G. (1995). Internal Ribosome Entry Sites and Dicistronic Rnas in Mammalian Transgenesis. *Trends in Genetics*, Vol. 11, No. 5, pp. 179-184

Mulloy, J.C.; Cammenga, J.; Berguido, F.J.; Wu, K.; Zhou, P.; Comenzo, R.L.; Jhanwar, S.; Moore, M.A. & Nimer, S.D. (2003). Maintaining the self-renewal and differentiation potential of human CD34+ hematopoietic cells using a single genetic element. *Blood*, Vol. 102, No. 13, pp. 4369-4376

Mulloy, J.C.; Cammenga, J.; MacKenzie, K.L.; Berguido, F.J.; Moore, M.A. & Nimer, S.D. (2002). The AML1-ETO fusion protein promotes the expansion of human hematopoietic stem cells. *Blood*, Vol. 99, No. 1, pp. 15-23

Naldini, L.; Blomer, U.; Gallay, P.; Ory, D.; Mulligan, R.; Gage, F.H.; Verma, I.M. & Trono, D. (1996). In vivo gene delivery and stable transduction of nondividing cells by a lentiviral vector. *Science*, Vol. 272, No. 5259, pp. 263-267

Naldini, L.; Montini, E.; Cesana, D.; Schmidt, M.; Sanvito, F.; Ponzoni, M.; Bartholomae, C.; Sergi, L.S.; Benedicenti, F.; Ambrosi, A.; Di Serio, C.; Doglioni, C. & von Kalle, C. (2006). Hematopoietic stem cell gene transfer in a tumor-prone mouse model uncovers low genotoxicity of lentiviral vector integration. *Nature Biotechnology*, Vol. 24, No. 6, pp. 687-696

Niebuhr, B.; Fischer, M.; Tager, M.; Cammenga, J. & Stocking, C. (2008). Gatekeeper function of the RUNX1 transcription factor in acute leukemia. *Blood Cells Mol Dis*, Vol. 40, No. 2, pp. 211-218

Okada, S.; Nakauchi, H.; Nagayoshi, K.; Nishikawa, S.; Miura, Y. & Suda, T. (1992). In vivo and in vitro stem cell function of c-kit- and Sca-1-positive murine hematopoietic cells. *Blood*, Vol. 80, No. 12, pp. 3044-3050

Osawa, M.; Hanada, K.; Hamada, H. & Nakauchi, H. (1996). Long-term lymphohematopoietic reconstitution by a single CD34-low/negative hematopoietic stem cell. *Science*, Vol. 273, No. 5272, pp. 242-245

Paschka, P.; Marcucci, G.; Ruppert, A.S.; Mrozek, K.; Chen, H.; Kittles, R.A.; Vukosavljevic, T.; Perrotti, D.; Vardiman, J.W.; Carroll, A.J.; Kolitz, J.E.; Larson, R.A. & Bloomfield, C.D. (2006). Adverse prognostic significance of KIT mutations in adult acute myeloid leukemia with inv(16) and t(8;21): a Cancer and Leukemia Group B Study. *J Clin Oncol*, Vol. 24, No. 24, pp. 3904-3911

Paschka, P.; Schlenk, R.F.; Gaidzik, V.I.; Habdank, M.; Kronke, J.; Bullinger, L.; Spath, D.; Kayser, S.; Zucknick, M.; Gotze, K.; Horst, H.A.; Germing, U.; Dohner, H. & Dohner, K. (2010). IDH1 and IDH2 mutations are frequent genetic alterations in acute myeloid leukemia and confer adverse prognosis in cytogenetically normal acute myeloid leukemia with NPM1 mutation without FLT3 internal tandem duplication. *J Clin Oncol*, Vol. 28, No. 22, pp. 3636-3643

Puccetti, E. & Ruthardt, M. (2004). Acute promyelocytic leukemia: PML/RARalpha and the leukemic stem cell. *Leukemia*, Vol. 18, No. 7, pp. 1169-1175

Rangarajan, A. & Weinberg, R.A. (2003). Opinion: Comparative biology of mouse versus human cells: modelling human cancer in mice. *Nat Rev Cancer*, Vol. 3, No. 12, pp. 952-959

Rego, E.M.; He, L.Z.; Warrell, R.P.; Wang, Z.G. & Pandolfi, P.P. (2000). Retinoic acid (RA) and As2O3 treatment in transgenic models of acute promyelocytic leukemia (APL) unravel the distinct nature of the leukemogenic process induced by the PML-RAR alpha and PLZF-RAR alpha oncoproteins. *Proceedings of the National Academy of Sciences of the United States of America*, Vol. 97, No. 18, pp. 10173-10178

Rhoades, K.L.; Hetherington, C.J.; Harakawa, N.; Yergeau, D.A.; Zhou, L.; Liu, L.Q.; Little, M.T.; Tenen, D.G. & Zhang, D.E. (2000). Analysis of the role of AML1-ETO in leukemogenesis, using an inducible transgenic mouse model. *Blood*, Vol. 96, No. 6, pp. 2108-2115

Rizo, A.; Horton, S.J.; Olthof, S.; Dontje, B.; Ausema, A.; van Os, R.; van den Boom, V.; Vellenga, E.; de Haan, G. & Schuringa, J.J. (2010). BMI1 collaborates with BCR-ABL in leukemic transformation of human CD34+ cells. *Blood*, Vol. 116, No. 22, pp. 4621-4630

Robinson, C.R. & Sauer, R.T. (1998). Optimizing the stability of single-chain proteins by linker length and composition mutagenesis. *Proc Natl Acad Sci U S A*, Vol. 95, No. 11, pp. 5929-5934

Roe, T.Y.; Reynolds, T.C.; Yu, G. & Brown, P.O. (1993). Integration of Murine Leukemia-Virus DNA Depends on Mitosis. *Embo Journal*, Vol. 12, No. 5, pp. 2099-2108

Ryan, M.D.; King, A.M.Q. & Thomas, G.P. (1991). Cleavage of Foot-and-Mouth-Disease Virus Polyprotein Is Mediated by Residues Located within a 19 Amino-Acid-Sequence. *Journal of General Virology*, Vol. 72, No. pp. 2727-2732

Sawyers, C.L. (1999). Chronic myeloid leukemia. *N Engl J Med*, Vol. 340, No. 17, pp. 1330-1340

Sawyers, C.L.; Hochhaus, A.; Feldman, E.; Goldman, J.M.; Miller, C.B.; Ottmann, O.G.; Schiffer, C.A.; Talpaz, M.; Guilhot, F.; Deininger, M.W.; Fischer, T.; O'Brien, S.G.; Stone, R.M.; Gambacorti-Passerini, C.B.; Russell, N.H.; Reiffers, J.J.; Shea, T.C.; Chapuis, B.; Coutre, S.; Tura, S.; Morra, E.; Larson, R.A.; Saven, A.; Peschel, C.; Gratwohl, A.; Mandelli, F.; Ben-Am, M.; Gathmann, I.; Capdeville, R.; Paquette, R.L. & Druker, B.J. (2002). Imatinib induces hematologic and cytogenetic responses in patients with chronic myelogenous leukemia in myeloid blast crisis: results of a phase II study. *Blood*, Vol. 99, No. 10, pp. 3530-3539

Schnittger, S.; Dicker, F.; Kern, W.; Wendland, N.; Sundermann, J.; Alpermann, T.; Haferlach, C. & Haferlach, T. (2011). RUNX1 mutations are frequent in de novo AML with noncomplex karyotype and confer an unfavorable prognosis. *Blood*, Vol. 117, No. 8, pp. 2348-2357

Schuringa, J.J.; van den Boom, V. & Horton, S.J. (2010). *Genetic & Epigenetic Alterations That Drive Leukemic Stem Cell Self-Renewal*, Nova Science Publishers Inc, ISBN 978-1-61728-379-6, New York, USA

Song, J.; Mercer, D.; Hu, X.; Liu, H. & Li, M.M. (2011). Common leukemia- and lymphoma-associated genetic aberrations in healthy individuals. *J Mol Diagn*, Vol. 13, No. 2, pp. 213-219

Szilvassy, S.J.; Bass, M.J.; Van Zant, G. & Grimes, B. (1999). Organ-selective homing defines engraftment kinetics of murine hematopoietic stem cells and is compromised by ex vivo expansion. *Blood*, Vol. 93, No. 5, pp. 1557-1566

Szymczak, A.L.; Workman, C.J.; Wang, Y.; Vignali, K.M.; Dilioglou, S.; Vanin, E.F. & Vignali, D.A. (2004). Correction of multi-gene deficiency in vivo using a single 'self-cleaving' 2A peptide-based retroviral vector. *Nature Biotechnology*, Vol. 22, No. 5, pp. 589-594

Takeda, A.; Goolsby, C. & Yaseen, N.R. (2006). NUP98-HOXA9 induces long-term proliferation and blocks differentiation of primary human CD34+ hematopoietic cells. *Cancer Res*, Vol. 66, No. 13, pp. 6628-6637

Terpe, K. (2003). Overview of tag protein fusions: from molecular and biochemical fundamentals to commercial systems. *Applied Microbiology and Biotechnology*, Vol. 60, No. 5, pp. 523-533

Trumpp, A. & Wiestler, O.D. (2008). Mechanisms of Disease: cancer stem cells--targeting the evil twin. *Nat Clin Pract Oncol*, Vol. 5, No. 6, pp. 337-347

Weber, K. (2007). Homepage of the Lentiviral Gene Ontology Vectors, Available from: http://www.lentigo-vectors.de/vectors.htm

Weber, K.; Bartsch, U.; Stocking, C. & Fehse, B. (2008). A multicolor panel of novel lentiviral " gene ontology" (LeGO) vectors for functional gene analysis. *Molecular Therapy*, Vol. 16, No. 4, pp. 698-706

Weber, K.; Mock, U.; Petrowitz, B.; Bartsch, U. & Fehse, B. (2010). Lentiviral gene ontology (LeGO) vectors equipped with novel drug-selectable fluorescent proteins: new building blocks for cell marking and multi-gene analysis. *Gene Therapy*, Vol. 17, No. 4, pp. 511-520

Wei, J.; Wunderlich, M.; Fox, C.; Alvarez, S.; Cigudosa, J.C.; Wilhelm, J.S.; Zheng, Y.; Cancelas, J.A.; Gu, Y.; Jansen, M.; Dimartino, J.F. & Mulloy, J.C. (2008). Microenvironment determines lineage fate in a human model of MLL-AF9 leukemia. *Cancer Cell*, Vol. 13, No. 6, pp. 483-495

Wichmann, C.; Becker, Y.; Chen-Wichmann, L.; Vogel, V.; Vojtkova, A.; Herglotz, J.; Moore, S.; Koch, J.; Lausen, J.; Mantele, W.; Gohlke, H. & Grez, M. (2010). Dimer-tetramer transition controls RUNX1/ETO leukemogenic activity. *Blood*, Vol. 116, No. 4, pp. 603-613

Wiernik, P.H. (2010). FLT3 inhibitors for the treatment of acute myeloid leukemia. *Clin Adv Hematol Oncol*, Vol. 8, No. 6, pp. 429-436, 444

Wu, X.L.; Li, Y.; Crise, B. & Burgess, S.M. (2003). Transcription start regions in the human genome are favored targets for MLV integration. *Science*, Vol. 300, No. 5626, pp. 1749-1751

Wunderlich, M.; Krejci, O.; Wei, J. & Mulloy, J.C. (2006). Human CD34+ cells expressing the inv(16) fusion protein exhibit a myelomonocytic phenotype with greatly enhanced proliferative ability. *Blood*, Vol. 108, No. 5, pp. 1690-1697

Xu, W.; Yang, H.; Liu, Y.; Yang, Y.; Wang, P.; Kim, S.H.; Ito, S.; Yang, C.; Wang, P.; Xiao, M.T.; Liu, L.X.; Jiang, W.Q.; Liu, J.; Zhang, J.Y.; Wang, B.; Frye, S.; Zhang, Y.; Xu, Y.H.; Lei, Q.Y.; Guan, K.L.; Zhao, S.M. & Xiong, Y. (2011). Oncometabolite 2-hydroxyglutarate is a competitive inhibitor of alpha-ketoglutarate-dependent dioxygenases. *Cancer Cell*, Vol. 19, No. 1, pp. 17-30

Yan, M.; Burel, S.A.; Peterson, L.F.; Kanbe, E.; Iwasaki, H.; Boyapati, A.; Hines, R.; Akashi, K. & Zhang, D.E. (2004). Deletion of an AML1-ETO C-terminal NcoR/SMRT-interacting region strongly induces leukemia development. *Proc Natl Acad Sci U S A*, Vol. 101, No. 49, pp. 17186-17191

Yan, M.; Kanbe, E.; Peterson, L.F.; Boyapati, A.; Miao, Y.; Wang, Y.; Chen, I.M.; Chen, Z.; Rowley, J.D.; Willman, C.L. & Zhang, D.E. (2006). A previously unidentified alternatively spliced isoform of t(8;21) transcript promotes leukemogenesis. *Nat Med*, Vol. 12, No. 8, pp. 945-949

Yang, L.; Bryder, D.; Adolfsson, J.; Nygren, J.; Mansson, R.; Sigvardsson, M. & Jacobsen, S.E. (2005). Identification of Lin(-)Sca1(+)kit(+)CD34(+)Flt3- short-term hematopoietic stem cells capable of rapidly reconstituting and rescuing myeloablated transplant recipients. *Blood*, Vol. 105, No. 7, pp. 2717-2723

Yu, S.F.; Vonruden, T.; Kantoff, P.W.; Garber, C.; Seiberg, M.; Ruther, U.; Anderson, W.F.; Wagner, E.F. & Gilboa, E. (1986). Self-Inactivating Retroviral Vectors Designed for Transfer of Whole Genes into Mammalian-Cells. *Proceedings of the National Academy of Sciences of the United States of America*, Vol. 83, No. 10, pp. 3194-3198

Zhang, X.W.; Yan, X.J.; Zhou, Z.R.; Yang, F.F.; Wu Z.Y.; Sun, H.B.; Liang, W.X.; Song, A.X.; Lallemand-Breitenbach, V.; Jeanne, M.; Zhang, Q.Y.; Yang, H.Y.; Huang, Q.H.; Zhou, G.B.; Tong, J.H.; Zhang, Y.; Wu, J.H.; Hu, H.Y.; de Thé, H.; Chen, S.J. & Chen, Z. (2010). Arsenic trioxide controls the fate of the PML-RAR alpha oncoprotein by directly binding PML (vol 328, pg 240, 2010). *Science*, Vol. 328, No. 5981, pp. 974-974

18

Acute Promyelocytic Leukemia: A Model Disease for Targeted Cancer Therapy

Emma Lång and Stig Ove Bøe
Oslo University Hospital, Oslo, Norway

1. Introduction

Acute promyelocytic leukemia (APL) is a distinct subtype of acute myeloid leukemia (AML) characterized by a severe bleeding tendency, accumulation of abnormal promyelocytes in the bone marrow and a reciprocal t(15;17) chromosomal translocation that fuses the gene encoding the promyelocytic leukemia protein (PML) to that encoding retinoic acid receptor alpha (RARA) (de Thé & Chen, 2010). During the past 30 years two therapeutic drugs have been introduced into the clinic that have dramatically improved the treatment outcome of this disease (Wang & Chen, 2008). The first of these components was all-trans retinoic acid (ATRA), a vitamin A derivative that significantly increased clinical remission and improved the 5-years disease-free survival rates from below 40% to more than 80% (Huang *et al.*, 1988). The second drug was arsenic trioxide (ATO), a component that was discovered to be remarkably effective in treating APL as a single agent (Sun *et al.*, 1992). Today, most hospitals employ ATRA in combination with chemotherapy as frontline therapy, while ATO is being used for refractory or relapsed patients. Recent clinical studies have also revealed a positive synergistic effect between the two drugs, suggesting that future therapy of newly diagnosed patients may involve a combination of the two reagents (Estey *et al.*, 2006; Hu *et al.*, 2009; Shen *et al.*, 2004; Wang *et al.*, 2004).

The success of using ATRA and ATO in APL therapy appears to be linked to the ability of these drugs to interact with the fusion oncoprotein PML/RARA, which is produced by the APL-associated t(15;17) translocation, and that causes the disease. ATRA contacts a ligand binding domain present within the RARA moiety of this chimeric protein and promotes differentiation of APL cells along the granulocyte linage (Huang *et al.*, 1988). ATO, on the other hand, has recently been shown to bind one or more cysteine rich motifs within the PML protein (Jeanne *et al.*, 2010; Zhang *et al.*, 2010) and contributes to the cure of APL through a mechanism that involves eradication of leukemic-initiating cells (LICs) (Nasr *et al.*, 2008; Ito *et al.*, 2008; Zheng *et al.*, 2007).

Due to the success of using ATRA and ATO in the clinic, and because of the ability of these drugs to promote clinical remission through a direct contact with PML/RARA, APL has become one of the most attractive model diseases for the development of targeted cancer therapy. The APL cure offers a proof of principle that a cancer can be cured through targeted inactivation of an oncoprotein, and it provides a rationale for the development of novel therapeutic strategies that target fusion oncoproteins produced by chromosomal translocations. In this chapter we will summarize the current knowledge of the biological properties of PML, RARA and PML/RARA with particular emphasis on tumorigenesis in APL patients and the molecular mechanisms that underlie the response to ATRA and ATO.

2. APL treatment – a historical perspective

2.1 The discovery of ATRA-based APL therapy

APL was first characterized as a distinct clinical entity in 1957 (Hillestad, 1957). Throughout the 1950s and 1960s, this disease had a 100% mortality rate and no effective treatment options. In 1973, chemotherapy by the topoisomerase inhibitor daunorubicin was shown to have some curative effect, yielding a complete remission (CR) rate of 55% (Bernard *et al.*, 1973), and in the early eighties induction therapy based on anthracyclins (daunorubicin, idarubicin among others) and the nucleocide analogue cytosine arabinoside (Ara-C) was found to yield CR rates of up to 80% in newly diagnosed patients (Cunningham *et al.*, 1989; Sanz *et al.*, 1988). However, the patients frequently suffered from one of the inherent drawbacks with induction therapy, namely the release of coagulation factors from dead leukemic cells, causing severe bleedings and increased risk of fatal outcome (Cordonnier *et al.*, 1985; Drapkin *et al.*, 1978; Ruggero *et al.*, 1977). Consequently, most APL patients required intensive platelet and fibrinogen support, and based on the criterion of 5-years disease-free survival (DFS), only 35-45% of the cases were cured (Fenaux *et al.*, 2007). The focus on APL therapy changed in 1978, as it became clear that leukemic cells undergo terminal differentiation upon treatment with differentiating-inducing agents, such as ATRA, Ara-C and 13-cis retinoic acid (Breitman *et al.*, 1981; Degos *et al.*, 1985; Gold *et al.*, 1983; Koeffler *et al.*, 1985; Sachs, 1978). Such differentiation therapy showed an advantage over induction therapy, with respect to incidences of severe bleedings, and led to reduced mortality rates. In 1985, the first attempt to treat APL patients with ATRA was made with promising results, but the percentage of patients with 5-years DFS was still relatively low (less than 50%) (Huang *et al.*, 1987; Huang *et al.*, 1988). Subsequently, optimization trials, combining ATRA with chemotherapy, raised the CR rates up to 90-95% and the 5-years DFS to 86% (Wang & Chen, 2008). In addition, the combination of ATRA and chemotherapy, which currently represents standard frontline APL therapy, helped reducing retinoic acid syndrome (RAS), a potentially fatal side effect caused by induction therapy and manifested in a burst of inflammatory cytokines released from malignant promyelocytes (de Botton *et al.*, 2003; Fenaux *et al.*, 1999; Sanz *et al.*, 1999; Tallman *et al.*, 1997).

2.2 The discovery of ATO-based APL therapy

Arsenic, in the form of arsenic trioxide (ATO), was first described as an agent that possesses antileukemic properties in the year 1878. In this study, Fowler's solution, a solution of ATO in potassium bicarbonate, was shown to dramatically reduce the number of white blood cells in a patient with chronic myelogenous leukemia (CML) (Cutler & Bradford, 1878). Subsequently, this remedy was used as a primary antileukemic agent until the discovery of radiation therapy in the early 20th century (Forkner & Scott, 1931; Kwong & Todd, 1997). In the 1970s, ATO reappeared as a therapeutic agent for APL as Chinese researchers showed that ailing-1, a mixture of ATO and crude herbal extracts, was effective in the treatment of both *de novo* as well as relapsed cases (Shen *et al.*, 1997; Sun *et al.*, 1992; Zhang *et al.*, 1996). Additional clinical studies showed that ATO, as a single agent, caused complete remission in up to 90% of patients and reduced the relapse rate for high risk patients (Niu *et al.*, 1999; Shen *et al.*, 1997). A research group in the United States confirmed these preliminary studies and further showed that ATO treatment induced partial differentiation of leukemic cells, caspase activation and subsequently apoptosis (Soignet *et al.*, 1998).

2.3 Present and future APL therapy

Currently, ATRA in combination with chemotherapy is being employed as frontline therapy for APL, whereas ATO primarily is being used for treatment of cases that are resistant to ATRA or patients suffering from frequent relapses. However, several clinical trials are now assessing the synergistic effect of combining ATRA and ATO with and without chemotherapy. These trials are conducted mainly on the basis of successful studies in animal models, showing a positive effect of ATRA/ATO combinations in APL mice (Jing *et al.*, 2001; Lallemand-Breitenbach *et al.*, 1999). The main conclusion so far from the ongoing clinical studies is that newly diagnosed patients are likely to benefit from ATRA/ATO combination treatment in addition to low-dose chemotherapy (Estey *et al.*, 2006; Hu *et al.*, 2009; Shen *et al.*, 2004; Wang *et al.*, 2004).

3. The mechanism of PML, RARA and PML/RARA

3.1 The role of PML/RARA in APL pathogenesis

The molecular hallmark of APL is the t(15;17) chromosomal translocation that expresses the fusion oncoprotein PML/RARA. While this genetic aberration is identified in more than 97% of all APL cases, the remaining patients diagnosed with this disease harbor variant translocations that all involve the *RARA* gene in fusion with alternative partners such as the genes encoding promyelocytic leukemia zinc finger (*PLZF*) (Chen *et al.*, 1993), nucleophosmin (*NPM*) (Redner *et al.*, 1996), nuclear matrix associated (*NUMA*) (Wells *et al.*, 1997), or signal transducer and activator of transcription 5b (*STAT5B*) (Arnould *et al.*, 1999). The most compelling evidence that PML/RARA alone can contribute directly to APL development comes from studies in mice showing that expression of this oncoprotein as a transgene leads to development of an APL-like disease. However, these experiments also show that a relatively long latency period is required prior to onset of disease, suggesting the involvement of acquired genetic aberrations in addition to the t(15;17) translocation (Brown *et al.*, 1997; Grisolano *et al.*, 1997).

3.2 The function of PML

The first component of the PML/RARA fusion, the PML protein, is a tumor suppressor (Bernardi *et al.*, 2006; Salomoni & Pandolfi, 2002; Trotman *et al.*, 2006) that functions in multiple cellular processes, including apoptosis (Wang *et al.*, 1998), differentiation (Ito *et al.*, 2008), DNA repair (Bøe *et al.*, 2006; Dellaire *et al.*, 2006a), senescence (Ferbeyre *et al.*, 2000; Pearson *et al.*, 2000), angiogenesis (Bernardi *et al.*, 2006) and virus defence (Everett & Maul, 1994). The human *PML* gene is located on chromosome 15, consists of nine exons and produces several alternatively spliced protein isoforms designated PML I through VII. All of these PML variants contain an identical tripartite (TRIM) motif in their N-terminal region, and a C-terminus that varies due to alternative splicing (Borden, 2002; Fagioli *et al.*, 1992; Jensen *et al.*, 2001; Jul-Larsen *et al.*, 2010; Reymond *et al.*, 2001). The TRIM motif, which comprises a RING finger, two B-boxes and a predicted coiled coil domain, has been shown to be important for PML multimerization, a feature responsible for one of the most striking properties of this protein, namely the ability to generate nuclear structures termed PML nuclear bodies (PML NBs) (Lallemand-Breitenbach & de The, 2010). These bodies are highly dynamic and change their morphology and biochemical composition in a cell cycle-dependent manner. For example, during entry into mitosis, several PML NB resident components, including Daxx, Sp100 and SUMO, are lost concomitant with formation of PML NB aggregates called mitotic assemblies of PML proteins (MAPPs), whereas transition from mitosis to G1-phase coincides with exclusion of PML NBs from the progeny nuclei and complex formation with nucleoporins and microtubule filaments to form cytoplasmic assemblies of PML and nucleoporins (CyPNs) (Chen *et al.*, 2008; Dellaire *et al.*, 2006b; Jul-Larsen *et al.*, 2009). Although, PML NBs have the capacity to recruit a large number of different protein components, PML is the only protein so far that has been shown to be required for their formation. For this reason, it is widely assumed that the ability to assemble these cellular compartments represents an integral part of PML biogenesis. It still remains, however, to clearly define the molecular mechanism involved in PML NB assembly and function.

3.3 The function of RARA

The second fusion partner, RARA, is a ligand binding transcription factor that contains a DNA binding motif in its central region and a retinoid binding domain at the C-terminus. To generate an active protein complex, this nuclear receptor forms a heterodimer with the RXR family of transcription factors. Upon direct binding to a RA responsive element (RARE) within the regulatory region of a target gene, RARA/RXR complexes promote transcriptional silencing by recruiting co-repressor proteins such as NCOR1, SMRT and histone deacetylase to the promoter-binding complexes. In the presence of physiological concentrations of ligand (i.e. retinoids), a conformational change occurs within the RARA/RXR heterodimer that leads to dissociation of co-repressors and concomitant recruitment of histone acetylases and components of the basic transcription machinery, thus transforming the protein complex from a gene silencer to a gene activator (Bastien & Rochette-Egly, 2004). RARA regulates several genes involved in myeloid progenitor cell differentiation, including c-myc (Bentley & Groudine, 1986; Gowda *et al.*, 1986), C/EBPβ (Duprez *et al.*, 2003), C/EBPε (Park *et al.*, 1999) and PU.1 (Mueller *et al.*, 2006), suggesting an important role of this protein in blood cell maturation.

3.4 The function of PML/RARA

Upon fusion between PML and RARA, the variable C-terminus of the PML protein is lost, whereas the constant N-terminal TRIM motif generally remains intact. In the case of RARA, fusion to PML leads to loss of the first 50 to 60 N-terminal amino acids, a deletion that does not appear to affect the DNA and ligand binding activities of this protein (de Thé *et al.*, 1991). Thus, PML/RARA retains the powerful protein-protein interaction domain of the PML protein, whereas the variable isoform-specific region is replaced by the trans-activating functions of RARA (Fig. 1.).

One of the gained PML/RARA functions that is thought to contribute largely to APL development is the ability of this chimeric protein to form stable transcription repression complexes that are irresponsive to physiological concentrations of retinoids. As a consequence, gene promoters that are targeted by PML/RARA become constitutively repressed, an observation that has led to the general assumption that this oncoprotein causes a block in blood cell differentiation through transcriptional inhibition of key genes involved in hematopoietic maturation. Consistent with a role in gene repression, PML/RARA has also been shown to recruit the histone methyl transferase SUV39H1 (Carbone *et al.*, 2006), members of the polycomb repressive complex 2 (PRC2) (Villa *et al.*, 2007) and DNA methyltransferases (DNMTs) (Di Croce *et al.*, 2002), proteins that are known to induce a repressive chromatin structure. In addition to increased repressor activity, the PML/RARA fusion also appears to possess a considerable expanded repertoire of target genes compared to the normal RARA protein. This notion is supported by *in vitro* binding studies showing that PML/RARA has a broader and more relaxed DNA binding specificity compared to RARA (Hauksdottir & Privalsky, 2001; Kamashev *et al.*, 2004), and by a genome wide screen revealing a wide range of PML/RARA target genes (Hoemme *et al.*, 2008). The altered DNA binding and transcription repression properties of PML/RARA are partially due to the ability of this chimeric protein to form homodimeres through protein-protein interactions mediated by the TRIM motif of PML (Jansen *et al.*, 1995; Perez *et al.*, 1993). In addition, this chimeric protein has also been shown to form functional complexes with other transcription factors such as RXR and Daxx, a feature that may further contribute to the expanded promoter binding capacity (Zeisig *et al.*, 2007; Zhu *et al.*, 2005; Zhu *et al.*, 2007).

PML/RARA is also thought to contribute to malignant transformation and development of APL through inhibition of PML tumor suppressor functions. A dominant negative effect of PML/RARA on this protein is evident by studies demonstrating disruption of nuclear PML bodies into a dispersed microspeckled pattern in cells expressing this oncoprotein (Dyck *et al.*, 1994; Koken *et al.*, 1994; Weis *et al.*, 1994). Interestingly, while disruption of PML NBs by PML/RARA in the nucleus is evident, this oncoprotein readily assembles into MAPPS and CyPNs, the mitotic and cytoplasmic versions of PML NBs, respectively (Jul-Larsen *et al.*, 2009). The disruption of PML NBs in the nucleus may reflect the role of this oncoprotein in repression of gene activity.

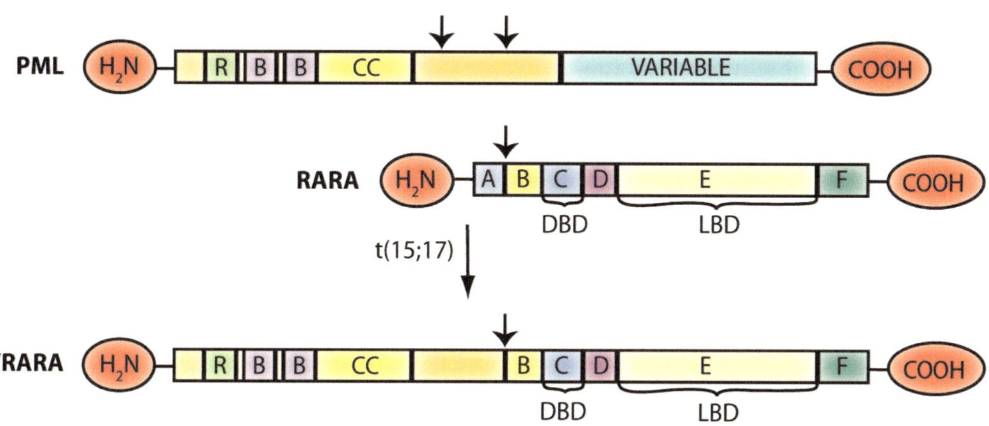

Fig. 1. Structural organization of PML, RARA and PML/RARA. PML contains a RING domain (R), two B boxes (B), a coiled coil (CC) and a variable C-terminus. RARA consists of six regulatory domains (A-F), of which domain C and E harbor the DNA binding domain (DBD) and the ligand binding domain (LBD), respectively. The t (15;17) translocation produces PML/RARA, which retains the N-terminal PML motifs as well as RARA DNA and ligand binding activity. Arrows indicate protein breakpoints.

While PML/RARA is constantly expressed in more than 97% of all APL patients, the reciprocal fusion protein RARA/PML, which contains the N-terminus of RARA and variable lengths of the PML C-terminus, is identified in only 70-80% of the cases (Alcalay *et al.*, 1992; Grimwade *et al.*, 1996). Not much is known about the role of this protein in the pathogenesis of APL. However, one study has described a possible link between RARA/PML fusion gene deletions and resistance to ATRA-based therapy (Subramaniyam *et al.*, 2006).

4. The mechanism of ATRA and ATO-mediated APL therapy

4.1 The mechanism of ATRA-based APL therapy

Phenotypically, pharmacological concentrations of ATRA lead to effective differentiation of immature APL cells to terminally differentiated granulocytes. From a therapeutic point of view this may be beneficial since the immature malignant cells progress from being highly proliferative and long-lived to arrested and short-lived. In addition, *in vitro* cell culture experiments have shown that ATRA-induced differentiation also coincides with activation of apoptosis (Altucci *et al.*, 2001; Grignani *et al.*, 1998; Martin *et al.*, 1990). The relative contribution of apoptotic cell death versus increased turnover of mature granulocytes to ATRA-induced clearance of tumorigenic cells is not clear. Although ATRA appears to be highly effective in clearing the bulk of proliferative tumor cells, a residual population of cells with detectable t(15;17) translocation almost invariably persist following treatment with this reagent alone, a feature that probably explains the additional need for chemotherapy in order to achieve complete remission (Chen *et al.*, 1991; Chomienne *et al.*, 1990; Huang *et al.*, 1988; Zhu *et al.*, 1995).

At the molecular level, therapeutic doses of ATRA reverse the differentiation block caused by PML/RARA through a direct interaction with the ligand binding site present on the RARA moiety. As for normal RARA, the ligand-receptor interaction induces a change in the PML/RARA protein structural conformation, which leads to release of transcription repressors and subsequent activation of the basal transcription machinery. Coincident with transcription activation, ATRA also induces recruitment of the proteasome to the ligand binding transcription activation domain AF2 of RARA, and subsequent proteasome-dependent degradation (Kopf *et al.*, 2000; Zhu *et al.*, 1999). A protein that has been proposed to participate in this pathway is the ubiquitin-activating enzyme E1-like (UBE1L) protein, which itself represents one of the ATRA-induced proteins (Kitareewan *et al.*, 2002). ATRA-mediated degradation appears to affect RARA and PML/RARA equally well and may be functionally linked to transcription activation, since mutations in RARA that impairs its DNA binding activity also inhibits ATRA-mediated catabolism (Zhu *et al.*, 1999). The relative contribution of transcriptional activation, differentiation and degradation on therapy remains to be fully elucidated.

4.2 The mechanism of ATO-based APL therapy

Compared to ATRA, ATO has a more limited ability to induce terminal differentiation of APL cells. *In vitro* studies using cultured cells have revealed a dose-dependent effect of this drug on differentiation and apoptosis (Chen *et al.*, 1997). At high concentrations (0.5-2.0 μM) ATO induced cell death by apoptosis, while at low concentrations (0.1-0.25 μM) this drug caused partial differentiation of APL cells along the granulocyte linage (Cai *et al.*, 2000; Chen *et al.*, 1997). The results from these experiments appear to be in good agreement with studies demonstrating ATO-induced partial differentiation and apoptosis in APL patients or animal models, where the effective serum concentrations of ATO generally ranges from 0.1 to 1.0 μM (Chen *et al.*, 1997; Lallemand-Breitenbach *et al.*, 1999). Interestingly, ATO-mediated differentiation has been shown to become dramatically enhanced in the presence of cyclic adenosine monophosphate (cAMP). The mechanism responsible for this synergistic effect was proposed to be the combined effect of ATO-induced PML/RARA degradation and cAMP-mediated inhibition of cell cycle progression (Guillemin *et al.*, 2002; Zhu *et al.*, 2002).

At the molecular level, ATO exerts its therapeutic effect on APL in part by initiating a cascade of biochemical alterations that primarily affect the PML moiety of PML/RARA. Firstly, the presence of arsenic in the cell culture medium has been shown to increase PML and PML/RARA multimerization, an effect that is manifested by decreased solubility of these proteins upon preparation of cell lysates and reduced mobility within PML NBs as determined by analysis of GFP-tagged PML in living cells (Jeanne *et al.*, 2010; Zhang *et al.*, 2010). Concomitant with increased aggregation, PML becomes extensively SUMOylated on at least three different lysine residues. All of the three different SUMO isoforms, including SUMO1, 2 and 3, appear to participate in this reaction, and both mono and poly-SUMOylation events have been reported (Lallemand-Breitenbach *et al.*, 2001; Lallemand-Breitenbach *et al.*, 2008; Muller *et al.*, 1998; Tatham *et al.*, 2008). Subsequent to SUMOylation, a protein called RNF4 binds SUMOylated residues on PML in order to catalyze poly-ubiquitination, a modification that directs PML and PML/RARA to the proteasome for degradation (Lallemand-Breitenbach *et al.*, 2008; Tatham *et al.*, 2008). Recently, a direct interaction between PML and ATO, that potentially triggers this SUMO-mediated degradation pathway, was mapped to cysteine residues located in the TRIM and B-box motifs of PML (Jeanne *et al.*, 2010; Zhang *et al.*, 2010).

In addition to affecting differentiation of leukemic cells, recent studies have also implicated ATO in clearance of leukemic-initiating cells (LICs), a small population of malignantly transformed cells with stem cell characteristics that frequently are refractory to cancer therapeutic drugs. Consistent with this, PML/RARA expression has been reported to support properties of self-renewal of LICs (Wojiski *et al.*, 2009), and certain characteristics of promyelocytic phenotypes provide the basic properties for the development of APL-initiating LICs (Guibal *et al.*, 2009). Furthermore, a recent study demonstrated LIC clearance in association with ATO-induced PML/RARA degradation by a mechanism that appeared to be uncoupled from the observed cell differentiation (Nasr *et al.*, 2008; Shao *et al.*, 1998). In addition, ATO has been reported to cause increased proliferation of LICs in a chronic myelogenous mouse model, hence sensitizing otherwise therapy-insensitive leukemic cells to Ara-C-based treatment (Ito *et al.*, 2008; Ito *et al.*, 2009).

The proapoptotic activity of ATO is not specific for APL cells (Akao *et al.*, 1998; Bachleitner-Hofmann *et al.*, 2001; Ishitsuka *et al.*, 1998; Perkins *et al.*, 2000; Rousselot *et al.*, 1999; Wang *et al.*, 1996; Zhang *et al.*, 1998; Zheng *et al.*, 1999), although non-APL tumor cells have been shown to be less sensitive to this drug (Huang *et al.*, 1999). ATO induces apoptosis by downregulation of the antiapoptotic protein Bcl-2, leading to a disturbance in the regulated balance between pro- and antiapoptotic proteins (Akao *et al.*, 1998; Chen *et al.*, 1996; Zhang *et al.*, 1998). In addition, ATO increases radioactive oxygen species (ROS) production in malignant cells. As a consequence, this drug leads to disruption of the mitochondrial membrane potential, followed by cytochrome c release, caspase activation and subsequent apoptotic cell death (Jing *et al.*, 1999).

4.3 The synergy between ATRA and ATO

While ATRA and ATO on their own are known to be effective in curing APL, it is also becoming increasingly clear that treatment regiments based on a combination of the two drugs leads to a quicker clinical remission, a more effective clearance of leukemic cells and a significantly longer period of relapse free survival (Estey *et al.*, 2006; Hu *et al.*, 2009; Shen *et al.*, 2004; Wang *et al.*, 2004). This synergistic effect may result due to the ability of both these drugs to cause PML/RARA degradation, a parameter that appears to be critical for the success of APL therapy. In addition, the combined effect of ATO and ATRA may also result due to the ability of the two agents to act on separate targets, both of which are important for disease remission. For example, ATO may be effective in eradicating self-renewable LICs through stimulated PML/RARA degradation, while ATRA represents a more effective differentiating agent, and hence may lead to a more complete clearance of undifferentiated APL cells.

5. Therapy-induced degradation of PML/RARA

ATRA and ATO-induced therapy of APL may be connected to the ability of these drugs to induce PML/RARA catabolism (Fig. 2.). In agreement with this, reduced PML/RARA expression can be observed in both ATRA and ATO-treated cells, and the two drugs synergize both for their ability to induce oncoprotein degradation as well as for their capacity to promote clinical remission (Hu *et al.*, 2009; Nasr *et al.*, 2008; Shen *et al.*, 2004). An important role of protein degradation for effective APL therapy is also supported by experiments in mice. For example, treatment of an APL mouse model with the proteasome inhibitor bortezomid led to reduced degradation of PML/RARA and concomitant resistance to ATRA and ATO-based therapy (Nasr *et al.*, 2008). In addition, PML/RARA mutated in critical SUMOylation target sites, were found to be more resistant to ATO-mediated degradation compared to unmodified PML/RARA (Lallemand-Breitenbach *et al.*, 2001; Lallemand-Breitenbach *et al.*, 2008).

In addition to proteasome-dependent degradation induced by ATRA and ATO, PML/RARA has also been shown to be amenable for degradation by the lysosome-dependent degradation pathway autophagy (Isakson *et al.*, 2010; Klionsky, 2007). This degradation mechanism appears to play a major role both for basal turnover as well as for therapy-induced catabolism of PML/RARA. Indeed, pharmacological inhibitors of autophagy were found to completely prevent ATRA and ATO-stimulated degradation of PML/RARA expressed in the APL cell line NB4 (Isakson *et al.*, 2010). In contrast to proteasome-dependent degradation, autophagy-mediated proteolyses of PML/RARA appears to be independent of a direct interaction between the drugs and the target protein. Instead, ATRA and ATO seem to stimulate autophagy in APL cells primarily through a mechanism that involves the mammalian target of rapamycin (mTOR) and Unc-51-like kinase 1 (ULK1) (Bøe & Simonsen, 2010; Isakson *et al.*, 2010). Furthermore, PML/RARA is highly aggregation prone and therefore a good substrate for this degradation pathway (Isakson *et al.*, 2010; Lallemand-Breitenbach *et al.*, 2001). Aggregates of PML/RARA may form during the process of protein synthesis. In agreement with this, synthesis of PML/RARA has been shown to be associated with endoplasmatic reticulum stress, a feature indicative of aberrant folding during protein synthesis (Khan *et al.*, 2004).

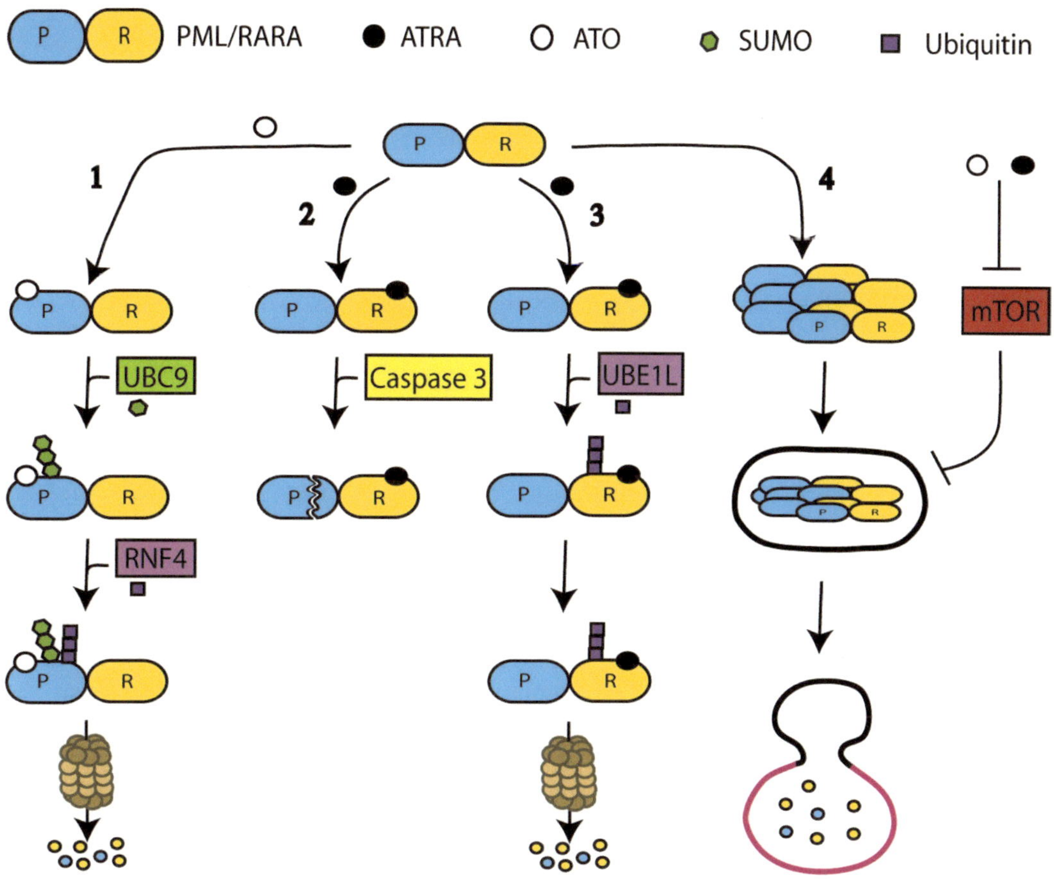

Fig. 2. Schematic overview of the four main ATRA and ATO-mediated PML/RARA degradation pathways: 1. ATO-induced proteasome-dependent degradation, 2. ATRA-induced caspase cleavage, 3. ATRA-induced proteasome-dependent degradation, 4. ATRA/ATO-induced autophagy-mediated degradation.

Two different types of proteases have also been implicated in PML/RARA proteolysis. First, PML/RARA has been shown to be susceptible to a caspase 3-like activity expressed in APL cells and that becomes induced by the presence of ATRA (Nervi *et al.*, 1998). The second protease shown to be involved is neutrophil elastase, a myeloid specific serine protease that is maximally expressed in promyelocytes (Lane & Ley, 2003). The contribution of this protease to APL development is unclear since one study showed enhanced penetrance of PML/RARA in a neutrophil elastase defective mice (Lane & Ley, 2003), while another demonstrated decreased tumorigenesis in a mouse model expressing a neutrophil elastase cleavage defective PML/RARA protein (Uy *et al.*, 2010).

PML turnover has also been shown to be regulated by a pathway that involves direct phosphorylation by the casein kinase 2 (CK2) and subsequent ubiquitin-mediated degradation, a mechanism that was proposed to cause decreased PML tumor suppressor activity in lung cancer (Scaglioni *et al.*, 2006). However, the significance of CK2-mediated PML phosphorylation in PML/RARA degradation and APL pathogenesis has not been elucidated.

6. The mechanism of APL therapy resistance

The second most common translocation associated with APL, the t(11;17) translocation that expresses PLZF/RARA fusion instead of PML/RARA, is generally insensitive to ATRA and ATO-based therapy (Chen *et al.*, 1993; Licht *et al.*, 1995). The poor response of these patients to ATO add support to studies showing that this drug primarily target PML, which is absent in PLZF/RARA. In the case of the poor response to ATRA, on the other hand, the underlying mechanism has been hypothesized to be due to enhanced co-repressor activity conferred by the PLZF moiety of the PLZF-RARA fusion (Grignani *et al.*, 1998; He *et al.*, 1998; Lin *et al.*, 1998). However, the notion that PLZF/RARA is irresponsive to ATRA stimulation has been contradicted in more recent studies demonstrating ATRA-induced gene expression and differentiation also in PLZF/RARA expressing APL cells (Nasr *et al.*, 2008; Petti *et al.*, 2002; Rice *et al.*, 2009). Thus, further work is needed in order to fully understand the mechanism underlying the insensitivity of PLZF/RARA positive APL cells to ATRA.

Resistance to ATRA-mediated therapy is also seen in APL patients that have relapsed following the first clinical remission. Such acquired resistance may be caused by a number of different physiological factors, including increased catabolism, reduced cellular uptake, or increased cytoplasmic sequestration of the therapeutic drugs (Freemantle *et al.*, 2003; Gallagher, 2002). In addition, *in vitro* cell culture experiments, using the APL cell line NB4, have revealed mutations within the PML/RARA gene of subclones with acquired resistance to ATRA. Interestingly, several of these mutations were found clustered at/or near the ligand binding domain of RARA leading to defects in ATRA binding. Since these mutants generally retain their capacity to form complex with RXR and to bind DNA, they have been suggested to act as dominant inhibitors of wild type RARA (Duprez *et al.*, 2000; Kitamura *et al.*, 1997; Nason-Burchenal *et al.*, 1998; Rosenauer *et al.*, 1996; Shao *et al.*, 1997). Mutations in PML/RARA have also been identified in a subset of ATRA-relapsed patients, and these mutations were found to be variably associated with inactivation of ATRA binding (Ding *et al.*, 1998; Gallagher *et al.*, 2006; Imaizumi *et al.*, 1998; Marasca *et al.*, 1999; Takayama *et al.*, 2001; Zhou *et al.*, 2002). Interestingly, one study identified mutations within the intact PML locus of APL patients with ATRA-resistance and poor prognosis (Gurrieri *et al.*, 2004).

Recently, PML/RARA mutations have also been discovered in two APL cases with poor response to ATO (Goto *et al.*, 2011). In both cases, the mutations were located within the second B-box motif of the PML protein. Since the amino acids affected by these mutations were close to a cysteine-rich region, previously proposed to bind ATO (Jeanne *et al.*, 2010), the authors of this paper hypothesized that these mutations may affect interactions between this drug and PML/RARA. Alternatively, the mutated protein may have defects in oligomerization, since the B-box domains are known to function in PML multimerization. Combined, the PML/RARA mutations that have been identified in ATRA and/or ATO–resistant APL cells support the notion that these drugs interact with separate moieties of the fusion protein to induce clinical remission.

7. Perspectives

During the past 30 years, APL has progressed from a deadly disease to a highly curable malignancy. In addition, the advances that have been made in understanding the pathology and cure of APL at the molecular level have led to the emergence of a highly attractive model disease for the development of targeted cancer therapy. For example, the case of APL clearly demonstrates the therapeutic effectiveness of targeting a defined oncoprotein, and since recurrent translocations and expression of fusion oncoproteins similar to that of PML/RARA is a common trait also among other types of cancers (including leukemias and sarcomas), a large number of malignancies, in addition to APL, may benefit from similar targeted therapies. Thus, it will be important to continue identifying therapeutic concepts that contribute to the success of APL therapy and to modulate these concepts for treatment of other cancers.

Since both ATRA and ATO have been shown to exert their therapeutic effects through interactions with specific regions of the PML/RARA oncoprotein, it may be assumed that these drugs will be effective only against APL. However, one should also keep in mind that the ability of ATRA and ATO to mediate cure of APL is regarded as a rather fortuitous discovery and not merely as a result of rational therapeutic design. For this reason, these drugs are likely to have other yet unidentified cellular targets, beside the APL-associated fusion portion, that are important for effective treatment. Evidence for this comes from one of the studies mentioned above showing that both ATRA and ATO-stimulated autophagic degradation of PML/RARA through a mTOR-dependent pathway that does not seem to involve direct interactions between drugs and the oncoprotein (Isakson *et al.*, 2010). In addition, it is also becoming increasingly clear that ATO has the potential to cure a subset of cancers that don't express PML/RARA. For example, induced clearance of LICs has been demonstrated both in PML/RARA positive as well as PML/RARA negative leukemic cells (Ito *et al.*, 2008; Nasr *et al.*, 2008). Furthermore, a phase II clinical study was recently published that showed promising results of using ATO in combination with interferon alpha and zidovudine for treatment of patients with chronic adult T cell leukemia (Kchour *et al.*, 2009), and finally, this drug was found to sensitize glucocorticoid-resistant acute lymphoblastic leukemia cells to dexamethasone (Bornhauser *et al.*, 2007). Thus, it is likely that APL for many years to come will continue to represent an important model disease for targeted and non-targeted effects of ATRA and ATO, while increased understanding of the molecular pathways involved may lead to discoveries of new therapies that are applicable for other types of cancers.

8. Acknowledgements

The work in our laboratory is funded by the Research Council of Norway, The Norwegian Cancer society and South-Eastern Norway Regional Health Authority.

9. References

Akao, Y., Mizoguchi, H., Kojima, S., Naoe, T., Ohishi, N. & Yagi, K. (1998). Arsenic induces apoptosis in B-cell leukaemic cell lines in vitro: activation of caspases and down-regulation of Bcl-2 protein. *British Journal of Haematology* 102, 1055-1060.

Alcalay, M., Zangrilli, D., Fagioli, M., Pandolfi, P. P., Mencarelli, A., Lo Coco, F., Biondi, A., Grignani, F. & Pelicci, P. G. (1992). Expression pattern of the RAR alpha-PML fusion gene in acute promyelocytic leukemia. *Proc Natl Acad Sci U S A* 89, 4840-4844.

Altucci, L., Rossin, A., Raffelsberger, W., Reitmair, A., Chomienne, C. & Gronemeyer, H. (2001). Retinoic acid-induced apoptosis in leukemia cells is mediated by paracrine action of tumor-selective death ligand TRAIL. *Nature Medicine* 7, 680-686.

Arnould, C., Philippe, C., Bourdon, V., Gr goire, M. J., Berger, R. & Jonveaux, P. (1999). The signal transducer and activator of transcription STAT5b gene is a new partner of retinoic acid receptor alpha in acute promyelocytic-like leukaemia. *Human Molecular Genetics* 8, 1741-1749.

Bachleitner-Hofmann, T., Gisslinger, B., Grumbeck, E. & Gisslinger, H. (2001). Arsenic trioxide and ascorbic acid: synergy with potential implications for the treatment of acute myeloid leukaemia? *British Journal of Haematology* 112, 783-786.

Bastien, J. & Rochette-Egly, C. (2004). Nuclear retinoid receptors and the transcription of retinoid-target genes. *Gene* 328, 1-16.

Bentley, D. L. & Groudine, M. (1986). A block to elongation is largely responsible for decreased transcription of c-myc in differentiated HL60 cells. *Nature* 321, 702-706.

Bernard, J., Weil, M., Boiron, M., Jacquillat, C., Flandrin, G. & Gemon, M. F. (1973). Acute promyelocytic leukemia: results of treatment by daunorubicin. *Blood* 41, 489-496.

Bernardi, R., Guernah, I., Jin, D. & other authors (2006). PML inhibits HIF-1alpha translation and neoangiogenesis through repression of mTOR. *Nature* 442, 779-785.

Borden, K. L. (2002). Pondering the promyelocytic leukemia protein (PML) puzzle: possible functions for PML nuclear bodies. *Molecular & Cellular Biology* 22, 5259-5269.

Bornhauser, B. C., Bonapace, L., Lindholm, D., Martinez, R., Cario, G., Schrappe, M., Niggli, F. K., Schafer, B. W. & Bourquin, J. P. (2007). Low-dose arsenic trioxide sensitizes glucocorticoid-resistant acute lymphoblastic leukemia cells to dexamethasone via an Akt-dependent pathway. *Blood* 110, 2084-2091.

Breitman, T. R., Collins, S. J. & Keene, B. R. (1981). Terminal differentiation of human promyelocytic leukemic cells in primary culture in response to retinoic acid. *Blood* 57, 1000-1004.

Brown, D., Kogan, S., Lagasse, E., Weissman, I., Alcalay, M., Pelicci, P. G., Atwater, S. & Bishop, J. M. (1997). A PMLRARalpha transgene initiates murine acute promyelocytic leukemia. *Proceedings of the National Academy of Sciences U S A* 94, 2551-2556.

Bøe, S. O., Haave, M., Jul-Larsen, A., Grudic, A., Bjerkvig, R. & Lonning, P. E. (2006). Promyelocytic leukemia nuclear bodies are predetermined processing sites for damaged DNA. *Journal of Cell Science* 119, 3284-3295.

Bøe, S. O. & Simonsen, A. (2010). Autophagic degradation of an oncoprotein. *Autophagy* 6, 964-965.

Cai, X., Shen, Y. L., Zhu, Q. & other authors (2000). Arsenic trioxide-induced apoptosis and differentiation are associated respectively with mitochondrial transmembrane potential collapse and retinoic acid signaling pathways in acute promyelocytic leukemia. *Leukemia* 14, 262-270.

Carbone, R., Botrugno, O. A., Ronzoni, S., Insinga, A., Di Croce, L., Pelicci, P. G. & Minucci, S. (2006). Recruitment of the histone methyltransferase SUV39H1 and its role in the oncogenic properties of the leukemia-associated PML-retinoic acid receptor fusion protein. *Molecular & Cellular Biology* 26, 1288-1296.

Chen, G. Q., Zhu, J., Shi, X. G. & other authors (1996). In vitro studies on cellular and molecular mechanisms of arsenic trioxide (As2O3) in the treatment of acute promyelocytic leukemia: As2O3 induces NB4 cell apoptosis with downregulation of Bcl-2 expression and modulation of PML-RAR alpha/PML proteins. *Blood* 88, 1052-1061.

Chen, G. Q., Shi, X. G., Tang, W. & other authors (1997). Use of arsenic trioxide (As2O3) in the treatment of acute promyelocytic leukemia (APL): I. As2O3 exerts dose-dependent dual effects on APL cells. *Blood* 89, 3345-3353.

Chen, Y. C., Kappel, C., Beaudouin, J., Eils, R. & Spector, D. L. (2008). Live cell dynamics of promyelocytic leukemia nuclear bodies upon entry into and exit from mitosis. *Molecular biology of the cell* 19, 3147-3162.

Chen, Z., Brand, N. J., Chen, A., Chen, S. J., Tong, J. H., Wang, Z. Y., Waxman, S. & Zelent, A. (1993). Fusion between a novel Kruppel-like zinc finger gene and the retinoic acid receptor-alpha locus due to a variant t(11;17) translocation associated with acute promyelocytic leukaemia. *The EMBO Journal* 12, 1161-1167.

Chen, Z. X., Xue, Y. Q., Zhang, R. & other authors (1991). A clinical and experimental study on all-trans retinoic acid-treated acute promyelocytic leukemia patients. *Blood* 78, 1413-1419.

Chomienne, C., Ballerini, P., Balitrand, N., Daniel, M. T., Fenaux, P., Castaigne, S. & Degos, L. (1990). All-trans retinoic acid in acute promyelocytic leukemias. II. In vitro studies: structure-function relationship. *Blood* 76, 1710-1717.

Cordonnier, C., Vernant, J. P., Brun, B. & other authors (1985). Acute promyelocytic leukemia in 57 previously untreated patients. *Cancer* 55, 18-25.

Cunningham, I., Gee, T. S., Reich, L. M., Kempin, S. J., Naval, A. N. & Clarkson, B. D. (1989). Acute promyelocytic leukemia: treatment results during a decade at Memorial Hospital. *Blood* 73, 1116-1122.

Cutler, E. G. & Bradford, E. H. (1878). Action of iron, cod-liver oil, and arsenic on the globular richness of the blood. *American Journal of Medical Sciences* 75, 74-84.

de Botton, S., Chevret, S., Coiteux, V. & other authors (2003). Early onset of chemotherapy can reduce the incidence of ATRA syndrome in newly diagnosed acute promyelocytic leukemia (APL) with low white blood cell counts: results from APL 93 trial. *Leukemia* 17, 339-342.

de Thé, H., Lavau, C., Marchio, A., Chomienne, C., Degos, L. & Dejean, A. (1991). The PML-RAR alpha fusion mRNA generated by the t(15;17) translocation in acute promyelocytic leukemia encodes a functionally altered RAR. *Cell* 66, 675-684.

de Thé, H. & Chen, Z. (2010). Acute promyelocytic leukaemia: novel insights into the mechanisms of cure. *Nature Reviews Cancer* 10, 775-783.

Degos, L., Castaigne, S., Tilly, H., Sigaux, F. & Daniel, M. T. (1985). Treatment of leukemia with low-dose ara-C: a study of 160 cases. *Seminars in Oncology* 12, 196-199.

Dellaire, G., Ching, R. W., Ahmed, K., Jalali, F., Tse, K. C., Bristow, R. G. & Bazett-Jones, D. P. (2006a). Promyelocytic leukemia nuclear bodies behave as DNA damage sensors whose response to DNA double-strand breaks is regulated by NBS1 and the kinases ATM, Chk2, and ATR. *The Journal of cell biology* 175, 55-66.

Dellaire, G., Eskiw, C. H., Dehghani, H., Ching, R. W. & Bazett-Jones, D. P. (2006b). Mitotic accumulations of PML protein contribute to the re-establishment of PML nuclear bodies in G1. *Journal of cell science* 119, 1034-1042.

Di Croce, L., Raker, V. A., Corsaro, M. & other authors (2002). Methyltransferase recruitment and DNA hypermethylation of target promoters by an oncogenic transcription factor. *Science* 295, 1079-1082.

Ding, W., Li, Y. P., Nobile, L. M., Grills, G., Carrera, I., Paietta, E., Tallman, M. S., Wiernik, P. H. & Gallagher, R. E. (1998). Leukemic cellular retinoic acid resistance and missense mutations in the PML-RARalpha fusion gene after relapse of acute promyelocytic leukemia from treatment with all-trans retinoic acid and intensive chemotherapy. *Blood* 92, 1172-1183.

Drapkin, R. L., Gee, T. S., Dowling, M. D., Arlin, Z., McKenzie, S., Kempin, S. & Clarkson, B. (1978). Prophylactic heparin therapy in acute promyelocytic leukemia. *Cancer* 41, 2484-2490.

Duprez, E., Benoit, G., Flexor, M., Lillehaug, J. R. & Lanotte, M. (2000). A mutated PML/RARA found in the retinoid maturation resistant NB4 subclone, NB4-R2, blocks RARA and wild-type PML/RARA transcriptional activities. *Leukemia* 14, 255-261.

Duprez, E., Wagner, K., Koch, H. & Tenen, D. G. (2003). C/EBPbeta: a major PML-RARA-responsive gene in retinoic acid-induced differentiation of APL cells. *Embo J* 22, 5806-5816.

Dyck, J. A., Maul, G. G., Miller, W. H., Jr., Chen, J. D., Kakizuka, A. & Evans, R. M. (1994). A novel macromolecular structure is a target of the promyelocyte-retinoic acid receptor oncoprotein. *Cell* 76, 333-343.

Estey, E., Garcia-Manero, G., Ferrajoli, A., Faderl, S., Verstovsek, S., Jones, D. & Kantarjian, H. (2006). Use of all-trans retinoic acid plus arsenic trioxide as an alternative to chemotherapy in untreated acute promyelocytic leukemia. *Blood* 107, 3469-3473.

Everett, R. D. & Maul, G. G. (1994). HSV-1 IE protein Vmw110 causes redistribution of PML. *The EMBO journal* 13, 5062-5069.

Fagioli, M., Alcalay, M., Pandolfi, P. P., Venturini, L., Mencarelli, A., Simeone, A., Acampora, D., Grignani, F. & Pelicci, P. G. (1992). Alternative splicing of PML transcripts predicts coexpression of several carboxy-terminally different protein isoforms. *Oncogene* 7, 1083-1091.

Fenaux, P., Chastang, C., Chevret, S. & other authors (1999). A randomized comparison of all transretinoic acid (ATRA) followed by chemotherapy and ATRA plus chemotherapy and the role of maintenance therapy in newly diagnosed acute promyelocytic leukemia. The European APL Group. *Blood* 94, 1192-1200.

Fenaux, P., Wang, Z. Z. & Degos, L. (2007). Treatment of acute promyelocytic leukemia by retinoids. *Current Topics in Microbiology & Immunology* 313, 101-128.

Ferbeyre, G., de Stanchina, E., Querido, E., Baptiste, N., Prives, C. & Lowe, S. W. (2000). PML is induced by oncogenic ras and promotes premature senescence. *Genes & development* 14, 2015-2027.

Forkner, C. E. & Scott, T. F. M. (1931). Arsenic as a therapeutic agent in chronic myelogenous leukemia. *Journal of the American Medical Association* 97, 3-5.

Freemantle, S. J., Spinella, M. J. & Dmitrovsky, E. (2003). Retinoids in cancer therapy and chemoprevention: promise meets resistance. *Oncogene* 22, 7305-7315.

Gallagher, R. E. (2002). Retinoic acid resistance in acute promyelocytic leukemia. *Leukemia* 16, 1940-1958.

Gallagher, R. E., Schachter-Tokarz, E. L., Zhou, D. C. & other authors (2006). Relapse of acute promyelocytic leukemia with PML-RARalpha mutant subclones independent of proximate all-trans retinoic acid selection pressure. *Leukemia* 20, 556-562.

Gold, E. J., Mertelsmann, R. H., Itri, L. M., Gee, T., Arlin, Z., Kempin, S., Clarkson, B. & Moore, M. A. (1983). Phase I clinical trial of 13-cis-retinoic acid in myelodysplastic syndromes. *Cancer Treatment Reports* 67, 981-986.

Goto, E., Tomita, A., Hayakawa, F., Atsumi, A., Kiyoi, H. & Naoe, T. (2011). Missense mutations in PML-RARA critical for the lack of responsiveness to arsenic trioxide treatment. *Blood*.

Gowda, S. D., Koler, R. D. & Bagby, G. C., Jr. (1986). Regulation of C-myc expression during growth and differentiation of normal and leukemic human myeloid progenitor cells. *The Journal of clinical investigation* 77, 271-278.

Grignani, F., De Matteis, S., Nervi, C. & other authors (1998). Fusion proteins of the retinoic acid receptor-alpha recruit histone deacetylase in promyelocytic leukaemia. *Nature* 391, 815-818.

Grimwade, D., Howe, K., Langabeer, S. & other authors (1996). Establishing the presence of the t(15;17) in suspected acute promyelocytic leukaemia: cytogenetic, molecular and PML immunofluorescence assessment of patients entered into the M.R.C. ATRA trial. M.R.C. Adult Leukaemia Working Party. *Br J Haematol* 94, 557-573.

Grisolano, J. L., Wesselschmidt, R. L., Pelicci, P. G. & Ley, T. J. (1997). Altered myeloid development and acute leukemia in transgenic mice expressing PML-RAR alpha under control of cathepsin G regulatory sequences. *Blood* 89, 376-387.

Guibal, F. C., Alberich-Jorda, M., Hirai, H. & other authors (2009). Identification of a myeloid committed progenitor as the cancer-initiating cell in acute promyelocytic leukemia. *Blood* 114, 5415-5425.

Guillemin, M. C., Raffoux, E., Vitoux, D. & other authors (2002). In vivo activation of cAMP signaling induces growth arrest and differentiation in acute promyelocytic leukemia. *Journal of Experimental Medicine* 196, 1373-1380.

Gurrieri, C., Nafa, K., Merghoub, T. & other authors (2004). Mutations of the PML tumor suppressor gene in acute promyelocytic leukemia. *Blood* 103, 2358-2362.

Hauksdottir, H. & Privalsky, M. L. (2001). DNA recognition by the aberrant retinoic acid receptors implicated in human acute promyelocytic leukemia. *Cell Growth Differ* 12, 85-98.

He, L. Z., Guidez, F., Tribioli, C., Peruzzi, D., Ruthardt, M., Zelent, A. & Pandolfi, P. P. (1998). Distinct interactions of PML-RARalpha and PLZF-RARalpha with co-repressors determine differential responses to RA in APL. *Nature Genetics* 18, 126-135.

Hillestad, L. K. (1957). Acute promyelocytic leukemia. *Acta Medica Scandinavica* 159, 189-194.

Hoemme, C., Peerzada, A., Behre, G. & other authors (2008).Chromatin modifications induced by PML-RARÎ± repress critical targets in leukemogenesis as analyzed by ChIP-Chip, pp. 2887-2895.

Hu, J., Liu, Y. F., Wu, C. F. & other authors (2009). Long-term efficacy and safety of all-trans retinoic acid/arsenic trioxide-based therapy in newly diagnosed acute promyelocytic leukemia. *Proceedings of the National Academy of Sciences U S A* 106, 3342-3347.

Huang, M. E., Ye, Y. C., Chen, S. R. & other authors (1987). All-trans retinoic acid with or without low dose cytosine arabinoside in acute promyelocytic leukemia. Report of 6 cases. *Chinese Medical Journal (Engl)* 100, 949-953.

Huang, M. E., Ye, Y. C., Chen, S. R., Chai, J. R., Lu, J. X., Zhoa, L., Gu, L. J. & Wang, Z. Y. (1988). Use of all-trans retinoic acid in the treatment of acute promyelocytic leukemia. *Blood* 72, 567-572.

Huang, X. J., Wiernik, P. H., Klein, R. S. & Gallagher, R. E. (1999). Arsenic trioxide induces apoptosis of myeloid leukemia cells by activation of caspases. *Medical Oncology* 16, 58-64.

Imaizumi, M., Suzuki, H., Yoshinari, M. & other authors (1998). Mutations in the E-domain of RAR portion of the PML/RAR chimeric gene may confer clinical resistance to all-trans retinoic acid in acute promyelocytic leukemia. *Blood* 92, 374-382.

Isakson, P., Bjørås, M., Bøe, S. O. & Simonsen, A. (2010). Autophagy contributes to therapy-induced degradation of the PML/RARA oncoprotein. *Blood* 116, 2324-2331.

Ishitsuka, K., Hanada, S., Suzuki, S. & other authors (1998). Arsenic trioxide inhibits growth of human T-cell leukaemia virus type I infected T-cell lines more effectively than retinoic acids. *British Journal of Haematology* 103, 721-728.

Ito, K., Bernardi, R., Morotti, A. & other authors (2008). PML targeting eradicates quiescent leukaemia-initiating cells. *Nature* 453, 1072-1078.

Ito, K., Bernardi, R. & Pandolfi, P. P. (2009). A novel signaling network as a critical rheostat for the biology and maintenance of the normal stem cell and the cancer-initiating cell. *Current Opinion in Genetics & Development* 19, 51-59.

Jansen, J. H., Mahfoudi, A., Rambaud, S., Lavau, C., Wahli, W. & Dejean, A. (1995). Multimeric complexes of the PML-retinoic acid receptor alpha fusion protein in acute promyelocytic leukemia cells and interference with retinoid and peroxisome-proliferator signaling pathways. *Proceedings in the National Academy of Sciences U S A* 92, 7401-7405.

Jeanne, M., Lallemand-Breitenbach, V., Ferhi, O. & other authors (2010). PML/RARA oxidation and arsenic binding initiate the antileukemia response of As2O3. *Cancer Cell* 18, 88-98.

Jensen, K., Shiels, C. & Freemont, P. S. (2001). PML protein isoforms and the RBCC/TRIM motif. *Oncogene* 20, 7223-7233.

Jing, Y., Dai, J., Chalmers-Redman, R. M., Tatton, W. G. & Waxman, S. (1999). Arsenic trioxide selectively induces acute promyelocytic leukemia cell apoptosis via a hydrogen peroxide-dependent pathway. *Blood* 94, 2102-2111.

Jing, Y., Wang, L., Xia, L., Chen, G. Q., Chen, Z., Miller, W. H. & Waxman, S. (2001). Combined effect of all-trans retinoic acid and arsenic trioxide in acute promyelocytic leukemia cells in vitro and in vivo. *Blood* 97, 264-269.

Jul-Larsen, A., Grudic, A., Bjerkvig, R. & Bøe, S. O. (2009). Cell-cycle regulation and dynamics of cytoplasmic compartments containing the promyelocytic leukemia protein and nucleoporins. *Journal of Cell Science* 122, 1201-1210.

Jul-Larsen, A., Grudic, A., Bjerkvig, R. & Bøe, S. O. (2010). Subcellular distribution of nuclear import-defective isoforms of the promyelocytic leukemia protein. *BMC Molecular Biology* 11, 89.

Kamashev, D., Vitoux, D. & De The, H. (2004). PML-RARA-RXR oligomers mediate retinoid and rexinoid/cAMP cross-talk in acute promyelocytic leukemia cell differentiation. *Journal of Experimental Medicine* 199, 1163-1174.

Kchour, G., Tarhini, M., Kooshyar, M. M. & other authors (2009). Phase 2 study of the efficacy and safety of the combination of arsenic trioxide, interferon alpha, and zidovudine in newly diagnosed chronic adult T-cell leukemia/lymphoma (ATL). *Blood* 113, 6528-6532.

Khan, M. M., Nomura, T., Chiba, T., Tanaka, K., Yoshida, H., Mori, K. & Ishii, S. (2004). The fusion oncoprotein PML-RARalpha induces endoplasmic reticulum (ER)-associated degradation of N-CoR and ER stress. *Journal of Biological Chemistry* 279, 11814-11824.

Kitamura, K., Kiyoi, H., Yoshida, H., Saito, H., Ohno, R. & Naoe, T. (1997). Mutant AF-2 domain of PML-RARalpha in retinoic acid-resistant NB4 cells: differentiation induced by RA is triggered directly through PML-RARalpha and its down-regulation in acute promyelocytic leukemia. *Leukemia* 11, 1950-1956.

Kitareewan, S., Pitha-Rowe, I., Sekula, D., Lowrey, C. H., Nemeth, M. J., Golub, T. R., Freemantle, S. J. & Dmitrovsky, E. (2002). UBE1L is a retinoid target that triggers PML/RARalpha degradation and apoptosis in acute promyelocytic leukemia. *Proceedings in the National Academy of Sciences U S A* 99, 3806-3811.

Klionsky, D. J. (2007). Autophagy: from phenomenology to molecular understanding in less than a decade. *Nature Reviews Molecular Cell Biology* 8, 931-937.

Koeffler, H. P., Hirji, K. & Itri, L. (1985). 1,25-Dihydroxyvitamin D3: in vivo and in vitro effects on human preleukemic and leukemic cells. *Cancer Treatment Reports* 69, 1399-1407.

Koken, M. H., Puvion-Dutilleul, F., Guillemin, M. C. & other authors (1994). The t(15;17) translocation alters a nuclear body in a retinoic acid-reversible fashion. *The EMBO Journal* 13, 1073-1083.

Kopf, E., Plassat, J. L., Vivat, V., de The, H., Chambon, P. & Rochette-Egly, C. (2000). Dimerization with retinoid X receptors and phosphorylation modulate the retinoic acid-induced degradation of retinoic acid receptors alpha and gamma through the ubiquitin-proteasome pathway. *Journal of Biological Chemistry* 275, 33280-33288.

Kwong, Y. L. & Todd, D. (1997). Delicious poison: arsenic trioxide for the treatment of leukemia. *Blood* 89, 3487-3488.

Lallemand-Breitenbach, V., Guillemin, M. C., Janin, A., Daniel, M. T., Degos, L., Kogan, S. C., Bishop, J. M. & de The, H. (1999). Retinoic acid and arsenic synergize to eradicate leukemic cells in a mouse model of acute promyelocytic leukemia. *Journal of Experimental Medicine* 189, 1043-1052.

Lallemand-Breitenbach, V., Zhu, J., Puvion, F. & other authors (2001). Role of promyelocytic leukemia (PML) sumolation in nuclear body formation, 11S proteasome recruitment, and As2O3-induced PML or PML/retinoic acid receptor alpha degradation. *Journal of Experimental Medicine* 193, 1361-1371.

Lallemand-Breitenbach, V., Jeanne, M., Benhenda, S. & other authors (2008). Arsenic degrades PML or PML-RARalpha through a SUMO-triggered RNF4/ubiquitin-mediated pathway. *Nature Cell Biology* 10, 547-555.

Lallemand-Breitenbach, V. & de The, H. (2010). PML nuclear bodies. *Cold Spring Harbor Perspectives in Biology* 2, a000661.

Lane, A. A. & Ley, T. J. (2003). Neutrophil elastase cleaves PML-RARalpha and is important for the development of acute promyelocytic leukemia in mice. *Cell* 115, 305-318.

Licht, J. D., Chomienne, C., Goy, A. & other authors (1995). Clinical and molecular characterization of a rare syndrome of acute promyelocytic leukemia associated with translocation (11;17). *Blood* 85, 1083-1094.

Lin, R. J., Nagy, L., Inoue, S., Shao, W., Miller, W. H., Jr. & Evans, R. M. (1998). Role of the histone deacetylase complex in acute promyelocytic leukaemia. *Nature* 391, 811-814.

Marasca, R., Zucchini, P., Galimberti, S., Leonardi, G., Vaccari, P., Donelli, A., Luppi, M., Petrini, M. & Torelli, G. (1999). Missense mutations in the PML/RARalpha ligand binding domain in ATRA-resistant As(2)O(3) sensitive relapsed acute promyelocytic leukemia. *Haematologica* 84, 963-968.

Martin, S. J., Bradley, J. G. & Cotter, T. G. (1990). HL-60 cells induced to differentiate towards neutrophils subsequently die via apoptosis. *Clinical & Experimental Immunology* 79, 448-453.

Mueller, B. U., Pabst, T., Fos, J., Petkovic, V., Fey, M. F., Asou, N., Buergi, U. & Tenen, D. G. (2006). ATRA resolves the differentiation block in t(15;17) acute myeloid leukemia by restoring PU.1 expression. *Blood* 107, 3330-3338.

Muller, S., Matunis, M. J. & Dejean, A. (1998). Conjugation with the ubiquitin-related modifier SUMO-1 regulates the partitioning of PML within the nucleus. *The EMBO Journal* 17, 61-70.

Nason-Burchenal, K., Allopenna, J., Begue, A., Stehelin, D., Dmitrovsky, E. & Martin, P. (1998). Targeting of PML/RARalpha is lethal to retinoic acid-resistant promyelocytic leukemia cells. *Blood* 92, 1758-1767.

Nasr, R., Guillemin, M. C., Ferhi, O. & other authors (2008). Eradication of acute promyelocytic leukemia-initiating cells through PML-RARA degradation. *Nature Medicine* 14, 1333-1342.

Nervi, C., Ferrara, F. F., Fanelli, M. & other authors (1998). Caspases mediate retinoic acid-induced degradation of the acute promyelocytic leukemia PML/RARalpha fusion protein. *Blood* 92, 2244-2251.

Niu, C., Yan, H., Yu, T. & other authors (1999). Studies on treatment of acute promyelocytic leukemia with arsenic trioxide: remission induction, follow-up, and molecular monitoring in 11 newly diagnosed and 47 relapsed acute promyelocytic leukemia patients. *Blood* 94, 3315-3324.

Park, D. J., Chumakov, A. M., Vuong, P. T., Chih, D. Y., Gombart, A. F., Miller, W. H., Jr. & Koeffler, H. P. (1999). CCAAT/enhancer binding protein epsilon is a potential retinoid target gene in acute promyelocytic leukemia treatment. *The Journal of clinical investigation* 103, 1399-1408.

Pearson, M., Carbone, R., Sebastiani, C. & other authors (2000). PML regulates p53 acetylation and premature senescence induced by oncogenic Ras. *Nature* 406, 207-210.

Perez, A., Kastner, P., Sethi, S., Lutz, Y., Reibel, C. & Chambon, P. (1993). PMLRAR homodimers: distinct DNA binding properties and heteromeric interactions with RXR. *The EMBO Journal* 12, 3171-3182.

Perkins, C., Kim, C. N., Fang, G. & Bhalla, K. N. (2000). Arsenic induces apoptosis of multidrug-resistant human myeloid leukemia cells that express Bcr-Abl or overexpress MDR, MRP, Bcl-2, or Bcl-x(L). *Blood* 95, 1014-1022.

Petti, M. C., Fazi, F., Gentile, M. & other authors (2002). Complete remission through blast cell differentiation in PLZF/RARalpha-positive acute promyelocytic leukemia: in vitro and in vivo studies. *Blood* 100, 1065-1067.

Redner, R. L., Rush, E. A., Faas, S., Rudert, W. A. & Corey, S. J. (1996). The t(5;17) variant of acute promyelocytic leukemia expresses a nucleophosmin-retinoic acid receptor fusion. *Blood* 87, 882-886.

Reymond, A., Meroni, G., Fantozzi, A. & other authors (2001). The tripartite motif family identifies cell compartments. *The EMBO Journal* 20, 2140-2151.

Rice, K. L., Hormaeche, I., Doulatov, S. & other authors (2009). Comprehensive genomic screens identify a role for PLZF-RARalpha as a positive regulator of cell proliferation via direct regulation of c-MYC. *Blood* 114, 5499-5511.

Rosenauer, A., Raelson, J. V., Nervi, C., Eydoux, P., DeBlasio, A. & Miller, W. H., Jr. (1996). Alterations in expression, binding to ligand and DNA, and transcriptional activity of rearranged and wild-type retinoid receptors in retinoid-resistant acute promyelocytic leukemia cell lines. *Blood* 88, 2671-2682.

Rousselot, P., Labaume, S., Marolleau, J. P., Larghero, J., Noguera, M. H., Brouet, J. C. & Fermand, J. P. (1999). Arsenic trioxide and melarsoprol induce apoptosis in plasma cell lines and in plasma cells from myeloma patients. *Cancer Research* 59, 1041-1048.

Ruggero, D., Baccarani, M., Guarini, A. & other authors (1977). Acute promyelocytic leukemia: results of therapy and analysis of 13 cases. *Acta Haematologica* 58, 108-119.

Sachs, L. (1978). Control of normal cell differentiation and the phenotypic reversion of malignancy in myeloid leukaemia. *Nature* 274, 535-539.

Salomoni, P. & Pandolfi, P. P. (2002). The role of PML in tumor suppression. *Cell* 108, 165-170.

Sanz, M. A., Jarque, I., Martin, G. & other authors (1988). Acute promyelocytic leukemia. Therapy results and prognostic factors. *Cancer* 61, 7-13.

Sanz, M. A., Martin, G., Rayon, C. & other authors (1999). A modified AIDA protocol with anthracycline-based consolidation results in high antileukemic efficacy and reduced toxicity in newly diagnosed PML/RARalpha-positive acute promyelocytic leukemia. PETHEMA group. *Blood* 94, 3015-3021.

Scaglioni, P. P., Yung, T. M., Cai, L. F., Erdjument-Bromage, H., Kaufman, A. J., Singh, B., Teruya-Feldstein, J., Tempst, P. & Pandolfi, P. P. (2006). A CK2-dependent mechanism for degradation of the PML tumor suppressor. *Cell* 126, 269-283.

Shao, W., Benedetti, L., Lamph, W. W., Nervi, C. & Miller, W. H., Jr. (1997). A retinoid-resistant acute promyelocytic leukemia subclone expresses a dominant negative PML-RAR alpha mutation. *Blood* 89, 4282-4289.

Shao, W., Fanelli, M., Ferrara, F. F. & other authors (1998). Arsenic trioxide as an inducer of apoptosis and loss of PML/RAR alpha protein in acute promyelocytic leukemia cells. *Journal of the National Cancer Institute* 90, 124-133.

Shen, Z. X., Chen, G. Q., Ni, J. H. & other authors (1997). Use of arsenic trioxide (As2O3) in the treatment of acute promyelocytic leukemia (APL): II. Clinical efficacy and pharmacokinetics in relapsed patients. *Blood* 89, 3354-3360.

Shen, Z. X., Shi, Z. Z., Fang, J. & other authors (2004). All-trans retinoic acid/As2O3 combination yields a high quality remission and survival in newly diagnosed acute promyelocytic leukemia. *Proceedings in the National Academy of Sciences U S A* 101, 5328-5335.

Soignet, S. L., Maslak, P., Wang, Z. G. & other authors (1998). Complete remission after treatment of acute promyelocytic leukemia with arsenic trioxide. *New England Journal of Medicine* 339, 1341-1348.

Subramaniyam, S., Nandula, S. V., Nichols, G., Weiner, M., Satwani, P., Alobeid, B., Bhagat, G. & Murty, V. V. (2006). Do RARA/PML fusion gene deletions confer resistance to ATRA-based therapy in patients with acute promyelocytic leukemia? *Leukemia* 20, 2193-2195.

Sun, H. D., Ma, L., Hu, X. C. & Zhang, T. D. (1992). Ai-Lin 1 treated 32 cases of acute promyelocytic leukemia. *Chinese Journal of Integrated Chinese Western Medicine* 12, 170-172.

Takayama, N., Kizaki, M., Hida, T., Kinjo, K. & Ikeda, Y. (2001). Novel mutation in the PML/RARalpha chimeric gene exhibits dramatically decreased ligand-binding activity and confers acquired resistance to retinoic acid in acute promyelocytic leukemia. *Experimental hematology* 29, 864-872.

Tallman, M. S., Andersen, J. W., Schiffer, C. A. & other authors (1997). All-trans-retinoic acid in acute promyelocytic leukemia. *New England Journal of Medicine* 337, 1021-1028.

Tatham, M. H., Geoffroy, M. C., Shen, L., Plechanovova, A., Hattersley, N., Jaffray, E. G., Palvimo, J. J. & Hay, R. T. (2008). RNF4 is a poly-SUMO-specific E3 ubiquitin ligase required for arsenic-induced PML degradation. *Nature Cell Biology* 10, 538-546.

Trotman, L. C., Alimonti, A., Scaglioni, P. P., Koutcher, J. A., Cordon-Cardo, C. & Pandolfi, P. P. (2006). Identification of a tumour suppressor network opposing nuclear Akt function. *Nature* 441, 523-527.

Uy, G. L., Lane, A. A., Welch, J. S., Grieselhuber, N. R., Payton, J. E. & Ley, T. J. (2010). A protease-resistant PML-RAR{alpha} has increased leukemogenic potential in a murine model of acute promyelocytic leukemia. *Blood* 116, 3604-3610.

Villa, R., Pasini, D., Gutierrez, A. & other authors (2007). Role of the polycomb repressive complex 2 in acute promyelocytic leukemia. *Cancer Cell* 11, 513-525.

Wang, G., Li, W., Cui, J. & other authors (2004). An efficient therapeutic approach to patients with acute promyelocytic leukemia using a combination of arsenic trioxide with low-dose all-trans retinoic acid. *Journal of Hematology & Oncology* 22, 63-71.

Wang, T. S., Kuo, C. F., Jan, K. Y. & Huang, H. (1996). Arsenite induces apoptosis in Chinese hamster ovary cells by generation of reactive oxygen species. *Journal of Cellular Physiology* 169, 256-268.

Wang, Z. G., Ruggero, D., Ronchetti, S., Zhong, S., Gaboli, M., Rivi, R. & Pandolfi, P. P. (1998). PML is essential for multiple apoptotic pathways. *Nature Genetics* 20, 266-272.

Wang, Z. Y. & Chen, Z. (2008). Acute promyelocytic leukemia: from highly fatal to highly curable. *Blood* 111, 2505-2515.

Weis, K., Rambaud, S., Lavau, C., Jansen, J., Carvalho, T., Carmo-Fonseca, M., Lamond, A. & Dejean, A. (1994). Retinoic acid regulates aberrant nuclear localization of PML-RAR alpha in acute promyelocytic leukemia cells. *Cell* 76, 345-356.

Wells, R. A., Catzavelos, C. & Kamel-Reid, S. (1997). Fusion of retinoic acid receptor alpha to NuMA, the nuclear mitotic apparatus protein, by a variant translocation in acute promyelocytic leukaemia. *Nature Genetics* 17, 109-113.

Wojiski, S., Guibal, F. C., Kindler, T., Lee, B. H., Jesneck, J. L., Fabian, A., Tenen, D. G. & Gilliland, D. G. (2009). PML-RARalpha initiates leukemia by conferring properties of self-renewal to committed promyelocytic progenitors. *Leukemia* 23, 1462-1471.

Zeisig, B. B., Kwok, C., Zelent, A., Shankaranarayanan, P., Gronemeyer, H., Dong, S. & So, C. W. (2007). Recruitment of RXR by homotetrameric RARalpha fusion proteins is essential for transformation. *Cancer Cell* 12, 36-51.

Zhang, P., Wang, S. Y. & Hu, X. H. (1996). Arsenic trioxide treated 72 cases of acute promyelocytic leukemia. *Chinese Journal of Hematology* 17, 58-62.

Zhang, W., Ohnishi, K., Shigeno, K., Fujisawa, S., Naito, K., Nakamura, S., Takeshita, K., Takeshita, A. & Ohno, R. (1998). The induction of apoptosis and cell cycle arrest by arsenic trioxide in lymphoid neoplasms. *Leukemia* 12, 1383-1391.

Zhang, X. W., Yan, X. J., Zhou, Z. R. & other authors (2010). Arsenic trioxide controls the fate of the PML-RARalpha oncoprotein by directly binding PML. *Science* 328, 240-243.

Zheng, J., Deng, Y. P., Lin, C., Fu, M., Xiao, P. G. & Wu, M. (1999). Arsenic trioxide induces apoptosis of HPV16 DNA-immortalized human cervical epithelial cells and selectively inhibits viral gene expression. *International Journal of Cancer* 82, 286-292.

Zheng, X., Seshire, A., Ruster, B., Bug, G., Beissert, T., Puccetti, E., Hoelzer, D., Henschler, R. & Ruthardt, M. (2007). Arsenic but not all-trans retinoic acid overcomes the aberrant stem cell capacity of PML/RARalpha-positive leukemic stem cells. *Haematologica* 92, 323-331.

Zhou, D. C., Kim, S. H., Ding, W., Schultz, C., Warrell, R. P., Jr. & Gallagher, R. E. (2002). Frequent mutations in the ligand-binding domain of PML-RARalpha after multiple relapses of acute promyelocytic leukemia: analysis for functional relationship to response to all-trans retinoic acid and histone deacetylase inhibitors in vitro and in vivo. *Blood* 99, 1356-1363.

Zhu, J., Shi, X. G., Chu, H. Y., Tong, J. H., Wang, Z. Y., Naoe, T., Waxman, S., Chen, S. J. & Chen, Z. (1995). Effect of retinoic acid isomers on proliferation, differentiation and PML relocalization in the APL cell line NB4. *Leukemia* 9, 302-309.

Zhu, J., Gianni, M., Kopf, E., Honore, N., Chelbi-Alix, M., Koken, M., Quignon, F., Rochette-Egly, C. & de The, H. (1999). Retinoic acid induces proteasome-dependent degradation of retinoic acid receptor alpha (RARalpha) and oncogenic RARalpha fusion proteins. *Proceedings in the National Academy of Sciences U S A* 96, 14807-14812.

Zhu, J., Zhou, J., Peres, L., Riaucoux, F., Honore, N., Kogan, S. & de The, H. (2005). A sumoylation site in PML/RARA is essential for leukemic transformation. *Cancer Cell* 7, 143-153.

Zhu, J., Nasr, R., Peres, L. & other authors (2007). RXR is an essential component of the oncogenic PML/RARA complex in vivo. *Cancer Cell* 12, 23-35.

Zhu, Q., Zhang, J. W., Zhu, H. Q. & other authors (2002). Synergic effects of arsenic trioxide and cAMP during acute promyelocytic leukemia cell maturation subtends a novel signaling cross-talk. *Blood* 99, 1014-1022.

19

The Association of the DNA Repair Genes with Acute Myeloid Leukemia: The Susceptibility and the Outcome After Therapy

Claudia Bănescu, Carmen Duicu and Minodora Dobreanu
Univ Med & Pharm Tg-Mures
România

1. Introduction

Acute myeloid leukemia (AML), the most common acute leukemia in adults, is a clonal hemopoietic disorder that is frequently associated with genetic instability characterized by a diversity of chromosomal and molecular abnormalities. There are a lot of reports that show that human cancer can be initiated by DNA damage caused by ultraviolet (UV), ionizing radiation, and environmental chemical agents. Many genes encode proteins that function to protect cells against genetic instability through numerous mechanisms, including deoxyribonucleic acid (DNA) repair pathways and protection against oxidative stress.

DNA repair pathways play an important role in maintaining the integrity of the genome, and it is obvious that defects in repair pathways are involved in many different types of diseases, including leukemia and cancer (Seedhouse, 2002).

DNA damage repair and cell-cycle checkpoints are the most important defense mechanisms against mutagenic exposures. The most important DNA-repair pathways in human cells are: direct repair, base excision repair (BER), nucleotide excision repair (NER), mismatch repair (MMR), Double Strand Break Repair (DSB repair) and translesion DNA synthesis (TLS). Each pathway repairs a different type of lession (D'Andrea, 2010). The NER pathway mainly removes bulky distortions in the shape of the DNA double helix. The BER pathway is responsible for removal of oxidized DNA bases that may arise endogenously or from exogenous agents. The DSB pathway is responsible for repairing double-strand breaks caused by a variety of exposures, including ionizing radiation. There are two distinct and complementary pathways for DSB repair-namely, homologous recombination (HR) and nonhomologous end joining (NHEJ).

Recent studies have suggested that DNA damage was related to the pathogenesis of some diseases such as AML. Therefore, some DNA repair genes may be involved in AML susceptibility (Allan, 2004; Kuptsova, 2007; Seedhouse, 2002, 2004; Voso, 2007).

Exposure to carcinogenic and genotoxic compounds causes DNA damage, and the cells have developed multiple DNA repair pathways to protect themselves from different types of DNA damage.

Polymorphisms in DNA repair genes, including those involved in base excision repair (BER), nucleotide excision repair, mismatch repair and double strand break repair have been implicated in carcinogenesis. Common polymorphisms in DNA repair genes may alter protein function and an individual's capacity to repair damaged DNA. Deficits in repair capacity may lead to genetic instability and tumorigenesis.

Studies have noted associations between risk of de novo AML and DNA repair gene polymorphisms (Matullo et al., 2006; Seedhouse et al., 2004). Increased risk of therapy-related AML was also linked to several gene polymorphisms in base excision repair (BER; XRCC1 Arg399Gln), nucleotide excision repair (NER; XPD Lys751Gln), and DSB repair (RAD51 G135C and XRCC3 Thr241Met) pathways (Allan et al. 2004; Seedhouse et al., 2002, 2004) and may be linked to secondary AML etiology through failure to recognize or excise accumulated DNA lesions.

2. Mechanism of DNA repair

DNA damage response pathways, some of the genes known to participate in each of these pathways, their modes of action are summarized in Table 1. These categories are not exclusive; there may be functional overlap between repair systems. For example, certain types of base damage can be repaired by base excision repair, nucleotide excision repair or homologous recombinational repair.

DNA repair genes may also have great implications in the therapeutic outcome of certain cancer treatments. Most antileukemic drugs interact with target cell DNA and exert their cytotoxic effects preferentially in replicating cells. In addition to the primary DNA lesions, secondary DNA alterations induced in the course of repair processes also contribute to the cytotoxic effects of DNA-reactive agents (Rajewsky &Müller, 2005).

Although there are several reports on associations between polymorphisms in DNA repair genes and cancer risk (Goode et al., 2002), fewer studies have been conducted to evaluate relationships between DNA repair gene polymorphisms and response to treatment.

2.1 Direct repair mechanism

This is the simplest repair mechanism compared to other repair system regarding number of molecules involved. It is an enzyme-catalyzed process used to correct the most frequent cause of point mutations in humans.

In direct repair mechanisms, the lesion is removed or reversed by a single step reaction restoring the local sequence to its original state. There are several direct repair enzymes, each having a different substrate. For example, O^6- methyl guanine DNA methyltransferase (O^6-MT, the product of the MGMT gene) repairs the alkylation damage. MGMT is important in the repair of alkylation damage. The alkyl group from the lesion is transferred to a cysteine residue in the active site of MGMT (Hazra et al., 1997). In 20% of human tumor cell lines the MGMT activity is decreased and the sensivity to alkylating agent is increased (Sancar, 1995), but there are few data which suggest that mutations in the MGMT gene contribute to cancer (Wang L et al, 1997; Yu Z et al, 1999).

The functional status of the O^6-MT pathway may be important in patients treated with alkylating agents, for O^6-methylation of guanine appears to be an important effect of some members of that class of drugs (Kaina & Christmann, 2002). High levels of O^6-MT are often found in AML blasts, which are thereby rendered resistant to certain alkylators (Gerson & Trey, 1988).

Pathway	Function	Genes Involved	References
Direct Repair Mechanism	Reverses damage to restore DNA integrity.	DNA photolyase, O^6-MGMT	Kaina et al., 2007; Mitra, 2007
Base Excision Repair (BER)	Repair of damaged bases or single-strand DNA breaks	OGG1, XRCC1, APE1, PARP,	Chaudhry, 2007; Yu et al., 1999; Hazra et al., 2007
Nucleotide Excision Repair (NER)	Excision of a variety of helix-distorting DNA lesions	XPA, XPB, XPC, XPD, XPE, XPF, XPG, RAD23, TFIIH, RPA1, RPA2, RPA3, PCNA	Kang et al., 2011; Reardon & Sancar, 2005; Yu et al., 1999
Mismatch Repair (MMR)	Repair of mispaired nucleotides	MSH2, MSH6, MSH4, PMS1, MLH1, PMS2, MLH3, PMS2L3, PCNA, RPA	Jiricny, 2006; Martin et al., 2010; Papouli et al., 2004; Surtees et al., 2004
Homologous recombination (HR)	Repair of double strand DNA break	RAD51, RAD51B, RAD51C, RAD51D, XRCC2, XRCC3, RAD52, RAD54, BRCA1, BRCA2, RAD50, NBS1, MRE11	Li & Heyer, 2008; Sung & Klein, 2006;
Nonhomologous End Joining (NHEJ)	Repair of double strand DNA breaks	XRCC4, XRCC5, XRCC6, XRCC7, LIG4, XLF,	Burma et al., 2006; Shrivastav et al., 2008
Translesion Synthesis (TLS)	Bypass of DNA adducts during DNA replication	POLK, POLI, POLZ, REV7, REV1, POLH,	Lehmann, 2006

Table 1. DNA Damage Response Pathways

2.2 Base Excision Repair

Base excision repair (BER) is the predominant DNA damage repair pathway for the processing of small base lesions, derived from ionizing radiation (Chen et al., 2010), oxidation, hydrolysis, or deamination and alkylation damages. The repair system involves three steps: removal of damaged bases from DNA by DNA glycosylases, then formed abasic site is removed and finally gap is filled by DNA polymerase.

In BER, the removal of a single modified base from one DNA strand is performed by DNA glycosylases, specialized enzymes. Some of these glycosylases show pronounced lesion specificity, others recognize multiple, and structurally different damaged bases. The apurinic/apyrimidinic (AP) site left behind after cleavage of the N-glycosylic bond is hydrolyzed by an AP endonuclease, and the 5'-deoxyribose phosphate is excised by a phosphodiesterase. The resulting single-nucleotide gap is then filled by polymerase β and ligated. Alternatives to this common BER pathway include the excision of a short oligonucleotide patch containing the AP site and filling of the gap by polymerase δ or ε. Base alterations caused by a large variety of agents and processes (e.g. spontaneous deamination, ionizing radiation, alkylating agents, DNA replication errors) are processed by BER. A common feature of the DNA lesions recognized by BER glycosylases is that they do not significantly distort the DNA helix (Yu, 2009).

Common single-nucleotide polymorphisms (SNPs) in the 8-oxoguanine glycosylase 1 (OGG1), X-ray repair cross-complementing group1 (XRCC1), and the apyrimidinic endonuclease-endonuclease 1 (APE1) genes in the BER pathway have been studied for their influences in induction of DNA damage (Chen et al., 2010).

XRCC1

X-ray repair cross-complementing group 1 (XRCC1) is required for repairing single-strand breaks and damaged bases in DNA. The XRCC1 protein interacts with DNA polymerase β, DNA ligase III and polyadenosine diphosphate-ribose polymerases (PARP) involved in excision and recombinational repair pathways (Cardecott, 2003). The XRCC1 has no known enzymatic activity (Thompson et al., 1990) and participates as a scaffold protein in both single-strand break repair and base excision repair activities. The human XRCC1 gene is located on chromosome 19q13.2 which contains 17 exons and encodes a protein of consisting 633 amino acids (Lindahl & Wood, 1999). More than 60 validated single-nucleotide XRCC1 polymorphisms are known. The most studied single nucleotide polymorphisms are Arg194Trp on exon 6, Arg280His on exon 9, and Arg399Gln on exon 10. All these polymorphisms were studied with association to different types of cancer.

The presences of the variant (399Gln and 194Trp) alleles have been shown to be associated with measurable reduced DNA repair capacity and increased risk of several types of cancers (Dufloth et al., 2005; Goode et al., 2002; Hu et al., 2005; Hung et al., 2005). In our study involving 43 patients with acute leukemia and 40 controls, for XRCC1 Arg194Trp and Arg399Gln polymorphism, we observed the relationship of XRCC1 polymorphisms with acute myeloid leukemia (our own unpublished data). Our cases with a codon 194 Trp/Trp homozygous variant as well as the heterozygous Arg/Trp variant had an increased risk of AML with a greater risk in the case of the homozygous codon 194 Trp/Trp allele (OR=2.28, 95% for Trp/Trp). There was a significantly high risk of AML among patients who were carriers of the variant allele 399Gln (OR=2.45, 95% for Gln/Gln and OR=1.90, 95% for Arg/Gln).

A study by Seedhouse et al. (2002) reported that the presence of at least one XRCC1 399Gln allele indicated a protective effect for the allele in controls compared with patients with AML, particularly therapy-related AML (t-AML) (odds ratio OR=0.44; 95% confidence interval CI=0.20~0.93). According to the same study patients who develop AML as a result of therapy for a primary malignancy are more likely to have the wild-type XRCC1 399 arginine allele. El-Din et al. (2010) reported that XRCC1 gene polymorphism is important in the pathogenesis of de novo AML. El-Din et al. (2010) observed that AML patients expressing XRCC1 Arg194Trp polymorphism are at high risk of developing AML; in addition, a significant risk in the development of AML was observed when XRCC1 Arg399Gln polymorphism was present. In a study of 372 patients with acute myeloid leukemia, Kuptsova et al. (2007) reported no significant associations between XRCC1 polymorphisms and treatment outcomes.

hOGG1

The human 8-oxoguanine DNA glycosylase 1 (hOGG1) encoded by the hOGG1 gene can remove 8-hydroxy-2-deoxyguanine (8-OHdG) from damaged DNA as a part of the base excision repair pathway (Kohno et al., 1998). The hOGG1 gene is located on chromosome 3p26.2 (Kohno et al., 1998). Although, several polymorphisms in the hOGG1 gene have been described, the most commonly studied polymorphism is an amino acid change from serine to cysteine at codon 326 (Ser326Cys). Several studies have reported that Ser326Cys polymorphism in OGG1 gene may increase susceptibility to for bladder (Arizono et al., 2008), lung (Park et al., 2004), oesophageal (Xing et al., 2001), gallbladder and gastric (Tsukino et al., 2004) cancer development.

Liddiard et al (2010) provided a study about the importance of 8-oxoguanine in AML including the genotyping of 174 AML patients for the hOGG1 Ser326Cys polymorphism. Using Affymetrix microarrays they showed that the prevalence rate of hOGG1 expression was 33% and correlated strongly with adverse cytogenetics. hOGG1-expressing patients had a worse relapse-free survival and overall survival and an increased risk of relapse at 5-years of follow-up. According to Liddiard et al. (2010) hOGG1 is an important prognostic marker that could be used to sub-stratify AML patients to predict those likely to fail conventional chemotherapies and those likely to benefit from novel therapeutic approaches that modulate DNA repair activity. In a recent study Stanczyk et al. (2011) have demonstrated that Cys/Cys variant of the OGG1 Ser326Cys polymorphism may increase the risk of ALL (OR=5.36, P<0.001).

APE1

The human apurinic/apyrimidinic endonuclease (APE1) plays a central role in the base excision repair pathway, which is the primary mechanism for the repair of DNA damage caused by oxidation and alkylation. The APE1 gene is located on chromosome 14q11.2–q12 and contains five exons. A total of 18 polymorphisms in APE1 have been reported, but the most extensively studied polymorphism is Asp148Glu (Gu et al., 2009). The damaged bases of purine and pyrimidine are recognized and excised by specific DNA glycosylases, leaving abasic sites. Apurinic/apyrimidinic endonuclease then incise the DNA 5' to the abasic sites; further repair proceeds to short-patch (when the gap is only one nucleotide) or long-patch (when the gap is two or more nucleotides) subpathways of base excision repair (Lo et al., 2009). In a hospital-based matched case-control study with 730 lung cancer cases and 730 cancer-free controls Lo et al. (2009) found that the -656T>G variant in the APE1 promoter was associated with a significantly decreased risk for lung cancer. In a study of 320 pediatric patients with acute leukemia, Krajinovic et al. (2002) reported no significant associations between polymorphic APE1 148Glu and XRCC1 194Trp variants and event-free survival. Ji et al. (2020) performed a meta-analysis to explore the association between the APE1 Asn148Glu gene polymorphisms and lung cancer risk. They suggested that the APE1 T1349G (Asp148Glu) polymorphism was not associated with lung cancer risk among Asians or Caucasians. But, the APE1 G allele was an increased risk factor for developing lung cancer among smokers. Pre-clinical and clinical data indicate a role for APE1 in the pathogenesis of cancer and in resistance to DNA-interactive drugs, particularly monofunctional alkylators and antimetabolites (Wilson & Simeonov, 2010).

2.3 Nucleotide Excision Repair

Nucleotide excision repair is the most studied DNA repair system in humans (de Laat et al., 1999). The NER pathway is responsible for repair of bulky distortions in the shape of the DNA double helix such as chemical adducts, pyrimidine dimers, and cross-links caused by endogenous and environmental lesions (Riedl et al., 2003; van der Wees et al., 2007; Wood, 1989). This pathway may also be important in conferring resistance to chemotherapeutic agents such as platinum-based chemotherapy (Kennedy & D'Andrea, 2006).

NER has five stages: recognition of the bulky damage which distorts the DNA helix; hydrolyzing a phosphodiester bond in the deoxyribose backbone on the 5' side of the lesion; excising the damage; filling in the resultant gap using the information from the complementary strand; closing the nicked DNA to generate intact strand (Yasbin, 2002).

NER can be divided into two subpathways (Transcription coupled NER and Global genomic NER) that differ only in their recognition of helix-distorting DNA damage (Hanawalt, 2002). Global genome repair is a slow process of inspecting the entire genome for damage (Kennedy & D'Andrea AD, 2006). Transcription-coupled repair is more rapid, highly specific and efficient and repairs DNA damage that blocks the progression of RNA polymerase II.

The actual repair mechanism appears to be identical in transcription-coupled and in global-genome repair. However, the damage recognition in global-genome repair does not involve the RNA polymerase, but is performed by the XPC and HHR23 proteins. Following lesion recognition, however, both repair systems use TFIIH components such as XPB and XPD, as well as the single-strand binding protein RPA and the XPA protein to fully unwind and mark the lesion. The damaged segment of DNA is excised through 5'-incision by the XPF endonuclease and 3'-incision by the XPG endonuclease. The DNA gap is filled by DNA polymerases δ or ε supported by PCNA and sealed by a DNA ligase, presumably DNA ligase I (Kennedy & D'Andrea, 2006; Yu et al., 1999).

XPD

The XPD gene (xeroderma pigmentosum group D, also known as ERCC2) encodes a DNA helicase involved in nucleotide excision repair pathway. The XPD gene maps to chromosome 19q13.3 and consists of 23 exons (Wang et al., 2008). Its protein is 761 amino acids in length. The XPD protein repairs a wide range of structurally unrelated lesions, such as bulky adducts and thymidine dimers (Braithwaite et al., 1999). The DNA repair process and gene transcription are coupled via activity of the TFIIH complex, a protein complex with functions including transcription, NER, transcription-coupled repair, apoptosis, and cell cycle regulation. XPD protein is involved in maintaining the stability of the TFIIH complex. The XPD gene product has an ATP-dependent DNA helicase activity (Laine et al, 2007).

Because of the biological significance of XPD, the XPD Lys751Gln (2251A>C) polymorphism has been a common subject of studies in different malignant diseases in the last years. Although the XPD 751Gln variant was associated with an increased risk of esophageal cancer and acute lymphoid leukemia (Wang et al., 2008) Allan et al. (2004) investigated XPD Lys751Gln polymorphism in 341 adult British AML patients and observed that the XPD codon 751 polymorphism is an independent prognostic marker for disease-free survival and overall survival in elderly AML patients treated with chemotherapy, and specifically that the glutamine variant was associated with a poorer prognosis relative to the lysine variant. In a pediatric study, Mehta et al. (2006) found no influence of XPD751 genotype on susceptibility to de novo AML in children. In another study, Kuptsova-Clarkson et al. (2010)

evaluated the role of XPD and XRCC1 gene polymorphic variation in response to induction chemotherapy, toxicities and survival in a population of 293 predominantly Caucasian adult patients treated for AML. Kuptsova-Clarkson et al. (2010) had reported that in AML, variation in the XPD gene may be associated with suboptimal DNA repair activity and may thus predispose to therapy-related AML development. In a UK study by Seedhouse et al. (2002), therapy-related AML was not associated with XPD genotypes.

There have been studies of XPD, involved in NER, and survival of patients with AML (Allan et al., 2004). In a study of elderly patients with AML conducted by researchers in the United Kingdom, modestly increased hazard ratio (HR) of 1.30 and 1.19 were found for disease-free and overall survival, respectively, by XPD variant genotypes. However, in a study of pediatric patients with acute myeloid leukemia conducted by the the Children's Oncology Group (Mehta et al., 2006) survival and treatment-related mortality were not associated with XPD codon 751 genotypes.

2.4 Mismatch repair

DNA mismatch repair (MMR) plays a critical role in maintaining genomic integrity. MMR is responsible for correction of mismatched basepairs which occurs through processes including misincorporations during DNA replication, formation of heteroduplexes, and secondary structure such as imperfect palindromes (Bishop et al., 1985).

In addition, MMR can also process some types of DNA damage. MMR deficient tumors display widespread alterations in simple repetitive DNA sequences, a phenomenon also called microsatellite instability; MSI (Li, 2008). The repair mechanism is similar to that of excision repair; a patch of nucleotides is removed from one strand, and followed by resynthesis and ligation processes.

There are two types of mismatch repair, long-patch and short-patch which have been found in human cells. In short-patch repair system there are three enzymes possessing nicking activities specific for mismatch repair; T/G specific (Wiebauer & Jiricny, 1989), A/G specific, and all type mismatch nicking enzymes (Yeh et al., 1991). That enzymes have different mode of action, but in either an A/G mismatch or a T/G mismatch, it is usually the guanine that remains untouched by mismatch specific glycosylases (Wiebauer & Jiricny, 1989).

Long patch can repair all types of mismatches. Long-patch MMR removes a patch of one of the DNA strands from an incision on the to-be-removed strand to 90~170 nucleotides beyond the mismatch (Fang & Modrich, 1993; Yu et al., 1999).

Defects in the MMR pathway significantly increase the mutation frequency and promote oncogenesis. It has been documented that defects in MMR genes, are the genetic basis for certain types of hereditary and sporadic cancers, including hereditary nonpolyposis colorectal cancer (Mao et al., 2008). There are some studies looking at the incidence of MMR deficiency (microsatellite instability; MSI) in AML (Mao et al., 2008). Genomic instability in AML has led to a search for MSI in AML patients, but the results are quite controversial. While several studies have reported MSI in AML (Das-Gupta et al., 2001; Sheikhha et al., 2002), a study of 132 cases failed to confirm the previous results (Rimsza et al., 2000). According to Rimsza et al. (2000) MMR deficiency was associated with all stages of AML, but the rate of the deficiency was much higher in patients with refractory and relapsed AML than in de novo AML patients, suggesting that the loss of MMR function could contribute to the refractory and relapsed disease.

2.5 Double Strand Break repair

Double strand break repair (DSB) is responsible for the repair of double strand DNA breaks. DNA double strand breaks represent the most important class of DNA damage because, if unrepaired, they can result in a loss of genetic material, chromosome abnormalities and possibly cell death. Moreover, the breaks are prone to nuclease attack with subsequent destruction (Rufer & Morgan, 1992). Double strand breaks (DSBs) can be produced by exogenous agents such as ionizing radiation, some chemotherapeutic drugs, endogenous formed reactive oxygen species. When DNA replication forks encounter DNA single strand breaks or other types of lesion, it might result in formation of DSBs. In addition, DSBs are generated to initiate recombination between homologues chromosomes during meiosis, and also during the immunoglobulin class-switch recombination. Repair of DSBs is more difficult than other type of DNA damage because there is no undamaged template available (Khanna & Jackson, 2001).

Direct DSBs are mainly repaired by non-homologous end joining (Sargent et al., 1997), whereas replication-associated DSBs are repaired by homologous recombination (HR) and related replication repair pathways (Iliakis et al., 2004).

2.5.1 Non-homologous End Joining

Non homologous end joining (NHEJ) is active in all phases of the cell cycle and is considered to be the most important DSB repair pathway in mammalian cells. The NHEJ pathway is simpler than HR and requires no complementary template. The protein components of NHEJ include the catalytic subunit of DNA protein kinase (DNA-PKCS), the two regulatory subunits of the DNA-PK complex Ku70 and Ku80, DNA ligase IV with its cofactor XRCC4 (the X-ray cross complementing group 4 protein) and the nuclease artemis (Drouet et al., 2005; Khanna & Jackson, 2001). The Ku70/Ku80 (Ku) heterodimer is the first protein to bind to the damaged DNA ends. When bound to the DSB, Ku recruits and activates DNA-PKcs. These proteins play an important role in DNA DSB repair and will act as tumor suppressors. However, either the DNA protein kinase complex, or its three subunits individually, can also act as oncogenes, depending on the compartment of the cell in which they are expressed and on the cell cycle phase (Gullo et al., 2006).

XRCC4

The X-ray cross-complementing group 4 (XRCC4) gene is one of the specific members of the NHEJ system. Some of the SNPs of XRCC4 have been found to be associated with the susceptibility to different types of cancer. Two single nucleotide polymorphisms (SNPs) of XRCC4, one splicing-site polymorphism (SNP14 rs1805377:A4G) and one intronic polymorphism (SNP1 rs2075685:G4T), have been studied, and the results are conflicting (Allen-Brady et al., 2006; Fu et al., 2003). The protein encoded by XRCC4 consists of 336 amino acid residues distributed among 8 exons, and has a long helical stem domain responsible for multimerization and interaction with DNA ligase IV (Junop et al., 2000). By forming a complex with DNA ligase IV and DNA-dependent protein kinase, XRCC4 functions in the repair of DNA double-strand breaks by non-homologous end joining (NHEJ) and the completion of V(D)J recombination events (Hayden et al, 2007). The NHEJ pathway is required not only for normal development but also for suppression of tumors. Since it is one of the ubiquitous NHEJ components, XRCC4 might be considered as a potential tumor suppressor gene in cancer and leukemia.

There have been several studies showing that variations of the XRCC4 gene are associated with prostate (Chang et al., 2008), gastric (Chiu et al., 2008), and breast cancer (Fu et al., 2003). Therefore, XRCC4 and the DNA double-strand break repair pathway may serve as a common mechanism of early carcinogenesis. In a recent study, Wu et al. (2008) investigated the association between XRCC4 gene polymorphisms and oral cancer. Their findings suggest that the presence of the A allele of XRCC4 codon 247 was associated with a higher susceptibility to oral cancer, and the A allele of XRCC4 codon 247 may be a useful novel marker in oral oncology for primary prevention and intervention.

XRCC5, XRCC6, XRCC7

A key component of the NHEJ pathway is the DNA-dependent Protein Kinase (DNA-PK), which consists of a heterodimeric DNA targeting subunit (i.e., Ku70/Ku80, encoded by XRCC6/XRCC5 genes) and a catalytic subunit DNA-PKcs, encoded by XRCC7 gene (Smith & Jackson, 1999).

XRCC5 (X-ray repair cross-complementing 5) is a gene involved in repair of DNA double-strand breaks. Abnormal expression of the XRCC5 protein is associated with genomic instability and an increased incidence of cancers. The XRCC5 gene mapped to chromosome 2q35, encodes the 80-kDa subunit of the Ku heterodimer protein, the DNA-binding component of the DNA-dependent protein kinase. The Ku80 is essential for maintaining genomic integrity through its ability to bind DNA double-strand breaks and to facilitate repair by the nonhomologous end-joining pathway in mammalian cells (Taccioli et al., 1994).

XRCC6 (X-ray repair complementing defective repair in Chinese hamster cells 6) is a helicase involved in DNA repair and chromatin remodeling. The XRCC6 gene (also called Ku70) maps to chromosome 22q13.2-q1. Ku70 plays an important role in the DNA double-strand breaks repair and maintenance of genomic integrity. Genetic variations within human Ku70 have been demonstrated to be associated with increased risk of several types of cancers (Wenshan et al., 2011).

XRCC7 (X-ray repair cross complementing group 7) is located on chromosome 8q12, span about 110-180 kb and contains 100 exons. The human XRCC7 gene encodes DNA-PKcs, which is recruited to the site of DSBs by the Ku70/Ku80 heterodimer to form an active DNA-PK complex (Sipley et al., 1995). The expression of Ku70 and XRCC7 is elevated in bladder tumor tissue and head and neck cancer cell lines, respectively (Stronati et al., 2001; Sturgis et al., 1999) and Ku70 may function as a caretaker gene for the development of T-cell lymphomas (Li et al., 1998). XRCC7 encodes DNA-PKcs, which also may have a caretaker role in colon carcinogenesis. Therefore, the variants of the Ku70 and XRCC7 genes could be expected to have an effect on DSB repair, and thus, on carcinogenesis. The Ku70 polymorphism is associated with risk of breast cancer (Fu et al., 2003), and the XRCC7 polymorphism is associated with risk of glioma (Wang et al., 2004). According to Wang et al. (2008) the XRCC7 polymorphism appears to be involved in the etiology of human bladder cancer. This data support the notion that the XRCC7 polymorphism is implicated in cancer risk.

Given the crucial roles of the NHEJ pathway in DNA repair (Gullo et al., 2006), it is possible that the XRCC5, XRCC6 and XRCC7 variants may modulate the risk of cancer, including leukemia. It has been shown that increased NHEJ activity is due to the presence of XRCC5 and XRCC6 protein, which results in genomic instability in myeloid leukemia cells (Gaymes et al., 2002). XRCC5 and XRCC6 may function as a caretaker gene for the development of T-cell lymphomas, while XRCC7 may have a caretaker role in colon carcinogenesis (Wang et al., 2009). In a recent study, Wang et al. (2009) have investigated the association between the X-ray repair cross complementing group XRCC5, XRCC6 and XRCC7 polymorphisms and risk of AML in Chinese population. In this case-control study in a southern Chinese population three polymorphisms, XRCC5 2R/1R/0R, XRCC6 -61C>G and XRCC7 6721G>T were investigated. For the XRCC7 6721G>T polymorphism among AML cases and controls no significant association was observed (P=0.68). Significant association was observed (P=0.04) for the XRCC6 -61C > G polymorphism. Their analysis revealed that compared with the XRCC6 -61CC wild type homozygote, the -61CG heterozygotes had a significant 43% decreased risk of AML (adjusted OR=0.57; 95% CI=0.35~0.92) and subjects carrying -61CG/GG variant genotypes had 45% decrease in risk of AML (adjusted OR=0.55; 95% CI=0.34~0.89). For the XRCC5 2R/1R/0R polymorphism, Wang et al. (2009) found that XRRC5 1R/0R genotype was associated with a 2.60-fold increase in risk of AML (95% CI=1.42~5.92) compared with the 2R/2R genotype. They found a significant association with the polymorphisms of XRCC5 2R/1R/0R, XRCC6 -61C>G and the risk of AML, but there was no evidence for an association between the XRCC7 6721G>T variants and AML.

2.5.2 Homologous recombination

Homologous recombination (HR) is one of the main pathways for the repair of DNA double strand breaks (DSBs). HR is thought to be particularly important in DNA repair occurring during cellular replication (Rollinson et al., 2007). Although HR is indispensable for maintaining genome integrity, it must be tightly regulated to avoid harmful outcomes. The repair process is complex and involves many proteins working coordinately. Key players include MRE11, RAD50, NBS1 (MRN), RAD51, RAD51B, RAD51C, RAD51D, XRCC2, XRCC3, RAD52, RAD54 and BRCA2 (Lieberman, 2008). A number of polymorphic genes involved in this pathway have been studied in AML.

Homologous recombination mechanism starts with degradation of the DNA next to the double-strand break, leaving single-strand ends. Next the single-strand end of the damaged strand invades and binds to its complementary DNA sequence on the homologous duplex. This is associated with the displacement of the cross-complementary strand toward the gap site, where it serves as a template for gap-filling DNA synthesis. The repair sequence is terminated by religation of the repair patches. This mechanism requires the presence of undamaged homologous DNA, and increased activity of this repair pathway has been observed.

RAD51 protein catalyzes homologous recombination through its homologous pairing and strand exchange activities. RAD52 may modulate these activities through its RAD51-interacting region. The ability of RAD52 to induce homologous recombination requires its binding to the p34 subunit of RPA. This RPA binding domain is at amino acids 221–280. Recall that RPA is also involved in NER—this may provide a linkage between these two repair systems (Yu Z et al., 1999).

XRRC3

The X-ray repair cross-complementing group 3 (XRCC3), codes for a protein participating in homologous recombination repair of DNA double-strand breaks. XRCC3 is a member of the RAD-51-related protein family. RAD-51-like proteins are known to participate in homologous recombination to maintain chromosome stability and repair DNA damage (Brenneman et al., 2000). XRCC3-deficient cells demonstrated genetic instability and increased sensitivity to DNA damaging agents (Griffin, 2002). The human XRCC3 gene is located on chromosome 14q32.3 and consists of 17870 bases. The protein product of XRCC3 gene contains 346 amino acids. According to NCBI SNP database, XRCC3 gene has 111 SNPs. The main polymorphism in this gene involves the change of threonine (Thr) to methionine (Met) at codon 241 in exon 7 (Shen et al., 1998). Little is known about the functional consequences of this variation, although some studies observed a positive relation between the Thr241Met polymorphism and an increased risk for skin (Winsey et al., 2000), bladder (Matullo et al., 2001), breast (Garcia-Closas et al., 2006) and lung (Jacobsen et al., 2004) cancers.

A meta-analysis of 48 case-control studies, including 24975 cancer patients and 34209 controls, investigated the associations of the three DNA repair gene XRCC3 polymorphisms (Thr241Met; 4541A4G; 17893A4G) with cancer risk (Han et al., 2006). According to this meta-analysis individuals carrying the XRCC3 Met/Met genotype have a smaller cancer risk compared with the individuals with the Thr/Thr or Thr/Met genotype (OR=1.07; P=0.008; 95% CI=1.02~1.13) (Han et al., 2006). For A4541G, a significantly increased risk was associated with the variant genotypes (G/G+A/G), compared with the wild homozygote A/A genotype (OR=1.09; P=0.004; 95% CI, 1.03~1.15). For A17893G, individuals with the variant genotypes (G/G+A/G) had a significantly decreased cancer risk, compared with individuals with the A/A genotype under a dominant genetic model (OR=0.92; P=0.0004; 95% CI=0.87~0.96). Han et al. (2006) consider that the XRCC3 could not be a major increased risk factor for cancer but it might represent a low-penetrance susceptible gene especially for cancer of breast, bladder, head and neck, and non-melanoma skin cancer

In their study Seedhouse et al. (2004) have observed that the presence of variant XRCC3 241Met was associated with an increase in the risk of developing therapy-related AML of more than 8 fold, whereas the increase in risk for the development of de novo AML was nearly 4 fold.

RAD 51

The RAD51 gene plays an important role in homologous recombination and in maintaining the genetic stability of the cell. In HR, RAD51 interacts with and is stabilized by XRCC3, during strand invasion and cross-strand resolution. RAD51 is a central protein in the HR repair pathway binding to DNA and promoting ATP-dependent homologous pairing and strand transfer reactions.

The RAD51 gene is located on chromosome 15q15.1 and consists of 36998 bases. The protein product of RAD51 has 6 domains, one for DNA binding, one for ATPase activity, and the other domains are specific to action of RAD51. According to NCBI SNP database, RAD51 gene has 296 SNPs. The most important polymorphism identified for RAD51 is G135C SNP in 5′ untranslated region. The RAD51 G135C polymorphism is associated with RAD51 protein over-expression (Richardson et al., 2004). Regarding the role of RAD51 in the homologous DNA repair mechanism, several studies have examined the relationship between RAD51 G135C polymorphism and risk of certain cancers. However the results from these studies are conflicting. Further studies are needed to establish the role of RAD51 G135C polymorphism in human carcinogenesis.

Voso et al. (2007) found an increased frequency of the RAD51 135C allele in AML, mainly in de novo AML, when compared with controls, but not between therapy-related AML (t-AML) and controls. Other reports found increased frequency of the RAD51 135C allele in

t-AML patients compared with controls (Seedhouse et al., 2004), suggesting an effect of RAD51 over-expression during leukemogenesis induced by chemotherapy or radiotherapy.
According to Bhatla et al. (2008) RAD51 gene polymorphism did not influence the outcome of AML therapy in the study of de novo AML patients. On the contrary, Liu et al. (2008) concluded that RAD51 gene polymorphism was significantly related to response to therapy, adverse effects, and prognosis of AML and reported that detection of the RAD51 gene polymorphism genotypes may be useful in selecting individual chemotherapy regimens for patients with AML. Also, Bolufer et al. (2007) reported that the RAD51 gene polymorphism showed significant unfavorable outcome among AML patients.
In their study, Bathla et al. (2008) observed a doubling of risk of AML in children with a RAD51 G135C variant allele and a wild-type XRCC3 Thre241Met genotype. In addition risk of AML was significantly increased in children with at least one variant XRCC3 Thr241Met allele. In antithesis, risk was not significantly elevated in children with variant alleles at both wild-type XRCC3 Thre241Met and RAD51 G135C. Liu et al. (2008) found that XRCC3 gene polymorphism was significantly related to response to therapy and prognosis of AML and reported that detection of the XRCC3 gene polymorphism genotypes may be useful in selecting individual chemotherapy regimens for AML patients.

2.6 Translesion synthesis

Translesion synthesis is an important mechanism by which cells replicate past DNA damage. The sliding clamp DNA polymerase processivity factors play a central role in this process. The clamps are dimeric in bacteria and trimeric in eukaryotes and archaea, raising the question of whether more than one polymerase can interact with the clamp simultaneously (Lehmann, 2006).

3. Inherited human disease with leukemia susceptibility

Several studies have demonstrated that the genes involved in DNA repair and maintenance of genome integrity are critically in protecting against mutations that lead to cancer and/or inherited human disease (Table 2).

Syndrome	Gene(s) involved	Chromosome	References
Fanconi anaemia (FA)	FANC-A to FANC-N	16q24.3	Levitus et al., 2004; Steensma, 2007;
Ataxia-telangiectasia (AT)	Ataxia-telangiectasia (AT)	11q22.3	Savitsky et al., 1995; Thompson & Schild, 2002
Nijmegen breakage syndrome (NBS)	NBS1 (Nibrin)	8p21	Digweed et al., 1999; Varon et al. 2003
Bloom syndrome (BLM)	BLM (RECQL3)	15q26.1	Ellis & German, 1996; Thompson & Schild, 2002
Seckel Syndrome	ATR	3q22-24	Casper et al., 2002;

Table 2. DNA repair defective syndromes

Several of these diseases include an inherent predisposition to hematologic malignancies, including AML. The clinical features and molecular characteristics of several of the inherited disorders with leukemia risk are described below.

Fanconi anemia (FA) is a rare disorder with a birth incidence around 3 per million. FA is an autosomal recessive and rarely X-linked syndrome which is characterised by congenital abnormalities, defective haemopoiesis (bone marrow failure) and a high risk of developing AML and certain solid tumours.

Affected individuals can have mild growth retardation, hypo- or hyperpigmented areas of the skin, skeletal defects including radial limb defects (absent thumb with or without radial aplasia), abnormalities of ribs and hips and scoliosis, cardiac and renal malformations, genital abnormalities (especially undescended testes, testicular agenesis, hypospadias). Other associated anomalies include micropthalmia and developmental delay (Grompe & D'Andrea, 2001). The phenotypic abnormalities are variable and there is marked variability between affected individuals in the same family (Alter, 1993).

The Fanconi anemia defect results from biallelic mutation of any one of thirteen known Fanconi anemia genes (A, B, C, D1, D2, E, F, G, I, J, L, M, N). The proteins encoded by these Fanconi anemia genes cooperate in a common DNA repair pathway, referred to as the Fanconi anemia /BRCA pathway. In this pathway, eight of the Fanconi anemia proteins (A, B, C, E, F, G, L, M) are assembled into a core complex that functions as an E3 ubiquitin ligase. This ligase activates in response to DNA damage from a crosslinking drug, adding a 76-amino acid moiety onto two other Fanconi proteins, D2 and I. This monoubiquinated D2/I complex is translocated into chromatin, where it interacts with the downstream Fanconi proteins BRCA2, N, and J. This combination of proteins mediates the DNA repair process. After the repair has occurred, there is another enzyme complex, called USP1, which removes the ubiquitin and inactivates the pathway. Knocking out any of the proteins in this pathway causes FA (D'Andrea, 2010).

FANCA, located on chromosome 16q24.3, is the most commonly mutated gene and is altered in 60-65% of FA patients (Steensma, 2007). FANCC and G mutations account for almost 25%, and FANCE and FANCF for a further 8%.

Approximately one third of patients homozygous for a Fanconi anemia gene mutation will develop a hematologic or solid tumors by the age of 40 years (Kennedy & D'Andrea, 2006). Fanconi anemia patients develop predominately myeloid malignancies (the most common hematologic maliganancy is AML), although numerous other cancers arise, including squamous cell carcinomas of the head and neck or gynecologic system, skin cancers, esophageal cancers and liver tumors (Alter, 2003; Rosenberg et al, 2008).

Fanconi anemia patients have a systemic DNA repair defect that results in a low tolerance for DNA damaging chemotherapeutic agents.

Ataxia-telangiectasia (AT) is a rare autosomal recessive disorder. This human disease is characterized by cerebellar degeneration, immunodeficiency, hypogonadism, growth retardation, genome instability, extreme sensitivity to radiation and predisposition to cancer (Taylor & Byrd, 2005). The disease is caused by homozygous mutations in the gene encoding the ATM protein kinase that plays a critical role in DNA damage detection and regulates DNA double-strand break repair (Mavrou et al, 2008). The ATM gene is located on chromosome 11q23. When ATM is dysfunctional or absent, cells are able to progress from G1 to S phase and initiate DNA replication in the presence of DNA damage.

Approximately one third of AT patients develop cancer, mainly leukemias and lymphomas which develop in childhood and are a common cause of death (Ball & Xiao, 2005; Gumy-Pause et al, 2004). Solid tumors in AT patients are usually adenocarcinoma of the stomach, dysgerminoma, gonadoblastoma and medulloblastoma (Mavrou et al, 2008).

Bloom's syndrome (BS) is a rare autosomal recessive syndrome of growth retardation, telangiectasia manifest by facial erythema, immunodeficiency, and skull abnormalities. BS patients also are predisposed to cancer, as they develop mostly leukemias and lymphomas in about half of the patients. This disorder is most commonly found in the Ashkenazi Jewish population resulting from a founder mutation (Ellis et al, 1998). It is characterised by low birth weight, growth deficiency, characteristic facies (long thin face, prominent nose) sun-sensitivity, immunodeficiency and infertility in males.

Bloom's syndrome arise through mutations in both copies of the BLM gene, which is located on chromosome 15 at 15q26.1. This gene encodes a member of the RecQ family of DNA helicases (BLM) that is important in maintaining appropriate DNA conformation during chromosomal recombination and repair. Together with topoisomerase III, BLM resolves Holliday junctions during homologous recombination (HR) by a mechanism called double-junction dissolution that is distinct from classical Holliday junction resolution and that prevents erroneous exchange of flanking sequences (Steensma, 2007).

Nijmegen breakage syndrome (NBS) is an autosomal recessive disorder that is most commonly found in Eastern Europe. NBS is caused by abnormalities in the NBN gene at 8p21 (Varon et al, 2003), which encodes the protein NBN (NBS1). Complete loss of this polypeptide is lethal. The NBS gene encodes a 95-kDa protein that binds with MRE11 and RAD50 to form a nuclease-containing protein complex that appears to be involved in homologous and nonhomologous recombination. Clinical features include growth retardation, microcephaly, skin findings such as vitiligo and café au lait spots, skeletal defects, immunodeficiency and propensity to infection. Radiation hypersensitivity is a hallmark of the disease, along with a predisposition to cancer, most notably lymphomas (Digweed et al, 1999). The most common cause of death for NBS patients is neoplasia (Steensma, 2007). Although the predominant neoplasm is lymphoma, both lymphoid and myeloid leukemia have been reported (Resnick et al, 2002).

Seckel syndrome (SCKL) is a rare autosomal recessive disorder associated with short stature, prenatal and postnatal growth retardation, characteristic craniofacial dysmorphism (bird-headed face including prominent beaked nose, micrognathia and malformed ears), mental deficiency, microcephaly, and skeletal defects (Faivre et al, 2002). Hematological abnormalities, including pancytopenia, myelodysplasia and acute myeloid leukemia, have been reported in some patients with Seckel syndrome (Chanan-Khan et al, 2003; Hayani et al,1994). A gene for Seckel syndrome was mapped on chromosome 3q22.1-q24. The ataxia-telancgiectasia and RAD3-related (ATR) gene is mutated in Seckel syndrome, and encodes an phosphotidylinositol-3-kinase-like kinase which has distinct, but overlapping functions with ATM in co-ordinating the response to DNA damage. ATR is activated by single stranded DNA whilst ATM responds to DNA double strand breaks (Casper et al, 2002; Steensma, 2007).

4. Conclusion

Genetic variations in genes involved in DNA repair may influence both cancer susceptibility and treatment response. However, in AML, the relevance of these genetic variations remains to be fully established. There is evidence that some polymorphisms in DNA repair genes play a role in carcinogenesis, notably hOGG1 Ser326Cys, XRCC1 Arg194Trp, XRCC3 Thr241Met, RAD51 G135C and XPD Lys751Gln. Additional studies of these and other DNA repair polymorphisms will provide essential information about the relationships between the DNA repair mechanisms and risk of AML.

5. Acknowledgement

This paper is partly supported by the Sectorial operational programme human resources development (SOP HRD), financed from the European social Fund and by the Romanian Government under the contract number POSDRU 60782.

6. References

Allan JM, Smith AG, Wheatley K, Hills RK, Travis LB, Hill DA, Swirsky DM, Morgan GJ, Wild CP. (2004). Genetic variation in XPD predicts treatment outcome and risk of acute myeloid leukemia following chemotherapy. *Blood*, Vol.104 (December 2004), pp. 3872–3877, ISSN: 1528-0020

Allen-Brady K, Cannon-Albright LA, Neuhausen SL, Camp NJ. (2006). A role for XRCC4 in age at diagnosis and breast cancer risk. *Cancer Epidemiol Biomarkers Prev*, Vol.15, No.7 (July 2006), pp. 1306–1310, ISSN: 1538-7755

Alter BP. (1993). Fanconi's anaemia and its variability. *Br J Haematol*, Vol.85, No.1 (1993 Sep), pp.9-14, ISSN: 1365-2141.

Alter BP. (2003). Cancer in Fanconi anemia, 1927-2001. *Cancer*, Vol. 97, No. 2 (January 2003), pp.425-440, ISSN: 1097-0142.

Arizono K, Osada Y, Kuroda Y. (2008). DNA repair gene hOGG1codon 326 and XRCC1 codon 399 polymorphisms and bladder cancer risk in a Japanese population. *Jpn J Clin Oncol*, Vol.38, No.3 (February 2008) pp.186–191, ISSN: 1465-3621

Ball LG, Xiao W. (2005). Molecular basis of ataxia telangiectasia and related diseases. *Acta Parmacologica Sinica*, Vol. 26, No.8 (August 2005), pp.897-907, ISSN: 1745-7254.

Bhatla D, Gerbing R, Alonzo T. (2008). DNA repair polymorphisms and outcome of chemotherapy for acute myelogenous leukemia: a report from the Children's Oncology Group. *Leukemia*, Vol.22, No.2 (February 2008), pp. 265–272, ISSN: 0887-6924

Bishop JO, Selman GG, Hickman J, Black L, Saunders RD, Clark AJ. (1985) The 45-kb unit of major urinary protein gene organization is a gigantic imperfect palindrome. *Mol Cell Biol*, Vol.5, No.7 (July 1985), pp.1591–1600, ISSN: 1098-5549

Bolufer P, Collado M, Barragán E, Cervera J, Calasanz MJ, Colomer D, Roman-Gómez J, Sanz MA. (2007). The potential effect of gender in combination with common genetic polymorphisms of drug-metabolizing enzymes on the risk of developing acute leukemia. *Haematologica*, Vol.92, No.3 (March 2007), pp. 308–314, ISSN: 1592-8721

Braithwaite E, Wu X, Wang Z.(1999). Repair of DNA lesions: mechanisms and relative repair efficiencies. *Mutat Res*, Vol. 424, No.1-2 (1999 Mar 8), pp.207–219, ISSN: 0027-5107

Brenneman MA, Weiss AE, Nickoloff JA, Chenet DJ. (2000). XRCC3 is required for efficient repair of chromosome breaks by homologous recombination. *Mutat Res*, Vol.459, No.2 (March 2000), pp. 89–97, ISSN: 1568-7864

Burma S, Chen BP, Chen DJ. (2006). Role of non-homologous end joining (NHEJ) in maintaining genomic integrity. *DNA Repair*, Vol.5, No.9-10 (September 2006), pp. 1042-1048, ISSN: 1568-7864

Cardecott KW.(2003). XRCC1 and DNA stand break repair. *DNA Repair*, Vol.2, No.9 (September 2003), pp. 955–969, ISSN: 1568-7864

Casper AM, Nghiem P, Arlt MF, Glover TW. (2002). ATR regulates fragile site stability. *Cell*, Vol.111, No.6 (December 2002), pp.779–789.

Chanan-Khan A, Holkova B, Perle MA, Reich E, Wu CD, Inghirami G, Takeshita K. (2003). T-cell clonality and myelodysplasia without chromosomal fragility in a patient with features of Seckel syndrome. *Haematologica*, Vol.88, No. 5 (May 2003), ECR14, ISSN: 1592-8721.

Chang CH, Chiu CF, Wu HC, Tseng HC, Wang CH, Lin CC, Tsai CW, Liang SY, Wang CL, Bau DT. (2008). Significant association of XRCC4 single nucleotide polymorphisms with prostate cancer susceptibility in Taiwanese males. *Mol Med Report*, Vol.1, No.4 (July 2008), pp.525–30, ISSN: 1791-3004

Chen PL, Yeh KT, Tsai YY, Koeh H, Liu YL, Lee H, Cheng YW. (2010). XRCC1, but not APE1 and hOGG1 gene polymorphisms is a risk factor for pterygium. *Mol Vis*, Vol.16 (June 2010), pp.991-996.

Chiu CF, Wang CH, Wang CL, Lin CC, Hsu NY, Weng JR, Bau DT. (2008). A novel single nucleotide polymorphism in XRCC4 gene is associated with gastric cancer susceptibility in Taiwan. *Ann Surg Oncol*, Vol.15, No.2 (February 2008), pp.514–518, ISSN: 1534-4681

D'Andrea AD. Targeting DNA repair pathways in AML. (2010). *Best Pract Res Clin Haematol*, Vol.23, No.4 (December 2010), pp.469–73, ISSN: 1521-6926

Das-Gupta EP, Seedhouse CH, Russell NH. (2001). Microsatellite instability occurs in defined subsets of patients with acute myeloblastic leukaemia. *Br J Haematol*, Vol.114, No.2 (August 2001), pp.307–312.

de Laat W L, Jaspers N G, Hoeijmakers J H.(1999). Molecular mechanism of nucleotide excision repair. *Genes & Dev*, Vol.13, pp.768–785, ISSN: 1549-5477

Digweed M, Reis A, Sperling K. (1999). Nijmegen breakage syndrome: consequences of defective DNA double strand break repair. *BioEssays*, Vol.21, No.8 (August 1999), pp.649–656, ISSN: 1521-1878

Drouet J, Delteil C, Lefrançois J, Concannon P, Salles B, Calsou P. (2005). DNA-dependent protein kinase and XRCC4-DNA ligase IV mobilization in the cell in response to DNA double strand breaks. *J Biol Chem*, Vol.280, No.8 (February 2005), pp.7060–7069, ISSN: 1521-1878

Dufloth RM, Costa S, Schmitt F, Zeferino LC. (2005). DNA repair gene polymorphisms and susceptibility to familial breast cancer in a group of patients from Campinas, Brazil. *Genet Mol Res*, Vol.4, No.4 (Decembrie 2005), pp.771–782.

El-Din M, Raslan H, Abdel-Hamid S, Makhlouf M. (2010). Detection of XRCC1 gene polymorphisms in Egyptian patients with acute myeloid leukemia. *Comparative Clinical Pathology* (November 2010), 1–9

Ellis NA, Ciocci S, Proytcheva M, Lennon D, Groden J, German I. (1998). The Ashkenazic Jewish Bloom syndrome mutation blmAsh is present in non-Jewish Americans of Spanish ancestry. *Am J Hum Genet*, Vol. 63, No. 6 (December 1998), pp.1685-1693, ISSN: 0002-9297.

Ellis NA, German J. (1996). Molecular genetics of Bloom's syndrome. *Hum Mol Genet*, Vol.5 Spec, pp.1457–1463, ISSN: 1460-208

Faivre L, Le Merrer M, Lyonnet S, Plauchu H, Dagoneau N, Campos-Xavier AB, Attia-Sobol J, Verloes A, Munnich A, Cormier-Daire V. (2002). Clinical and genetic heterogeneity of Seckel syndrome. *Am J Med Genet*, Vol.112, No.4 (November 2002), pp.379-83, ISSN: 1552-4833.

Fang WH, Modrich P. (1993). Human strand-specific mismatch repair occurs by a bidirectional mechanism similar to that of the bacterial reaction. J Biol Chem, Vol.268, (June 1993), pp.11838 –11844, ISSN: 1083-351X

Fu YP, Yu JC, Cheng TC, Lou MA, Hsu GC, Wu CY, Chen ST, Wu HS, Wu PE, Shen CY. (2003). Breast cancer risk associated with genotypic polymorphism of the nonhomologous end-joining genes: a multigenic study on cancer susceptibility. *Cancer Res*, Vol.63 (May 2003), pp.2440–2446, ISSN: 1538-7445

Garcia-Closas M, Egan KM, Newcomb PA, Brinton LA, Titus-Ernstoff L, Chanock S, Welch R, Lissowska J, Peplonska B, Szeszenia-Dabrowska N, Zatonski W, Bardin-Mikolajczak A, Struewing JP. (2006). Polymorphisms in DNA double-strand break repair genes and risk of breast cancer: two population-based studies in USA and Poland, and meta-analyses. *Hum Genet*, Vol.119, No.4 (May2006), pp.376–88, ISSN: 0014-4266

Gaymes TJ, Mufti GJ, Rassool FV. (2002). Myeloid leukemias have increased activity of the nonhomologous end-joining pathway and concomitant DNA misrepair that is dependent on the Ku70/86 heterodimer. *Cancer Res*, Vol.62, No.10 (May 2002), pp.2791–2797, ISSN: 1538-7445

Gerson SL, Trey JE. 1988. Modulation of nitrosourea resistance in myeloid leukemias. *Blood*, Vol.71, No.5 (May 1988), pp.1487–1494, ISSN: 1528-0020

Goode EL, Ulrich CM, Potter JD. (2002). Polymorphisms in DNA repair genes and associations with cancer risk. *Cancer Epidemiol Biomarkers Prev*, Vol.11 (December 2002), pp.1513–1530, ISSN: 1538-7755

Griffin CS. (2002). Aneuploidy, centrosome activity and chromosome instability in cells deficient in homologous recombination repair. *Mutat Res*, Vol.504, No.1-2 (July 2002,), pp.149– 155, ISSN: 0027-5107

Grompe M, D'Andrea A. (2001). Fanconi anemia and DNA repair. *Hum Mol Genet*, Vol. 10, No. 20 (October 2001), pp.2253-2259, ISSN 1460-2083.

Gu D, Wang M, Wang M, Zhang Z, Chen J. (2009). The DNA repair gene APE1 T1349G polymorphism and cancer risk: a meta-analysis of 27 case-control studies. *Mutagenesis*, Vol. 24, No. 6 (November 2009), pp.507-512, ISSN 1464-3804

Gullo C, Au M, Feng G, Teoh G. (2006). The biology of Ku and its potential oncogenic role in cancer. *Biochim Biophys Acta*, Vol.1765, No.2 (April 2006), pp.223–234, ISSN: 0304-419X

Gumy-Pause F, Wacker P, Sappino AP. (2004). ATM gene and lymphoid malignancies. *Leukemia*, Vol.18, (November 2003), pp.238-242, ISSN: 1476-555.

Han S, Zhang HT, Wang Z, Xie Y, Tang R, Mao Y, Li Y. (2006). DNA repair gene XRCC3 polymorphisms and cancer risk: a meta-analysis of 48 case-control studies. *Eur J Hum Genet*, Vol.14, No.10 (June 2006), pp.1136–1144, ISSN: 1018-4813

Hanawalt PC. (2002). Subpathways of nucleotide excision repair and their regulation. *Oncogene*, Vol.21, No.58 (December 2002), pp.8949–8956, ISSN: 0950-9232

Hayani A, Suarez CR, Molnar Z, LeBeau M, Godwin. (1994). Acute myeloid leukaemia in a patient with Seckel syndrome. *J Med Genet*, Vol.31, No.2 (February 1994), pp.148–149, ISSN: 0022-2593

Hayden PJ, Tewari P, Morris DW, Staines A, Crowley D, Nieters A, Becker N, de Sanjosé S, Foretova L, Maynadié M, Cocco PL, Boffetta P, Brennan P, Chanock SJ, Browne PV, Lawler M. (2007). Variation in DNA repair genes XRCC3, XRCC4, XRCC5 and susceptibility to myeloma. *Hum Mol Genet*, Vol.16, No.24 (December 2007), pp.3117–3127, ISSN: 0964-6906

Hazra TK, Das A, Das S, Choudhury S, Kow YW, Roy R. (2007). Oxidative DNA damage repair in mammalian cells: a new perspective. *DNA Repair*, Vol.6, No.4 (April 2007), pp.470–80, ISSN: 1568-7864

Hazra TK, Roy R, Biswas T, Grabowski DT, Pegg AE, Mitra S. (1997). Specific recognition of O6-methylguanine in DNA by active site mutants of human O6-methylguanine-DNA methyltransferase. *Biochemistry*, Vol.36, No.19 (May 1997), pp.5769 –5776, ISSN: 0006-2960

He W, Luo S, Huang T, Ren J, Wu X, Shao J, Zhu Q. (2011). The Ku70 -1310C/G promoter polymorphism is associated with breast cancer susceptibility in Chinese Han population. *Mol Biol Rep*. May 10. [Epub ahead of print], ISSN: 1573-4978.

Hu Z, Ma H, Chen F, Wei Q, Shen H. (2005). XRCC1 polymorphisms and cancer risk: a meta-analysis of 38 case-control studies. *Cancer Epidemiol Biomarkers Prev*, Vol.14, No.7 (July 2005), pp.1810–1818, ISSN: 1538-7755

Hung RJ, Hall J, Brennan P, Boffetta P. (2005). Genetic polymorphisms in the base excision repair pathway and cancer risk: a HuGE review. *Am J Epidemiol*, Vol.162, No.10 (November 2005), pp.925–942, ISSN: 1476-6256

Iliakis G, Wang H, Perrault AR, Boecker W, Rosidi B, Windhofer F, Wu W, Guan J, Terzoudi G, Pantelias G. (2004). Mechanisms of DNA double strand break repair and chromosome aberration formation. *Cytogenet Genome Res*, Vol.104, No.1-4, pp.14–20.

Jacobsen NR, Raaschou-Nielsen O, Nexo B, Wallin H, Overvad K, Tjonneland A, Vogel U. (2004). XRCC3 polymorphisms and risk of lung cancer. Cancer Lett, Vol.213, No.1 (September 2004) pp.67–72, ISSN: 0304-3835

Ji YN, Zhan P, Wang J, Qiu LX, Yu LK. (2010). APE1 Asp148Glu gene polymorphism and lung cancer risk: a meta-analysis. *Mol Biol Rep*, Epub December 2010 Dec,

Jiricny J. (2006). The multifaceted mismatch-repair system. *Nat Rev Mol Cell Biol*, Vol.7, No.5 (May2006), pp.335–346, ISSN: 1471-0072

Junop MS, Modesti M, Guarne A, Ghirlando R, Gellert M, Yang W. (2000). Crystal structure of the Xrcc4 DNA repair protein and implications for end joining. *EMBO J*, Vol.19, No.22 (November 2000), pp.5962–5970.

Kaina B, Christmann M, Naumann S, Roos WP. MGMT: key node in the battle against genotoxicity, carcinogenicity and apoptosis induced by alkylating agents. *DNA Repair*, Vol.6, No.8 (August 2007), pp.1079–1099, ISSN: 1568-7864

Kaina B, Christmann M. (2002). DNA repair in resistance to alkylating anticancer drugs. *Int J Clin Pharmacol Ther*, Vol.40, No.8 (August 2002), pp.354–367, ISSN: 0946-1965

Kang TH, Reardon JT, Sancar A. (2011). Regulation of nucleotide excision repair activity by transcriptional and post-transcriptional control of the XPA protein. *Nucleic Acids Res*, Vol.39, No.8 (December 2010), pp.3176–87, ISSN: 0305-1048

Kennedy RD, D'Andrea AD.(2006). DNA repair pathways in clinical practice: lessons from pediatric cancer susceptibility syndromes. *J Clin Oncol*, Vol.24, No.23 (August 2006), pp.3799–3808, ISSN: 0732-183X

Khanna KK, Jackson SP. (2001). DNA double-strand breaks: signaling, repair and the cancer connection. *Nat Genet*, Vol.27, No.3 (March 2001), pp.247–254, ISSN: 1061-4036

Kohno T, Shinmura K, Tosaka M, Tani M, Kim SR, Sugimura H, Nohmi T, Kasai H, Yokota J. (1998). Genetic polymorphisms and alternative splicing of the hOGG1 gene, that is involved in the repair of 8-hydroxyguanine in damaged DNA. *Oncogene*, Vol.16, No.25 (June 1998), pp.3219–3225, ISSN: 0950-9232

Krajinovic M, Labuda D, Mathonnet G, Labuda M, Moghrabi A, Champagne J, Sinnett D. (2002). Polymorphisms in genes encoding drugs and xenobiotic metabolizing enzymes, DNA repair enzymes, and response to treatment of childhood acute lymphoblastic leukemia. *Clin Cancer Res*, Vol. 8, No.2 (March 2002), pp.802-810, ISSN: 1557-3265.

Kuptsova N, Kopecky KJ, Godwin J, Anderson J, Hoque A, Willman CL, Slovak ML, Ambrosone CB. (2007). Polymorphisms in DNA repair genes and therapeutic outcomes of AML patients from SWOG clinical trials. *Blood*, Vol.109, No.9 (May2007), pp.3936–3944, ISSN: 1528-0020

Kuptsova-Clarkson N, Ambrosone CB, Weiss J, Baer MR, Sucheston LE, Zirpoli G, Kopecky KJ, Ford L, Blanco J, Wetzler M, Moysich KB. (2010). XPD DNA nucleotide excision repair gene polymorphisms associated with DNA repair deficiency predict better treatment outcomes in secondary acute myeloid leukemia. *Int J Mol Epidemiol Genet*, Vol.1, No.4 (August2010), pp.278–294, ISSN: 1948-1756

Laine JP, Mocquet V, Bonfanti M, Braun C, Egly JM, Brousset P. (2007). Common XPD (ERCC2) polymorphisms have no measurable effect on nucleotide excision repair and basal transcription. *DNA Repair*, Vol.6, No.9 (September 2007),pp.1264 -1270, ISSN: 1568-7864

Lehmann AR. (2006). Clubbing together on clamps: The key to translesion synthesis. *DNA Repair*, Vol.5, No.3 (March 2006), pp.404–407, ISSN: 1568-7864

Levitus M, Rooimans MA, Steltenpool J, Cool NF, Oostra AB, Mathew CG, Hoatlin ME, Waisfisz Q, Arwert F, de Winter JP, Joenje H. (2004). Heterogeneity in Fanconi anemia: evidence for 2 new genetic subtypes. *Blood*, Nol.103, No.7 (April 2004), pp.2498–2503, ISSN: 1528-0020

Li GC, Ouyang H, Li X, Nagasawa H, Little JB, Chen DJ, Ling CC, Fuks Z, Cordon-Cardo C. (1998). Ku70: a candidate tumor suppressor gene for murine T cell lymphoma. *Mol Cell*, Vol.2, No.1(July 1998), pp.1–8.

Li GM. (2008). Mechanisms and functions of DNA mismatch repair. *Cell Res*, Vol.18, No.1 (January 2008), pp.85–98, ISSN: 1001-0602

Li X, Heyer WD. (2008). Homologous recombination in DNA repair and DNA damage tolerance. *Cell Res*, Vol.18, No.1 (January 2008), pp.99–113, ISSN: 1001-0602

Liddiard K, Hills R, Burnett AK, Darley RL, Tonks A. (2010). OGG1 is a novel prognostic indicator in acute myeloid leukaemia. *Oncogene*, Vol.29, No.13 (April 2010), pp.2005-2012 ISSN: 0950-9232

Lieberman HB.(2008). DNA damage repair and response proteins as targets for cancer therapy. *Curr Med Chem*, Vol.15, No.4 (February 2008), pp.360-367, ISSN 0929-8673

Lindahl T, Wood RD. (1999). Quality control by DNA repair. *Science*, Vol.286, No.5446 (December 1999), pp.1897–905, ISSN: 0036-8075

Liu L, Yang L, Zhang Y, Wei J, Zou Z, Qian X, Nakamura T, Ding Y, Feng J, Yu L. (2008). Polymorphisms of RAD51 (G135C) and XRCC3 (C241T) genes and correlations there of with prognosis and clinical outcomes of acute myeloid leukemia. *Mol. Cell*, Vol.88, No.6 (February 2008), pp.378–382

Lo YL, Jou YS, Hsiao CF, Chang GC, Tsai YH, Su WC, Chen KY, Chen YM, Huang MS, Hu CY, Chen CJ, Hsiung CA. (2009). A polymorphism in the APE1 gene promoter is associated with lung cancer risk. *Cancer Epidemiol Biomarkers Prev*, Vol. 18, No. 1 (Jabuary 2009), pp.223-229, ISSN: 1538-7755

Mao G, Yuan F, Absher K, Jennings CD, Howard DS, Jordan CT, Gu L. (2008). Preferential loss of mismatch repair function in refractory and relapsed acute myeloid leukemia: potential contribution to AML progression. *Cell Res*, Vol.18, No.2 (February 2008), pp.281–289, ISSN: 1001-0602

Martin SA, Lord CJ, Ashworth A. (2010). Therapeutic targeting of the DNA mismatch repair pathway. *Clin Cancer Res*, Vol.16, No.21(November 2010), pp.5107–5113, ISSN: 1557-3265

Matullo G, Dunning AM, Guarrera S, Baynes C, Polidoro S, Garte S, Autrup H, Malaveille C, Peluso M, Airoldi L, Veglia F, Gormally E, Hoek G, Krzyzanowski M, Overvad K, Raaschou-Nielsen O, Clavel-Chapelon F, Linseisen J, Boeing H, Trichopoulou A, Palli D, Krogh V, Tumino R, Panico S, Bueno-De-Mesquita HB, Peeters PH, Lund E, Pera G, Martinez C, Dorronsoro M, Barricarte A, Tormo MJ, Quiros JR, Day NE, Key TJ, Saracci R, Kaaks R, Riboli E, Vineis P. (2006). DNA repair polymorphisms and cancer risk in non-smokers in a cohort study. *Carcinogenesis*, Vol.27, No.5 (May 2006), pp.997–1007, ISSN: 1460-2180

Matullo G, Guarrera S, Carturan S, Peluso M, Malaveille C, Davico L, Piazza A, Vineis P. (2001). DNA repair gene polymorphisms, bulky DNA adducts in white blood cells and bladder cancer in a case-control study. *Int J Cancer*, Vol.92, No.4 (May 2001), pp.562–567, ISSN: 1097-0215

Mavrou A, Tsangaris GT, Roma E, Kolialexi A. (2008). The ATM gene and ataxia telangiectasia. *Anticancer Res*, Vol. 28, No. 1B (February 2008), pp.401-405, ISSN: 1791-7530.

Mehta PA, Alonzo TA, Gerbing RB, Elliott JS, Wilke TA, Kennedy RJ, Ross JA, Perentesis JP, Lange BJ, Davies SM. (2006). XPD Lys751Gln polymorphism in the etiology and outcome of childhood acute myeloid leukemia: a Children's Oncology Group report. *Blood*, Vol.107, No.1 (January 2007), pp.39–45, ISSN: 1528-0020

Mitra S. (2007). MGMT: a personal perspective. *DNA Repair*, Vol.6, No.8 (August 2007), pp.1064–1670, ISSN: 0036-8075

NCBI, http://www.ncbi.nlm.nih.gov, last accessed on 20/05/2011

Papouli E, Cejka P, Jiricny J. (2004). Dependence of the cytotoxicity of DNA-damaging agents on the mismatch repair status of human cells. *Cancer Res*, Vol.64, No. 10 (May 2004), pp.3391–3394, ISSN: 1538-7445

Park J, Chen L, Tockman MS, Elahi A, Lazarus P. (2004). The human 8-oxoguanine DNA N-glycosylase 1 (hOGG1) DNA repair enzyme and its association with lung cancer risk. *Pharmacogenetics*. Vol.14, No.2 (February 2004), pp. 103-109, ISSN: 1744-6880

Rajewsky MF, Müller R. (2005). DNA Repair and the Cell Cycle as Targets in Cancer Therapy in *The Cancer Handbook* 1st Ed, Malcolm R. Alison, John Wiley & Sons, Ltd, Available from:< http://hasdl.kau.edu.sa/encyclopedia/2/h6 20archive/24.pdf>

Reardon JT, Sancar A. (2005). Nucleotide excision repair. *Prog Nucleic Acid Res Mol Biol*, Vol.79 (August 2005), pp.183–235, ISBN: 10: 0-12-540066-7

Resnick IB, Kondratenko I, Togoev O, Vasserman N, Shagina I, Evgrafov O, Tverskaya S, Cerosaletti KM, Gatti RA, Concannon P. (2002). Nijmegen breakage syndrome: clinical characteristics and mutation analysis in eight unrelated Russian families. *J Pediatr*, Vol. 140, No. 3 (March 2002), pp. 355-361.

Richardson C, Stark JM, Ommundsen M, Jasin M. (2004). Rad51 overexpression promotes alternative double-strand break repair pathways and genome instability. *Oncogene*, Vol. 23, No.2 (January 2004), pp.546–553, ISSN: 0950-9232

Riedl T, Hanaoka F, Egly JM. (2003). The comings and goings of nucleotide excision repair factors on damaged DNA. *EMBO J*, Vol.22, No.19 (October 2003), pp.5293–5303.

Rimsza LM, Kopecky KJ, Ruschulte J, Chen IM, Slovak ML, Karanes C, Godwin J, List A, Willman CL. (2000). Microsatellite instability is not a defining genetic feature of acute myeloid leukemogenesis in adults: results of a retrospective study of 132 patients and review of the literature. *Leukemia*, Vol.14, No.6 (June 2000), pp.1044–1051, ISSN: 0887-6924

Rollinson S, Smith AG, Allan JM, Adamson PJ, Scott K, Skibola CF, Smith MT, Morgan GJ. (2007). RAD51 homologous recombination repair gene haplotypes and risk of acute myeloid leukaemia. *Leuk Res*, Vol.31, No.2 (February 2007), pp.169–74, ISSN: 0145-2126

Rosenberg PS, Alter BP, Ebell W. (2008). Cancer risks in Fanconi anemia: findings from the German Fanconi Anemia Registry. *Haematologica*, Vol. 93, No. 4 (Aprilie 2008), pp. 511-517, ISSN: 1592-8721.

Rufer JT, Morgan WF. (1992). Potentiation of DNA damage by inhibition of poly (ADP-ribosyl)ation: A test of the hypothesis for random nuclease action. *Exp Cell Res*, Vol.200, No.2 (June 1992), pp.506–512, ISSN: 0014-4827

Sargent RG, Brenneman MA, Wilson JH. (1997). Repair of site-specific double-strand breaks in a mammalian chromosome by homologous and illegitimate recombination. Mol *Cell Biol*, Vol.17, No.1 (January 1997), pp.267–277, ISSN: 1098-5549

Savitsky K, Bar-Shira A, Gilad S, Rotman G, Ziv Y, Vanagaite L, Tagle DA, Smith S, Uziel T, Sfez S, Ashkenazi M, Pecker I, Frydman M, Harnik R, Patanjali SR, Simmons A, Clines GA, Sartiel A, Gatti RA, Chessa L, Sanal O, Lavin MF, Jaspers NG, Taylor AM, Arlett CF, Miki T, Weissman SM, Lovett M, Collins FS, Shiloh Y. (1995). A single ataxia telangiectasia gene with a product similar to PI-3 kinase. *Science*, Vol.268, No.5218 (June 1995), pp.1749–1753, ISSN: 1095-9203

Seedhouse C, Bainton R, Lewis M, Harding A, Russell N, Das-Gupta E. (2002). The genotype distribution of the XRCC1 gene indicates a role for base excision repair in the development of therapy-related acute myeloblastic leukemia. *Blood*, Vol.100, No.10 (November 2002), pp.3761–66, ISSN: 1528-0020

Seedhouse C, Faulkner R, Ashraf N, Das-Gupta E, Russell N. (2004). Polymorphisms in genes involved in homologous recombination repair interact to increase the risk of developing acute myeloid leukemia. *Clin Cancer Res;* Vol.10, No.8 (April 2004), pp.2675–2680, ISSN: 1557-3265

Sheikhha MH, Tobal K, Liu Yin JA. (2002). High level of microsatellite instability but not hypermethylation of mismatch repair genes in therapy-related and secondary acute myeloid leukaemia and myelodysplastic syndrome. *Br J Haematol*, Vol.117, No.2 (May 2002), pp.359–365, ISSN: 1365-2141

Shen MR, Jones IM, Mohrenweiser H. (1998). Nonconservative amino acid substitution variants exist at polymorphic frequency in DNA repair genes in healthy humans. *Cancer Res*, Vol.58, No.4 (february 1998), pp.604–608, ISSN: 1538-7445

Shrivastav M, De Haro LP, Nickoloff JA. (2008). Regulation of DNA double-strand break repair pathway choice. *Cell Res*, Vol.18, No.1 (December 2007), pp.134–47, ISSN: 1001-0602

Sipley JD, Menninger JC, Hartley KO, Ward DC, Jackson SP, Anderson CW. (1995). Gene for the catalytic subunit of the human DNA-activated protein kinase maps to the site of the XRCC7 gene on chromosome 8. *Proc Natl Acad Sc. USA*, Vol.92, pp.7515–19.

Smith GC, Jackson SP. (1999). The DNA-dependent protein kinase. *Genes Dev*, Vol.13, No.8 (April 1999), pp.916–934, ISSN: 1549-5477

Stanczyk M, Sliwinski T, Cuchra M, Zubowska M, Bielecka-Kowalska A, Kowalski M, Szemraj J, Mlynarski W, Majsterek I. (2011). The association of polymorphisms in DNA base excision repair genes XRCC1, OGG1 and MUTYH with the risk of childhood acute lymphoblastic leukemia. *Mol Biol Rep*,Vol.38, No.1 (January, 2011), pp.445-451, n.d.

Steensma DP. (2007). The DNA Damage Response, DNA Repair, and AML. In: *Acute Myelogenous Leukemia*. Karp JE. pp.97-132, Humana Press, ISBN-13: 978-1-58829-621 1, Totowa, New Jersey

Stronati L, Gensabella G, Lamberti C, Barattini P, Frasca D, Tanzarella C, Giacobini S, Toscano M, Santacroce C, Danesi DT. (2001). Expression and DNA binding activity of the Ku heterodimer in bladder carcinoma. *Cancer*, Vol.92, No.9 (November 2001), pp.2484–2492, ISSN: 1097-0142

Sturgis EM, Clayman GL, Guan Y, Guo Z, Wei Q. (1999). DNA repair in lymphoblastoid cell lines from patients with head and neck cancer. *Arch Otolaryngol Head Neck Surg*, Vol.125, No.2 (February 1999), pp.185–90.

Sung P, Klein H. (2006). Mechanism of homologous recombination: mediators and helicases take on regulatory functions. *Nat Rev Mol Cell Biol*, Vol.7, No.10 (October 2006), pp.739–50, ISSN: 1471-0072

Surtees JA, Argueso JL, Alani E. (2004). Mismatch repair proteins: key regulators of genetic recombination. *Cytogenet Genome Res*, Vol.107, No.3-4, pp.146–59.

Taccioli GE, Gottlieb TM, Blunt T, Priestley A, Demengeot J, Mizuta R, Lehmann AR, Alt FW, Jackson SP, Jeggo PA. (1994). Ku80: product of the XRCC5 gene and its role in DNA repair and V(D)J recombination. *Science*, Vol.265, No.5177 (September 1994):1442–1445, ISSN: 0036-8075

Taylor AM, Byrd PJ. (2005). Molecular pathology of ataxia telangiectasia. *J Clin Pathol*, Vol.58, no. 10 (October 2005), pp.1009-1015, ISSN: 1472-4146.

Thompson LH, Brookman KW, Jones NJ, Allen SA, Carrano AV. (1990). Molecular cloning of the human XRCC1 gene, which corrects defective DNA strand break repair and sister chromatid exchange. *Mol Cell Biol*, Vol.10, No.12 (December 1990), pp.6160–6171 ISSN: 1098-5549

Thompson LH, Schild D. (2002). Recombinational DNA repair and human disease. *Mutat Res*; Vol.509, No.1-2 (November 2002), pp.49–78, ISSN: 0027-5107

Tsukino H, Hanaoka T, Otani T, Iwasaki M, Kobayashi M, Hara M, Natsukawa S, Shaura K, Koizumi Y, Kasuga Y, Tsugane S. (2004). hOGG1 Ser326Cys polymorphism, interaction with environmental exposures, and gastric cancer risk in Japanese populations. *Cancer Sci*, Vol.95, No.12 (December 2004), pp.977–83, ISSN: 1349-7006

van der Wees C, Jansen J, Vrieling H, van der LaarseA, Van Zeeland A, Mullenders L. (2007). Nucleotide excision repair in differentiated cells. *Mutat Res*, Vol.614, No.1-2 (January 2007), pp.16–23, ISSN: 0027-5107

Varon R, Schoch C, Reis A, Hiddemann WC, Sperling K, Schnittger S. (2003). Mutation analysis of the Nijmegen breakage syndrome gene (NBSl) in nineteen patients with acute myeloid leukemia with complex karyotypes. *Leuk Lymphoma*, Vol.44, No.11 (January 2003), pp.1931–1934, ISSN: 1042-8194

Voso MT, Fabiani E, D'Alo' F, Guidi F, Di Ruscio A, Sica S, Pagano L, Greco M, Hohaus S, Leone G. (2007). Increased risk of acute myeloid leukemia due to polymorphisms in detoxification and DNA repair enzymes. *Ann Oncol*, Vol.18, No.9 (September 2007), pp.1523–1528, ISSN: 1569-8041

Wang F, Chang D, Hu FL, Sui H, Han B, Li DD, Zhao YS. (2008). DNA repair gene XPD polymorphisms and cancer risk: a metaanalysis based on 56 case-control studies. Cancer Epidemiol Biomarkers Prev, Vol.17, No.3 (March 2008), pp.507–517, ISSN: 1538-7755

Wang G, Wang S, Shen Q, Yina S, Li C, Lia A, Li J, Zhoua J, Liu Q. (2009). Polymorphisms in XRCC5, XRCC6, XRCC7 genes are involved in DNA double-strand breaks (DSBs) repair associated with the risk of acute myeloid leukemia (AML) in Chinese population. *Journal of Nanjing Medical University*, Vol.23, No.2 (March 2009), pp.93–99, ISSN: 1007-4376

Wang L, Zhu D, Zhang C, Mao X, Wang G, Mitra S, Li BF, Wang X, WuM. (1997). Mutations of O6-methylguanine-DNA methyltransferasegene in esophageal cancer tissues from Northern China. *Int J Cancer*, Vol.7, No. 5 (May 1997), pp.719 -723, ISSN: 1097-0215.

Wang LE, Bondy ML, Shen H, El-Zein R, Aldape K, Cao Y, Pudavalli V, Levin VA, Yung WK, Wei Q. (2004). Polymorphisms of DNA repair genes and risk of glioma. *Cancer Res*, Vol.64, No.16 (August 2004), pp.5560–5563, ISSN: 1538-7445

Wang SY, Peng L, Li CP, Li AP, Zhou JW, Zhang ZD, Liu QZ. (2008). Genetic variants of the XRCC7 gene involved in DNA repair and risk of human bladder cancer. *Int J Urol*, Vol.15, No.6 (June 2008):, pp.534–539, ISSN: 1442-2042

Wenshan He, Sijia Luo, Tao Huang, Jinghua Ren, Xiaoling Wu, Jun Shao. Qingyao Zhu. (2011). The Ku70 −1310C/G promoter polymorphism is associated with breast cancer susceptibility in Chinese Han population. *Mol Biol Rep*, (May 2011), n.d.

Wiebauer K, Jiricny J. (1990). Mismatch-specific thymine DNA glycosylase and DNA polymerase beta mediate the correction of G.T mispairs in nuclear extracts from human cells. *Proc Natl Acad Sci USA*, Vol.87, No.15 (August 1990), pp.5842–5845

Wilson DM 3rd, Simeonov A. (2010). Small molecule inhibitors of DNA repair nuclease activities of APE1. *Cell Mol Life Sci*, Vol.67, No.21 (November 2010), pp. 3621-3631, ISSN: 1420-682X

Winsey SL, Haldar NA, Marsh HP, Bunce M, Marshall SE, Harris AL, Wojnarowska F, Welsh KI. (2000). A variant within the DNA repair gene XRCC3 is associated with the development of melanoma skin cancer. *Cancer Res*, Vol.60, No.20 (Octombrie 2000), pp.5612–5616, ISSN: 1538-7445

Wood RD. (1989). Repair of pyrimidine dimer ultraviolet light photoproducts by human cell extracts. Biochemistry, Vol.28, No.21 (October 1989), pp.8287–8292, ISSN: 0006-2960

Wu CN, Liang SY, Tsai CW, Bau DT. (2008). The role of XRCC4 in carcinogenesis and anticancer drug discovery. *Recent Pat Anticancer Drug Discov*, Vol.3, No.3 (November 2008), pp.209–219, ISSN: 1574-8928

Xing DY, Tan W, Song N, Lin DX. (2001). Ser326Cys polymorphism in hOGG1 gene and risk of esophageal cancer in a Chinese population. *Int J Cancer*, Vol.95, No.3 (May 2001), pp.140–143, ISSN: 1097-0215

Yasbin RE. (2002). DNA repair mechanism and Mutagenesis, In: *Modern Microbial Genetics*, Second Edition. Streips UN, Yasbin RE, 24-46, Wiley-Liss Inc, ISBN: 0-471-22197-X, New York, USA.

Yeh YC, Chang DY, Masin J, Lu AL. (1991). Two nicking enzyme systems specific for mismatch-containing DNA in nuclear extracts from human cells. *J Biol Chem*, Vol.266, No.10 (April 1991), pp.6480–6484, ISSN: 0021-9258

Yu JJ. (2009). Unlocking the Molecular Mechanisms of DNA Repair and Platinum Drug Resistance in Cancer Chemotherapy. *Current Drug Therapy*, Vol 4, No 1 (January 2009) , pp.19-28, ISSN: 1574-8855

Yu Z, Chen J, Ford BN, Brackley ME, Glickman BW. (1999). Human DNA repair systems: an overview. *Environ Mol Mutagen*, Vol.33, No.1 (February 1999), pp.3–20, ISSN: 0893-6692

20

Apoptosis and Apoptosis Modulators in Myeloid Leukemia

Maha Abdullah and Zainina Seman
University Putra Malaysia
Malaysia

1. Introduction

Acute myeloid leukemia (AML) is one of the most common types of leukemia in adults (American Cancer Society, 2010) however overall survival rate remain poor despite advancement in treatment modality.

Since the last 50 years, systemic chemotherapy has greatly improved outcome in many types of cancers. The use of continuous infusion Arabinosylcytosine (Ara-C) combined with another agent, usually an anthracycline or anthracenedione, the "3+7" regimen, has been the backbone of induction therapy for AML cases (Yates et al., 1973). An attempt to add other drugs (Preisler et al., 1987) and intensification of the Ara-C dose (Schiller et al., 1992; Weick et al., 1996) to this approach has achieved some degree of success. Currently more work is attempted at improving patient outcome by intensifying the doses of anthracyclines (Lowenberg et al., 2010a) or by adding targeted therapies like gemtuzumabozogamicin (Lowenberg et al., 2010b; Nabhan et al., 2005).

For consolidation therapy, the use of Ara-C with or without other agents has been employed to maintain remission and cure. Allogeneic hematopoietic cell transplantation (HCT) based on initial cytogenetic (Cornelissen et al., 2007; Koreth et al., 2009) and molecular studies (Castaigne et al., 2004) have been proposed as an alternative consolidation therapies.

Induction therapy aims to produce complete remission (CR) defined as a marrow with less than 5% blast, a neutrophil count greater than 1000/mm^3 and a platelet count greater than 100,000/mm^3 (Cheson et al., 2003). Majority of younger patients (65-75%) will achieve CR after receiving induction treatment while CR in elderly group is much lower (40-50%).

Patients who do not respond to induction treatment display chemotherapy resistance (Estey et al., 1996). In trials done by the Southwest Oncology Group (SWOG), resistant disease was found in about 33% (patients younger than 56) out of 404 patients' enrolled into the studies, 62% for patients in between 56-65 year old, 61% for patients between 66-75 years old and 57% for age more than 75 year old (Frederick et al., 2006).

Resistance is also common at relapse (Estey et al., 1996). Relapse itself could be due to resistance to treatment in a subgroup of leukaemic cells which survived induction therapy despite CR. Patients usually relapse within two to three years after achieving CR.

2. Multi-drug resistance protein as a mechanism of drug resistance

Development of drug resistance is a major problem in AML therapy. It will eventually occur in most haematological malignancies treated with chemotherapy. Classically, drug resistance is divided into extrinsic and intrinsic (Jean-Pierre et al., 2003). Extrinsic resistance (host factors) refers to the inability of the drug to reach the tumour cell. It occurs when the bioavailability of the oral form varies from patient to patient like poor absorption resulting in low serum levels.

Intrinsic (cellular) resistance is due to properties of the tumour cell. It can be classified as simple resistance, when cells are resistant to only one particular drug, or as multidrug resistance (MDR) when cross resistance is observed among chemotherapeutic drugs with different biochemical targets. Multidrug resistance is more common than simple resistance and it can be due to several mechanisms. The most common pharmacological mechanism involved is due to an active efflux of drugs from the tumour cells or enhanced drug metabolism which prevented the drug from reaching its target in the nucleus.

The most important protein described in MDR cells is P-glycoprotein (P-gp), a transmembrane energy-dependent drug efflux pump, which is most efficient at transporting naturally occurring substances. It is encoded by the MDR1/ABCB1 gene and belongs to a superfamily of ABC (ATP binding cassette) transporters. P-gp expression in AML at initial presentation has been reported to be 20% to 40% (Motoji T et al., 2000). Increase in P-gp expression in leukaemic cells causes reduced intracellular concentration of cytotoxic drugs. There are many drugs used in AML that are transported by P-gp including anthracyclines and anthracenediones like daunorubicin and mitoxantrone, the vinca alkaloids (vincristine and vinblastine) and the epipodophyllotoxins (etoposide and teniposide).

Other ABC transport proteins that have been implicated in MDR include the multi-drug resistance associated proteins (MRP1/ABCC1) and the breast cancer resistance protein (BCRP/ABCG2). All these proteins are not unique to drug resistance cells but expressed in tissue with excretory and secretory functions. However, many studies have found that overexpression of these proteins correlate with poor treatment response (Damiani et al., 2010; Bendarra et al., 2005).

A non-ABC protein, found widely expressed in P-gp negative multidrug resistant cancer cell termed initially as lung resistance related protein (LRP) and now known as major vault protein (MVP) also has been implicated in drug resistance mechanism (Izquierdo et al., 1996; Huh et al., 2006). This protein is involved in bidirectional transportation of a variety of substrates between nucleus and cytoplasm. It is present in many cells and seems to be upregulated in cancer cells and has been found to be an adverse prognostic factor in AML (Styczynski et al., 2007). The expression of P-gp (Leith et al., 1999), MRP and LRP in AML was also found to correlate with advanced age (>60 years) and high white cell count (van delHeuvel et al., 2007). It also correlates with high risk of relapse (Daniela et al., 2007).

There have been extensive trials conducted on AML therapy to circumvent drug resistance like reversion of P-gp, targeted agents against DNA replication and repair, cell cycling and apoptosis.

With the extensive knowledge on P-gp efflux mechanism and its contribution to drug resistance in AML, quinine and cyclosporine were tested to reverse the P-gp action. However, these substances did not significantly improve the response rate in AML (Eric et al., 2003; Solary et al., 1996; Liu et al., 1998; Tallman et al., 1995). Combination of tetrandrine, a potent inhibitor of the MDR-1 efflux pump, with induction therapy also showed no significant difference in response between P-gp positive and P-gp negative patients (Wen et al., 2006). Nevertheless, an early study revealed by using P-gp reversal modulators, the emergence of drug resistance could be prevented (Futscher et al., 1996). However, a recent randomized phase III trial involving 302 newly diagnosed AML patients, evaluated the effect of P-gp inhibitor valspodar (PSC-833) showed no difference in overall disease survival (Jonathan et al., 2010). Similar result was obtained in another phase III randomized trial involving poor risk AML patients when valspodar was added in the induction therapy (Peter et al., 2004)

3. Molecular 'signatures' in AML

AML is characterized by a high degree of heterogeneity with respect to chromosome abnormalities, gene mutations and expression of multiple genes. The heterogeneous nature of AML has significant clinical impact as there are marked differences in survival following intensive chemotherapy (explained in detail elsewhere in this book). The World Health Organization (WHO) classifies AML by cytogenetics, morphology, immunophenotype and clinical features (Swerdlow et al., 2008). Diagnostic karyotype emerges as the most significant prognostic factor as determined in multivariable analyses that take into account age, type of AML (*de novo* or secondary) and presenting white blood cell count (WBC), and accordingly provides the framework for current risk stratified treatment approaches (Grimwade, 2007). Nevertheless as cytogenetic and molecular genetic aberrations are not mutually exclusive the expression of downstream target genes that encode proteins involved in complex biologic networks are affected (Mrozek et al., 2009) and may alter predictability of standard prognostic markers. Microarray genome-wide gene-expression profiling (GEP) and microRNA-expression profiling assays have revealed AML signatures and may be readily applicable for diagnosis and outcome class prediction in AML (Mrozek et al., 2009). Many of the molecules involved are known mediators of signal transduction pathways and apoptosis.

4. Apoptotic molecules in AML

Apoptosis occurs principally via two separate yet interlinked signaling mechanisms: the extrinsic pathway, activated by proapoptotic receptor signals at the cellular surface (members of tumor necrosis factor, TNF, family), and the intrinsic pathway (members of Bcl-2 family), activated by mitochondrial signals from within the cell. These pathways converge through "effector" caspases, which orchestrate the apoptotic program. Nevertheless, each requires different initiation caspases to begin the process. The *extrinsic* pathway is activated by engagement of death receptors on the cell membrane. The death receptors involved in the extrinsic apoptotic pathway belong to the TNF receptor superfamily that include Fas (CD95 or Apo1), TNFR1 (TNF receptor 1), death receptor 3 (DR3/Wsl-1/APO-3/TRAMP/LARD), death receptor 4 (DR4/TRAIL-R1), death receptor 5 (DR5/TRAIL-R2) and DR6. These receptors are characterized by an intracellular death domain. There are also decoy receptors (i.e. DcR1 and DcR2) that contain no death domain or a truncated death domain and can bind ligand but cannot signal. Therefore, these decoy receptors function as antagonists to inhibit death ligand/death receptor-induced apoptosis. Binding of ligands, such as FasL, tumor necrosis factor-alpha (TNF-alpha) and TNF-related apoptosis-inducing ligand (TRAIL) to their respective membrane receptors Fas, TNF-R and

TRAIL-R induces trimerization of the receptors and recruitment of adaptor proteins such as the Fas-associated death domain (FADD) to the death domain. This then recruits procaspase-8 which then leads to the formation of the oligomeric death-induced signaling complex (DISC). DISC in turn promotes activation of caspase-8 and a cascade of other caspase enzymes that culminates with cell death (reviewed in Elrod and Sun, 2008).

The *intrinsic* pathway is triggered by various extracellular and intracellular stresses, including growth factor deprivation, DNA damage, oncogene induction, hypoxia and cytotoxic drugs. Cellular signals originated by various mechanisms by these different stresses converge on a cellular target represented by mitochondria. Mitochondrial membrane permeability is controlled by pro-apoptotic (Bax, Bak, Bad, Bid, Bim, Bmf, NOXA, PUMA, Bok, Bcl-G, Bfk) and anti-apoptotic (Bcl-2, Bcl-L, Mcl-1, Bcl-w, A1) members of the Bcl-2 family, inducing or preventing heterodimerization of pro-apoptotic members. A series of biochemical events is induced that lead to damage of the outer mitochondrial membrane, with the consequent release of cytochrome c and other pro-apoptotic molecules, such as Smac/DIABLO, from the inner membrane into the cytosol enabling the formation of the apoptosome, a large molecular complex formed by cytochrome c, apoptotic protease activating factor 1 (APAF-1) and caspase-9, and massive activation of caspases. These proteins all play crucial roles for cell survival and the loss of any of these proteins causes major deregulation of survival of some cell types (reviewed in Ashkenazi and Herbst, 2008).

Dysregulation of apoptosis plays an important role in the development of a variety of human pathologies, including cancer and particularly leukemia. The evasion of programmed cell death has been regarded as one of the six essential alterations in cellular physiology that dictate the growth of cancer cells and is a hallmark of virtually all cancers. Moreover, tumors that have alterations in proteins involved in cell death signaling are very frequently resistant to chemotherapy and are difficult to treat with chemotherapeutic agents that primarily act by inducing apoptosis (Testa et al., 2007).

Fas, DR4 and DR5 are generally expressed in both normal and malignant cells. An examination of patients with de novo AML revealed Fas was expressed on eight of nine (89%) patients tested (Tourneur et al., 2004). Another study showed expression of Fas on 62% of 29 AML patients (Min et al., 2004). Fas mutation was observed in 4/28 CML cases and none of the six AML cases tested (Rozenfeld-Granot et al., 2001). DR4 and DR5 mutations detected in cancers including chronic myelogenous leukemia were very low (0–10.6%) (Liu et al., 2005). On the other hand, DR4 and DR5 receptors were positive in 20 (69%) and 29 (100%) patients, respectively. This study also showed, relapse-free survival was significantly prolonged in patients with CD95-positive AML cells compared with patients with CD95-negative AML cells (73% versus 38% at 3 years; $p = 0.047$) using univariate analysis (Min et al., 2004). This was however not supported by another study on 99 AML patients where multivariate analysis showed no correlation with overall survival and disease free survival (Brouwer et al., 2001).

Three ligands (TNF-α, FasL and TRAIL) of the TNF-family and their respective four receptors (TNF-R1, Fas, TRAIL-R1 and TRAIL-R2) are potentially important as anti-cancer therapeutics. The demonstration that TNF-α selectively kills tumor cells but not normal cells, set it up for the first molecules to be studied. Unfortunately, marked pro-inflammatory effects precluded its systemic administration (Buzzoni and Butler, 1996). Fas was also excluded as agonistic antibodies triggering Fas activation was highly hepatotoxic causing death in mouse models (Ogasarawa et al., 1993). In contrast, TRAIL and agonistic anti-

TRAIL-R1/TRAIL-R2 antibodies appear to be well tolerated *in vivo*. TRAIL/Apo-2L exhibited potent anti-tumor activity and induces little cytotoxic effects in immunodeficient mice xenograft models implanted with several human tumor cell lines (Ashkenazi et al., 1999). However, the *in vivo* half-life of the TRAIL-ligand is very short (<4 minutes) (Kelley et al., 2001). Agonistic TRAIL-R1 and TRAIL-R2 antibodies do not bind to TRAIL decoy receptors, TRAIL-R3 and TRAIL-R4, which are frequently expressed on the membrane of tumor cells.

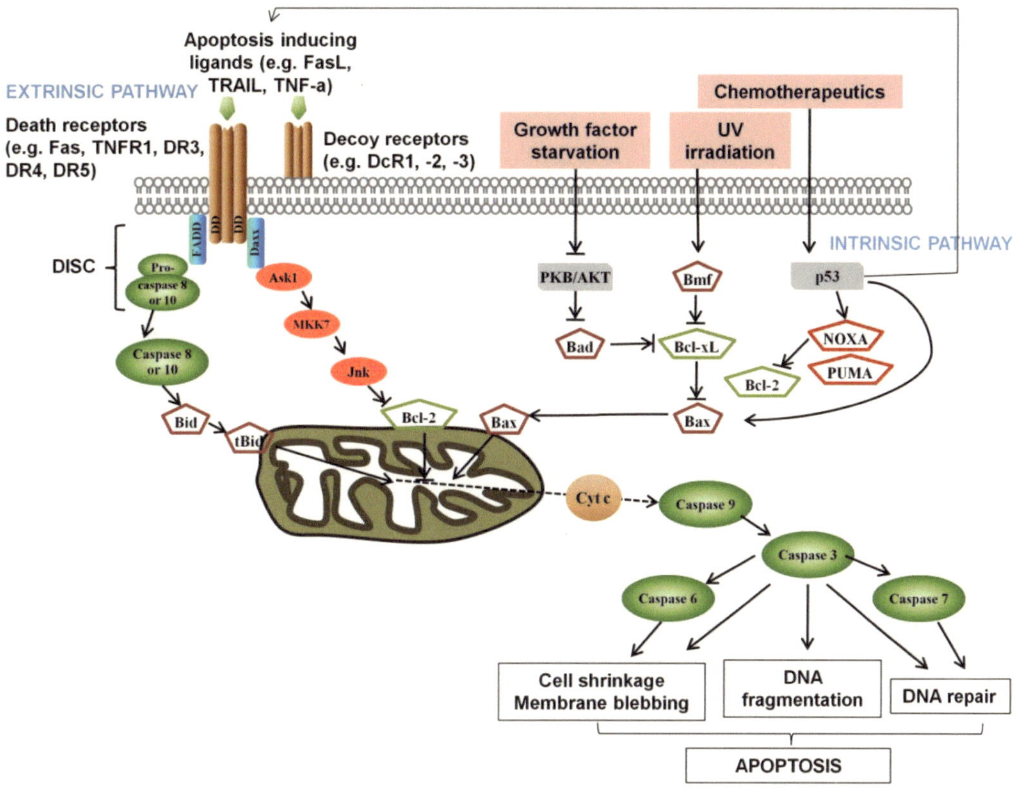

Fig. 1. Extrinsic and intrinsic pathways in apoptosis (see text for further details).

Antisense therapies involved the use of sequences of single-stranded DNA to complement and bind specific coding regions on mRNA hence forming DNA–mRNA which is then degraded by a ribonuclease, therefore gene expression and translation are prevented. Most widely studied were with XIAP (X-linked inhibitor of apoptosis) and antiapoptotic proteins Bcl-2.

Sufficient evidence exists to show that Bcl-2 was overexpressed in AML patients and predictive of worst outcome (Campos et al., 1993; Andreef and Konopleva, 2002). It seemed conceivable that Bcl-2 downregulation might lower the apoptotic threshold of leukemic cells and, through this mechanism, favor response to chemotherapy. Much success has been achieved. A phase I study using oblimersen, an antisense to Bcl-2, added during induction and then consolidation therapy, in elderly AML patients, induced remission in 14/27 patients, of which seven relapsed within 12.6 months (Marcucci et al., 2005); In a multicenter phase II trial, 12/39 relapsed AML patients treated with oblimersen and gentuzamab (anti-

CD33) achieved complete remission of which 10/12 survived for more than 6 months (Moore et al., 2004).

XIAP binds and inhibits caspases 3, 7, and 9, mediators of the apoptotic cascade. Downregulation of XIAP using multiple approaches (e.g., antisense, RNAi, knock-out animals and cell lines, immuno-depletion) in vitro and in vivo conditions resulted in increased caspase activation and/or cell death. Antitumor activity was also observed with the use of second generation anti-sense compound, AEG35156, in xenograft models of cancer (Lacasse et al., 2005) Results from clinical trials however, have been variable. While one study on five phase 1 (12–350mg/m2 AEG35156) and eight phase 2 (350 mg/m2 AEG35156) patients showed increased apoptotic cells and increase response (Bing et al., 2011) another study on 27 patients randomized to receive high dose Ara-C and idarubicin with or without AEG35156 (650 mg) found a lower overall response rate in the group which received the anti-XIAP drug (Schimmer et al., 2011).

The analysis of Mcl-1 protein expression in AML showed great heterogeneity, but the levels of the protein do not seem to correlate with response to standard chemotherapy (Kaufmann et al., 1998). Bad and Bcl-xL have been shown to be expressed in normal and leukemic hematopoietic precursor cells. Immature hematopoietic cells do not express Bcl-2 but do express Bcl-xL. CD34 positive cells express Bcl-2, Bcl-xL and Bad. Bcl-2 expression is higher on CD34 positive cells than on AML cells. Phosphorylated Bad was expressed in AML (Andreef et al., 1999).

Potential abnormalities of the various initiator caspases in AML have been explored. Levels of caspase-8, caspase-2 and caspase-3 are heterogeneous in AML. AML with an immature phenotype (i.e., M0 and M1 AML) predominantly express caspase-8L (Mohr et al., 2005).The significance of caspases as prognostic indicators in AML are unclear as current reports are still controversial may be due to the different format of molecules examined (Svingen et al., 2000; Estrov et al., 1998; Holleman et al., 2005).

Expression of pro- and anti-apoptotic molecules continues to be studied in AML to correlate its mutated state, expression, activity or methylated state with treatment outcome (Testa et al., 2007). At present, the prognostic utility of measurements of pro- and antiapoptotic molecules for predicting clinical outcome and response to chemotherapy is uncertain.

5. Drug modulation of signaling, differentiation and apoptotic pathways

The study of cancer cell biology in predicting treatment outcome cannot stop at the presentation stage as cells continue to be modified by the microenvironment and are ultimately subjected to chemotherapy. While remarkable progress have been achieved in targeted therapies, for most tumors chemo- or radiotherapy is likely to remain in the near future. Both chemo- and radiotherapy are designed to kill cancer cells by damaging nuclear DNA. DNA damage triggers the DNA damage response (DDR) which have three critical goals: (i) halting cell cycle progression and division to prevent transfer of DNA damage to progeny cells; (ii) increasing accessibility of the damage sites to- and engagement of- the DNA damage repair machinery, and (iii) triggering apoptosis to exterminate cells whose damaged DNA cannot successfully be repaired (reviewed in Darzynkiewicz et al., 2009).

Chemotherapeutic drugs such as cisplatin, mitomycin, methotrexate, mitoxantrone, adriamycin, and bleomycin induce Fas expression in human cancer cells, primarily through a p53-dependent mechanism (Muller et al., 1998). Adriamycin, etoposide, Ara-C, cisplatin and camptosar were shown to induce the expression of DR4 and DR5 or only DR5 expression, through either p53-dependent, or p53-independent mechanisms (Wu et al., 1997; Guan et al., 2001; Sheikh et al., 1998). Etoposide was shown to induce DR5 expression in human acute leukemia cells (Wen et al., 2000).

To complete induction of cell death, chemotherapeutic drugs have to suppress survival mediators in activated signaling pathways. Paclitaxel treatment of transfected MDA MB-435 human breast carcinoma cell line was observed to downregulate phosphorylated Akt (Klos et al., 2003). Nevertheless, chemotherapy induction of cell death is not equal in all cells. Adriamycin produced differential responses in Akt phosphorylation and kinase activity in a panel of breast cancer cell lines. While MCF7, MDA468 and T47D cells showed a dose dependent increase in p-Akt levels; in contrast, SKBR3 and MDA231 cells showed a dose-dependent decrease and no or minimal change was detected in MDA361, MDA157 and BT474 cells (Li et al., 2005). The diversity in response may also be predictive of a heterogeneity in treatment outcome.

Other signaling molecules are activated by chemotherapeutic drugs leading to cell death. Ara-C induced apoptosis in HL-60 cell lines through the activation of p38 (Stadheim et al., 2000). Adriamycin was shown to activate Jnk in a T cell leukemia cell line (Yu et al., 1999). Leukemia cell lines (TF-1 and K562) primed for apoptosis were also revealed to stimulate Jnk and p38 phosphorylation (Tucker et al., 2004)

Certain cytokines have apoptotic activity. TNF-alpha and IFN-gamma induced the expression of DR5 in a number of cancer cell lines (Meng and El-Deiry, 2000). IFN-gamma had differential effect on induction of death receptors in colon carcinoma cell lines. While it raised the levels of CD95 membrane 6 - 8-fold, it had no effect on the TRAIL-receptors (DR4, DR5, DcR1 and DcR2) (van Geelan et al., 2003). Interferon-alpha was also reported to increase DR5 expression in human hepatoma (Shigeno et al., 2003).

In contrast some cytokines exert protective effect from chemotherapeutic drug induced cell death, decreasing the effectiveness of cancer radiotherapy and chemotherapy. Normal hematopoietic cells, like other normal cell types, die by the process of apoptosis when deprived of viability inducing cytokines that include colony stimulating factors (CSFs) and various other cytokines. Induction of apoptosis by cancer chemotherapy such as vincristine, adriamycin, methotrexate and Ara-C was suppressed by IL (interleukin)-6, IL-3, granulocyte-CSF (G-CSF), granulocyte-monocyte CSF (GM-CSF) and IFN-gamma in myeloid leukemia cells (reviewed in Lotem and Sachs, 2002). These cytokines upregulate pro-survival molecules such as Bcl-2 [IL-2, IL-3, stem cell factor (SCF), IFN-gamma], Bcl-xL [IL-3, IL-6, IL-7, IL15, GM-CSF, IFN-gamma and erythropoietin (EPO)] and other apoptosis suppressing genes such as Survivin (Carter et al., 2001), X-linked inhibitor of apoptosis protein (XIAP) and cellular inhibitor of apoptosis 2 (cIAP2) (Digicylioglu and Lipton, 2001) that are caspase inhibitors and FLICE-like inhibitory protein (FLIP), that may disrupt the ability of cell surface molecules such as Fas to activate apoptosis (Kovalovich et al., 2001) Some myeloid leukemic cells are autonomous and do not require an exogenous source of cytokines for viability (Griffin and Lowenberg,1986), while others do. Thus, it is possible to suppress leukemia not only by cytotoxic agents or by induction of terminal differentiation, but also by decreasing the in vivo supply of apoptosis suppressing cytokines or the response of leukemic cells to these cytokines (reviewed in Sachs, 1996).

A characteristic abnormality of leukemia cells is that they are blocked at an early stage of their development. Myeloid leukemic cells however can be induced to differentiate to non dividing mature granulocytes and macrophages by different cytokines, including cytokine independent myeloid leukemic cells that were induced to differentiate with IL-6. Different myeloid leukemic clones however have different blocks and ability to undergo differentiation by cytokines. Our own work on in vitro cultured AML blasts exhibited different degrees of spontaneous apoptosis. Univariate analysis of 13 AML patients revealed blasts with lower levels of cell viability after 72h culture was significantly correlated with a longer disease free survival . Within a smaller number of samples (n=7) we observed blasts with lower levels of cell viability were associated with reduced levels CD34 and higher levels of CD16, indicating an increased level of cell differentiation (Maha et al., 2008). The observations may indicate an abnormal developmental program in leukemic cells which may be reprogrammed epigenetically by appropriate differentiation inducing cytokines. Constitutive expression of transcription factors such as c-myc, c-myb and E2F1 (Gonda and Metcalf, 1984; Blatt et al., 1992; Melamed et al., 1993) as well as others such as the homeobox gene Hox B8 (Hox 2.4) (Blatt et al., 1992) or GATA-1 (Tanaka et al., 2000), disrupted the ability of cells to undergo cytokine induced differentiation (reviewed in Lotem and Sachs, 2002)

Cytokines as a differentiation treatment against leukemia however has been disappointing. Hematopoietic leukemia cell lines of myeloid origin such as K562, U937, HL-60, CS-1, KG-1, MUTZ-3, or ex vivo AML or chronic myeloid leukemia (CML) blasts were modestly permissive to induction of in vitro differentiation by EPO, G-CSF, GM-CSF, IL-4, IL-6, SCF, or synergistic combinations of several cytokines (Leung et al., 2005; Koss et al., 1996; Goliaei et al. 1998; Kamano et al., 1994; Kamijo et al., 1990). A niche for hematopoietic cytokines in differentiation therapy exists in the treatment of congenital neutropenia disorder. The administration of G-CSF to patients has overcome a block of myeloid differentiation leading to a substantial prolongation of their survival (Berliner, 2008).

Clinically, differentiation therapy has been most successful in acute promyelocytic leukemia (APL) using all-trans-retinoic acid (ATRA) as the inducer. This targeted APL cells carrying the chromosomal translocation between chromosomes 15 and 17 [t(15;17)(q22;q21)]. Subsequently, APL therapy was improved with the combination regimen of ATRA with cytotoxic chemotherapy. Currently, complete remission rates of up to 90% to 95% are achievable using ATRA/ATO (arsenic trioxide) and anthracycline-based chemotherapy (Niu et al., 1999; Soignet et al., 2001; Raffoux et al., 2003; Ghavamzadeh et al., 2006; Mathews et al., 2006; Estey et al., 2006; Sanz et al., 2008).

Another targeted treatment with tyrosine kinase inhibitor (TKI) imatinib for the treatment of CMLalso achieved better success. Gefinitib and erlotinib which inhibit the intracellular tyrosine kinase activity of epidermal growth factor receptor (EGFR), induce a differentiation program in myeloid leukemia cells that corresponds to neutrophil maturation (Stegmaier et al., 2005; Boehrer et al., 2008a; Boehrer et al., 2008b).

These results together emphasize further not only the heterogeneity of leukemias but also complexity of host-cancer interaction and its influence on outcome in survival and also during induction of cell death.

6. In vivo drug induced molecular profiles: Potential predictor of drug resistance

The in vivo molecular changes in acute myeloid leukemia cells early after start of conventional genotoxic chemotherapy are incompletely understood, and it is not known if early molecular modulations reflect clinical response. As increasing evidence is proposing tumor-host mechanisms as important for effective chemotherapy, there is an immediate need to investigate these issues in vivo in human cancer (Oyan et al., 2009)

For that purpose, blasts from patients undergoing chemotherapy were collected as a 'natural' and rich source to study response of these cells to the myriad of signals they were subjected to. Even though cells undergo cell death, as white blood cell counts may decline at early stages of chemotherapy, very low percentages of apoptotic cells were detected. Oyan et al. (2009) comparing treated ('3+7', idarubicin + Ara-C) with untreated AML cells from seven patients, observed upregulation of 113 genes (23 of unknown function) at early time points (2 – 4 hours) and 108 genes at late time points (18 – 24 hours). Among the 113 genes a substantial number (31 genes) were related to the tumor suppressor p53 (Oyan et al., 2009). p53 is implicated to affect a variety of cellular processes, the most undisputed roles of p53 are to induce growth arrest and to induce apoptosis (Bates and Vousden, 1996). p53 is the most commonly mutated gene in a variety of human cancers (Greenblatt et al., 1994). In AML however, mutations of p53 are rare, occurring in approximately 5% to 10% (Fenaux et al., 1992) but in these cases it correlates with worse outcome (Wattel et al., 1994). Wild-type p53 appears to change the balance in expression of apoptosis-inducing versus apoptosis-suppressing genes in favor of the former and thus induce apoptosis.

In tune with the above, a significant increase in gene expression of the apoptosis facilitators PUMA and Bax and a decrease in the Bcl-2 /Bax ratio as well as Bcl-2 /PUMA were observed for most of the AML samples. The mRNA profile of three other pro-apoptotic mediators Bad , Bak1 and Bim did not change significantly during the first hours, but the level of gene expression varied across patients. Altogether five tumor necrosis factor-related receptor genes were modulated 2–4 h after induction therapy (Oyan et al., 2009).

Induction of ligand to death receptor during chemotherapy was also supported by Devemy et al. (2001) who observed increased TNF transcripts in treated AML cells. We also studied molecular changes in paired AML samples at diagnosis and during chemotherapy (Ara-C + daunorubicin). We showed increased TNF-alpha was significantly higher in chemo-sensitive patients. Thus, expression of TNF-alpha early during chemotherapy may be a marker to predict good treatment outcome. In chemo-resistant cases, a higher, though not significant, percentage of cases expressed IL-1beta and IL-18 (Maha et al., 2009).

We observed a significantly higher percentage of chemo-responsive AML patients with blasts cells increased for the expression of IL-6. This was consistent with Devemy et al (2001) who reported that increase of IL-6 transcripts during remission induction therapy of AML patients was accompanied by a fall in blood count and bone marrow cellularity. The role of cytokines in the induction of cell differentiation is well established. Oyan et al (2009) also observed several receptors expressed on monocytic/macrophage lineage cells were upregulated, probably related to chemotherapy induced differentiation of the leukemic cells. Thus, induction of cytokines expression in drug responsive AML patients may be due to induction of cell differentiation.

Comparing blasts profiles before and during early chemotherapy also revealed upregulation of genes potentially involved in interaction between AML blasts and the host microenvironment. Chemokine receptors CXCR4 and CX3CR1 were upregulated in the late phase after start of chemotherapy indicating intention to home into a microenvironment that favours their growth and survival. This supports the hypothesis that the host response in chemotherapy is crucial for persistent remission (Oyan et al., 2009).

We further examined activation of signaling molecules in AML blasts. Chemotherapy increased the percentage of cases showing phosphorylation of the Akt molecules and Forkhead transcription factor (FKHR) but no significant differences were observed between chemo-resistant and chemo-sensitive cases. We however, observed a significantly higher percentage of chemo-resistant cases showing phosphorylation and inactivation of the pro-apoptotic Bad molecule. A higher percentage of chemo-sensitive cases were phosphorylated for p38, and Jnk (Maha et al., 2009). In summary, we were able to show in chemo-sensitive cases, chemotherapy stimulated IL-6, induced apoptosis by up-regulating TNF-alpha and downregulated phosphorylated Bad. In reverse, in chemo-resistant cases, cells survived by maintaining high levels of phosphorylated Bad maybe through protective role of IL-1b and IL-18 cytokines (Maha et al., 2009).

Most anticancer drugs exert their effects by the induction of apoptosis and/or interfering with cell cycle progression. Often these drugs give rise to specific patterns of cell death and cell cycle arrest that vary according to the drug used and the molecular status of the target cell. Simple in vitro methods may aid in this investigation. Drug cytotoxicity and sensitivity of individual tumor samples was demonstrated by combining cytochrome c and propidium iodide staining of DNA content and detected on flowcytometry. This method elucidated mitochondrial resistance mechanisms which may prove useful in identifying the apoptosis-sensitive cell cycle phase for a given tumor sample/anticancer drug combination. It offers the opportunity to design personalized drug regimens and to identify new combined treatment modalities (Mohr et al., 2004).

7. Conclusion

The heterogeneity in AML continues to elude the best methods to characterize them. Genome and proteome-wide analysis has further revealed complexity in the makeup of the leukemic cell. The rapid advancement in targeted therapies implied the urgent need for alternative therapy and the readiness of the community to embrace it. Nevertheless so far, combinatorial medicine still holds out as the best option for successful treatment. If targeted therapies remain the way forward it will eventually bank deeply on the ability to identify molecular signatures in the individual leading to the establishment of personalized medicine.

In the meantime, the mechanisms in leukemogenesis, drug resistance and relapse remain an area of much research. From cell biology to cytogenetics to molecular defects to signaling pathways, all have contributed to a better understanding of cancer biology. New knowledge in epigenetics and microRNA remain to be elucidated.

Current diagnostic and prognostication are based on the assumption that the phenotype of the leukemic cell is static and thus definitive. There is much evidence that suggest otherwise. Activation of oncogenes leads to constitutive expression of signal transduction pathways involved in cell survival and anti-apoptotic activities. These pathways are multiple and made up of a myriad of molecules that are receptive to the environment. The host-cancer microenvironment is a dynamic microcosm of interacting signals and cascading molecules that constantly respond to stimuli in the surrounding to find a balance that maintains survival. In the course of treatment, blast cells are exposed to DNA damaging cytotoxic agents which trigger a gamut of other signaling mediators to exert the opposite effect. It would appear that a struggle ensues in which the strength of the victor determines whether the blast cell would maintain life or be pushed off-balance and replaced with a new profile signaling cell death. This new phenotype corresponded to a sensitive response to chemotherapy. On the other hand, cells may strengthen on pro-survival features which corresponded with resistance to chemotherapy. A few reports, including ours, are lending support to this hypothesis.

Unsurprisingly, chemotherapy-induce phenotype is not confined purely to either a survival or an apoptosis profile but a complex mix of conflicting signals to survive or die in addition to triggers to shut down cell proliferation, induce terminal differentiation or activate inflammatory responses. Thus, further elucidation of these profiles would involve assignment of each of the modulated molecule to its rightful pathway.

The immaturity feature in leukemias will undoubtedly be a factor that will further compound the heterogeneity in results obtained. An example is the striking correlations found between lower Bax/Bcl-2 ratio and higher progenitor marker expression, such as CD34, CD117 and CD133 antigens, confirming the link between this apoptotic index and the maturation pathways (Del Principe et al., 2005). Attempts to induce cell death by triggering death receptors has so far achieved mix results with the use of TNF-alpha, Fas ligands and the tumor necrosis factor-related apoptosis-inducing ligand (TRAIL) (i.e., DR4 and DR5). These molecules also selectively kill cancer cells while sparing normal cells (reviewed in Elrod and Sun, 2008). These results indicate a preferential expression of specific death receptors on different tissues.

Selection of lab methods for prognostication depends on the ability to identify lineage, maturation stages, genetic aberrations and activated signal transduction pathways. This feat may include the difficult task of combining surface markers, cytokines (secreted proteins) and phosphorylated proteins (unstable intracellular proteins) in the same tube on the same platform such as flowcytometry. Furthermore many of these proteins such as TNF-a, IL-6, p38 and Jnk have dual function of pro-survival and pro-apoptosis capabilities depending on the stimulating conditions cells are exposed to at that period of time. Precise markers will be required to differentiate these situations. Altogether, all of these add up to an interesting and exciting field of research for the immediate future.

8. References

[1] American Cancer Society. Cancer facts & figures 2010. American Cancer Society Web site. http://www.cancer.org. Accessed June 29, 2010.

[2] Andreeff M, Jiang S, Zhang X, Konopleva M, Estrov Z, Snell VE et al. Expression of Bcl-2 related genes in normal and AML progenitors: changes induced by chemotherapy and retinoic acid. Leukemia 1999; 11: 1881–1892.

[3] Andreef M, Konopleva M. Mechanisms of drug resistance in AML. Cancer Treat Res 2002;112: 237-262.

[4] Ashkenazi A, Herbst RS. To kill a tumor cell: the potential of proapoptotic receptor agonists. J Clin Invest. 2008 Jun;118(6):1979-1990.

[5] Ashkenazi A, Pai RC, Fong S, Leung S, Lawrence DA, Marsters SA, et al. Safety and antitumor activity of recombinant soluble Apo2 ligand. J Clin Invest 1999;104:155-162.

[6] Bates, S., and Vousden, K. H. p53 in signaling checkpoint arrest or apoptosis. Curr. Opin. Genet. Dev. 1996; 6: 1-7.

[7] Bazzoni F, Butler B. The tumor necrosis factor ligand and receptor families N Engl J Med 1996;334: 1717-1725.

[8] Berliner N. Lessons from congenital neutropenia: 50 years of progress in understanding myelopoiesis. *Blood.* 2008;111:5427–5432.
[9] Bing ZC, Duncan HM, Stephen JM, et al. XIAP antisense oligonucleotide (AEG35156) achieves target knockdown and induces apoptosis preferentially in CD34+38 cells in a phase 1/2 study of patients with relapsed/refractory AML. Apoptosis;2011: 16:67–74.
[10] Blatt C, Lotem J and Sachs L. Inhibition of specific pathways of myeloid cell differentiation by an activated Hox-2.4 homeobox gene. Cell Growth Differ. 1992; 3, 671-676.
[11] Boehrer S, Ades L, Galluzzi L, et al. Erlotinib and gefitinib for the treatment of myelodysplastic syndrome and acute myeloid leukemia: a preclinical comparison. *BiochemPharmacol.* 2008a;76:1417–1425.
[12] Boehrer S, Ades L, Braun T, et al. Erlotinib exhibits antineoplastic off-target effects in AML and MDS: a preclinical study. *Blood.* 2008b;111:2170–2180.
[13] Byrd JC, Mrozek K, Dodge RK, et al. Pretreatment cytogenetic abnormalities are predictive of induction success, cumulative incidence of relapse, and overall survival in adult patients with de novo acute myeloid leukemia: results from Cancer and Leukemia Group B (CALGB 8461). Blood. 2002;100:4325–4336.
[14] Campos L, Rouault JP, Sabido O. High expression of bcl-2 protein in acute myeloid leukemia cells is associated with poor response to chemotherapy. Blood 1993;81: 3091-3096.
[15] Carter BZ, Miella M, Altieri DC and Andreef M. Cytokine-regulated expression of survivin in myeloid leukemia. Blood. 2001; 97, 2784 2790.
[16] Castaigne S, Chevret S, Archimbaud E, et al. Randomized comparison of double induction and timed-sequential induction to a "37" induction in adults with AML: long-term analysis of the Acute Leukemia French Association (ALFA) 9000 study. Blood. 2004;104:2467-2474.
[17] Cheson B, Bennett J, Kopecky K et al. Revised recommendations of the International Working Group for diagnosis, standardization of response criteria, treatment outcomes, and reporting standards for therapeutic trials in acute myeloid leukemia, J ClinOncol. 2003;21:4642–4649.
[18] Cornelissen JJ, van Putten WL, Verdonck LF, et al. Results of a HOVON/SAKK donor versus no-donor analysis of myeloablative HLA-identical sibling stem cell transplantation in first remission acute myeloid leukemia in young and middle-aged adults: benefits for whom? Blood. 2007;109:3658 –3666.
[19] Damiani D, Tiribelli M, Michelutti A et al. Fludarabine-based induction therapy does not overcome the negative effect of ABCG2 (BCRP) over-expression in adult acute myeloid leukemia patients. Leuk Res. 2010;34(7):942-945.
[20] Daniela D, Mario T, Donatella R et al. The role of MDR-related proteins in the prognosis of adult acute myeloid leukaemia (AML) with normal karyotype. HematolOncol 2007; 25: 38–43.
[21] Darzynkiewicz Z, Traganos F, Wlodkowic D. Impaired DNA damage response--an Achilles' heel sensitizing cancer to chemotherapy and radiotherapy. Eur J Pharmacol. 2009;625(1-3):143-150.

[22] Del Principe MI, Del Poeta G, Venditti A, Buccisano F, Maurillo L, Mazzone C, Bruno A, Neri B, IrnoConsalvo M, Lo Coco F,Amadori S. Apoptosis and immaturity in acute myeloid leukemia. Hematology. 2005;10(1):25-34.
[23] Devemy E, Li B, Tao M *et al.* Poor prognosis acute myelogenousleukemia: 3—biological and molecular biological changes during remission induction therapy. Leuk Res 2001; 25(9):783-791.
[24] Digicaylioglu M and Lipton SA. Erythropoietin-mediated neuroprotection involves cross-talk between Jak2 and NF-kappaBsignalling cascades. Nature. 2001; 412, 641 - 647.
[25] Dohner H, Estey EH, Amadori S, et al. Diagnosis and management of acute myeloid leukemia in adults: recommendations from an international expert panel, on behalf of the European LeukemiaNet. *Blood*. 2010;115:453– 474
[26] Dufour A, Schneider F, Metzeler KH, et al. Acute myeloid leukemia with biallelic CEBPA gene mutations and normal karyotype represents a distinct genetic entity associated with a favorable clinical outcome. *J ClinOncol*. 2010;28:570 –577.
[27] Eric S, Bernard D, Lydia C et al. Quinine as a multidrug resistance inhibitor: a phase 3 multicentric randomized study in adult de novo acute myelogenousleukemia. Blood.2003;102:1202-1210.
[28] Estey E, Kornblau S, Pierce S et al. A stratification system for evaluating and selecting therapies in patients with relapsed or primary refractory acute myeloid leukaemia. Blood 1996;88:756.
[29] Estey E, Garcia-Manero G, Ferrajoli A, et al. Use of all-trans retinoic acid plus arsenic trioxide as an alternative to chemotherapy in untreated acute promyelocyticleukemia. *Blood.* 2006;107:3469–3473.
[30] Estrov Z, Thall PF, Talpaz M, Estey EH, Kantarjian HM, Harris D, et al. Caspase 2 and caspase 3 protein levels as predictors of survival in acute myelogenousleukaemia.Blood 1998; 92:3090-3097.
[31] Falini B, Mecucci C, Tiacci E, et al. Cytoplasmic nucleophosmin in acute myelogenousleukemia with a normal karyotype. *N Engl J Med.* 2005;352:254 –266.
[32] Fenaux P, Preudhomme C, Quiquandon I, et al. Mutations of the p53 gene in acute myeloid leukaemia. Br J Haematol. 1992;80:178-183.
[33] Frederick R A, Holly G, David R H, et al. Age and acute myeloid leukemia. Blood. 2006 107: 3481-3485.
[34] Futscher BW, Foley NE, Gleason-Guzman MC, Meltzer PS, Sullivan DM, Dalton WS. Verapamil suppresses the emergence of P-glycoproteinmediated multi-drug resistance. Int J Cancer. 1996;66:520-525.
[35] Ghavamzadeh A, Alimoghaddam K, Ghaffari SH, et al. Treatment of acute promyelocyticleukemia with arsenic trioxide without ATRA and/or chemotherapy. *Ann Oncol.* 2006;17:131–134.
[36] Gibson BE, Wheatley K, Hann IM, et al. Treatment strategy and long-term results in paediatric patients treated in consecutive UK AML trials. Leukemia. 2005;19:2130-2138.
[37] Goliaei B, Deizadji A. Effects of hyperthermia and granulocyte-macrophage colony-stimulating factor on the differentiation of human leukemic cell line U937. *Leuk Res.* 1998;22:705–710.

[38] Gonda TJ and Metcalf D. Expression of myb, myc and fos proto-oncogenes during the differentiation of a murine myeloid leukaemia. Nature. 1984; 310, 249- 251.

[39] Greenblatt, M. S., Benneu, W. P., Hollstein, M., and Harris, C. C. Mutations in the p53 tumorsuppressorgene: clues to cancer etiology and molecular pathogenesis. Cancer Res. 1994; 54: 4855-4878.

[40] Griffin JD and Lowenberg B. (1986).Clonogenic cells in acute myeloblastic leukemia. Blood. 1986; 68, 1185-1195

[41] Grimwade D. Impact of cytogenetics on clinical outcome in AML. In: Karp JE, ed. Acute MyelogenousLeukemia. Totowa, New Jersey: Humana Press; 2007:177-192.

[42] Grimwade D, Hills RK. Independent prognostic factors for AML outcome.Hematology Am SocHematolEduc Program. 2009:385-395.

[43] Grimwade D, Hills RK, Moorman AV, et al. Refinement of cytogenetic classification in acute myeloid leukemia: determination of prognostic significance of rare recurring chromosomal abnormalities amongst 5,876 younger adult patients treated in the UK Medical Research Council trials. *Blood*. 2010;116:354–365.

[44] Guan B, Yue P, Clayman GL, Sun SY. Evidence that the death receptor DR4 is a DNA damage-inducible, p53-regulated gene. J Cell Physiol 2001; 188:98-105.

[45] Holleman A, Den Boer M, Kazemeier KM, Beverloo HB, Von Bergh A, Janka-Schaub GE, et al. Decreased PARP and procaspase-2 protein levels are associated with cellular drug resistance in childhood lymphoblastic leukemia. Blood 2005;106:1817-1823.

[46] Huh HJ, Park CJ, Jang S et al. Prognostic significance of multidrug resistance gene 1 (MDR1), multidrug resistance-related protein (MRP) and lung resistance protein (LRP) mRNA expression in acute leukemia. J Korean Med Sci. 2006 Apr;21(2):253-258.

[47] Izquierdo M, Scheffer G, Flens M et al. Major vault protein LRP-related multidrug resistance. Eur J Cancer. 1996;32A:979-984.

[48] Jean-Pierre M, Ollivier L. Drug resistance in acute leukaemia and reversion. Turk J Med Sci. 2003;33:271-279.

[49] Jonathan EK, Stephen LG, Guido M et al. P-glycoprotein inhibition using valspodar (PSC-833) does not improve outcomes for patients younger than age 60 years with newly diagnosed acute myeloid leukemia: Cancer and Leukemia Group B study 19808. *Blood* 2010 116: 1413-1421.

[50] Kamano H, Tanaka T, Ohnishi H, et al. Effects of the antisense myb expression on hemin- and erythropoietin-induced erythroid differentiation of K562 cells. *BiochemMolBiol Int.* 1994;34:85–92

[51] Kamijo R, Takeda K, Nagumo M, Konno K. Effects of combinations of transforming growth factor-beta 1 and tumor necrosis factor on induction of differentiation of human myelogenous leukemic cell lines. *J Immunol.* 1990;144:1311–1316.

[52] Kaufmann SH, Karp JE, Svingen PA, Kraiewski S, Burke PJ, Gore SD, Reed JC. Elevated expression of the apoptotic regulator Mcl-1 at the time of leukemic relapse. Blood 1998;91: 991-1000.

[53] Kelley S, Harris L, Xie D, DeForge L, Totpal K, Bussiere J, et al. Preclinical studies to predict the disposition of Apo2L/tumor necrosis factor-related apoptosis-inducing ligand in humans: characterization on in vivo efficacy, pharmacokinetics, and safety. J PharmacolExpTher 2001;299: 31-38.

[54] Klos KS, Zhou X, Lee S, Zhang L, Yang W, Nagata Y, Yu D. Combined trastuzumab and paclitaxel treatment better inhibits ErbB-2-mediated angiogenesis in breast carcinoma through a more effective inhibition of Akt than either treatment alone. Cancer. 2003;98(7):1377-1385.

[55] Koreth J, Schlenk R, Kopecky KJ, Honda S, Sierra J, Djulbegovic BJ, Wadleigh M, DeAngelo DJ, Stone RM, Sakamaki H, Appelbaum FR, Döhner H, Antin JH, Soiffer RJ, Cutler C. Allogeneic stem cell transplantation for acute myeloid leukemia in first complete remission: systematic review and meta-analysis of prospective clinical trials. JAMA. 2009;301(22):2349-2361.

[56] Koss A, Lucero G, Koziner B. Granulocyte-colony stimulating factor, granulocyte-macrophage colony stimulating factor and interleukin 4 induce differentiation in the U-937 human monocyticleukemia cell line. *Leuk Lymphoma*. 1996;22:163–171. follow. 186, color plate XIV-V.

[57] Kovalovich K, Li W, DeAngelis R, Greenbaum LE, Ciliberto G and Taub R. Interleukin-6 protects against Fas-mediated death by establishing a critical level of anti-apoptotic hepatic proteins FLIP, Bcl-2, and Bcl-xLJ. Biol. Chem. 2001; 276, 26605-26613.

[58] Krauter J, Wagner K, Schäfer I, Marschalek R, Meyer C, Heil G, Schaich M, EhningerG,Niederwieser D, Krahl R, Büchner T, Sauerland C, Schlegelberger B, Döhner K, DöhnerH,Schlenk RF, Ganser A. Prognostic factors in adult patients up to 60 years old with acute myeloid leukemia and translocations of chromosome band11q23: individual patient data-based meta-analysis of the German Acute Myeloid Leukemia Intergroup. J ClinOncol. 2009; 27(18):3000-3006.

[59] Lacasse EC, Kandimalla ER, Winocour P, et al. Application of XIAP antisense to cancer and other proliferative disorders: development of AEG35156/ GEM640. Ann N Y Acad Sci. 2005;1058:215–234.

[60] Lamba JK, Crews KR, Pounds SB, Cao X, Gandhi V, Plunkett W, Razzouk BI, Lamba V, Baker SD, Raimondi SC, Campana D, Pui CH, Downing JR, Rubnitz JE, Ribeiro RC. Identification of predictive markers of cytarabine response in AML by integrative analysis of gene-expression profiles with multiple phenotypes. Pharmacogenomics. 2011;12(3):327-339.

[61] Leith CP, Kopecky KJ, Chen IM, Eijdems L, Slovak ML, McConnell TS, Head DR, Weick J, Grever MR,Appelbaum FR, Willman CL. Frequency and clinical significance of the expression of the multidrug resistance proteins MDR1/P-glycoprotein, MRP1, and LRP in acute myeloid leukemia: a Southwest Oncology Group Study. Blood. 1999;94(3):1086-99.

[62] Leung KN, Mak NK, Fung MC. Cytokines in the differentiation therapy of leukemia: from laboratory investigations to clinical applications.Crit Rev Clin Lab Sci. 2005;42(5-6):473-514.

[63] Li X, Lu Y, Liang K, Liu B, Fan Z. Differential responses to doxorubicin-induced phosphorylationand activation of Akt in human breast cancer cells. Breast Cancer Res. 2005;7(5):R589-597.

[64] Liu YJ, Wheatley K, Rees J et al. Comparison of two chemotherapy regimen with or without cyclosporine A in relapse/refractory acute myeloid leukaemia: result of the UK Medical Research Council AML-R Trial. Blood 1998;92:231a.

[65] Liu LG, Tanaka H, Ito K, Ito T, Sultana TA, Kyo T, Kimura A. Absence of gene mutation in TRAIL receptor 1 (TRAIL-R1) and TRAIL receptor 2 (TRAIL-R2) in chronic myelogenousleukemia and myelodysplastic syndrome, and analysis of mRNA Expressions of TRAIL and TRAIL-related genes in chronic myelogenousleukemia. ActaHaematol 2005; 113:113-123.

[66] Lowenberg, B., Ossenkoppele, G.J., van Putten, W.,etal.High dose daunorubicin in older patients with acute myeloid leukemia.NEng J Med. 2010a;361:1235–1248.

[67] Lowenberg B, Beck J, GrauxC,et al. Gemtuzumabozogamicin as postremission treatment in AML at 60 years of age or more: results of a multicenter phase 3 study. Blood. 2010b; 115: 2586–2591.

[68] Maha A, Cheong SK, Leong CF, Seow HF. Cell viability of acute myeloid leukaemia blasts in culture correlates with treatment outcome.Hematology. 2008;13(1):13-20.

[69] Maha A, Cheong SK, Leong CF, Seow HF. Molecular responses during chemotherapy in acute myeloid leukemias in predicting poor-response to standard chemotherapy.Malays J Pathol. 2009 Dec;31(2):81-91.

[70] Marcucci G, Stock W, Dai G, Klisovic RB, Liu S, Klisovic MI, Blum W, Kefauver C, Sher DA, Green M,Moran M, Maharry K, Novick S, Bloomfield CD, Zwiebel JA, Larson RA, Grever MR, Chan KK, Byrd JC. Phase I study of oblimersen sodium, an antisense to Bcl-2, in untreated older patients with acute myeloid leukemia: pharmacokinetics, pharmacodynamics, and clinical activity. J Clin Oncol. 2005 May 20;23(15):3404-11.

[71] Mathews V, George B, Lakshmi KM, et al. Single-agent arsenic trioxide in the treatment of newly diagnosed acute promyelocyticleukemia: durable remissions with minimal toxicity. *Blood*.2006;107:2627–2632.

[72] Melamed D, Tiefenbrun N, Yarden A and Kimchi A. Interferons and interleukin-6 suppress the DNA-binding activity of E2F in growth-sensitive hematopoietic cells. Mol. Cell. Biol. 1993; 13, 5255-5265.

[73] Meng RD, El-Deiry WS. p53-independent upregulation of KILLER/DR5 TRAIL receptor expression by glucocorticoids and interferon-gamma. Exp Cell Res. 2001;262(2):154-169.

[74] Min YJ, Lee JH, Choi SJ, Chi HS, Lee JS, Kim WK, Lee KH. Prognostic significance of Fas (CD95) and TRAIL receptors (DR4/DR5) expression in acute myelogenousleukemia. Leukemia research 2004; 28:359-365.

[75] Mohr A, Zwacka RM, Debatin KM and Stahnke K. A novel method for the combined flow cytometric analysis of cell cycle and cytochrome c release. Cell Death and Differentiation (2004) 11, 1153–1154.

[76] Mohr A, Zwacka RM, Jarmy G, Buneker C, Schrezenmeier H, Dohner K, et al. Caspase-8L expression protects CD34+ hematopoietic progenitor cells and leukemic cells from CD95-mediated apoptosis. Oncogene 2005; 24:2421-2429.

[77] Moore LO, Seiter K, Kolitz JE, Stock W, Yu R, Frankel SR. Phase 2 study of oblimersen sodium (G31\39; Bcl-2 antisense; Gena sense) plus gentuzumabozogamicin (Myelotarg) in elderly patients with relapsed acute myeloid leukemia (AML). Blood 2004;104:247a.

[78] Motoji T, Motomura S, Wang YH. Multidrug resistance of acute leukemia and a strategy to overcome it. Int J Hematol 2000 Dec;72(4):418-24.

[79] Mrozek K, Radmachera MD, Bloomfield CD and Marcucci G. Molecular signatures in acute myeloid leukemia. CurrOpinHematol 16:64–69

[80] Muller M, Wilder S, Bannasch D, Israeli D, Lehlbach K, Li-Weber M, Friedman SL, Galle PR, Stremmel W, Oren M, Krammer PH. p53 activates the CD95 (APO-1/Fas) gene in response to DNA damage by anticancer drugs. J Exp Med 1998; 188:2033-2045.

[81] Nabhan C, Rundhaugen LM, Riley MB, et al. Phase II pilot trial of gemtuzumabozogamicin (GO) as first line therapy in acute myeloid leukemia patients age 65 or older. Leukemia Research.2005;29:53–57

[82] Niu C, Yan H, Yu T, et al. Studies on treatment of acute promyelocyticleukemia with arsenic trioxide: remission induction, follow-up, and molecular monitoring in 11 newly diagnosed and 47 relapsed acute promyelocyticleukemia patients. *Blood.* 1999;94:3315–3324.

[83] Nowak D, Stewart D, Koeffler HP. Differentiation therapy of leukemia: 3 decades of development. Blood. 2009;113(16):3655-3665.

[84] O'Donnell MR, Appelbaum FR, Coutre SE, et al. Acute myeloid leukemia: NCCN clinical practice guidelines in oncology, v.2.2010. National Comprehensive Cancer Network On-Line. http://wwwnccnorg. Accessed April 18, 2010.

[85] Ogasarawa J, Watanabe-Fukunaga R, Adachi M, Matsuzawa A, Kasugai T, Kita mura Y, et al. Lethal effect of the anti-Fas antibody in the mice. Nature 1993; 364: 806-809.

[86] Øyan AM, Anensen N, Bø TH, Stordrange L, Jonassen I, Bruserud Ø, Kalland KH, Gjertsen BT. Genes of cell-cell interactions, chemotherapy detoxification and apoptosis are induced during chemotherapy of acute myeloid leukemia.BMC Cancer. 2009; 9:77.

[87] Paschka P, Marcucci G, Ruppert AS, et al. Adverse prognostic significance of KIT mutations in adult acute myeloid leukemia with inv(16) and t(8;21): a Cancer and Leukemia Group B Study. *J ClinOncol.* 2006;24:3904 -3911.

[88] Peter L. Greenberg, Sandra J. Lee, Ranjana Advani, Martin S. Tallman, Branimir I. Sikic, Louis Letendre, Kathleen Dugan, Bert Lum, David L. Chin, Gordon Dewald, Elisabeth Paietta, John M. Bennett, and Jacob M. Rowe. Mitoxantrone, Etoposide, and Cytarabine With or Without Valspodar in Patients With Relapsed or Refractory Acute Myeloid Leukemia and High-Risk Myelodysplastic Syndrome: A Phase III Trial (E2995). J Clin Oncol 2004;22:1078-1086.

[89] Preisler H, Davis RB, Kirshner J, et al. Comparison of three remission induction regimens and two postinduction strategies for the treatment of acute nonlymphocyticleukemia: a cancer and leukemia group B study. Blood. 1987;69:1441–1449.

[90] Raffoux E, Rousselot P, Poupon J, et al. Combined treatment with arsenic trioxide and all-trans-retinoic acid in patients with relapsed acute promyelocyticleukemia. *J ClinOncol.* 2003;21:2326–2334.

[91] Rowe JM. Optimal induction and post-remission therapy for AML in first remission. Hematology Am SocHematolEduc Program. 2009:396-405.

[92] Rozenfeld-Granot G, Toren A, Amariglio N, Brok-Simoni F, Rechavi G. Mutation analysis of the FAS and TNFR apoptotic cascade genes in hematological malignancies. Exp Hematol. 2001;29(2):228-33.

[93] Sachs L. The control of hematopoiesis and leukemia: from basic biology to the clinic. Proc. Natl. Acad. Sci. USA. 1996; 93, 4742- 4749.

[94] Sanz MA, Grimwade D, Tallman MS, et al. Guidelines on the management of acute promyelocyticleukemia: recommendations from an expert panel on behalf of the European LeukemiaNet. *Blood.* Prepublished on September 23, 2008.

[95] Schiller G, Gajewski J, Nimer S, et al. A randomized study of intermediate versus conventional-dose cytarabine as intensive induction for acute myelogenous leukaemia. Br J Haematol. 1992;81:170 –177.

[96] Schlenk RF, Dohner K, Krauter J, et al. Mutations and treatment outcome in cytogenetically normal acute myeloid leukemia. *N Engl J Med.* 2008;358:1909 –1918.

[97] Schnittger S, Kohl TM, Haferlach T, et al. KIT-D816 mutations in AML1-ETO-positive AML are associated with impaired event-free and overall survival. *Blood.* 2006;107:1791–1799.

[98] Sheikh MS, Burns TF, Huang Y, Wu GS, Amundson S, Brooks KS, FornaceJr AJ, el-Deiry WS. p53-dependent and -independent regulation of the death receptor KILLER/DR5 gene expression in response to genotoxic stress and tumor necrosis factor alpha. Cancer Res 1998; 58:1593-1598.

[99] Shigeno M, Nakao K, Ichikawa T, Suzuki K, Kawakami A, Abiru S, Miyazoe S, Nakagawa Y, Ishikawa H, Hamasaki K, Nakata K, Ishii N, Eguchi K. Interferon-alpha sensitizes human hepatoma cells to TRAIL-induced apoptosis through DR5 upregulation and NF-kappa B inactivation. Oncogene 2003; 22:1653-1662.

[100] Schimmer AD, Herr W, Hänel M, Borthakur G, Frankel A, Horst HA, Martin S, Kassis J, Desjardins P, Seiter K, Fiedler W, Noppeney R, Giagounidis A, Jacob C, Jolivet J, Tallman MS, Koschmieder S. Addition of AEG35156 XIAP Antisense Oligonucleotide in Reinduction Chemotherapy Does Not Improve Remission Rates in Patients With Primary Refractory Acute Myeloid Leukemia in a Randomized Phase II Study. Clin Lymphoma Myeloma Leuk. 2011;11(5):433-8.

[101] Solary E, Witz F, Caillot D, et al. Combination of quinine as a potential reversing agent with mitoxantrone and cytarabine for the treatment of acute leukemias: a randomized multicentric study. Blood. 1996;88:1198-1205.

[102] Soignet SL, Frankel SR, Douer D, et al. United States multicenter study of arsenic trioxide in relapsed acute promyelocyticleukemia. *J ClinOncol.* 2001;19:3852–3860.

[103] Stadheim TA, Saluta GR, Kucera GL. Role of c-Jun N-terminal kinase/p38 stress signaling in 1-beta-D-arabinofuranosylcytosine-induced apoptosis. BiochemPharmacol 2000; 59(4):407-418.

[104] Stegmaier K, Corsello SM, Ross KN, Wong JS, Deangelo DJ, Golub TR. Gefitinib induces myeloid differentiation of acute myeloid leukemia. *Blood.* 2005;106:2841–2848.

[105] Stelljes M, Beelen DW, Braess J, Sauerland MC, Heinecke A, Berning B, Kolb HJ, Holler E,Schwerdtfeger R, Arnold R, Spiekermann K, Müller-Tidow C, Serve HL, Silling G, HiddemannW,Berdel WE, Büchner T, Kienast J; German AML Cooperative Group (AMLCG). Allogeneic transplantation as post-remission therapy for cytogenetically high-risk acute myeloid leukemia: landmark analysis from a single prospective multicenter trial. Haematologica. 2011;96(7):972-979.

[106] Styczynski J, Wysocki m, Debski R et al. Predictive value of multidrug resistance proteins and cellular drug resistance in childhood relapsed acute lymphoblastic leukemia. J Cancer Res ClinOncol. 2007;133(11):875-93.

[107] Svingen PA, Karp JE, Kraiewski S, Mesner PW, Gore SD, Burke PJ, et al. Evaluation of Apaf-1 and procaspases-2, -3, -7, and -9 as potential prognostic markers in acute leukaemia. Blood 2000;96:3922-3931.

[108] Swerdlow SH, Campo E, Harris NL, et al, eds.WHO Classification of Tumours of Haematopoietic and Lymphoid Tissues. Lyon, France: IARC Press; 2008.

[109] Tallman MS, Lee S, SikicBl et al. Mitoxantrone, etoposide and cytarabine plus cyclosporine for patients with relapse or refractory acute myeloid leukaemia: an Eastern Cooperative Oncology Group pilot study. Cancer .1999;85:358-367.

[110] Tanaka H, Matsumura I, Nakajima K, Daino H, Sonoyama J, Yoshida H, Oritani K, Machii T, Yamamoto M, Hirano T and Kanakura Y. GATA-1 blocks IL-6-induced macrophage differentiation and apoptosis through the sustained expression of cyclin D1 and bcl-2 in a murine myeloid cell line M1. Blood. 2000; 95, 1264-1273.

[111] Testa U and Riccioni R. Deregulation of apoptosis in acute myeloid leukemia. Haematologica 2007; 92:81-94

[112] Tourneur L, Delluc S, Lévy V, Valensi F, Radford-Weiss I, Legrand O, Vargaftig J, BoixC,Macintyre EA, Varet B, Chiocchia G, Buzyn A. Absence or low expression of fas-associated protein with death domain in acute myeloid leukemia cells predicts resistance to chemotherapy and poor outcome. Cancer Res. 2004 Nov 1;64(21):8101-8108.

[113] Tucker SJ, Rae C, Littlejohn AF, Paul A, MacEwan DJ. Switching leukemia cell phenotype between life and death. ProcNatlAcadSci U S A 2004; 101(35):12940-5.

[114] Van del Heuvel E, van der Holt B, Burnette AK et al. CD34-related coexpression of MDR1 and BCRP indicates a clinically resistant phenotype in patients with acute myeloid leukemia (AML) of older age. Ann Hematol. 2007;86(5):329-337.

[115] van Geelen CM, de Vries EG, Le TK, van Weeghel RP, de Jong S. Differential modulation of the TRAIL receptors and the CD95 receptor in colon carcinoma cell lines. Br J Cancer. 2003;89(2):363-373.

[116] Vardiman JW, Thiele J, Arber DA, et al. The 2008 revision of the World Health Organization (WHO) classification of myeloid neoplasms and acute leukemia: rationale and important changes. *Blood*. 2009;114:937–951.

[117] Wattel E, Preudhomme C, Hecquet B, et al. p53 mutations are associated with resistance to chemotherapy and short survival in hematologic malignancies. Blood. 1994;84:3148-3157.

[118] Wen LX, Hui LS, Zhong FA et al. Combination of tetrandrine as a potential-reversing agent with daunorubicin, etoposide and cytarabine for the treatment of refractory and relapsed acute myelogenousleukemia. Leuk Res. 2006;30(4):407-413.

[119] Wen J, Ramadevi N, Nguyen D, Perkins C, Worthington E, Bhalla K. Antileukemic drugs increase death receptor 5 levels and enhance Apo-2L-induced apoptosis of human acute leukemia cells. Blood 2000; 96:3900-3906.

[120] Weick JK, Kopecky KJ, Appelbaum FR, et al. A randomized investigation of high-dose versus standard-dose cytosine arabinoside with daunorubicin in patients with previously untreated acute myeloid leukemia: a Southwest Oncology Group study. Blood. 1996;88:2841–2851.

[121] Wu GS, Burns TF, McDonald IIIrd ER, Jiang W, Meng R, Krantz ID, Kao G, Gan DD, Zhou JY, Muschel R, Hamilton SR, Spinner NB, Markowitz S, Wu G, el-Deiry WS. KILLER/DR5 is a DNA damage-inducible p53-regulated death receptor gene. Nat Genet. 1997; 17:141-143.
[122] Yates JW, Wallace HJ Jr, Ellison RR, Holland JF. Cytosine arabinoside (NSC-63878) and daunorubicin (NSC-83142) therapy in acute nonlymphocyticleukemia. Cancer Chemother Rep. 1973;57:485 - 488.
[123] Yu R, Shtil AA, Tan TH, Roninson IB, Kong AN. Adriamycin activates c-Jun N-terminal kinase in human leukemia cells: a relevance to apoptosis. Cancer Letter 1999; 107(1):73-81.

21

Role of Signaling Pathways in Acute Myeloid Leukemia

Maha Abdullah and Zainina Seman
Immunology Unit, Department of Pathology
Faculty of Medicine and Health Sciences
Universiti Putra Malaysia
Malaysia

1. Introduction

Acute myeloid leukemia (AML) is a cancer wherein dysregulated differentiation, uncontrolled growth and inhibition of apoptosis lead to accumulation of immature myeloid progenitor cells and progression of oncogenic expression (Lowenberg et al., 1999). AML is now seen to be initiated and maintained from a small, self-renewing population of leukemic stem cells (LSCs), which give rise to a progeny of more mature and highly cycling progenitors (colony forming unit-leukemia, CFU-L). CFU-Ls do not self-renew, however they are committed to proliferation and limited differentiation. By doing so, they originate a population of blast cells which constitute the majority of leukemic cells in both the bone marrow and peripheral blood of patients. The exact phenotype of LSCs is still debated, but they are comprised in the CD34+/CD38-/low population (Lane et al., 2009). CD34+/CD38+ leukemic cells were unable to initiate leukemia in immunodeficient mice. It should be noted that only about 50% of AML are able to initiate leukemia in NOD/SCID mice (Testa et al., 2007)

2. Leukemogenesis

The pathogenesis of leukemia may be explained by two classes of alterations of oncogenic genes as a result of chromosomal aberrations. *Class I* mutations confers a proliferative and/or survival advantage to the cells. The current list of known leukemogenic class I mutations consists of more than 10 different protein tyrosine kinases (PTK) that undergo constitutive activation either by being fused to different N-terminal partner proteins providing an oligomerization domain, or by activating mutations such as point mutations in their kinase domain or internal tandem repeats (length mutations) in the juxtamembrane domain (Flt3, Kit). Most of these alterations are associated with chronic myeloproliferative disorders such as chronic myeloid leukemia/chronic myelomonocytic leukemia (CML/CMML) or Philadelphia negative myeloproliferative disorders, except activating mutations of Flt3 and Kit which are found almost exclusively in acute leukemia. Flt3 ITD (internal tandem duplication) mutants constitutively activate MAPK, AKT and STAT5, leading to Pim-1 activation and Bcl-xL (B-cell lymphoma) hyperexpression (Minami et al., 2003; Kim et al., 2005). Extracellular c-Kit mutations resulted in c-Kit receptor

hyperactivation in response to Kit ligand, with subsequent strong activation of MAPK and PI3K, while codon 816 c-Kit mutations induced constitutive STAT-3 activation and upregulation of Bcl-xL and c-myc (Schnittger et al., 2006)). Other class I alterations are gain of function mutations of the three main RAS isoforms (N-Ras, Ki-Ras, Ha-Ras) which are frequently seen in different myeloid malignancies (Beaupre and Kurzrock, 1999). N-Ras mutations lead to increased activity of the Ras pathway, resulting in increased proliferation and decreased apoptosis (Testa et al., 2007). Overexpression of *class I* mutations is generally sufficient to transform hematopoietic cells to growth-factor independence *in vitro* and to induce a lethal *leukemialike* myeloproliferative disorder in mice (Ilaria, 2004).
(Flt- FMS-Like Tyrosine Kinase 3, STAT- Signal Transducer and Activator of Transcription, MAPK-Mitogen-Activated Protein Kinase)
In contrast to class I mutations, there is a large group of genetic alterations mostly associated with acute leukemia, referred to as *class II* mutations, which impair differentiation of hematopoietic cells and subsequent apoptosis but do not directly provide proliferative and/or survival advantage. Many of them are loss of function mutations (either through fusion formation or point mutations) of transcriptional regulators that are critical for normal hematopoietic development and differentiation. Transcription factor fusion genes include CBF, RAR, MLL, HOX and CBP while loss of function mutations occur in AML1, CEBP/a, PU.1, GATA1 and IKAROS (reviewed in Chalandon and Schwaller, 2005). Via mediators of apoptosis, fusion proteins send anti-apoptotic signals that favor the preferential survival of leukemic cells:PML/RAR-α or CBF/SMMHC through the p53 pathway and AML1/ETO through the Bcl2-related pathway (Klampfer et al., 1996; Britos-bray et al., 1998; Pandolfi, 2001). PML/RARα fusion protein was also shown to exert an anti-apoptotic activity by downmodulating the expression of some death-inducing genes, such as TNF-R1 (Testa et al., 1998) and TRAIL-R1/-R2 (Ricioni et al., 2005). Nucleophosmin acts as a cellular p53 negative regulator to protect hematopoietic cells from stress-induced apoptosis (Lambert and Buckle, 2006). These mutations are usually not sufficient to mimic the human disease in transgenic mice since they do not readily induce a leukemia phenotype. However, after a long latency period, signs of myelodysplasia are often seen with a variable propensity to develop an immature and clonal hematologic disorder closely resembling human AML (reviewed in Chalandon and Schwaller, 2005). Additional mutations, occurring at the level of signal transduction molecules (the receptor tyrosine kinases Flt3 or c-Kit, NRas and Ki-Ras), are required for the generation of disease (reviewed in Testa et al., 2007). This hypothesis is supported by the analysis of unselected blood samples from neonates which showed that about 1% have class II genetic alterations that are detectable by PCR (Greaves et al., 2003).
(CBF-core binding factor, RAR –retinoic acid receptor, MLL-mixed lineage leukemia, HOX-homeobox, CBP-CREB binding protein, CEBP/a-CCAAT/enhancer binding protein, PML-promyelocyte leukemia, SMMHC-smooth muscle myosin heavy chain, TRAIL-tumor necrosis factor–related apoptosis-inducing ligand)
In the same light, being a heterogeneous disease, relapsed AML is unlikely to emanate from one predominant mechanism; instead, there are likely to be multiple biologic factors at play that allow for clinical relapse to occur. These factors likely include multidrug resistance proteins, aberrant signal transduction pathways, survival of leukemia stem cells, microenvironmental interactions, and immune tolerance. Many conditions in the environment select for the development of these target mechanisms, ranging from chemotherapeutic modalities, to signal transduction inhibitors, to upregulation of antileukemic immune responses (reviewed in Lancet and Karp, 2009)

PTK involved	Fusion gene	Chromosomal aberration	Disease phenotype
A. Fusion genes			
ABL (9q34)	BCR/ABL	t(9;22)(q34;q11)	CML
(ABL1)	TEL/ABL	t(9;12)(q34;p13)	Atypical CML
ARG (1q24)	BCR/ARG	t(1;22)(q24;q11)	Atypical CML
(ABL2)	TEL/ARG	t(1;12)(q24;p13)	Atypical CML
PDGF R (5q33)	TEL/PDGF R	t(5;12)(q33;p13)	CMML, atypical CML
	HIP1/PDGF R	t(5;7)(q33;q11)	CMML, atypical CML
	RAB5/PDGF R	t(5;17)(q33;p13)	CMML, atypical CML
	H4/PDGF R	t(5;10)(q33;q21)	CMML,atypical CML
	Myomegalin/PDGF R	t(1;5)(q23;q33)	CMML,atypical CML
	CEV14/PDGF R	t(5;14)(q33;q32)	relapse AML
	NIN1/PDGF R	t(1;5)(q23;q33)	atypical CML
	HCMOGT/PDGF R	t(5;17)(q33;p11)	juvenile CMML
	TP53BP1/PDGF R	t(5;15)(q33;q22)	atypical CML
PDGF R (4q12)	BCR/PDGF R	t(4;22)(q12;q11)	Atypical CML
AK2 (9p24)	BCR/JAK2	t(9;22)(p24;q11)	CML, atypical CML
	TEL/JAK2	t(9;12)(p24;p13)	Atypical CML, ALL, AML
	PCM1/JAK2	t(8;9)(p21-22;p23-24)	Atypical CML, AML, ALL
TRKC (15q25)	TEL/TRKC	t(12;15)(p13;q25)	AML
GFR3 (4p16)	TEL/FGFR3	t(4;12)(p16;p13)	AML
FRK(6q21)	TEL/FRK	t(6;12)(q21;p13)	AML
B. Gain of function mutations			
FLT3 (13q12)	ITD (80%), activation loop kinase domain (15%)		AML
KIT (4q12)	JM region, activation loop kinase domain		AML
JAK2 (9p21)	JAK2 V617F mutation	9pLOH	PV, ET, myelofibrosis
C. Deregulated expression			
FLT3 (13q12)	Overexpression	MLL alterations	ALL/AML

CML: chronic myeloid leukemia; AML: acute myeloid leukemia; ALL: acute lymphoblastic leukemia; CMML: chronic myelomonocytic leukemia; EMS; ITD: internal tandem duplication; JM: juxtamembrane; PV: polycythemia vera; ET: essential thrombocythemia; LOH: loss of heterozygosity

Table 1. Deregulated protein tyrosine kinases in myeloid leukemias (taken from Chalandon and Schwaller, 2005)

3. Signal Transduction Pathways (STP)

Signal transduction is the primary means by which eukaryotic cells respond to external signals from their environment and coordinate complex cellular changes. Extracellular signal is transduced into the cell through ligand-receptor binding, followed by the activation of intracellular signaling pathways that involve a series of protein phosphorylation and dephosphorylation, protein-protein interaction, and protein-small molecules interaction (Liu and Zhou, 2004). Cytokines interact with cell-surface receptors initiating signaling cascades that promote cell growth and division, while inhibiting the pathways of apoptotic cell death. The JAK/STAT, Raf/ MEK/ERK and PI3K/Akt signaling pathways are activated by a variety of cytokines that function to potentiate or inhibit hematopoiesis. These include IL (interleukin)-3, IL-7, SCF (stem cell factor), G (granulocyte)-CSF, type I interferons (IFN) and TGF- (transforming growth factor)- beta (Steelman et al., 2004).

The phosphatidylinositol 3-kinase (PI3K)

PI3K /protein kinase B (Akt)/mammalian target of rapamycin (mTOR) (a family of lipid kinases) signaling cascade is crucial to many widely divergent physiological processes which include cell cycle progression, transcription, translation, differentiation, apoptosis, motility, and metabolism (Yuan and Cantley, 2008). The family of PI3K enzymes phosphorylates inositol lipids and comprises three different classes, I, II, and III. Phosphorylated phosphatidylinositol 3,4,5trisphosphate [PtdIns (3,4,5)P3] recruits to the plasma membrane pleckstrin homology (PH) domain-containing proteins, which include phosphoinositide-dependent protein kinase 1 (PDK1) and Akt. The phospholipid products of PI3K activate downstream targets, including PDK, Akt and PKC (Palmer et al., 1995; Toker et al., 1994; Nakanishi et al., 1993).
Class I PI3K is further classified as A [activated by receptor tyrosine kinases (RTKs), Ras, and G-protein coupled receptors (GPCRs)] and B (activated by GPCRs) subtype. Class IA and 1B PI3Ks are heterodimeric enzymes composed of a regulatory and of catalytic subunits (Martelli et al., 2010).

Phosphoinositide-dependent kinase (PDK)

PDK requires the phospholipid product of PI3K for activation. There are believed to be two members of the PDK family - PDK1 and PDK2. Association of Akt with phosphoinositides produces a conformational change allowing Ser473 to be phosphorylated by PDK1 (Scheid et al., 2002).

Protein kinase B (Akt)

Akt is a 57-kDa serine/threonine protein kinase central to cell signaling downstream of growth factors, cytokines, and other cellular stimuli. Activated Akt was originally isolated from cells of the leukemia and lymphoma prone AKR strain of mice (Staal, 1987). It comprises three highly conserved isoforms: Akt1/α, Akt2/β, and Akt3/γ which are functionally different (Staal, 1987; Nicolson and Anderson, 2002; Staal et al., 1988). Once Akt is recruited at the plasma membrane, its activation loop is phosphorylated on Thr308 by PDK1 while the mTOR complex 2 (mTORC2), activated by RTK, phosphorylates Ser473 in the Akt COOH-terminus. Full Akt activation requires both phosphorylation steps. Active Akt migrates to both the cytosol and the nucleus. Nuclear Akt may fulfill important anti-apoptotic roles. So far, over 100 Akt substrates have been identified (Manning and Cantley, 2007). Of these, about 40 which mediate the pleiotropic Akt functions have been characterized, including Bad, caspase-9, murine double minute 2 (MDM2), IκB kinase (IKK) α, proline-rich Akt substrate 40-kDa (PRAS40) 40, the Foxo family of Forkhead box-o transcription factors, apoptosis signal-regulated kinase 1 [ASK1, a negative regulator of pro-apoptotic c-Jun N-terminal kinase (JNK)], Raf, p27Kip1, p21Cip1, glycogen synthase kinase

3β (GSK3β). Each of these substrates has a key role in the regulation of cell survival and proliferation, either directly or through an intermediary.

The antiapoptotic effects of Akt occur through its phosphorylation of a wide variety of targets. The first antiapoptotic target identified was Bad, a member of the Bcl-2 family. Phosphorylation of Bad at S136 by Akt allows phosphorylated Bad to interact with 14-3-3 proteins, promoting cell survival (Datta et al., 1997; Andreeff et al., 1999). Interaction of Bad with 14-3-3 proteins inhibits the ability of Bad to interact with Bcl-2 and Bcl-xL. This allows Bcl-xL to bind to proapoptotic Bax molecules and prevent the formation of proapoptotic Bax homodimers. However, Bad is also phosphorylated on different sites by members of the Raf/MEK/ERK (S112) and PKA (S112, S155) pathways.

In human cells, Akt phosphorylates and inactivates caspase-9. Overexpression of Akt inhibits cytochrome c-induced activation of caspase-9 (Cardone et al., 1998). Phosphorylation of the Foxo family of transcription factors is also attributed to Akt (Biggs et al 1999); Brunet et al., 1999; Rena et al., 1999; Tang et al., 1999).This phosphorylation results in forkhead transcription factors translocation to the cytoplasm, thus inhibiting transcription of pro-apoptotic genes such as FasL (Brunet et al., 1999). Akt activates transcription of antiapoptotic genes through phosphorylation of IKK and regulation of nuclear factor-kappa B (NF-kB) (Ozes et al., 1999). Akt also promotes cell survival and cell cycle progression by its ability to phosphorylate MDM2 and GSK-3 (Fukumoto et al., 2001; Zhou et al., 2001). Once phosphorylated by Akt, MDM2 translocates to the nucleus and interacts with p300. p300 dissociates from p19ARF, resulting in the degradation of p53 and cell cycle progression. Akt phosphorylates GSK-3, inhibiting its activity. The decreased GSK-3 activity increases stability of catenin and enhances its association with lymphoid enhancer factor/T cell factor (LEF/TCF) (Fukumoto et al., 2001). The catenin–LEF/TCF complex increases transcription of proteins such as cyclin D1 and c-myc, promoting cell cycle progression (Fukumoto et al., 2001). Clearly, Akt can affect both cell cycle progression and apoptosis (reviewed in Steelman et al., 2004).

MTORC1 is a critical regulator of translation initiation and ribosome biogenesis and plays an evolutionarily conserved role in cell growth control (Wullschleger et al., 2006). The enhanced sensitivity of cancer cells and mouse tumor models exhibiting oncogenic activation of the PI3K-Akt pathway to mTORC1 inhibitors, such as rapamycin, illustrates the importance of mTORC1 activation downstream of Akt (Sabatini, 2006). One of the best-conserved functions of Akt is its role in promoting cell growth (i.e., an increase in cell mass). The predominant mechanism appears to be through activation of mTOR complex 1 (mTORC1 or the mTOR-raptor complex), which is regulated by both nutrients and growth factor signaling. mTORC1 signaling integrates environmental clues (growth factors, hormones, nutrients, stressors) and information from the cell metabolic status. Thus, mTORC1 controls anabolic processes for promoting protein synthesis and cell growth (Manning and Cantley, 2007).

Janus kinase/Signal Transducer and Activator of Transcription (JAK/STAT)

The JAK/STAT pathway consists of three families of genes: the JAK, or Janus family of tyrosine kinases, the STAT (signal transducers and activators of transcription) family and the CIS/SOCS family, which serves to downregulate the activity of the JAK/STAT pathway (Silvennoinen et al., 1993; Kisseleva et al., 2002; Krebs and Hilton, 2002; Fujitani et al., 1997). The JAK/STAT pathway involves signaling from the cytokine receptor to the nucleus. JAKs are stimulated by activation of a cytokine receptor. Stimulation of JAKs results in STAT transcription factor activity. JAKs are a family of large tyrosine kinases, having molecular weights in the range of 120–140 kDa (1130–1142 aa). Four JAKs (JAK1, JAK2, JAK3 and Tyk2) have been identified in mammals. JAK3 expression is limited to hematopoietic cells (Steelman et al., 2004).

The STAT gene family consists of seven proteins (STAT1,STAT2, STAT3, STAT4, STAT5a, STAT5b and STAT6). Upregulation of STAT3 is detected with high frequency inhuman cancer. STAT3 is activated not only by cytokine receptors, such as the receptor for the IL-6 family cytokines, but also growth receptor tyrosine kinases, such as the EGFR family including Her2/Neu, and non-receptor tyrosine kinases such as Src and Abl(Turkson et al., 1998), and is also activated in response to stimulation of G-protein-coupled receptors (GPCR) (Pelletier et al., 2003). Classically, the receptor stimulation by ligand induces STAT3 binding to phosphotyrosine residues of receptors through its SH2 domain and its phosphorylation on a critical tyr705 residue by the receptor itself, or by associated Janus kinase (JAK, Jak1-3, Tyk2) or Src family tyrosine kinases (Yu et al., 2004).

Ras/Raf/MAPK kinase/extracellular signal-regulated kinase pathway
(Ras/Raf/MEK/ERK)

The Ras/Raf/MEK/ERK pathway is a central signal transduction pathway, which transmits signals from multiple cell surface receptors to transcription factors in the nucleus (Chang et al., 2003a; Chang et al., 2003b; Chang et al., 2003c). This pathway is frequently referred to as the MAP kinase pathway as MAPK stands for mitogen-activated protein kinase indicating that this pathway can be stimulated by mitogens, cytokines and growth factors. The pathway can be activated by Ras stimulating the membrane translocation of Raf. This pathway also interacts with many different signal transduction pathways including PI3K/Akt and JAK/STAT.

Ras is a small GTP-binding protein, which is the common upstream molecule of several signaling pathways including Raf/MEK/ERK, PI3K/Akt and RalEGF/Ral (Chang et al., 2003a; Chang et al., 2003b; Chang et al., 2003c). There are three different Ras family members: Ha-Ras, Ki-Ras and N-Ras. The Ras proteins show varying abilities to activate the Raf/MEK/ERK and PI3K/Akt cascades, as Ki-Ras has been associated with Raf/MEK/ERK while Ha-Ras is associated with PI3K/Akt activation.

The Raf protein family consists of A-Raf, B-Raf and Raf-1, which are involved in the regulation of proliferation, differentiation and apoptosis induced after cytokine stimulation (Blalock et al., 1999; Mercer et al., 2003; Naumann et al., 1007, Pritchard et al., 1996; Mercer et al., 2002).Raf-1 has many effects on the regulation of apoptosis. Some of these effects occur at the mitochondrial membrane and are independent of MEK and ERK activity. It was observed that overexpression of activated A-Raf abrogates the cytokine dependence of hematopoietic cells. Overexpression of B-Raf in Rat-1 cells results in decreased apoptosis due to inhibition of caspase activity. Raf-1 has important roles in apoptosis as it phosphorylates and inactivates Bad (Wang et al., 1996). Raf-1 phosphorylates and co-immunoprecipitates with Bcl-2, as well as regulates Bag and Bad expression, in BCR/ABL-expressing cells (Salomoni et al., 1998). The ability of Raf proteins to phosphorylate MEK1 varies from B-Raf, Raf-1, A-Raf. The ability of Raf to abrogate cytokine dependency is inversely proportional to their MEK1 activity, with A-Raf, Raf-1, B-Raf (McCubrey et al., 1998; Hoyle et al., 2000). Stimulation of Raf activates MEK1 and ERK resulting in phosphorylation of transcription factors, proliferation, and inhibition of apoptosis (Steelman et al., 2004).

Raf-1 is also phosphorylated by Akt which has been associated with inhibition of Raf-1 activity (Wojknowski et al., 1997; Rommel et al., 1999). CAMP-dependent protein kinase (PKA) inhibits Raf-1 (Wu et al., 1993; Schramm et al., 1994; Dumaz et al., 2002). Protein kinase C isoforms (a, b and g) stimulates Raf-1 activity (Sozeri t al., 1992). Raf-1 has been postulated to have important roles in cell cycle progression, activation of the p53 and NF-kB transcription factors and the prevention of apoptosis (reviewed in Steelman et al., 2004)
Interactions between the Raf and PI3K/Akt pathways, or crosstalk, is an area of intense research Recently, it was demonstrated that it is more effective to inhibit the growth of Raf- and MEK1-transformed hematopoietic cells with inhibitors that target both the Raf/MEK/ERK and PI3K/Akt pathways (Navolanic et al., 2004).

MEK

MEK proteins are the primary downstream targets of Raf. The MEK family of genes consists of five genes: MEK1, MEK2, MEK3, MEK4 and MEK5. The structure of MEK consists of an amino-terminal negative regulatory domain and a carboxy-terminal MAP kinase-binding domain, which is necessary for binding and activation of ERKs (Huang et al., 1995; Tanoue et al., 2001; Crews et al., 1992). Deletion of the regulatory MEK1 domain results in constitutive MEK1 and ERK activation. Activated MEK1 could abrogate cytokine dependency of certain hematopoietic cells. Constitutive activity of MEK1 inhibits NF-kB transcription by negatively regulating p38MAPK activity (Carter et al., 2000).

ERK

The main physiological substrates of MEK are the members of the ERK (extracellular signal-regulated kinase) or MAPK (mitogen activated protein kinase) family of genes. The ERK family consists of four distinct groups of kinases: ERK, Jun amino terminal kinases (JNK1/2/3), p38MAPK (p38 a/b/g/d) and ERK5. In addition, there are ERK3, ERK4, ERK6, ERK7 and ERK8 kinases, which while related to ERK1 and ERK2 have different modes of activation, and their biochemical roles are not as well characterized. Downstream targets of ERK include the p90Rsk kinase and the CREB, c-Myc and other transcription factors. ERK and p90Rsk can enter the nucleus to phosphorylate transcription factors which can lead to their activation (reviewed in Steelman et al., 2004).

Nuclear factor kappa B (NFkB)

Cilloni et al. (2007) have presented a comprehensive review on NF-kB. NF-kB proteins are a small group of related and evolutionarily conserved proteins which in mammals consists of five members: Rel (c-Rel), RelA/p65, RelB, p50, and p52 (Ghosh et al., 1998; Hayden et al., 2004).In resting cells, NF-kB proteins arepredominantly cytoplasmic, associating with members of the inhibitory IkB family such as IkBa, IkBb and Ikbe (Ghosh et al., 1998).These interact with NF-kB through multiple ankyrin repeats and as a result inhibit its DNA binding activity. Two NF-kB activation pathways exist; the first is normally triggered in response to infections or exposure to pro-inflammatorycytokines that activate the IkB kinase (IKK) complex leading to phosphorylation-induced IkB degradation, the other pathway leads to selective activation of p52: RelB dimers. This pathway is triggered by certain membersof the tumor necrosis factor (TNF)cytokine family through selective activation of IKKa by the upstream kinase, NF-kappa B-inducing kinase (NIK).In response to many stimuli such as inflammatorycytokines, bacterial lipopolysaccharide, phorbol esters, viral infection or stress, IkB are phosphorylated on two critical serine residues (Senftleben et al., 2001).

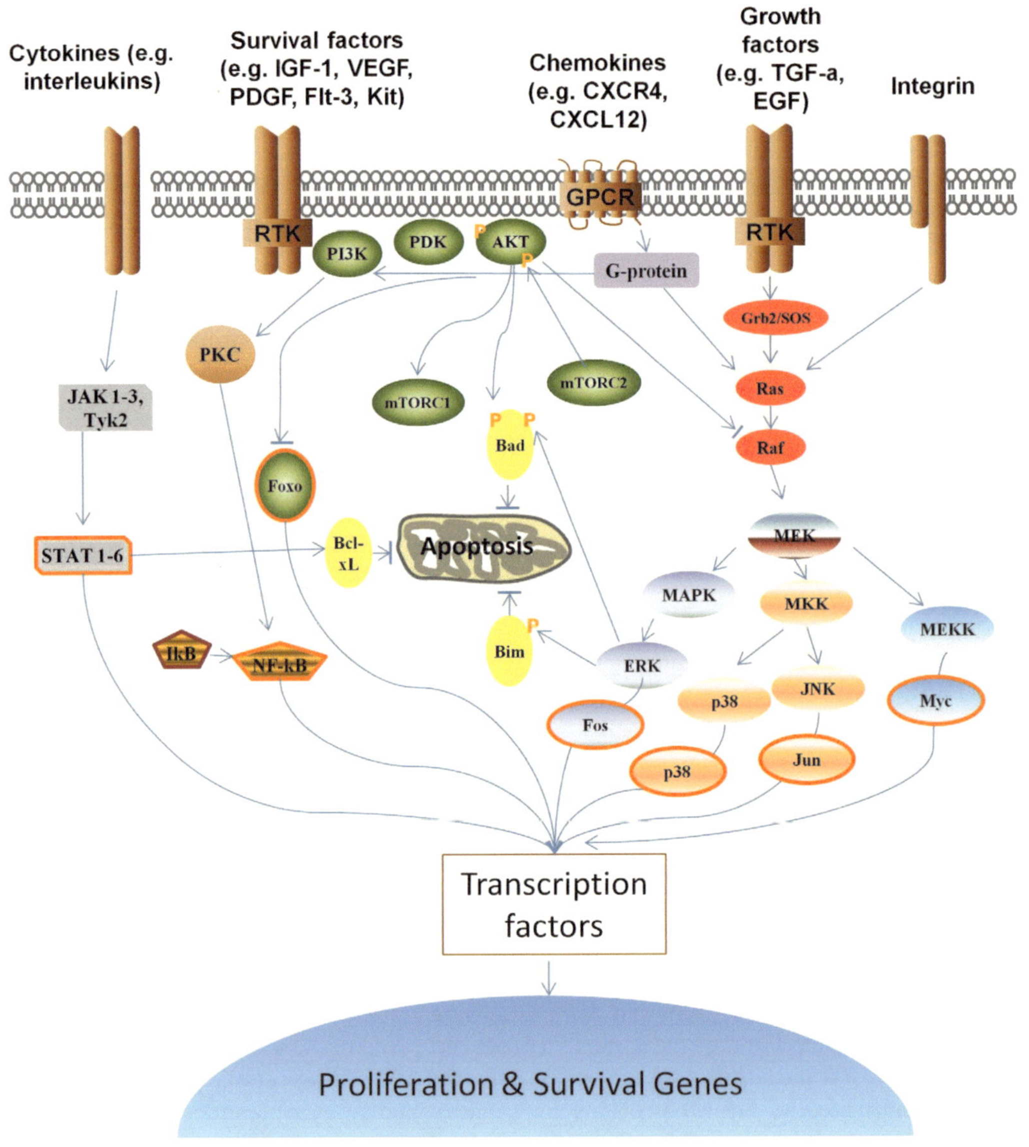

Fig. 1. Signal transduction pathways (refer text for details)

This modification triggers IkB ubiquitination and destruction via the 26Sproteasome degradation machinery. As a consequence, NF-kBis freed to enter the nucleus and regulate transcription of over 150 genes encoding cell adhesion molecules, cytokines, growth factors, components of the immune systems and anti-apoptotic genes such as FLIP (FLICE inhibitory protein), cIAPs (inhibitor of apoptosis), Bcl-2 and Bcl-xL (Aggarwall, 2004). It is also implicated in the regulation of cell proliferation by controlling D-type cyclins (Takebayashi et al., 2003).

The three main signaling pathways are kept in check by naturally occurring inhibitors or tumor suppressor proteins. For example, the JAK/STAT pathway has the SOCS/CIS family of proteins, which serve to limit its effects by a negative feedback pathway. The Raf/MEK/ERK pathway can be negatively regulated by the PI3K/Akt cascade as well as the MKP1 phosphatase, which inactivates phosphorylated ERK. The PI3K/Akt pathway has the PTEN and SHIP phosphatases, which serve to fine-tune its antiapoptotic effects (reviewed in Steelman et al., 2004).

4. Aberrant STP and drug resistance in AML

Genetic events that give rise to leukemic transformation occur through activation of components of receptor tyrosine kinase (RTK) signaling pathways (Liu and Zhou, 2004). These include fusion proteins or gene mutations such as seen with activated TEL-JAK, STAT5A and BCR-ABL. Transforming activity of oncogenic PTK is mediated by parallel activation of several downstream signaling pathways. Final downstream mediators of this complex signaling network are phosphoproteins that translocate to the nucleus and act as transcriptional regulators activating a distinct group of target genes. The oncogenic activity of a given PTK is mediated by several signaling pathways including JAK/STAT, Ras/MAPK, PI3K/AKT, or NF-kB.

Oncogenic activity severs dependence of transformed cell on external stimulation for survival. TEL-JAK fusion proteins contain the oligomerization domain of TEL and the tyrosine kinase domains of JAK1, JAK2, JAK3, or TYK2. These efficiently substitute for the survival and mitogenic signals controlled by IL-3, without concomitant activation of the IL-3 receptor. STAT5 are constitutively active in TEL-JAK2- and TEL-JAK1-expressing cells (Lacronique et al., 2000). The BCR-ABL oncogene produces an activated tyrosine kinase fusion protein and gain independence from IL-3 for cell growth (Mandanas et al., 1992). Activated forms of Ras, Raf, MEK, PI3K and Akt however, show significant differences in the ability to abrogate cytokine dependence (Steelman et al., 2004).

TEL/JAK2 isoforms, depending on the location of the breakpoints in the JAK2 gene, have been described in acute lymphoblastic leukemia of the B-cell type and atypical CML (Lacronique et al., 1997). Somatically acquired JAK2 mutation (V617F) was detected in 472/944 (50%) of patients with Ph-negative chronic myeloproliferative disorders [including polycythemia vera (PV), idiopathic myelofibrosis (IMF) and essential thrombocytosis (ET)] with predominance in PV (66%) followed by IMF (42%) and ET (26%) (Jones et al., 2005). Recent investigation of novel mutations in JAK2 revealed a higher incidence, ~99% and 55% in PV and ET, respectively (Tefferi, 2010).

Flt-3 mediates its proliferative and antiapoptotic effects through several signaling pathways including the STAT5, Ras/MAPK and PI3K/AKT pathways. Overexpression of Flt-3 was detected in 73% of AML and 78% of ALL patients (Nakao et al., 1996). Flt-3 *length mutations* (internal tandem duplications (ITD) in the juxtamembrane domain) (Nakao et al., 1996), is observed in more than 20% of adult and more than 10% of pediatric AML patients harbor an Flt-3-ITD (reviewed in Testa et al., 2007). In general, patients with mutant FLT3 show higher cell counts and decreased overall survival. Absence of the wild-type allele in patients with Flt-3-ITD predicted poor prognosis in 82 adult *de novo* AML cases with otherwise normal cytogenetics who received uniform high-dose therapy. Of the the 23 (28%) patients with Flt3-ITD, disease-free survival (DFS) was inferior ($P = 0.03$), yet overall survival (OS) was not different ($P = 0.14$) (Whitman et al., 2001). In cytogenetic normal AML patients aged > 60 years treated on Cancer and Leukemia Group B frontline trials, FLT3-ITD remained associated with shorter disease-free survival ($P < .001$; hazard ratio 2.10) and overall survival ($P < .001$; hazard Ratio 1.97) in multivariable analyses (Whitman et al., 2010). Flt3 kinase domain point mutants is mutated in about 35% of AML (Stirewalt et al., 2003). In a study of 481 patients, FLT3 mutation did not have an impact on event-free survival (EFS) in patients with CBF-AML ($P = .84$) and poor-risk AML ($P = .37$). However, while event-free survival was worse in the FLT3-internal tandem duplication (ITD) group (20 weeks vs 41 weeks; P < .00,001) this was not observed for the FLT3-tyrosine kinase domain (TKD) point mutation group (61 weeks vs 41 weeks; $P = .15$) (Santos et al., 2011).

The profiles of signal transduction that correlated with poor response to chemotherapy showed potentiated STAT5 and STAT3 phosphorylations as well as attenuated STAT1 phosphorylation following cytokine stimulation (Irish et al., 2004)

Ras mutations are frequently observed in certain hematopoietic malignancies including myelodysplastic syndromes, juvenile myelomonocytic leukemia and acute myeloid leukemia (Bartram et al., 1988; Flotho et al., 1999; Stirewalt et al., 2001). It has been shown to activate both the Raf/MEK/ERK and the PI3K/Akt pathways. Thus, mutations at Ras should theoretically activate both pathways simultaneously. Consequence of this activation may be the increased expression of growth factors that can potentially further activate this cascade by an autocrine loop. Many cytokine and growth factor gene promoters contain binding sites for transcription factors (Ets, Elk, Jun, Fos, CREB) whose activities are often activated by the Raf/MEK/ERK cascade (reviewed in Steelman et al., 2004).

There is increasing evidence that activation of the PI3K/AKT signaling pathway leading to downstream inactivation of Foxo transcription factors, activation of the mammalian target of rapamycin (mTOR), or induction of Skp2 (leading to degradation of the cell cycle inhibitor p27), plays a central role in transformation by several mutated PTK such as BCR/ABL, mutated FLT3 or KIT (Scheijen et al., 2004; Andreu et al., 2005). Emerging evidence suggests that activation of NF-kB involves crosstalk between the PI3K and Ras/MAPK pathways (Gelfanov et al., 2001; Kirchner et al., 2003). Several NF-kB target genes, such as cIAP1/cIAP2, Bcl-xL, or Mcl-1, are well-known inhibitors of apoptosis that may co-mediate the antiapoptotic effect of a constitutively activated PTK (Aichberger et al., 2005).

Expression of transcription factor fusions like AML1/ETO and PML/RARa in leukemic cells leads to induction of several genes associated with WNT signaling (Muller-Tidow et al., 2004). WNT signaling activation was found in a significant fraction of leukemic blasts from patients with AML-M0 (Zheng et al., 2004).

Other causes of PI3K/Akt/mTOR activation in AML may be the result of several factors, including low levels of PP2A, autocrine/paracrine secretion of growth factors such as IGF-1 and VEGF (reviewed in Martelli et al., 2010). Interactions between leukemic cells and bone marrow stromal cells through CXCR4 (a GPCR) which is abundantly expressed on leukemic cell surface where it is up-regulated by hypoxic conditions and its physiological ligand, (Fierro et al., 2009; Fiegl et al., 2009) CXCL12, produced by stromal cells, (Fiegl et al., 2009; Ayala et al., 2009) could result in PI3K/Akt/mTOR activation (Zeng et al., 2009). Furthermore, interactions between β1 integrins on AML cells and stromal fibronectin could lead to pathway activation, (Matsunaga et al., 2003; Matsunaga et al., 2008) possibly through up-regulation of integrin-linked kinase 1 (ILK1) which is involved in Akt phosphorylation on Ser473 in a PI3K-dependent manner in AML cells (Tabe et al., 2007).

PI3K/Akt/ mTOR pathway influences proliferation, survival, and drug resistance of AML cells.

From 50% to 80% of patients with AML display Akt phosphorylated on either Thr308 or Ser473 (or both) (Xu et al., 2003; Min et al., 2003). Univariate analysis of 146 AML patients revealed those with low levels of pAKT had somewhat better CR rates (60% versus 50%; *P*=0.21), longer median CR durations (71 versus 32 weeks; *P*=0.13), and statistically significant longer median survival times (59 versus 30 weeks; *P*=0.02) compared with those with high levels of pAKT. In another study, single analysis of Akt phosphorylated at threonine 308 (Thr308) and serine 473 (Ser473) showed AktThr308(high) patients had significantly shorter overall survival (11 vs 47 months; P=0.01), event-free survival (9 vs 26 months; P=0.005) and relapse-free survival (10 months vs not reached; P=0.02) than Thr308(low) patients. This was not observed for Akt Ser473 (Gallay et al., 2009). Poor prognosis of AML patients with elevated PI3K/Akt/mTOR signaling could be also related to the fact that this pathway controls the expression of the membrane ATP binding cassette (ABC) transporter, multidrug resistance-associated protein 1, associated with a lower survival rate (Tazzari et al., 2007; Schaich et al., 2005). Nevertheless, a more recent report has highlighted that constitutive activation of PI3K/Akt/mTOR signaling could be a favourable prognostic factor in de novo cases of AML. One hypothesis for the lower relapse rate in patients with enhanced PI3K/Akt/mTOR signaling is that it could drive immature leukemic cells (LSCs and CFU-L) into S phase, thus rendering them more susceptible to polychemotherapy (Tamburini et al., 2005)

The AKT pathway was among the signaling cascades whose simultaneous activation with other pathways, such as PKCα and ERK, was found to confer a poor prognosis in AML (Altman et al., 2011). Eventhough often mutated in human cancer, MMAC1/PTEN gene are infrequent as genetic aberrations in myeloid leukaemia (Aggerholm et al., 2000)

NF-kB has been found to be activated in CD34+/CD38– blast cells derived from patients with *de novo* AML (Guzman et al., 2001; Baumgartner et al., 2002). Leukemic stem cells residing in this population are quiescent or slowly cycling and therefore less sensitive to chemotherapy. They are therefore likely to be responsible for disease relapse and represent the target for future innovative therapies (Bonnett et al.,1997; Lowenberg et al., 1999; Jordan, 2002). Activation of NF-kB in leukemia patients has been well documented though NF-kB activation is not uniform among AML patients. Forty percent of AML patients evaluated presented with increased NF-kB DNA binding activity. These patients are characterized by increased white cell counts at diagnosis and increased blast percentages in the bone marrow suggesting a link between NF-kB and cell proliferation. In particular, cyclin D1, whose expression is regulated by NF-kB. Alternatively, NF-kB action could be due to the induction of genes coding for AML growth factors such as GM-CSF or granulocyte colony-stimulating factor (G-CSF) (Cilloni et al., 2007).

The majority of LSCs are quiescent and insensitive to traditional chemotherapeutic drugs. This latter feature explains, at least in part, the difficulties in eradicating this cell population by conventional polychemotherapy. Thus, novel therapeutic strategies for AML eradication should also target LSCs (Misaghian et al., 2009). In AML, aberrant activation of several signal transduction pathways strongly enhances the proliferation and survival of both LSCs and CFU-Ls (McCubrey et al., 2008; Steelman et al., 2008). Therefore, these signaling networks are attractive targets for the development of innovative therapeutic strategies in AML (Scholl et al., 2008).

5. Conclusion

Expression of STP proteins is heterogenous and of prognostic value in AML (Kornblau et al., 2009). These signaling pathways in AML may in the future help rationally select targeted therapies in individual patients (Foran, 2010). While current classification schemes have prognostic relevance they generally do not alter therapeutic recommendations. As knowledge of mutated genes in cancersim proves, our ability to treat patients afflicted with certain diseases will increase substantially. The genetic mutation may affect multiple signal transduction pathways. Targeting multiple pathways may be more efficacious as this approach may suppress or eliminate tumor growth at lower concentrations of the drugs than that required to inhibit growth by targeting a single pathway (Steelmanet al., 2004).

The heterogeneity in AML continues to elude the best methods to characterize them. Genome and proteome-wide analysis has further revealed complexity in the makeup of the leukemic cell. The rapid advancement in targeted therapies implied the urgent need for alternative therapy and the readiness of the community to embrace it. Nevertheless so far, combinatorial medicine still holds out as the best option for successful treatment. If targeted therapies remain the way forward it will eventually bank deeply on the ability to identify molecular signatures in the individual leading to the establishment of personalized medicine.

Novel array technologies enabled the analysis of numerous features at the level of DNA for gene copy number variation, mutations, methylation in addition to mRNA transcription and regulatory microRNA. Emerging technologies to assess protein expression and phosphorylation levels within cells e.g. cytokine and chemokine arrays to assess external forces acting on leukemic cells and phosphoproteins in apoptosis, cell-cycle, and signal-transduction pathways, are highly needed. Protein expression and posttranslational modifications, either alone or in concert with other profiling approaches, could provide independent or complementary information not captured by transcriptional profiles. Protein signature groups, with prognostic information distinct from cytogenetics may reveal underlying similarities indistinguishable by cytogenetics (Kornblau et al., 2009).

Quantitative flow cytometry appears well suited for identifying predictive markers in AML patients because it offers obvious advantages over other techniques (western blot, for example), including rapidness, a much lower number of cells required to perform the assay, and the possibility of identifying different subclones in the leukemic population by coimmunostaining with multiple antibodies to surface antigens (Martelli et al., 2010). The mechanisms in leukemogenesis, drug resistance and relapse remain an area of much research. From cell biology to cytogenetics to molecular defects to signaling pathways, all have contributed to a better understanding of the cancer. New knowledge in epigenetics and microRNA remain to be elucidated.

6. References

[1] Aggarwall BB. Nuclear factor-kB: the enemy within cancer. Cancer Cell 2004;6:203-208.

[2] Aggerholm A, Grønbaek K, Guldberg P, Hokland P. Mutational analysis of the tumour suppressor gene MMAC1/PTEN in malignant myeloid disorders.Eur J Haematol. 2000(2):109-113.

[3] Aichberger KJ, Mayerhofer M, Krauth MT, Skvara H, Florian S, Sonneck K, et al. Identification of mcl-1 as a BCR/ABL dependent target in chronic myeloid

leukemia (CML): evidence for cooperative antileukemic effects of imatinib and mcl-1 antisense oligonucleotides. Blood 2005;105:3303-3311.
[4] Andreeff M, Jiang S, Zhang X, Konopleva M, Estrov Z, Snell VE et al. Expression of Bcl-2 related genes in normal and AML progenitors: changes induced by chemotherapy and retinoic acid. Leukemia 1999; 11: 1881–1892
[5] Andreu EJ, Lledo E, Poch E, Ivorra C, Albero MP, Martinez-Climent JA, et al. BCR-ABL induces the expression of Skp2 through the PI3K pathway to promote p27Kip1 degradation and proliferation of chronic myelogenousleukemia cells. Cancer Res 2005;65:3264-3272.
[6] Altman JK, Sassano A, Platanias LC. Targeting mTOR for the treatment of AML. New agents and new directions.Oncotarget. 2011;2(6):510-517.
[7] Ayala F, Dewar R, Kieran M, Kalluri R. Contribution of bone microenvironment to leukemogenesis and leukemia progression. Leukemia 2009;23:2233–2241.
[8] Blalock WL, Weinstein-Oppenheimer C, Chang F, HoylePE,Wang XY, Algate PA et al. Signal transduction, cell cycle regulatory, and anti-apoptotic pathways regulated by IL-3 in hematopoietic cells: possible sites for intervention with antineoplastic drugs. Leukemia 1999; 13: 1109–1166.
[9] Bartram CR. Mutations in ras genes in myelocyticleukemias and myelodysplastic syndromes. Blood Cells 1988; 14:533–538.
[10] Baumgartner B, Weber M, Quirling M, Fischer C, Page S, Adam M, et al. Increased IkB kinase activity is associated with activated NF-kB in acute myeloid blasts. Leukemia 2002;12: 2062-2071.
[11] Bonnet D, Dick J. Human acute myeloid leukaemia is organized as a hierarchy that originates from a primitive hematopoietic cell. Nat Med 1997;3:730-737.
[12] Beaupre DM, Kurzrock R. RAS and leukemia: from basic mechanisms to gene directed therapy. J ClinOncol 1999; 17:1071-9.Greaves MF, Wiemels J. Origins of chromosome translocations in childhood leukaemia.Nat Rev Cancer 2003;3:639-649.
[13] Biggs III WH, Meisenhelder J, Hunter T, Cavenee WK, Arden KC. Protein kinase B/Akt-mediated phosphorylation promotes nuclear exclusion of the winged helix transcription factor FKHR1. ProcNatlAcadSci USA 1999; 96: 7421–7426.
[14] Britos-Bray M, Ramirez M, Cao W, Wang X, Liu PP, Civin CI, Friedman AD. CBF-SMMHC, expressed in M4eo acute myeloid leukaemia,reduces p53 induction and slows apoptosis in hematopoietic cells exposed to DNA-damaging agents. Blood 1998;92:4344-4352.
[15] Brunet A, Bonni A, Zigmond MJ, Lin MZ, Juo P, Hu LS et al. Akt promotes cell survival by phosphorylating and inhibiting a Forkhead transcription factor. Cell 1999; 96: 857–868.
[16] Cardone MH, Roy N, Stennicke HR, Salvesen GS, Franke TF, Stanbridge E et al. Regulation of cell death protease caspase-9 by phosphorylation. Science 1998; 282: 1318–1321.
[17] Carter AB, Hunninghake GW. A constitutive active MEK-ERK pathway negatively regulates NF-kappa B-dependent gene expression by modulating TATA-binding protein phosphorylation. J BiolChem 2000; 275: 27858–27864.
[18] Chalandon Y, Schwaller J. Targeting mutated protein tyrosine kinases and their signaling pathways in hematologic malignancies.Haematologica. 2005 Jul;90(7):949-968.

[19] Chang F, Lee JT, Navolanic PM, Steelman JG, Blalock WL, Franklin RA et al. Involvement of PI3K/Akt pathway in cell cycle progression, apoptosis, and neoplastic transformation: a target for cancer chemotherapy. Leukemia 2003a; 17: 590–603.

[20] Chang F, Steelman LS, Shelton JG, Lee JT, Navolanic PN, Blalock WL et al. Regulation of cell cycle progression and apoptosis by the Ras/Raf/MEK/ERK pathway. Int J Oncol 2003b; 22: 469–480.

[21] Chang F, Steelman LS, Lee JT, Shelton JG, Navolanic PM, Blalock WL et al. Signal transduction mediated by the Ras/Raf/MEK/ERK pathway from cytokine receptors to transcription factors: potential targeting for therapeutic intervention. Leukemia 2003c;17: 1263–1293.

[22] Cilloni D, Martinelli G, Messa F, Baccarani M, Saglio G. Nuclear factor kB as a target for new drug development in myeloid malignancies.Haematologica. 2007 Sep;92(9):1224-1229.

[23] Crews CM, Alessandrini A, Erikson RL. The primary structure of MEK, a protein kinase that phosphorylates the ERK gene product. Science 1992; 258: 478–480.

[24] Datta SR, Dudek H, Tao X, Masters S, Fu H, Gotoh Y et al. Akt phosphorylation of BAD couples survival signals to the cell intrinsic death machinery. Cell 1997; 91: 231–241.

[25] Dumaz N, Light Y, Marais R. Cyclic AMP blocks cell growth through Raf-1-dependent and Raf-1-independent mechanisms. Mol Cell Biol 2002; 22: 3717–3728.

[26] Fierro FA, Brenner S, Oelschlaegel U, Jacobi A, Knoth H, Ehninger G, Illmer T, Bornhauser M. Combining SDF-1/CXCR4 antagonism and chemotherapy in relapsed acute myeloid leukemia. Leukemia 2009;23:393–396.

[27] Fiegl M, Samudio I, Clise-Dwyer K, Burks JK, Mnjoyan Z, Andreeff M. CXCR4 expression and biologic activity in acute myeloid leukemia are dependent on oxygen partial pressure. Blood 2009;113:1504–1512.

[28] Flotho C, Valcamonica S, Mach-Pascual S, Schmahl G, Corral L, Ritterbach J et al. RAS mutations and clonality analysis in children with juvenile myelomonocyticleukemia (JMML).Leukemia 1999; 13: 32–37.

[29] Fujitani Y, Hibi M, Fukada T, Takahashi-Tezuka M, Yoshida H, Yamaguchi T et al. An alternative pathway for STAT activation that is mediated by the direct interaction between JAK and STAT. Oncogene 1997; 14: 751–761.

[30] Fukumoto S, Hsieh CM, Maemura K, Layne MD, Yet SF, Lee KH et al. Akt participation in the Wntsignaling pathway through Dishevelled. J BiolChem 2001; 276: 17479–17483.

[31] Gallay N, Dos Santos C, Cuzin L, Bousquet M, SimmonetGouy V, Chaussade C, Attal M, Payrastre B, Demur C, Recher C. The level of AKT phosphorylation on threonine 308 but not on serine 473 is associated with high-risk cytogenetics and predicts poor overall survival in acute myeloid leukaemia. Leukemia 2009;23:1029–1038.

[32] Gelfanov VM, Burgess GS, Litz-Jackson S, King AJ, Marshall MS, Nakshatri H, et al. Transformation of interleukin-3-dependent cells without participation of Stat5/bcl-xL: cooperation of akt with raf/erk leads to p65 nuclear factor kB mediated antiapoptosis involving c-IAP2. Blood 2001;98:2508-2517.

[33] GhoshS, May MJ, Kopp EB. NF-kB ad Rel proteins: evolutionary conserved mediators of immune responses. Annu Rev Immunol 1998; 16:225-60. 3. Hayden MS, Ghosh S. Signaling to NF-kB. Genes Dev 2004;18: 2195-2224.
[34] Guzman M, Neering S, Upchurch D,Grimes B, Howard DS, Rizzieri DA, et al. Nuclear factor kB is constitutivelyactivated in primitive human acute myelogenous leukaemia cells. Blood 2001;98:2301-2307.
[35] Hoyle PE, Moye PW, Steelman LS, Blalock WL, Franklin RA,Pearce M et al. Differential abilities of the Raf family of protein kinases to abrogate cytokine dependency and prevent apoptosis in murine hematopoietic cells by a MEK1-dependent mechanism. Leukemia 2000; 14: 642–656.
[36] Huang W, Kessler DS, Erikson RL. Biochemical and biological analysis of Mek1 phosphorylation site mutants. MolBiol Cell 1995; 6: 237–245.
[37] Ilaria RL Jr. Animal models of chronic myelogenous leukemia. Hematol Oncol Clin North Am. 2004;18:525-543.
[38] Irish JM, Hovland R, Krutzik PO, Perez OD, Bruserud Ø, Gjertsen BT, Nolan GP. Single cell profiling of potentiated phospho-protein networks in cancer cells.Cell. 2004 Jul 23;118(2):217-228.
[39] Jones AV, Kreil S, Zoi K, Waghorn K, Curtis C, Zhang L, Score J, Seear R, Chase AJ, Grand FH, White H, Zoi C, Loukopoulos D, Terpos E, Vervessou EC, Schultheis B, Emig M, Ernst T,Lengfelder E, Hehlmann R, Hochhaus A, Oscier D, Silver RT, Reiter A, Cross NC. Widespread occurrence of the JAK2 V617F mutation in chronicmyeloproliferative disorders. Blood. 2005;106(6):2162-2168.
[40] Jordan C. Unique molecular and cellular features of acute myelogenous leukaemia stem cells. Leukemia 2002;16:559-562.
[41] Kim KT, Baird K, Ahn JY, Meltzer P, Lilly M, Levis M, et al. Pim-1 is upregulated by constitutively activated FLT3 and plays a role in FLT3-mediated cell survival. Blood 2005;105:1759-177
[42] Kisseleva T, Bhattacharya S, Braunstein J, Schindler CW. Signaling through the JAK/STAT pathway, recent advances and future challenges. Gene 2002; 285: 1–24.
[43] Kirchner D, Duyster J, Ottmann O, Schmid RM, Bergmann L, Munzert G. Mechanisms of Bcr-Abl-mediated NFkB/Rel activation. ExpHematol 2003;31:504-511.
[44] Klampfer L, Zhang J, Zelenetz AO, Uchida H, Nimer SD. The AML1/ETO fusion protein activates transcription of BCL-2. ProcNatlAcadSci USA 1996;95:11863-11868.
[45] Kornblau SM, Womble M, Qiu YH, Jackson CE, Chen W, Konopleva M, Estey EH, Andreeff M. Simultaneous activation of multiple signal transduction pathways confers poor prognosis in acute myelogenousleukemia. Blood 2006;108:2358–2365.
[46] Kornblau SM, Tibes R, Qiu YH, Chen W, Kantarjian HM, Andreeff M, Coombes KR, Mills GB. Functional proteomic profiling of AML predicts response and survival. Blood 2009;113:154–164.
[47] Krebs DL, Hilton DJ. SOCS proteins: negative regulators of cytokine signaling. Stem Cells 2001; 19: 378–387.
[48] Lacronique V, Boureux A, Valle VD, Poirel H, Quang CT, Mauchauffe M, et al. A TEL-JAK2 fusion protein with constitutive kinase activity in human leukemia. Science 1997;278:1309-1312.

[49] Lacronique V, Boureux A, Monni R, Dumon S, Mauchauffé M, Mayeux P, Gouilleux F, Berger R,Gisselbrecht S, Ghysdael J, Bernard OA. Transforming properties of chimeric TEL-JAK proteins in Ba/F3 cells. Blood. 2000;95(6):2076-2083.
[50] Lambert B, Buckle M. Characterization of the interface between nucleophosmin (NPM) and p53:potential role in p53 stabilization. FEBS Lett 2006;6580:345-350.
[51] Lane SW, Scadden DT, Gilliland DG. The leukemic stem cell niche: current concepts and therapeutic opportunities. Blood 2009;114:1150–1157.
[52] Liu Y and Zhao H. A computational approach for ordering signal transduction pathway components from genomics and proteomics Data *BMC Bioinformatics* 2004, 5:158
[53] Lowenberg B, Downing J, Burnett A. Acute myeloid leukaemia. N Engl J Med 1999;341:1051-1062.
[54] Mandanas RA, Boswell HS, Lu L, Leibowitz D. BCR/ABL confers growth factor independence upon a murine myeloid cell line. Leukemia. 1992;6(8):796-800.
[55] Martelli AM, Evangelisti C, Chiarini F, McCubrey JA . The phosphatidylinositol 3-kinase/Akt/mTOR signaling network as a therapeutic target in acute myelogenous leukemia patients.Oncotarget. 2010 Jun;1(2):89-103.
[56] Matsunaga T, Takemoto N, Sato T, Takimoto R, Tanaka I, Fujimi A, Akiyama T, Kuroda H,Kawano Y, Kobune M, Kato J, Hirayama Y, et al. Interaction between leukemic-cell VLA-4 and stromal fibronectin is a decisive factor for minimal residual disease of acute myelogenousleukemia. Nat Med 2003;9:1158–65.
[57] Matsunaga T, Fukai F, Miura S, Nakane Y, Owaki T, Kodama H, Tanaka M, Nagaya T, Takimoto R, Takayama T, Niitsu Y. Combination therapy of an anticancer drug with the FNIII14 peptide of fibronectin effectively overcomes cell adhesion-mediated drug resistance of acute myelogenousleukemia. Leukemia 2008;22:353–360.
[58] McCubrey JA, Steelman LS, Hoyle PE, Blalock WL, Weinstein-Oppenheimer C, Franklin RA et al. Differential abilities of activated Rafoncoproteins to abrogate cytokine dependency, prevent apoptosis and induce autocrine growth factor synthesis in human hematopoietic cells. Leukemia 1998; 12:1903–1929.
[59] McCubrey JA, Abrams SL, Ligresti G, Misaghian N, Wong EW, Steelman LS, Basecke J, Troppmair J, Libra M, Nicoletti F, Molton S, McMahon M, et al. Involvement of p53 and Raf/MEK/ERK pathways in hematopoietic drug resistance. Leukemia 2008;22:2080–2090.
[60] Mercer K, Chiloeches A, Huser M, Kiernan M, Marais R, Pritchard C. ERK signalling and oncogene transformation are not impaired in cells lacking A-Raf. Oncogene 2002; 21: 347–355.
[61] Mercer KE, Pritchard CA. Raf proteins and cancer: B-Raf is identified as a mutational target. BiochimBiophysActa 2003; 1653: 25–40.
[62] Min YH, Eom JI, Cheong JW, Maeng HO, Kim JY, Jeung HK, Lee ST, Lee MH, Hahn JS, Ko YW. Constitutive phosphorylation of Akt/PKB protein in acute myeloid leukemia: its significance as a prognostic variable. Leukemia 2003;17:995–997.
[63] Minami Y, Yamamoto K, Kiyoi H, Ueda R, Saito H, Naoe T. Different antiapoptotic pathways between wild-type and mutated FLT3: insights into therapeutic targets in leukemia. Blood 2003;102:2969-2975.

[64] Misaghian N, Ligresti G, Steelman LS, Bertrand FE, Basecke J, Libra M, Nicoletti F, Stivala F, Milella M, Tafuri A, Cervello M, Martelli AM, et al. Targeting the leukemic stem cell: the Holy Grail of leukemia therapy. Leukemia 2009;23:25–42.
[65] Muller-Tidow C, Steffen B, Cauvet T, Tickenbrock L, Ji P, Diederichs S, et al. Translocation products in acute myeloidleukemia activate the Wntsignaling pathway in hematopoietic cells. Mol Cell Biol 2004;24:2890-2904.
[66] Nakao M, Yokota S, Iwai T, Kaneko H,Horiike S, Kashima K, et al. Internal tandem duplication of the flt3 gene found in acute myeloid leukemia. Leukemia 1996;10:1911-198.
[67] Naumann U, Eisenmann-Tappe I, Rapp UR. The role of Raf kinases in development and growth of tumors. Recent Results Cancer Res 1997; 143: 237–244.
[68] Navolanic PM, Lee JT, McCubrey JA. Docetaxol cytotoxicity is enhanced by inhibition of the Raf/MEK/ERK pathway. Cancer BiolTher 2004; 3: 29–30.
[69] Nicolson KM, Anderson NG. The protein kinase B/Aktsignaling pathway in human malignancy. Cell Signal 2002; 14: 381–395.
[70] Ozes ON, Mayo LD, Gustin JA, Pfeffer SR, Pfeffer LM, Donner DB. NF-kappaB activation by tumour necrosis factor requires the Akt serine–threonine kinase. Nature 1999; 401: 82–85.
[71] Pandolfi PP. Oncogenes and tumor suppressors in the molecular pathogenesis of acute promyelocytic leukaemia. Hum Mol Genet 2001;10:769-775.
[72] Pelletier S, Duhamel F, Coulombe P, Popoff MR, Meloche S. Rho family GTPases are required for activation of Jak/STAT signaling by G protein-coupled receptors. Mol Cell Biol. 2003; 23:1316–1333.
[73] Pritchard CA, Bolin L, Slattery R, Murray R, McMahon M. Post-natal lethality and neurological and gastrointestinal defects in mice with targeted disruption of the A-Raf protein kinase gene. CurrBiol 1996; 6: 614–617.
[74] Rena G, Guo S, Cichy SC, Unterman TG, Cohen P. Phosphorylation of the transcription factor forkhead family member FKHR by protein kinase B. J BiolChem 1999; 274: 17179–17183.
[75] Riccioni R, Pasquini L, Mariani G, Saulle E, Rossini A, Diverio D, et al. TRAIL decoy receptors mediate resistance of acute myelo id leukemia cells to TRAIL. Haematologica 2005; 90:612-624.
[76] Rommel C, Clarke BA, Zimmermann S, Nunez L, Rossman R, Reid K et al. Differentiation stage-specific inhibition of the Raf–MEK–ERK pathway by Akt. Science 1999; 286: 1738–1741.
[77] Sabatini, D.M. (2006). mTOR and cancer: insights into a complex relationship.Nat. Rev. Cancer *6*, 729–734.
[78] Salomoni P, Wasik MA, Riedel RF, Reiss K, Choi JK, Skorski T et al. Expression of constitutively active Raf-1 in the mitochondria restores antiapoptotic and leukemogenic potential of a transformation-deficient BCR/ABL mutant. J Exp Med 1998; 187: 1995–2007.
[79] Santos FP, Jones D, Qiao W, Cortes JE, Ravandi F, Estey EE, Verma D, Kantarjian H, Borthakur G. Prognostic value of FLT3 mutations among different cytogenetic subgroups in acute myeloid leukemia. Cancer. 2011;117(10):2145-2155.

[80] Schaich M, Soucek S, Thiede C, Ehninger G, Illmer T. MDR1 and MRP1 gene expression are independent predictors for treatment outcome in adult acute myeloid leukaemia. Br J Haematol 2005;128:324–332.

[81] Scheijen B, Ngo HT, Kang H, Griffin JD. FLT3 receptors with internal tandem duplications promote cell viability and proliferation by signaling through Foxo proteins. Oncogene 2004;23:3338-3349.

[82] Schnittger S, Kohl TM, Haferlach T, Kern W, Hiddemann W, Spiekemann K, et al. KIT-816 mutations in AML1-ETO-positive AML are associated with impaired event-free and overall survival. Blood 2006;107:1790-1799.

[83] Scholl C, Gilliland DG, Frohling S. Deregulation of signaling pathways in acute myeloid leukemia. SeminOncol 2008;35:336–345.

[84] Schramm K, Niehof M, Radziwill G, Rommel C, Moelling K. Phosphorylation of c-Raf-1 by protein kinase A interferes with activation. BiochemBiophys Res Commun 1994; 201: 740–747.

[85] Senftleben U Cao Y, Xiao G, Greten FR, Krahn G, Bonizzi G, et al. Activation of IKKa of a second, evolutionary conserved NF-kBsignaling pathway. Science 2001;293:1495-1499.

[86] Steelman LS, Pohnert SC, Shelton JG, Franklin RA, Bertrand FE, McCubrey JA. JAK/STAT, Raf/MEK/ERK, PI3K/Akt and BCR-ABL in cell cycle progression and leukemogenesis. Leukemia. 2004; 18(2):189-218.

[87] Steelman LS, Abrams SL, Whelan J, Bertrand FE, Ludwig DE, Basecke J, Libra M, StivalaF, Milella M, Tafuri A, Lunghi P, Bonati A, et al. Contributions of the Raf/MEK/ERK, PI3K/PTEN/Akt/mTOR and Jak/STAT pathways to leukemia. Leukemia 2008;22:686–707.

[88] Silvennoinen O, Witthuhn BA, Quelle FW, Cleveland JL, Yi T,Ihle JN. Structure of the murine Jak2 protein-tyrosine kinase and its role in interleukin 3 signal transduction. ProcNatlAcadSci USA 1993; 90: 8429–8433.

[89] Sozeri O, Vollmer K, Liyanage M, Frith D, Kour G, Mark III GE et al. Activation of the c-Raf protein kinase by protein kinase C phosphorylation. Oncogene 1992; 7: 2259–2262.

[90] Staal SP. Molecular cloning of the akt oncogene and its human homologues AKT1 and AKT2: amplification of AKT1 in a primary human gastric adenocarcinoma. ProcNatlAcadSci USA 1987;84: 5034–5037.

[91] Staal SP, Huebner K, Croce CM, Parsa NZ, Testa JR. The AKT1proto-oncogene maps to human chromosome 14, band q32. Genomics 1988; 2: 96–98.

[92] Stirewalt DL, Kopecky KJ, Meshinchi S, Appelbaum FR, Slovak ML, Willman CL et al. FLT3, RAS, and TP53 mutations in elderly patients with acute myeloid leukemia. Blood 2001; 97:3589–3595.

[93] Stirewalt DL, Radich JP. The role of FLT3 in hemopoietic malignancies. Nat Rev Cancer 2003;3:650-665.

[94] Tabe Y, Jin L, Tsutsumi-Ishii Y, Xu Y, McQueen T, Priebe W, Mills GB, Ohsaka A, Nagaoka I, Andreeff M, Konopleva M. Activation of integrin-linked kinase is a critical prosurvival pathway induced in leukemic cells by bone marrow-derived stromal cells. Cancer Res 2007;67:684–694.

[95] Takebayashi T, Higashi H, Sudo H, Ozawa H, Suzuki E, Shirado O, et al.NF-kB-dependent induction of cyclin D1 by retinoblastoma protein (pRB) family proteins and tumor derived pRB mutants. J BiolChem 2003;278:14897-14905.
[96] Tamburini J, Elie C, Bardet V, Chapuis N, Park S, Broet P, Cornillet-Lefebvre P, Lioure B, Ugo V, Blanchet O, Ifrah N, Witz F, et al. Constitutive phosphoinositide 3-kinase/Akt activation represents a favorable prognostic factor in de novo acute myelogenousleukemia patients. Blood 2007;110:1025–1028.
[97] Tang ED, Nunez G, Barr FG, Guan KL. Negative regulation of the forkhead transcription factor FKHR by Akt. J BiolChem 1999; 274: 16741–16746.
[98] Tanoue T, Maeda R, Adachi M, Nishida E. Identification of a docking groove on ERK and p38 MAP kinases that regulates the specificity of docking interactions. EMBO J 2001; 20:466–479.
[99] Tazzari PL, Cappellini A, Ricci F, Evangelisti C, Papa V, Grafone T, Martinelli G, Conte R, Cocco L, McCubrey JA, Martelli AM. Multidrug resistance-associated protein 1 expression is under the control of the phosphoinositide 3 kinase/Akt signal transduction network in human acute myelogenousleukemia blasts. Leukemia 2007;21:427–438.
[100] Tefferi A. Novel mutations and their functional and clinical relevance in myeloproliferative neoplasms: JAK2, MLP, TET2, ASXL1,CBL, IDH and IKZF1. Leukemia. 2010;24:1128-1138.
[101] Testa U, Grignani F, Samoggia P, Zanetti C, Riccioni R, Lo Coco F, et al. The PML/RARa fusion protein inhibits tumor necrosis factor-a-induced apoptosis in U937 cells and acute promyelocyticleukemia blasts. J Clin Invest 1998;101:2278-2289.
[102] Testa U and Riccioni R. Deregulation of apoptosis in acute myeloid leukemia. Haematologica. 2007;92(1):81-94.
[103] Turkson J, Bowman T, Garcia R, Caldenhoven E, de Groot RP, Jove R. Stat3 activation by Src induces specific gene regulation and is required for cell transformation. Mol Cell Biol. 1998;18:2545–2552
[104] Wang HG, Rapp UR, Reed JC. Bcl-2 targets the protein kinase Raf-1 to mitochondria. Cell 1996; 87: 629–638.
[105] Whitman SP, Archer KJ, Feng L. Absence of the wild-type allele predicts poor prognosis in adult de novo acute myeloid leukemia with normal cytogenetics and the internal tandem duplication of FLT3: a cancer and leukemia group B study. Cancer Res 2001;61: 7233-7239.
[106] Whitman SP, Maharry K, Radmacher MD, Becker H, Mrózek K, Margeson D, Holland KB, Wu YZ, Schwind S, Metzeler KH, Wen J, Baer MR, Powell BL, Carter TH, Kolitz JE, Wetzler M, Moore JO, Stone RM, Carroll AJ, Larson RA, Caligiuri MA, Marcucci G, Bloomfield CD. FLT3 internal tandem duplication associates with adverseoutcome and gene- and microRNA-expression signatures in patients 60 years of age or older with primary cytogenetically normal acute myeloid leukemia: a Cancer and Leukemia Group B study. Blood. 2010;116(18):3622-3266.
[107] Wojnowski L, Zimmer AM, Beck TW, Hahn H, Bernal R, Rapp UR, Zimmer A. Endothelial apoptosis in Braf-deficient mice. Nat Genet 1997; 16: 293–297.

[108] Wu J, Dent P, Jelinek T, Wolfman A, Weber MJ, Sturgill TW. Inhibition of the EGF-activated MAP kinase signaling pathway by adenosine 30,50-monophosphate. Science 1993; 262: 1065–1069.

[109] Wullschleger S, Loewith R, Hall MN. TOR signaling in growth and metabolism. Cell. 2006 Feb 10;124(3):471-484.

[110] Xu Q, Simpson SE, Scialla TJ, Bagg A, Carroll M. Survival of acute myeloid leukemia cells requires PI3 kinase activation. Blood 2003;102:972–980.

[111] Yu H, Jove R. The STATs of cancer—new molecular targets come of age. Nat Rev Cancer. 2004; 4:97–105.

[112] Zhou BP, Liao Y, Xia W, Zou Y, Spohn B, Hung MC. HER-2/neu induces p53 ubiquitination via Akt-mediated MDM2 phosphorylation. Nat Cell Biol 2001; 3: 973–982.

[113] Zeng Z, Shi YX, Samudio IJ, Wang RY, Ling X, Frolova O, Levis M, Rubin JB, Negrin RR, Estey EH, Konoplev S, Andreeff M, et al. Targeting the leukemia microenvironment by CXCR4 inhibition overcomes resistance to kinase inhibitors and chemotherapy in AML. Blood 2009;113:6215–6224.

[114] Zheng X, Beissert T, Kukoc-Zivojnov N, Puccetti E, Altschmied J, Strolz C, et al. -catenin contributes to leukemogenesis induced by AML-associated translocation products by increasing the self renewal of very primitive progenitor cells. Blood 2004;103:3535-3543.

22

Epigenetic Changes Associated with Chromosomal Translocation in Leukemia

Soraya Gutierrez[1], Amjad Javed[2], Janet Stein[3], Gary Stein[3], Sandra Nicovani[4], Valentina Fernandez[1], Ricardo Alarcon[1], Marcela Stuardo[1], Milka Martinez[1], Marcela Hinojosa[1] and Boris Rebolledo-Jaramillo[1]

[1]*Universidad de Concepcion, Departamento de Bioquimica y Biologia Molecular,*
[2]*University of Alabama Department of Oral and Maxillofacial Surgery*
[3]*University of Massachusetts*
[4]*Universidad Santo Tomás;*
[1,4]*Chile,*
[2.3]*USA*

1. Introduction

Chromosome translocation reflects an abnormality caused by rearrangement of DNA fragments between non-homologous chromosomes. These rearrangements can be visualized by cytogenetic analysis of affected cells. Non-random chromosomal translocations are frequently associated with a variety of cancers, particularly hematological malignancies and childhood sarcomas although recent evidence demonstrates that such translocations are also common in epithelial tumors (Aplan, 2006; Mitelman et al., 2005). Initially considered as random events that get selected, it has become increasingly apparent that chromosomal translocations are influenced by cell type, cell stage and genomic context. Most commonly, these non-random chromosomal translocations are associated with specific hematopoietic cell types. Such chromosomal translocations are commonly used as diagnostic tool and are increasingly utilized to guide therapeutic decisions. Although, the mechanism that causes chromosomal translocations remains largely unknown, it is commonly accepted that they arise from DNA double strand breaks (DSBs) that are misrepaired (Aplan, 2006; Digweed and Sperling, 2004; Betti et al., 2003; Povirk, 2006). For a translocation to occur there are several mechanistic factors required: First there needs to be at least two DSBs in different chromosomes. Second the DSBs must arise close enough both in three-dimensional space and in time. Finally, DNA repair pathways must be available to join the two broken DNA fragments to form the translocation. It is estimated that everyday a normal cell in our body is exposed to approximately 20,000 DNA damaging events (Ames and Shigenaga, 1992). A major source of DNA damage is oxygen free radicals; however there are other endogenous and exogenous sources of DNA damage such as replication, transcription, and genotoxic stress. All of these processes can induce DSBs, but for two DNA fragments to be joined they must necessarily come in close proximity of each other (less than 1.3μm) (Chen et al., 1996;

Misteli, 2010). These requirements are accommodated in two competing models to explain DSBs proximity in the nucleus: the position first and the breakage first (Figure 1). The position first model suggests that the DNA regions involved in the translocation are in close proximity before DSBs generation. Support for this model comes from the observation that translocation frequencies differ among tissues and is paralleled by tissue-specific organization of the involved chromosomes (Mitelman et al., 2007). For example, the frequency of c-myc translocations to IgH, Igκ, or Igλ locus in Burkitt's lymphomas correlates with reciprocal distance (Roix et al., 2003). In contrast, the breakage first model proposes that DSBs are produced far apart and then move into close proximity to be repaired. In yeast for example, independent DNA lesions move and colocalize in repair factories (Lisby et al., 2003a; Lisby et al., 2003b). In mammalian cells experimental evidence, ranging from no or limited movement to an extensive movement and clustering of these DSBs breaks, provides support for both models (Kruhlak et al., 2006).

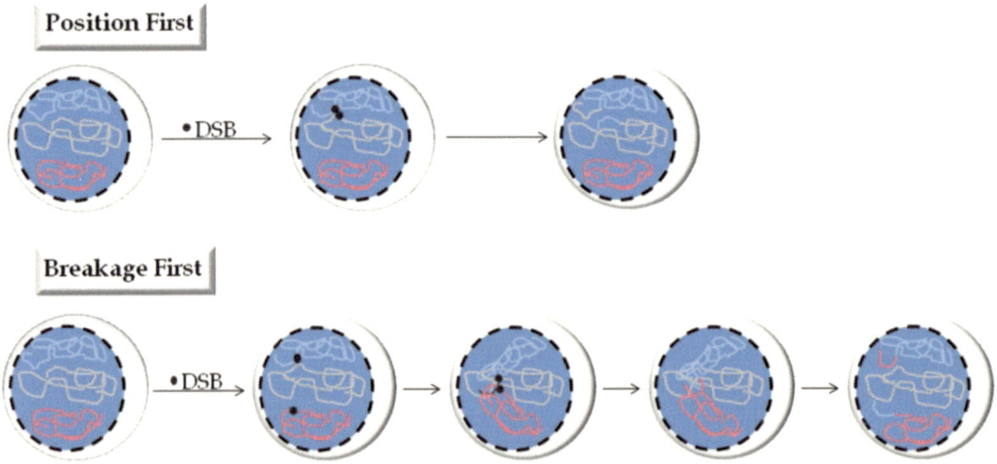

Fig. 1. **Models for Chromosomal Translocation Formation.** In the position first model two DSB that are nearby in the nuclei can be erroneously repair and give rise to a chromosomal translocation. In the breakage first model two DSB that are far apart in the nuclei are brought close together, probably to be repaired, resulting in a translocation.

In eukaryotic cells, DSBs are repaired by two different repair pathways: homologous recombination (HR) and non-homologous end joining (NHEJ) (Figure 2). HR is a relative error-free repair pathway that required information from a template sequence to repair the damage. This pathway is active during S and G2 phases of the cell cycle when the sister chromatid template is easily available and it can also take place during both mitosis and meiosis. NHEJ is a template independent DSBs repair mechanism. It is an error-prone pathway active throughout the cell cycle and the most commonly used DBSs repair pathway in multicellular eukaryotes. NHEJ is subdivided in classical (C-NHEJ) and alternate (A-NHEJ). The C-NHEJ is responsible for individual intrachromosomal DSBs repair in an homology independent manner, while A-NHEJ works in a micro-homology dependent manner, is more error-prone and seems to be the primary pathway responsible for the generation of chromosomal translocations (Simsek and Jasin, 2010; Boboila et al., 2010).

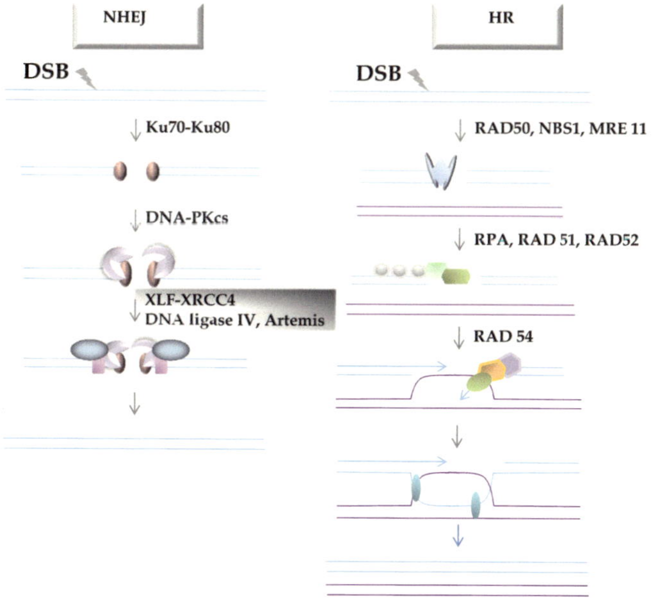

Fig. 2. **DNA Double Strand Break Repair Pathways**. Schematic representation of the two main DNA repair pathways: non homologous end joining (NHEJ) and homologous recombination (HR). The key regulatory proteins involved at multiple stages of each pathway are indicated.

Most of the chromosome translocations that have been analyzed to date show no consistent homologous sequences at the breakpoints regions. However, several structural features like DNase I hypersensitivity, topoisomerase II cleavage sites, DNA fragile sites and matrix or scaffold attachment regions (MARs or SARs) often colocalize with the mapped breakpoints. These observations suggest that chromatin organization may play a role in generation of translocations (Zhang et al., 2002; Strissel et al., 1998; Tanabe et al., 1996; Felix et al., 1995; Stanulla et al., 1997; Zhang and Rowley, 2006). Moreover, chromatin organization also has a prominent role in DNA repair process and therefore may influence both the selection of a DNA repair pathway and the eventual outcome of the DNA repair (Fernandez-Capetillo et al., 2004; Verger and Crossley, 2004; Tsukuda et al., 2005; Murr et al., 2006; Falk et al., 2008; Falk et al., 2010; Misteli and Soutoglou, 2009). Here we will focus on the current knowledge of the role that genomic structural features may have on formation of chromosomal translocations. Particularly we will analyze epigenetic marks associated with chromosome breakpoint regions and unusual DNA conformations among other structural features that may alter genomic structural stability.

2. Higher-order genome organization and translocations

The higher order organization of genomes architecture during interphase of the cell cycle forms chromosomes territories; which are defined as the nuclear space occupied by the DNA of a given chromosome (Cremer and Cremer, 2001; Cremer et al., 2006; Meaburn and Misteli, 2007; Misteli, 2007). Individual chromosomes are organized into open and closed chromatin domains that occupy different spatial compartments. A similar concept of nonrandom nuclear positioning applies to single loci and may be relevant to their translocation potential. For example the BCR and ABL genes, located on chromosomes 9 and 22, whose translocation leads to formation of a fusion protein involved in leukemia, are located in close proximity in normal hematopoietic cells at much higher frequency than would be expected based on a random distribution (Lukasova et al., 1997; Neves et al., 1999; Bartova et al., 2000). The same is true for the human chromosomes 12 and 16, which are frequently translocated in liposarcoma and are found in close proximity in differentiated adipocytes (Kuroda et al., 2004). Similarly, the frequency of c-myc translocations to IgH, Igκ or Igλ locus in Burkitt's lymphomas correlates with reciprocal nuclear distance. However, it is important to note that clonal oncogenic translocations in tumors are highly selected and therefore cannot be used to unequivocally determine the actual translocation frequency. More unbiased examinations may yet reveal translocations between loci that are not frequently in close proximity. The proximity of two particular loci within the interphase nucleus can be cell-type or tissue-specific. In this context, substantial colocalization of IgH and Igλ occurs in activated splenic B cells but not in embryonic stem cells or thymocytes (Wang et al., 2009). Notably, colocalization with IgH is not a characteristic of the entire chromosome 16 on which Igλ locus resides. In fact, about 15Mb sequences on either side of Igλ do not colocalize; therefore, proximity can be determinant in the context of more narrow areas around specific genes and not with broad chromosome territories.

The internal structure of the chromosomal territories is poorly understood but most probably is formed by a network of looping chromatin fibers. This relatively open structure allows access to gene regulatory factors while simultaneously protect the DNA from the continuous attack of damaging agents. Supporting this view, data from several different loci involved in genomic rearrangements exhibit an altered chromatin conformation in their breakpoint regions. For example, the MLL gene exhibits a strong topoisomerase II cleavage site near exon 12 where genomic breakpoint from therapy related AML (t-AML) patients and infant leukemia patient with MLL translocation have been mapped. Moreover, the same region also exhibit hypersensitivity to DNaseI and is cleaved by S1 and Mung Bean nuclease which specifically recognize and cleave single-strand regions in supercoiled DNA (Strissel et al., 1998; Felix et al., 1995; Stanulla et al., 1997). These features however are not exclusive to MLL gene, as topoisomerase II and DNaseI hypersensitive sites has also been found at the breakpoint regions of AF9, BCL, ABL, *RUNX1*, ETO and CBP among other genes (Greaves, 1996; Zhang et al., 2002; Strissel et al., 1998; Aplan et al., 1996; Relling et al., 1998; Strick et al., 2006; Sperry et al., 1989). However, not all breakpoint regions identified to date for genes involved in translocations colocalize with either topoisomeraseII cleavage sites or DHS, suggesting that other chromatin structural properties maybe involved in determining the location of chromosome breakage.

3. Chromatin organization and DNA repair

Higher order chromatin structure is not only important for global susceptibility of DNA to damage but may also be relevant for DNA repair. It is well documented that the earliest response to a DSB is the phosphorylation of the histone H2A variant histone H2AX on its C-terminus. Within seconds of DSB formation, the phosphorylated H2AX is present over surrounding regions, spanning thousand to millions of base pairs (Rogakou et al., 1998; Rogakou et al., 1999; Leatherbarrow et al., 2006; Kinner et al., 2008). H2AX is not present in lower eukaryote, but the domain that is phosphorylated in response to DSB is present in the C-terminus of other H2A-family members like H2A in S. cerevisiae and H2AZ in D. melanogaster (Downs et al., 2007). Although loss of H2AX does not abrogate DNA-damage checkpoints or repair, it impairs the joining of programmed DNA lesions during immunoglobulin class-switch recombination. These observations suggest that chromatin modifications at a distance are required for bringing together the DNA ends (Petersen et al., 2001; Reina-San-Martin et al., 2003). Moreover, failing to rejoin these programmed DSB in the absence of H2AX result in frequent chromosomal abnormalities (Franco et al., 2006; Ramiro et al., 2006). In addition to phosphorylation, H2A is also modified by acetylation in its N-terminal tail by NuA4, a histone acetyl transferase (HAT). Acetylation seems to be important for the ability of cells to survive after DNA damage (Bird et al., 2002).

The findings that DSB induces a rapid local decrease in the density of the chromatin fiber (Kruhlak et al., 2006) and that nearby nucleosomes are repositioned (Shim et al., 2007) support the idea that ATP-dependent chromatin remodeling factors have an early role in the DNA damage response. Indeed, several reports have demonstrated that the ATP-dependent chromatin remodeling complexes RSC (Remodels the Structure of Chromatin), SWI/SNF (SWItch/Sucrose NonFermenting), INO80 (INOsitol requiring) and SWR (Sick with Rat8 ts) are recruited to DSB, although at different time after the DNA damage. The first complex recruited to the DSB is RSC, which mobilize the nucleosomes near a DSB to new positions. Interestingly, in the absence of RSC the phosphorylation of H2AX is delayed. The other three chromatin remodeling complexes, SWI/SNF, INO80 and SWR, are enriched at sites of DSB at later times suggesting that they are not required for the initial detection or signaling of the DSB, but for the subsequent stages of the repair process.

Additionally, acetylation of conserved residues in the N-terminal tails of H3 and H4 has been found to contribute to both homologous and non-homologous recombination processes. For example, in mammalian cells, the TIP60 and the HAT cofactor TRRAP (transformation/transcription-domain associated protein) are recruited to sites of DSB, where they induce acetylation of H4 and facilitate homologous recombination. Similarly, another HAT, MOF (also known as MYST1) contributes to irradiation-induced acetylation of H4 at lysine 16 (H4K16). Defects on H3 and H4 acetylation have been linked to sensitivity to ionizing radiation and alteration in cell cycle checkpoints (Gupta et al., 2005). Complexes catalyzing the reverse process, i.e. histone deacetylation, have been shown to be enriched at late times at the DSB regions. If the acetylation of histones in the vicinity of DNA damage facilitate the repair process, then it is possible that the role of these histone deacetylase complexes might be to restore the chromatin to its original state once the DNA has been repaired.

4. Histone post-translational modifications in chromosomal rearrangements

The role of histone modifications on genomic rearrangements has been extensively studied in the V(D)J recombination process. This assembly process depends on a series of site-specific recombination reactions that are initiated by DSBs produced by RAG1 and RAG2 complex (Bassing et al., 2002). Each rearranging gene segment is flanked by a recombination signal sequence (RSS). The recombinase complex recognizes pair of compatible RSS, introduce DSBs and then channel the reaction products to a DNA repair pathway. Aberrant targeting of RAG proteins can produce chromosomal translocations that are associated with many forms of leukemia or lymphoma. In general, genes segments within recombinationally active loci are mark by the same histone modifications that characterize transcriptionally active genes, i.e. H3 and H4 acetylation as well as H3 trimethylation at lysine 4 (H3K4me3). More recently, it has become evident that the predominant effect of these histone modifications is to recruit the RAG complex to the RSS. In fact, RAG2 through its PHD domain specifically binds to H3K4me3 and mutations that abolish this binding results in greatly impaired V(D)J recombination activity (Liu et al., 2007; Matthews et al., 2007). Additional support for the epigenetic role on V(D)J recombination comes from the observation that in V genes H3 acetylation, although lower than in J genes, exhibit a gradient of enrichment that mirrored the rearrangement frequency. Interestingly, a reciprocal pattern is observed for the repressive modification H3 dimethylation at lysine 9 (H3K9me2) (Espinoza and Feeney, 2005; Espinoza and Feeney, 2007).

H3 trimethylation at lysine 4 (H3K4me3) is also implicated in meiotic recombination. In fact PRDM9, a zinc finger protein that catalyze the trimethylation of H3 at lysine 4, has recently been identified as a major determinant of sequence-specific meiotic recombination (Cheung et al., 2010).

Another histone modification, H3 methylation at lysine 79 (H3K79me), is associated with recombinationally active loci both in yeast and mammalian cell lines (Ng et al., 2003). Moreover, overexpression of DOT1L (a H3K79me specific methyltransferase) together with genotoxic stress and dihydrotestosterone significantly increases formation of chromosomal rearrangement involving the ETS genes, which are a distinguishing feature of prostate cancer (Kumar-Sinha et al., 2008; Lin et al., 2009).

Lin and colleagues (Lin et al., 2009), using prostate cancer as a model to study translocation mechanisms, have shown that after irradiation far more translocations are formed in androgen treated than in control cells. They also demonstrated that the translocation regions, TMPRSS2, ERG and ETV all contain binding sites for the androgen receptor (AR) near their breakpoints and that, after treatment with androgen, there is a rapid recruitment of AR to these sites. Moreover, AR recruitment induces changes in higher-order chromatin structure and epigenetic modifications establishing an open chromatin conformation characteristic of transcribed genes. Another consequence of AR binding was the recruitment of the activation-induced cytidine deaminase (AID), a key factor in somatic hypermutation (SHM) and class switch recombination (CSR) where it contributes to formation of DSB during the process of generating antibody diversity.

Additional data supporting the role of chromatin structure in genomic rearrangements comes from the analysis of the mechanisms involved in formation of t(2;5), a chromosomal translocation associated with anaplastic large cell lymphoma (ALCL). Mathas et al (Mathas et al., 2009) found up-regulation of several genes located near the ALCL translocation breakpoint, regardless of the presence of t(2;5) in the tumor. Moreover, their increased transcriptional activity promotes cell survival and repression of T-cell specific gene expression programs, both characteristics are a hallmark of ALCL (Mathas et al., 2009). Interestingly, cells isolated from ALCL patients lacking t(2;5) were more susceptible to form the (2;5) translocation than control cells. Together these data suggest that deregulation of breakpoint-proximal genes occurs before the formation of translocations and that similar to V(D)J recombination, transcriptional activity and altered chromatin structure predispose cells to chromosomal translocation.

This pattern of highly accessible chromatin structure characterized by H3 and H4 acetylation is also found at the breakpoint regions of other genes involved in translocations like MLL (Khobta et al., 2004), *RUNX1* (Stuardo et al., 2009) and ETO (our unpublished data). Using chromatin immunoprecipitation assays (ChIPs) we analyzed the chromatin structure at intrón 5 of the *RUNX1* gene, where all the translocation points for the (8;21) translocation has been mapped (Figure 3). Our results demonstrate that chromatin organization at intron 5 is completely different in HL-60 hematopoietic cells than in a non-hematopoietic cell (Stuardo et al., 2009). In fact, two distinct features mark the intron 5 in HL-60: a complete lack or significantly reduced levels of histone H1 and an increased association of hyperacetylated histone H3.

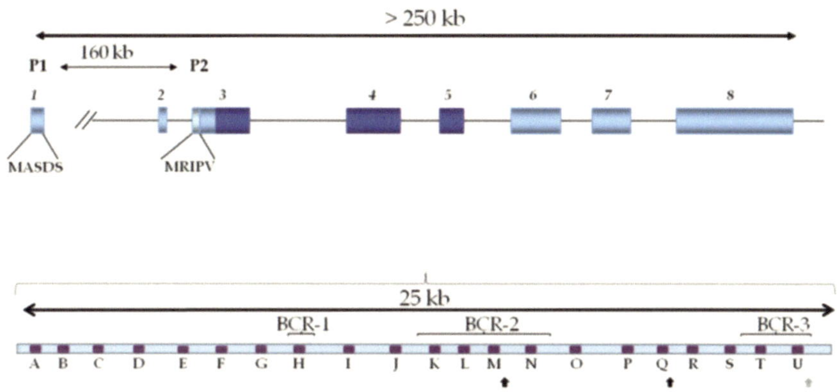

Fig. 3. **Diagrammatic representation of the *RUNX1* gene.** Top panel show the exon-intron organization of the gene as well as the two promoters that regulate its expression. Bottom panel show a magnification of intron 5 of the *RUNX1* gene. The three breakpoint clusters (BCR) are indicated as well as the amplification fragments analyzed by ChIP assays (purple blocks labeled A-U). Dark gray arrows indicate topoisomerase II sites and light gray arrow DNase I hypersensitive site.

The decreased association of histone H1, may indicate an overall enhanced accessibility and hence an increased availability to nucleases or DNA damaging agents. Notably, the region where the DNaseI hypersensitive site has been mapped presents one of the lowest rates of association of histone H1 in myeloid HL-60 cells (Figure 4, region U). Although the complete intron 5 is enriched in acetylated histone H3 (Figure 5), the chromatin organization is not homogeneous throughout the intron, suggesting that particular regions of intron 5 may play a regulatory role in transcription, subnuclear localization or compaction of the *RUNX1* gene. Interestingly, the chromatin organization at intron 5 resembles the chromatin structure adopted by the V(D)J gene segment. During V(D)J recombination, gene segments encoding the variable regions for immunoglobulins and T-cell receptors (TCR) are recombined and assembled in a new configuration. The same recombinase is present in both T and B cells, however recombination of immunoglobulins loci happens only in B cells while TCR loci rearrange only in T cells. Targeting of recombinase activity to specific gene segments is controlled largely by changes in chromatin accessibility in a spatio-temporal manner, and acetylation of histone tails has been shown to be a key event in this process. In fact, acetylation of histone H3 or H4 is elevated in B or T cell type at gene segments that can recombine, and reduced at segments that do not undergo recombination (Maes et al., 2006;

Maes et al., 2001; McMurry and Krangel, 2000). Moreover, hyperacetylation induced by inhibitors of histone deacetylase complexes (HDAC) rescues recombination defects caused by the elimination of extracellular signals that induce recombination (Durum et al., 1998). These studies suggest that histone hyperacetylation precedes recombination by opening chromatin and promoting access to the recombinase. Thus regardless of the molecular mechanism involved, it seems that an open chromatin conformation is a common requirement for a translocation to take place (Figure 6).

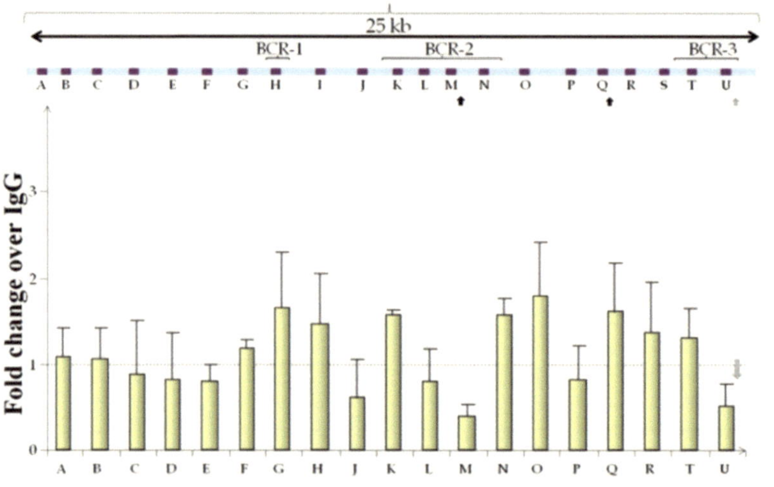

Fig. 4. **Intron 5 of *RUNX1* gene exhibit decreased association of histone H1.** Chromatin immunoprecipitation assays were performed with formaldehyde cross-linked chromatin isolated form HL-60 cells. Real-time PCR amplification of ChIP-DNA is shown as fold change over IgG in bar graph for immunoprecipitation with anti H1 antibody. Light gray arrow indicates DNaseI hypersensitive site.

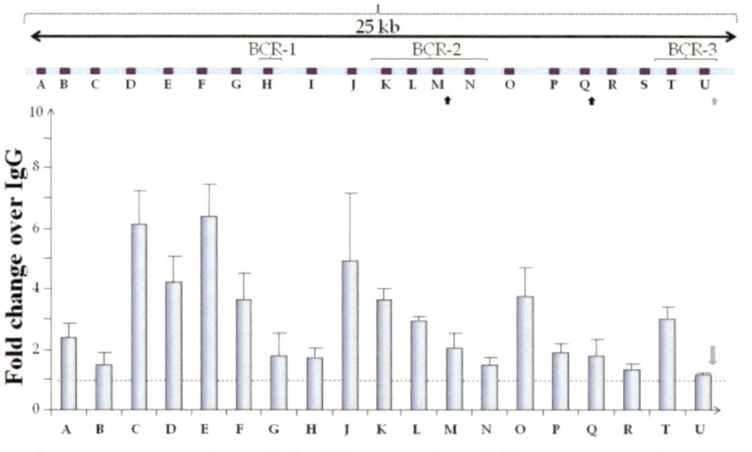

Fig. 5. **Intron 5 of *RUNX1* gene is enriched in acetylated histone H3.** Chromatin immunoprecipitation assays were performed with formaldehyde cross-linked chromatin isolated form HL-60 cells. Real-time PCR amplification of ChIP-DNA is shown as fold change over IgG for immunoprecipitation with anti acetylated H3 antibody. Light gray arrow indicates DNaseI hypersensitive site.

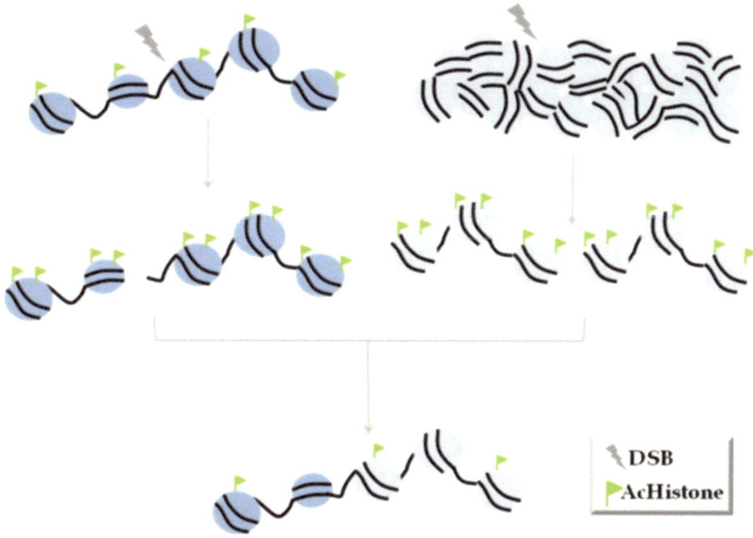

Fig. 6. **Summary of chromatin structure and histone modification in the regions involed in chromosomal translocation.** DSB can occur either in euchromatin or heterochromatin, but they must arise close enough both in time and in space to give rise to a chromosomal translocation. In both cases the regions surrounding the DSB will exhibit an open chromatin conformation either due to its presence in euchromatin or as result of the DNA repair process.

5. DNA conformation

In addition to the classical B-DNA structure described by Watson and Crick (Watson and Crick, 1953), more than 10 different DNA conformations are documented to date. These alternative DNA conformations include Z-DNA, hairpins/cruciforms, H-DNA (triplexes), slipped DNA and sticky DNA among others (Felsenfeld and RICH, 1957; Wang et al., 1979; Lilley, 1980; Panayotatos and Wells, 1981; Lyamichev et al., 1983; Sen and Gilbert, 1988; Mirkin, 2008). Several studies have shown that these non-canonical DNA structures affect DNA replication and transcription, and contribute to genome instability. For example non-B forming sequences located in c-MYC and BCL-2 genes localize with translocation breaking points. Studies have demonstrated that the H-DNA structure from the human c-MYC gene can induce DSBs in mammalian cells and stimulate genomic instability on mouse chromosomes in transgenic mice (Wang et al., 2008). However, the same sequences are not mutagenic in bacteria, suggesting a requirement for host-specific trans-acting factors to generate genomic instability.
Palindromic sequences, including palindromic AT-rich repeats (PATRRs), have the potential to form stem-loop structures by intrastrand base pairing within single-stranded DNA. In fact, PATRRs mapped on chromosome 22q11 and other chromosomes, such as 11q23 and 17q11, were found to cause non random chromosomal translocation in sperm cells in the general population (Kato et al., 2006) as well as in cell culture (Inagaki et al., 2009). Polymorphisms within the PATRRs affect the susceptibility to translocation *in vitro*, with longer and more symmetric PATRRs showing a stronger predisposition to translocation events (Kato et al., 2006; Kogo et al., 2007; Inagaki et al., 2009). Therefore, it has been

proposed that the secondary structures adopted by palindromic DNA induce a greater susceptibility to DSBs thus leading to translocations in human (Kurahashi et al., 2000).

There have also been identified chromosomal fragile sites, which are genomic regions especially susceptible to DNA breakage. These fragile sites are non-random specific loci that are stable under normal conditions, but under conditions of partial replication stress can form visible gaps or breaks in metaphase chromosomes (Durkin and Glover, 2007; Richards, 2001). Many different studies have established a connection between DNA fragile sites and the formation of cancer-specific genome rearrangements. However, only recently there has been direct evidence linking breakage at DNA fragile sites to the formation of a cancer specific translocation. Using as model RET/PTC rearrangements; which are commonly found in the papillary thyroid carcinoma (PTC) and in all cases result in the fusion of the tyrosine kinase domain of RET (rearranged in transformation) to the 5′ portion of various unrelated genes (Nikiforov, 2008) Gandhi et al (Gandhi et al., 2010) demonstrate that fragile site-inducing chemicals can create DNA breaks within the RET/PTC partner genes and ultimately lead to the formation of RET/PTC rearrangements. Moreover, aphidicolin induced DNA breaks at RET gene were located within intron 11, which is the breakpoint cluster region identified in thyroid cells. Clinical studies have shown that two different rearrangements, RET/PTC1 and RET/PTC3, are more frequent in sporadic and radiation-induced tumors respectively (Fenton et al., 2000; Fugazzola et al., 1995; Nikiforov et al., 1997; Motomura et al., 1998). Interestingly, treatment of cells with aphidicolin (APH), 2-aminopurine (2-AP) and 5-bromodeoxyuridine (BrdU) resulted in the generation of RET/PTC1 but not RET/PTC3 suggesting that sporadic PTC tumors may result from breakage at fragile sites. Although no consensus sequence have been identified in the fragile sites until now, the majority of them can form highly stable non-B DNA structures.

6. Concluding remarks

Traditionally it has been assumed that translocations arise randomly by stochastic DSB and that enrichment of particular translocations was result of the survival advantage acquired by the cells bearing the translocation. However, more recent results suggest that breaks in the genome occur in a nonrandom fashion and that higher-order chromatin organization maybe, at least in part, responsible for the formation of recurrent translocations. Although, significant progresses have been made in understanding formation of chromosomal translocation, particularly in the area of VDJ recombination, many more questions remain unanswered. For instance, it is still not known what proteins or pathways are involved in formation and maintenance of structure at the breakpoint regions, if these regions have a role in some cellular processes and what signaling pathways or environmental conditions promote chromosomal translocations. The response to these basic research questions may greatly improve diagnostic and therapeutic and may help to develop preventive measures for disorders associated with genomic instability such as chromosomal translocations.

7. Acknowledgments

This work has been supported by Fondo Nacional de Desarrollo Cientifico y Tecnologico (FONDECYT, Grant 1100670) (to SEG);National Institute of Health (Grant R03 TW007170-01A2) (JLS and SEG).

8. References

Ames, B.N. and Shigenaga, M.K. (1992). Oxidants are a major contributor to aging. Ann. N. Y. Acad. Sci. *663*, 85-96.

Aplan, P.D., Chervinsky, D.S., Stanulla, M., and Burhans, W.C. (1996). Site-specific DNA cleavage within the MLL breakpoint cluster region induced by topoisomerase II inhibitors. Blood *87*, 2649-2658.

Aplan, P.D. (2006). Causes of oncogenic chromosomal translocation. Trends in Genetics *22*, 46-55.

Bartova, E., Kozubek, S., Kozubek, M., Jirsova, P., Lukasova, E., Skalnikova, M., and Buchnickova, K. (2000). The influence of the cell cycle, differentiation and irradiation on the nuclear location of the abl, bcr and c-myc genes in human leukemic cells. Leuk. Res *24*, 233-241.

Bassing, C.H., Swat, W., and Alt, F.W. (2002). The mechanism and regulation of chromosomal V(D)J recombination. Cell *109 Suppl*, S45-S55.

Betti, C.J., Villalobos, M.J., Diaz, M.O., and Vaughan, A.T. (2003). Apoptotic stimuli initiate MLL-AF9 translocations that are transcribed in cells capable of division. Cancer Res *63*, 1377-1381.

Bird, A.W., Yu, D.Y., Pray-Grant, M.G., Qiu, Q., Harmon, K.E., Megee, P.C., Grant, P.A., Smith, M.M., and Christman, M.F. (2002). Acetylation of histone H4 by Esa1 is required for DNA double-strand break repair. Nature *419*, 411-415.

Boboila, C., Jankovic, M., Yan, C.T., Wang, J.H., Wesemann, D.R., Zhang, T., Fazeli, A., Feldman, L., Nussenzweig, A., Nussenzweig, M., and Alt, F.W. (2010). Alternative end-joining catalyzes robust IgH locus deletions and translocations in the combined absence of ligase 4 and Ku70. Proc. Natl. Acad. Sci. U. S. A *107*, 3034-3039.

Chen, A.M., Lucas, J.N., Hill, F.S., Brenner, D.J., and Sachs, R.K. (1996). Proximity effects for chromosome aberrations measured by FISH. Int. J Radiat. Biol *69*, 411-420.

Cheung, V.G., Sherman, S.L., and Feingold, E. (2010). Genetics. Genetic control of hotspots. Science *327*, 791-792.

Cremer, T. and Cremer, C. (2001). Chromosome territories, nuclear architecture and gene regulation in mammalian cells. Nat. Rev. Genet. *2*, 292-301.

Cremer, T., Cremer, M., Dietzel, S., Muller, S., Solovei, I., and Fakan, S. (2006). Chromosome territories--a functional nuclear landscape. Curr. Opin. Cell Biol *18*, 307-316.

Digweed, M. and Sperling, K. (2004). Nijmegen breakage syndrome: clinical manifestation of defective response to DNA double-strand breaks. DNA Repair (Amst) *3*, 1207-1217.

Downs, J.A., Nussenzweig, M.C., and Nussenzweig, A. (2007). Chromatin dynamics and the preservation of genetic information. Nature *447*, 951-958.

Durkin, S.G. and Glover, T.W. (2007). Chromosome fragile sites. Annu. Rev Genet *41*, 169-192.

Durum, S.K., Candeias, S., Nakajima, H., Leonard, W.J., Baird, A.M., Berg, L.J., and Muegge, K. (1998). Interleukin 7 receptor control of T cell receptor gamma gene rearrangement: role of receptor-associated chains and locus accessibility. J Exp. Med *188*, 2233-2241.

Espinoza, C.R. and Feeney, A.J. (2005). The extent of histone acetylation correlates with the differential rearrangement frequency of individual VH genes in pro-B cells. J Immunol. *175*, 6668-6675.

Espinoza, C.R. and Feeney, A.J. (2007). Chromatin accessibility and epigenetic modifications differ between frequently and infrequently rearranging VH genes. Mol Immunol. *44*, 2675-2685.

Falk, M., Lukasova, E., and Kozubek, S. (2008). Chromatin structure influences the sensitivity of DNA to gamma-radiation. Biochim. Biophys. Acta *1783*, 2398-2414.

Falk, M., Lukasova, E., and Kozubek, S. (2010). Higher-order chromatin structure in DSB induction, repair and misrepair. Mutat. Res *704*, 88-100.

Felix, C.A., Lange, B.J., Hosler, M.R., Fertala, J., and Bjornsti, M.A. (1995). Chromosome band 11q23 translocation breakpoints are DNA topoisomerase II cleavage sites. Cancer Res *55*, 4287-4292.

Felsenfeld, G. and RICH, A. (1957). Studies on the formation of two- and three-stranded polyribonucleotides. Biochim. Biophys. Acta *26*, 457-468.

Fenton, C.L., Lukes, Y., Nicholson, D., Dinauer, C.A., Francis, G.L., and Tuttle, R.M. (2000). The ret/PTC mutations are common in sporadic papillary thyroid carcinoma of children and young adults. J Clin. Endocrinol. Metab *85*, 1170-1175.

Fernandez-Capetillo, O., Lee, A., Nussenzweig, M., and Nussenzweig, A. (2004). H2AX: the histone guardian of the genome. DNA Repair (Amst) *3*, 959-967.

Franco, S., Gostissa, M., Zha, S., Lombard, D.B., Murphy, M.M., Zarrin, A.A., Yan, C., Tepsuporn, S., Morales, J.C., Adams, M.M., Lou, Z., Bassing, C.H., Manis, J.P., Chen, J., Carpenter, P.B., and Alt, F.W. (2006). H2AX prevents DNA breaks from progressing to chromosome breaks and translocations. Mol Cell *21*, 201-214.

Fugazzola, L., Pilotti, S., Pinchera, A., Vorontsova, T.V., Mondellini, P., Bongarzone, I., Greco, A., Astakhova, L., Butti, M.G., Demidchik, E.P., and . (1995). Oncogenic rearrangements of the RET proto-oncogene in papillary thyroid carcinomas from children exposed to the Chernobyl nuclear accident. Cancer Res *55*, 5617-5620.

Gandhi, M., Dillon, L.W., Pramanik, S., Nikiforov, Y.E., and Wang, Y.H. (2010). DNA breaks at fragile sites generate oncogenic RET/PTC rearrangements in human thyroid cells. Oncogene *29*, 2272-2280.

Greaves, M.F. (1996). Infant leukaemia biology, aetiology and treatment. Leukemia *10*, 372-377.

Gupta, A., Sharma, G.G., Young, C.S., Agarwal, M., Smith, E.R., Paull, T.T., Lucchesi, J.C., Khanna, K.K., Ludwig, T., and Pandita, T.K. (2005). Involvement of human MOF in ATM function. Mol Cell Biol *25*, 5292-5305.

Inagaki, H., Ohye, T., Kogo, H., Kato, T., Bolor, H., Taniguchi, M., Shaikh, T.H., Emanuel, B.S., and Kurahashi, H. (2009). Chromosomal instability mediated by non-B DNA: cruciform conformation and not DNA sequence is responsible for recurrent translocation in humans. Genome Res *19*, 191-198.

Kato, T., Inagaki, H., Yamada, K., Kogo, H., Ohye, T., Kowa, H., Nagaoka, K., Taniguchi, M., Emanuel, B.S., and Kurahashi, H. (2006). Genetic variation affects de novo translocation frequency. Science *311*, 971.

Khobta, A., Carlo-Stella, C., and Capranico, G. (2004). Specific histone patterns and acetylase/deacetylase activity at the breakpoint-cluster region of the human MLL gene. Cancer Res *64*, 2656-2662.

Kinner, A., Wu, W., Staudt, C., and Iliakis, G. (2008). Gamma-H2AX in recognition and signaling of DNA double-strand breaks in the context of chromatin. Nucleic Acids Res *36*, 5678-5694.

Kogo, H., Inagaki, H., Ohye, T., Kato, T., Emanuel, B.S., and Kurahashi, H. (2007). Cruciform extrusion propensity of human translocation-mediating palindromic AT-rich repeats. Nucleic Acids Res *35*, 1198-1208.

Kruhlak, M.J., Celeste, A., Dellaire, G., Fernandez-Capetillo, O., Muller, W.G., McNally, J.G., Bazett-Jones, D.P., and Nussenzweig, A. (2006). Changes in chromatin structure and mobility in living cells at sites of DNA double-strand breaks. J Cell Biol *172*, 823-834.

Kumar-Sinha, C., Tomlins, S.A., and Chinnaiyan, A.M. (2008). Recurrent gene fusions in prostate cancer. Nat Rev Cancer *8*, 497-511.

Kurahashi, H., Shaikh, T.H., Hu, P., Roe, B.A., Emanuel, B.S., and Budarf, M.L. (2000). Regions of genomic instability on 22q11 and 11q23 as the etiology for the recurrent constitutional t(11;22). Hum. Mol Genet *9*, 1665-1670.

Kuroda, M., Tanabe, H., Yoshida, K., Oikawa, K., Saito, A., Kiyuna, T., Mizusawa, H., and Mukai, K. (2004). Alteration of chromosome positioning during adipocyte differentiation. J Cell Sci *117*, 5897-5903.

Leatherbarrow, E.L., Harper, J.V., Cucinotta, F.A., and O'Neill, P. (2006). Induction and quantification of gamma-H2AX foci following low and high LET-irradiation. Int. J Radiat. Biol *82*, 111-118.

Lilley, D.M. (1980). The inverted repeat as a recognizable structural feature in supercoiled DNA molecules. Proc. Natl. Acad. Sci. U. S. A *77*, 6468-6472.

Lin, C., Yang, L., Tanasa, B., Hutt, K., Ju, B.G., Ohgi, K., Zhang, J., Rose, D.W., Fu, X.D., Glass, C.K., and Rosenfeld, M.G. (2009). Nuclear receptor-induced chromosomal proximity and DNA breaks underlie specific translocations in cancer. Cell *139*, 1069-1083.

Lisby, M., Antunez, d.M., Mortensen, U.H., and Rothstein, R. (2003a). Cell cycle-regulated centers of DNA double-strand break repair. Cell Cycle *2*, 479-483.

Lisby, M., Mortensen, U.H., and Rothstein, R. (2003b). Colocalization of multiple DNA double-strand breaks at a single Rad52 repair centre. Nat Cell Biol *5*, 572-577.

Liu, Y., Subrahmanyam, R., Chakraborty, T., Sen, R., and Desiderio, S. (2007). A plant homeodomain in RAG-2 that binds Hypermethylated lysine 4 of histone H3 is necessary for efficient antigen-receptor-gene rearrangement. Immunity. *27*, 561-571.

Lukasova, E., Kozubek, S., Kozubek, M., Kjeronska, J., Ryznar, L., Horakova, J., Krahulcova, E., and Horneck, G. (1997). Localisation and distance between ABL and BCR genes in interphase nuclei of bone marrow cells of control donors and patients with chronic myeloid leukaemia. Hum. Genet *100*, 525-535.

Lyamichev, V.I., Panyutin, I.G., and Frank-Kamenetskii, M.D. (1983). Evidence of cruciform structures in superhelical DNA provided by two-dimensional gel electrophoresis. FEBS Lett. *153*, 298-302.

Maes, J., Chappaz, S., Cavelier, P., O'Neill, L., Turner, B., Rougeon, F., and Goodhardt, M. (2006). Activation of V(D)J recombination at the IgH chain JH locus occurs within a 6-kilobase chromatin domain and is associated with nucleosomal remodeling. J Immunol. *176*, 5409-5417.

Maes, J., O'Neill, L.P., Cavelier, P., Turner, B.M., Rougeon, F., and Goodhardt, M. (2001). Chromatin remodeling at the Ig loci prior to V(D)J recombination. J Immunol. *167*, 866-874.

Mathas, S., Kreher, S., Meaburn, K.J., Johrens, K., Lamprecht, B., Assaf, C., Sterry, W., Kadin, M.E., Daibata, M., Joos, S., Hummel, M., Stein, H., Janz, M., Anagnostopoulos, I., Schrock, E., Misteli, T., and Dorken, B. (2009). Gene deregulation and spatial genome reorganization near breakpoints prior to formation of translocations in anaplastic large cell lymphoma. Proc. Natl. Acad. Sci. U. S. A *106*, 5831-5836.

Matthews, A.G.W., Kuo, A.J., Ramon-Maiques, S., Han, S., Champagne, K.S., Ivanov, D., Gallardo, M., Carney, D., Cheung, P., Ciccone, D.N., Walter, K.L., Utz, P.J., Shi, Y., Kutateladze, T.G., Yang, W., Gozani, O., and Oettinger, M.A. (2007). RAG2 PHD finger couples histone H3 lysine 4 trimethylation with V(D)J recombination. Nature *450*, 1106-1110.

McMurry, M.T. and Krangel, M.S. (2000). A role for histone acetylation in the developmental regulation of VDJ recombination. Science *287*, 495-498.

Meaburn, K.J. and Misteli, T. (2007). Cell biology: chromosome territories. Nature *445*, 379-781.

Mirkin, S.M. (2008). Discovery of alternative DNA structures: a heroic decade (1979-1989). Front Biosci. *13*, 1064-1071.

Misteli, T. (2007). Beyond the sequence: cellular organization of genome function. Cell *128*, 787-800.

Misteli, T. (2010). Higher-order genome organization in human disease. Cold Spring Harb. Perspect. Biol *2*, a000794.

Misteli, T. and Soutoglou, E. (2009). The emerging role of nuclear architecture in DNA repair and genome maintenance. Nat Rev Mol Cell Biol *10*, 243-254.

Mitelman, F., Mertens, F., and Johansson, B. (2005). Prevalence estimates of recurrent balanced cytogenetic aberrations and gene fusions in unselected patients with neoplastic disorders. Genes Chromosomes. Cancer *43*, 350-366.

Mitelman, F., Johansson, B., and Mertens, F. (2007). The impact of translocations and gene fusions on cancer causation. Nat Rev Cancer *7*, 233-245.

Motomura, T., Nikiforov, Y.E., Namba, H., Ashizawa, K., Nagataki, S., Yamashita, S., and Fagin, J.A. (1998). ret rearrangements in Japanese pediatric and adult papillary thyroid cancers. Thyroid *8*, 485-489.

Murr, R., Loizou, J.I., Yang, Y.G., Cuenin, C., Li, H., Wang, Z.Q., and Herceg, Z. (2006). Histone acetylation by Trrap-Tip60 modulates loading of repair proteins and repair of DNA double-strand breaks. Nat Cell Biol *8*, 91-99.

Neves, H., Ramos, C., da Silva, M.G., Parreira, A., and Parreira, L. (1999). The nuclear topography of ABL, BCR, PML, and RARalpha genes: evidence for gene proximity in specific phases of the cell cycle and stages of hematopoietic differentiation. Blood *93*, 1197-1207.

Ng, H.H., Ciccone, D.N., Morshead, K.B., Oettinger, M.A., and Struhl, K. (2003). Lysine-79 of histone H3 is hypomethylated at silenced loci in yeast and mammalian cells: a potential mechanism for position-effect variegation. Proc. Natl. Acad. Sci. U. S. A *100*, 1820-1825.

Nikiforov, Y.E. (2008). Thyroid carcinoma: molecular pathways and therapeutic targets. Mod. Pathol. *21 Suppl 2*, S37-S43.

Nikiforov, Y.E., Rowland, J.M., Bove, K.E., Monforte-Munoz, H., and Fagin, J.A. (1997). Distinct pattern of ret oncogene rearrangements in morphological variants of radiation-induced and sporadic thyroid papillary carcinomas in children. Cancer Res *57*, 1690-1694.

Panayotatos, N. and Wells, R.D. (1981). Cruciform structures in supercoiled DNA. Nature *289*, 466-470.

Petersen, S., Casellas, R., Reina-San-Martin, B., Chen, H.T., Difilippantonio, M.J., Wilson, P.C., Hanitsch, L., Celeste, A., Muramatsu, M., Pilch, D.R., Redon, C., Ried, T., Bonner, W.M., Honjo, T., Nussenzweig, M.C., and Nussenzweig, A. (2001). AID is required to initiate Nbs1/gamma-H2AX focus formation and mutations at sites of class switching. Nature *414*, 660-665.

Povirk, L.F. (2006). Biochemical mechanisms of chromosomal translocations resulting from DNA double-strand breaks. DNA Repair (Amst) *5*, 1199-1212.

Ramiro, A.R., Jankovic, M., Callen, E., Difilippantonio, S., Chen, H.T., McBride, K.M., Eisenreich, T.R., Chen, J., Dickins, R.A., Lowe, S.W., Nussenzweig, A., and Nussenzweig, M.C. (2006). Role of genomic instability and p53 in AID-induced c-myc-Igh translocations. Nature *440*, 105-109.

Reina-San-Martin, B., Difilippantonio, S., Hanitsch, L., Masilamani, R.F., Nussenzweig, A., and Nussenzweig, M.C. (2003). H2AX is required for recombination between immunoglobulin switch regions but not for intra-switch region recombination or somatic hypermutation. J Exp. Med. *197*, 1767-1778.

Relling, M.V., Yanishevski, Y., Nemec, J., Evans, W.E., Boyett, J.M., Behm, F.G., and Pui, C.H. (1998). Etoposide and antimetabolite pharmacology in patients who develop secondary acute myeloid leukemia. Leukemia *12*, 346-352.

Richards, R.I. (2001). Fragile and unstable chromosomes in cancer: causes and consequences. Trends Genet *17*, 339-345.

Rogakou, E.P., Boon, C., Redon, C., and Bonner, W.M. (1999). Megabase chromatin domains involved in DNA double-strand breaks in vivo. J Cell Biol *146*, 905-916.

Rogakou, E.P., Pilch, D.R., Orr, A.H., Ivanova, V.S., and Bonner, W.M. (1998). DNA double-stranded breaks induce histone H2AX phosphorylation on serine 139. J Biol Chem. *273*, 5858-5868.

Roix, J.J., McQueen, P.G., Munson, P.J., Parada, L.A., and Misteli, T. (2003). Spatial proximity of translocation-prone gene loci in human lymphomas. Nat Genet *34*, 287-291.

Sen, D. and Gilbert, W. (1988). Formation of parallel four-stranded complexes by guanine-rich motifs in DNA and its implications for meiosis. Nature *334*, 364-366.

Shim, E.Y., Hong, S.J., Oum, J.H., Yanez, Y., Zhang, Y., and Lee, S.E. (2007). RSC mobilizes nucleosomes to improve accessibility of repair machinery to the damaged chromatin. Mol Cell Biol *27*, 1602-1613.

Simsek, D. and Jasin, M. (2010). Alternative end-joining is suppressed by the canonical NHEJ component Xrcc4-ligase IV during chromosomal translocation formation. Nat Struct Mol Biol *17*, 410-416.

Sperry, A.O., Blasquez, V.C., and Garrard, W.T. (1989). Dysfunction of chromosomal loop attachment sites: illegitimate recombination linked to matrix association regions and topoisomerase II. Proc. Natl. Acad. Sci. U. S. A *86*, 5497-5501.

Stanulla, M., Wang, J., Chervinsky, D.S., Thandla, S., and Aplan, P.D. (1997). DNA cleavage within the MLL breakpoint cluster region is a specific event which occurs as part of higher-order chromatin fragmentation during the initial stages of apoptosis. Mol Cell Biol *17*, 4070-4079.

Strick, R., Zhang, Y., Emmanuel, N., and Strissel, P.L. (2006). Common chromatin structures at breakpoint cluster regions may lead to chromosomal translocations found in chronic and acute leukemias. Hum. Genet *119*, 479-495.

Strissel, P.L., Strick, R., Rowley, J.D., and Zeleznik, L. (1998). An in vivo topoisomerase II cleavage site and a DNase I hypersensitive site colocalize near exon 9 in the MLL breakpoint cluster region. Blood *92*, 3793-3803.

Stuardo, M., Martinez, M., Hidalgo, K., Montecino, M., Javed, A., Lian, J.B., Stein, G.S., Stein, J.L., and Gutierrez, S.E. (2009). Altered chromatin modifications in AML1/RUNX1 breakpoint regions involved in (8;21) translocation. J Cell Physiol *218*, 343-349.

Tanabe, S., Bohlander, S.K., Vignon, C.V., Espinosa, R., III, Zhao, N., Strissel, P.L., Zeleznik, L., and Rowley, J.D. (1996). AF10 is split by MLL and HEAB, a human homolog to a putative Caenorhabditis elegans ATP/GTP-binding protein in an invins(10;11)(p12;q23q12). Blood *88*, 3535-3545.

Tsukuda, T., Fleming, A.B., Nickoloff, J.A., and Osley, M.A. (2005). Chromatin remodelling at a DNA double-strand break site in Saccharomyces cerevisiae. Nature *438*, 379-383.

Verger, A. and Crossley, M. (2004). Chromatin modifiers in transcription and DNA repair. Cell Mol Life Sci. *61*, 2154-2162.

Wang, A.H., Quigley, G.J., Kolpak, F.J., Crawford, J.L., van Boom, J.H., van der, M.G., and Rich, A. (1979). Molecular structure of a left-handed double helical DNA fragment at atomic resolution. Nature *282*, 680-686.

Wang, G., Carbajal, S., Vijg, J., DiGiovanni, J., and Vasquez, K.M. (2008). DNA structure-induced genomic instability in vivo. J Natl. Cancer Inst. *100*, 1815-1817.

Wang, J.H., Gostissa, M., Yan, C.T., Goff, P., Hickernell, T., Hansen, E., Difilippantonio, S., Wesemann, D.R., Zarrin, A.A., Rajewsky, K., Nussenzweig, A., and Alt, F.W. (2009). Mechanisms promoting translocations in editing and switching peripheral B cells. Nature *460*, 231-236.

Watson, J.D. and Crick, F.H. (1953). Molecular structure of nucleic acids; a structure for deoxyribose nucleic acid. Nature *171*, 737-738.

Zhang, Y. and Rowley, J.D. (2006). Chromatin structural elements and chromosomal translocations in leukemia. DNA Repair (Amst) *5*, 1282-1297.

Zhang, Y., Strissel, P., Strick, R., Chen, J., Nucifora, G., Le Beau, M.M., Larson, R.A., and Rowley, J.D. (2002). Genomic DNA breakpoints in AML1/RUNX1 and ETO cluster with topoisomerase II DNA cleavage and DNase I hypersensitive sites in t(8;21) leukemia. Proc. Natl. Acad. Sci. U. S. A *99*, 3070-3075.

23

Myeloid Leukemia: A Molecular Focus on Etiology and Risk Within Africa

Muntaser E. Ibrahim and Emad-Aldin I. Osman
Department of Molecular Biology, Institute of Endemic Diseases, University of Khartoum, Khartoum, Sudan

1. Introduction

The developing world, Africa included, is witnessing an alarming upsurge of cancer incidence. The annual number of new cancer cases is expected to double by 2020 and up to 70% of the 20 million new cases of cancer predicted to occur yearly will be in the developing world (Jones et al., 1999; Ferlay et al., 2003; Yach et al., 2004).

One startling disparity, however, between cancer in the developing and developed worlds is that although the overall incidence of cancer in the developing world is half of that observed in the developed world, survival rates in the developing world are often less than one third of site-specific cancers in the developed world (Sener et al., 2005). This emphasizes the duality of the cancer problem in Africa, for being largely a disease of modern life style, occurring against a background of socio-economic disparities and greater burden of communicable diseases.

The study of genetic epidemiology of cancers in Africa hence entails the study of peculiar features of gene-environment interaction that may be largely private to Africa. In addition to the state of socio-economic underdevelopment that applies almost to the majority of African states, there is the plethora of extreme environments, wide range of climatic conditions and cultures, but most of all the transition state of the African communities from rural subsistent into urban market oriented life style. Furthermore one has to consider the notorious prevalence of infectious and non infectious diseases that may have a bearing both on the initiation of myeloid leukemia, its prognosis and management, e.g. tuberculosis (Omoti et al., 2009), malaria, other chronic infections, sickle cell disease (Ahmed et al., 2008) and common adaptive traits that could modulate the course of the disease, as well as the role of oncogenic viruses discussed below.

One interesting example of a potential trade-off between malignancies and parasitic diseases is CD36 a multiligand receptor associated with a broad array of physiological processes, believed to be under selective pressure from *Plasmodium falciparum,* and deficient or polymorphic in several African populations. The role of CD36 in sickle cell crises and cerebral malaria is debatable. As a receptor for thrombospondin 1, CD36 plays a role in the regulation of angiogenesis, which may be a therapeutic strategy for controlling the dissemination of malignant neoplasm. Moreover, it is commonly expressed on blasts in acute monocytic leukemia, megakaryoblastic leukemia, and erythroleukemia (Ge and

Elghetany, 2005). However, CD36 negative AML cells could be found especially in those populations that usually do not express CD36 (like in several African populations). CD36 negative cells appeared less susceptible to trombospondin-1 induced apoptosis, which make leukemic cells less vulnerable to death through this promising therapeutic strategy (Li et al., 2003).

On the other hand, due to the transition state, a number of risk factors believed to represent etiologic determinants of leukemia like use of pesticides, radiation etc. are not yet commonplace in Africa or at least its rural environment and may explain the differential distribution and the focal nature of hematological malignancies in the continent or/and individual countries. The potential impact of transition to a modern life style with the accompanying risks on the emergence and distribution of these diseases is worth our utmost attention.

Cancers in their complex etiology makes an ideal arena for the classical gene versus environment controversy. Those who favor an upper hand for the environment had their views strengthened by results of studies showing that people who migrate from one country to another generally acquire the cancer rates of the new host country, suggesting that environmental or lifestyle factors rather than genetic factors are the key determinants of the international variation in cancer rates. As far as Africa is concerned, African Americans´ disease data, represent a working model to test the role of changing environment and the effect of life style in complex diseases. Interestingly both sides of the argument seem to find support. Chronic myeloid leukemia (CML) patients show worse survival for African American and Hispanics compared to Americans of European origin (Lee et al., 2009). Although the difference in ethnicity data might be argued to reflect socio-economic differences, the current advances in genomics enable the implication of particular genomic regions and genes that explain the ethnic differences in susceptibility to infectious and chronic diseases.

Environmental determinants also falls short of explaining neither the "focality" of cancer types nor the aggressive course of some cancers in Sudan like the breast cancer, a feature that has been claimed to exist across Africa and even among African American women (reviewed by Morris and Mitchell, 2008).

Nutritional factors have also been implicated, adding an extra layer of complexity to the desperately compound picture of cancer etiology. Data on nutrition is greatly deficient in Africa similar to other aspects of genetic epidemiology, although differences in nutritional practices and culture may be key in providing vital clues to the contribution of life style. A study in China (Zhang et al., 2008), for example, suggested that a higher intake of green tea is associated with a reduced risk of adult leukemia. Furthermore, a study by Ross et al. which involved 35.221 older women provided evidence that increased vegetable consumption may decrease the risk of adult leukemia (Ross et al., 2002). Moreover, AML risk was negatively associated with milk intake among women and tea, and positively associated among women with beer, wine and beef (Li et al., 2006). A prospective cohort study by Ma et al. (2009) showed that smoking and total meat intake were risk factors for AML and those who did not drink coffee appeared to have a higher risk of AML.

Africa is still contains one of the last and few enclaves on the planet to harbor communities with distinctive patterns of traditional life styles that once used to characterize human existence. Farmers, pastoralists and hunter-gatherers- like societies do preserve their life style and culture and often coexist in shared terrains. These communities adopt fundamentally contrasting life styles and their food cultures are different. The significance of such disparity to all aspects of health and disease is of interest and the study of potential preponderance of these community members to chronic diseases including hematological malignancies should be investigated.

2. Incidence and epidemiology

The lowest rates of leukemia reported in sub-Saharan Africa probably represent failure of diagnosis or reporting to some extent (Davies, 1973; Fleming, 1993 and Parkin et al., 2005). We should therefore use caution, when drawing conclusions based on the varying prevalence and incidence, as an indication of clustering of cases or an environmental or genetic effect, as this may simply be due to the deficiency of statistics in Africa. The disparity could also be a reflection of the research milieu and capacity of individual countries or research groups, which indeed seem to be the case as most of the current reports on leukemia emerges from countries with well established science capacities.

Even with the scattered and available data, however, the difference from European and global trends could be observed as well as the evolution of the problem of leukemia. An early report from Uganda found that African children in Uganda showed a great and genuine deficiency of leukemia and an excess of solid lympho-reticular tumors (Davies et al., 1965).

In subsequence, the situation seems to change, a study of pediatric leukemia in Cameroon, showed that Acute Lymphoblastic Leukemia (ALL) comprised 78.6%, while AML 21.4% of all pediatric acute leukemia (Obama et al., 1995). In Egypt, the lymphatic and haemopoietic cancer incidence in 2001 have increased approximately 11-fold compared with the incidence in 1972. Moreover, the incidence of leukemia among infant less than 5 years increased exponentially with a higher incidence among boys (Hosny et al., 2002). In Kenya, leukemia in children below the age of 15 years comprised 37% of leukemia in all ages. Childhood acute leukemia formed 52.3% of all the acute leukemia. AML and ALL occurred, in almost equal proportions 42 % and 46 % respectively (Kasili, 1990). In Ethiopia, a report by Shamebo (1990) showed that the commonest type of leukemia was CML 57.8%, acute leukemia and chronic lymphatic leukemia (CLL) accounted for 21.1% each. Of the acute leukemia, 53.3% were ALL while 46.7% were AML (Shamebo, 1990). A recent study in south Nigeria showed that AML comprises 12.3% and CML 23.9% of all leukemia, with a mean age at diagnosis of 25.6 years and 35.2 years respectively (Nwannadi et al., 2011). In the last 25 years in Sudan CML became the predominant cancer in men, while lymphomas remained the second most common cancer. In women, breast, cervical and ovarian cancer remained the three most common cancers over both time periods, but there was also an increase in the incidence of CML among women (Hamad, 2006), the causes of this high incidence of CML are not known.

In Europe AML presents as mainly an adult's disease with a median age at presentation of 64 years, accounting for around 30% of all leukemia in adults, and ~18 000 new patients are diagnosed in Europe each year, representing ~0.6% of all cancers. The annual incidence rate in Europe ranges from two per 100 000/year to four per 100 000/year. In the past decade, the trend in overall incidence of AML has generally been stable or slowly increasing in most European countries, while most cases of CML occur in adults with a median age at presentation around age 60. CML comprises only around 2%-3% of all the leukemia diagnosed in patients <20 years of age but the incidence increases with age slowly until the mid-40s, then more rapidly from about one per 1000 000/year in children <10 years to two per 100 000 in people in the fifth decade to one per 10 000 at age 80. The disease is more common in males. There is no clear evidence of to geographic or ethnic background that predisposes to CML; however, in the United States the incidence is slightly higher in Caucasians than in Blacks or Hispanics (Lee et al., 2009), and it exhibits a male preponderance, in South African Coloured and Black people, and African Americans in comparison to whites but the reason for this is unexplained. (Jacobs et al., 1983). Furthermore, several reports showed an increased incidence of CML during the first 2 decades of life in African subjects (Haddock , 1967; Lowe et al., 1971; Lowenthal et al., 1975), but other reports by Leibowitz et al., (1976) and Jacobs et al., (1983) disagree with this. Jacobs et al. reported that in comparison with Whites and Coloureds, however, the peak incidence for Blacks was lower, lying between the 3rd and 4th decades. The peak incidence for Coloureds was in the 4th and 5th decades, and that for Whites in the 5th and 6th (Jacobs et al., 1983.)

An interesting study in United Arab Emirate (UAE) found that the rate of AML among UAE female nationals was higher than in nationals male and expatriates. The study proposed that chemicals in henna dye, which is used to decorate the body, as well as a lack of sunlight could be behind the increased incidence (Hassan et al., 2009). Henna is applied in many African countries especially Sudan where it is used by vast majority of Sudanese married women.

3. Molecular etiology

Leukemia in common with other cancers arises from mutations in a single cell, which enable the cell to reproduce excessively, emerging as a dominant clone. A large number of different mutant genes contribute to leukaemogenesis singly or, more often, in combination and many are leukemia sub-type specific (Greaves, 1986). The number of genetic abnormalities is believed to reflect the number of genes that control distinct developmental stages of blood formation and the multiple routes to clonal dominance. These include changes not only in proliferative activity, but in ability to differentiate, in resistance to cell death, in DNA repair activity and in general stability of the genes. Whether any particular mutant genes, or hot spots' for mutations within a gene, are linked to particular DNA damaging agents is a topic of considerable relevance to the molecular epidemiology of cancer in general. For these changes to happen some culprit agents has to come into action namely ionizing radiation, chemicals such as polycylic hydrocarbons and certain drugs, and viruses.

The way how these extrinsic factors affect the cell genetically and epigenetically is the core of the functional research in cancer. Although multiple risk factors have been linked to the development of leukemia, however these known risk factors account for only a small number of observed cases. Few epidemiological studies have explored the relation between lifestyle, dietary factors and the incidence of adult Leukemia, and almost none has addressed the molecular and genetic aspects of these interactions.

3.1 Role of viruses

For several reasons pertaining to ecology and the human history in Africa, several pathogens have gained access into human genomes through the African gate. This includes major parasites, viral and bacterial diseases. It is not coincidence that the first well proven case of viral oncogenesis that of Epstein Barr Virus (EBV) was established in Africa. EBV is a highly prevalent infection in the adult population in Africa and has been associated with a heterogeneous group of lymphomas, including Burkitt's lymphoma (especially the endemic form in Africa), Hodgkin's disease, NK, and T malignancies with cytotoxic phenotypes, and lymphomas in the immune-compromised patient (congenital immunodeficiency, organ transplantation, AIDS). (Rodriguez-Abreu et al., 2007) but not unequivocally with leukemia. Of the oncogenic retroviruses, the Human T-cell leukemia virus (HTLV) type 1 and type 2 have been identified as being related to the development of rare types of leukemia and lymphoma. HTLV-1 is endemic in certain areas including central Africa, and is associated with the development of adult T-cell leukemia or lymphoma (ATLL), which accounts for about half of the lymphoid malignancies in the endemic areas. The virus is transmitted mainly from mother to child, especially by breastfeeding. Sexual transmission and blood transfusion are minor routes of infection and cell-free blood products are not infectious (Rodriguez-Abreu et al., 2007).

The importance of oncogenic viruses stems not only from their transforming oncogenic properties but also from the potential methylating properties of selfish DNA.

Environmental determinant including infection with high-risk viruses are necessary but not sufficient alone in the development of cancer, as most infections regress without intervention. Thus, genetic host factors and cellular immune responses could be potential modifiers for the risk of developing cancer. In particular, p53 and Rb are considered as the most critical tumor suppressor genes involved in regulating cell division. The polymorphism on p53, which encodes either a Proline or an Arginin amino acid residue at codon 72, has been reported as a possible risk factor for several cancers including breast and cervical cancer in Sudan (Eltahir et al, submitted.).

3.2 Population and ethnic diversity

In the last decade the importance of ethnicity, socio-economic and gender differences in relation to disease incidence, diagnosis, and prognosis has been realised. Gender and ethnic differences in these areas should have a focus in health policy in Africa. A study by Lee et al. examined the demographic and clinical features of CML in an ethnically diverse population and found that Hispanic patients present with lower risk profile CML and achieve better treatment responses compared to non-Hispanic patients. The vast majority of their non-Hispanic patients were African American or Asian. This study proposed that biological/genetic factor can contributes to this observed ethnic differences in disease presentation and behavior. Hispanic ethnic group is thought to be the least diverse ethnic group, at the opposite site the African descent is the most diverse ethnic group. African populations are characterized by greater levels of genetic diversity, extensive population substructure, and less linkage disequilibrium (LD) among loci compared to non-African populations (Reich et al., 2001; Campbell and Tishkoff, 2008). Due to the long evolutionary history in Africa there is more genetic diversity within and between populations in the African continent, than between Africans and other peoples in the world (Cavalli-Sforza, 1997). African populations thus vary considerably in their genes. Moreover Africa shows a wide range of environments, climatic, vegetative and zoological. Thus human cancer patters are expected to show a similar degree of diversity, the study of which would contribute to our understanding of their causes.

The majority of cancers as genetic disease of complex nature involve a multiplicity of genetic loci that cooperates to make the disease happen (the multiple -hit theory). It is expected that such genetic component will be influenced by the genetic background of the population at risk. In one of the few studies on a cancer susceptibility genes background mutational profile in different populations, Africans were found to harbor more mutations in their BRCA2 than populations from the rest of the world (Wagner et al., 1999.) which is expected given their larger effective population size.

Africans also possess a number of genetic adaptations that have evolved in response to diverse climates and diets, as well as exposure to infectious disease (Campbell & Tishkoff, 2008), that diversity may carry great challenge in leukemia presentation and behavior/ prognosis and treatment. Moreover, experimental studies using synthetic peptides identical to the BCR-ABL fusion region in CML patients region have revealed the capability of specific peptides to bind to human leukocyte antigen (HLA) class I molecules (HLA-A2, A3, A11, B8) and class II molecules (HLA-DR1, DR2, DR3, DR4 and DR11). Individuals expressing HLA-A3, B8 or DR4 have a diminished risk for the development of CML in Caucasian populations. A statistically significant increase in the frequency of Cw3 and Cw4 antigens in Caucasians and European CML patients has been reported. Another report in Indian population showed that expression of HLA-Cw6 may result in a protective effect on CML acquisition (Chhaya, 2006). A study in Chinese population indicated that the expression of HLA-A*30, DRB1*07 might imply a protective effect on CML acquisition, while B*81 might be associated with CML susceptibility factors in that population (Miao et al., 2007). These results suggest that the development of CML is apparently associated with HLA phenotypes specific to each population. These data is missed in Africa and we intend to investigate this in Sudanese population.

Common polymorphism like the codon 72 in p53 has been argued to unlikely have major genetic effect since polymorphism in loci with major deleterious nature will not be selected for to reach such frequencies unless it is a balanced polymorphism. (i.e. selected for under the influence of the other allele possessing an favorable adaptive trait). Interestingly It has been proposed that the p53 polymorphism at times when the risk of tumors was not a Human concern, gave a reproductive leverage by increasing reproductive success (Kang et al., 2008). The cost of such trade off will not be visible as long as the conditions that predispose for tumors are absent. In fact the derived allele (arginine), almost reached fixation in some populations.

The p53 codon 72 was studied both in normal Sudanese (Bereir et al., 2002) and in the distribution of the polymorphism in different cancers in Sudan, (not including leukemia). The results show that the different alleles pose different risk ratios in different cancer. The Arg allele which is known to be more resistant to cell death was overrepresented breast carcinoma patients from different linguistic groups as compared to controls with an Odd ratio of 19.44 CI 6.6 - 78.3 $P<0.0001$. In cervical cancer the homozygous Arg genotype was detected in 42.3% (33/78) in cervical cancer patients while the heterozygous arg/pro in 38.5% (30/78) and only 19.2% (15/78) had the pro/pro genotype, with an allele effect of 2.4 (CI 1.12 - 5.33, P 0.015). In Burkitt´s lymphoma the opposite seems to be true with a major effect from the Pro allele, where the homozygous Arg accounted for only 6.9%, (OR 0.18 CI 0.02 - 0.89, P= 0.018) while the Arg/Pro was 51.7% and pro/pro 41.4% (OR: 0.57, CI 0.23-1.42, P= 0.1). Possibly indicating the different biological pathways of tumorigenesis (Eltahir et al., submitted).

3.3 Gene and chromosomal rearrangements

Cancers as a group of diseases display the entire range of inheritance modes from the single gene like disorder to the complex inheritance pattern seen in chronic diseases. The paucity of genetic investigation in Africa of cancer susceptibility genes and chromosomal aberrations linked to cancer, makes the picture even more opaque. The few examples discussed above and below demonstrate the great relevance of studying the genetic population structure of African populations and establishing the frequencies of the individual SNPs, Ins/dels and chromosomal abnormalities associated with diseases that may be necessary to define the molecular etiological basis of each cancer. In fact both molecular and genetic abnormalities became an important factor for characterising, treating and risk stratifying of myeloid leukemia. In 2002 the WHO classification of Myeloid Neoplasms showed that AML classification includes specific genetic subcategories; thus, determination of genetic features of the neoplastic cells must be performed if possible. Many recurring genetic abnormalities in the myeloid neoplasms can be identified by advanced molecular and cytogenetic techniques. In the WHO classification, the blast threshold for the diagnosis of AML is reduced from 30% to 20% blasts in the blood or marrow. In addition, patients with the clonal, recurring cytogenetic abnormalities t(8;21)(q22;q22), inv(16)(p13q22) or t(16;16)(p13;q22), and t(15;17)(q22;q12) should be considered to have AML regardless of the blast percentage. On the other hand, according to the WHO classification, CML is defined specifically as a myeloproliferative disease that is characterized by the invariable presence of the Philadelphia (Ph) chromosome or the BCR-ABL fusion gene. Although in most cases the diagnosis is easily made from morphologic evaluation of the blood smear, confirmation by genetic studies is essential, particularly in view of the advent of therapy that targets the BCR-ABL fusion protein (Vardiman et al., 2002)

Despite their diagnostic and prognostic values, studies on gene and chromosomal rearrangements associated malignancies is greatly lacking on the African continent, and in spite of the mandatory genotyping of the BCR-ABL as a prerequisite of administering the drug imatinib, in several African countries, there are very few reports on its frequencies. Among the few reports on its association with other leukemias, a multi-country study comprising 181 children with newly diagnosed ALL were tested in laboratories in India, Pakistan, Myanmar, and Sudan, following a common protocol. Across the four countries, the ETV6-RUNX1 (TEL-AML1) fusion gene was present in only 5% of cases. All the positive samples were from children aged 1 to 10 years, in whom the prevalence of this fusion gene, which is associated with good prognosis, was 7.4% (9 out of 121 samples), a much lower rate than reported from Western populations. In the 18 ALL cases tested in Sudan, a notable excess of MLL-AF4 (17%) and BCR-ABL1 (22%) fusion genes was found (Siddiqui et al., 2010).

The significance of studying the frequency of these rearrangements and their relation to pathology, is to establish the level of culpability of the molecular events. A study on Nigerian breast cancer patients suggest that while BRCA1 genomic rearrangement exists, it does not contribute significantly to BRCA1-associated risk in the Nigerian population (Zhang et al., 2011).

Chromosomal translocations in myeloid leukemia yield hybrid RNAs capable of encoding fusion chimeric proteins. The unique amino acid sequences found in these oncogenic fusion proteins represent true tumor-specific antigens that are potentially immunogenic. Although these leukemia-specific fusion proteins have an intracellular location, they might be recognized immunologically by T lymphocytes if peptides derived from the unique sequences are capable of presentation by the major histocompatibility complex (MHC) molecules on Leukemic cells (Bocchia *et al.*, 1995). The ability of a series of synthetic peptides corresponding to the junctional sequences of CML-derived BCR-ABL fusion proteins spanning the b3a2 and b2a2 breakpoints to bind to purified class I molecules was studied by Bocchia *et al.* Four peptides derived from b3a2 CML breakpoint bound with high or intermediate affinity to HLA A3, A11, and B8. None of the CML b2a2 junctional peptides showed affinity of this magnitude for the HLA class I molecules tested. Which draw another important conclusion on the significance of the types of BCR-ABL fusion transcripts among populations in relation to vaccine development? The frequencies of the types of the fusion transcript in Ecuadorian population for example consist of 95% b2a2 (Paz-y-Mino et al., 2002) indicating that they may not benefit much from such vaccine.

Several studies estimated the types of BCR-ABL fusion transcript in CML in different populations. The distribution of transcript type has been studied in European and some other populations (Eisenberg et al., 1988; Lee et al., 1989) with frequencies for b2a2 and b3a2 transcripts being roughly of the order of 40% and 55%, and that for co-expression of b3a2 and b2a2 representing 5% of the cases. A study on an Ecuadorian population, however, registered very different frequencies: 5% for b3a2 and 95% for b2a2 (Paz-y-Mino et al., 2002). In our report in Sudanese patients (Osman et al., 2010), a frequency of 53.5% and 41.9% for b2a2 and b3a2, respectively, was reported, values that are relatively closer to those from a Mexican population (Arana- Trejo et al., 2002). This difference in frequencies may be due to the genetic differences of the populations. Many Controversial reports about the clinical significant of the transcript type in CML were published; however it has a considerable importance in the diagnosis and follow up.

Recently, a polymorphic base in exon 13 of the BCR gene (exon b2 of the major breakpoint cluster region) has been identified in the eighth position before the junctional region of BCR-ABL cDNA. Cytosine replaces thymidine; the corresponding triplets are AAT (T allele) and AAC (C allele), respectively, both coding for asparagine. Therefore, this polymorphism has no implication in the primary structure of BCR and BCR-ABL proteins.

Co-expression of b2a2 and b3a2 transcripts has been linked to two polymorphisms, T to C at exon 13 and A to G at intron 13 (Meissner et al., 1998; Branford et al., 2002). However, in our study by Osman et al. (2010) six PCR products from four patients were sequenced to confirm the products of four b2a2 and two b3a2 and one was found to harbor T to C at exon 13 and expressed only b2a2 transcript which might indicate that this exonic polymorphism is not obligatory for co-expression, as reported by Mondal et al. (2006). Moreover, this polymorphism has no implication on the primary structure of BCR and BCR-ABL proteins. However, since the alteration is located close to the fusion region, it may have a significant influence on the annealing of PCR primers, probes for real time PCR, and antisense oligonucleotides. This polymorphism could be also a useful marker for the differentiation of normal and rearranged BCR alleles in heterozygotes patients and during follow up of minimal residual disease. The allele frequency for this SNP varied markedly between different world populations, with European attaining intermediate values between African and Asians (Table 1)

The molecular basis of CML is well defined and highly consistent, yet prognosis varies considerably. This could reflect the biological diversity occurring in normal populations.

Population	T allele	C allele
African American	0.55	0.45
Sub-Saharan African	0.425	0.575
Asians	0.922	0.078
Chinese	0.91	0.09
Japanese	0.98	0.02
European	0.70	0.30

Data from NCBI/dbSNP/Short Genetic Variations

Table 1. The frequencies of T and C alleles of BCR exon 13 SNP in different populations andethnic groups

The study by Gordon et al 2003 suggest that variation among normal individuals may contribute to inter patient heterogeneity in CML. Differences in behaviour of haemopoietic progenitor cells from different normal individuals may be attributable to genetic diversity or other variables. de Haan et al. (2002) concluded that the expression levels of a large number of genes might be responsible for controlling stem cell behaviour. These collections of genes may be analogous to those responsible for the inter-individual diversity in progenitor cell behavior

In CML, the occurrence of additional specific cytogenetic and molecular changes subsequent to the initiation of t(9;22) translocation herald disease progression prior to haematologic and clinical manifestation. These events occur in 50 to 80 percent of patients during the transition from the chronic phase of the disease to the accelerated and blast phases. Minor cytogenetic changes include monosomies of chromosomes 7, 17, and Y; trisomies of chromosomes 17 and 21; and translocation t(3;21)(q26;q22) (Mitelman, 1993). Major changes include trisomy 8, isochromosome i(17q), trisomy 19, and an extra Ph chromosome (double Ph). Trisomy 8 is most common, and isochromosome i(17q) occurs almost exclusively in the myeloid type blast phase (Kantarjian et al., 1987; Derderian et al., 1993; Mitelman, 1993).

Molecular abnormalities may correspond to cytogenetic changes. These include abnormalities in p53 (on chromosome 17p13); RB1 (13q14); c-MYC (8q24); p16INK4A (9p21); RAS; and AML-EVI-1, a fusion protein resulting from translocation t(3;21) (q26;q22). Alterations of p53 (deletions, rearrangements, and mutations) occur in 20 to 30 percent of patients with CML in the blast phase (Ahuja et al.,1989) and are associated exclusively with myeloid transformation (Stuppia et al., 1997), whereas abnormalities of RB1 are associated more with lymphoid transformation, although the association is weaker than it was between p53 and myeloid transformation. Mutations of p53 in the progression of CML are associated with an aberrant methylation status of CML cells (Guinn et al., 1997). The introduction of a methyl group causing transcriptional silencing of the calcitonin gene has been found in the transition of chronic-phase CML to blast-phase CML (Malinen et al., 1991). Altered methylation was also described within the M-bcr of cells from patients with chronic-phase CML (Litz et al., 1996). Up to 50 percent of patients with lymphoid transformation have homozygous deletion of p16INK4A (Sill et al., 1995). Alterations of RB1, amplifications of c-MYC, and mutations of RAS are less frequent (Faderl et al., 1999).

The genetic variation in Africa is poised to constitute major challenge for diagnosis and management. In a world where the diagnosis and prognosis of diseases and particularly cancer is increasingly dependent on molecular approaches such diversity might constitute a hurdle for future intervention against cancer in general. The anticancer drug imatinib has shown remarkable success in treatment of CML. Though a variety of resistance mechanisms can arise, in the majority of patients resistance coincides with reactivation of the tyrosine kinase activity of the BCR-ABL fusion oncoprotein. This can result from gene amplification and, more importantly, point mutations that disrupt the bind of imatinib to BCR-ABL itself (Nardi et al., 2004). Although there are no indication of resistance so far in Sudan (Alkhatib, 2011), perhaps due to the limited use of the drug, the risk of resistance is proportional to the number of mutations that exist within the kinase domain and even outside the domain which are expected to be higher in Africa given the increased genetic diversity of African populations. The risk of resistance increases with the identification of Novel potential signaling pathways associated with drug resistance (Duy et al., 2011).

The significance of population genetic background extends to diagnostic and prognostic markers that may be applied to populations and to individuals. This is expected to form a trend in the management of diseases of complex inheritance as we learn more of the biological networks in function during diseases and the role of each individual molecule. In a study by Elamin et al., (submitted), aimed at developing biomarkers for breast cancer, Peroxyredoxin V turned to be a potentially useful marker both as a prognostic and treatment marker in Sudanese breast cancer but not among Chinese.

3.4 Drug metabolizing enzymes

The drug metabolizing enzymes system has been shown to influence the susceptibility, sequel and outcome of cancer treatment. These systems include the Glutathione transferases a family member of genes encoding enzymes involved in the metabolism of many chemicals and shown to be polymorphic with *GSTM1* and *GSTT1* being deleted in proportion of individuals where in the homozygous state results in a phenotypic absence of the corresponding enzyme. These enzymes are considerably important in the detoxification of many environmental compounds and reactive oxygen species, and hence may constitute important cancer predisposition genes.

It includes also the cytochrome P450 enzymes one of the best studied for risk association with cancer (Aqundez, 2004). The P450 shows conflicting and variable degree of association with cancer, possibly reflecting, variation in the role played by these enzymes in carcinogenesis and the genetic background of the population.

In some populations like those of the Indian subcontinent, the frequencies of homozygous 3/3 genotype and CYP3A5*3 allele were elevated significantly in the CML group compared to controls (χ^2=93.15, df=2, p=0.0001) (Sailaja et al., 2010).

In India also, a statistically significant difference between an AML group and normal control was observed in the case of glutathione-S-transferase M1 null (odds ratio 3.25, 95% confidence interval 1.9-5.58, P<0.001) and N-acetyl transferase 2*6B (odds ratio 3.04, 95% confidence interval 1.79-5.16, P<0.001) genotypes. Combined deficiency of N-acetyl transferase 2 and glutathione-S-transferase M1 genes produced an odds ratio of 11.91 (95% confidence interval 4.06-34.96, P<0.001). Those with glutathione-S-transferase M1 null genotype and N-acetyl transferase 2*6B allele are at increased risk of developing AML, and the risk is considerably enhanced in persons with both glutathione-S-transferase M1 and N-acetyl transferase 2 deficiency (Majumdar et al., 2008).

Increased risk of AML has also been reported for combined polymorphisms in detoxification and DNA repair enzymes (Voso et al., 2007), and patients that achieved complete molecular response following administration of imatinib showed significantly (p=0.013) higher in vivo CYP3A activity than patients achieving partial molecular response (Green et al., 2010).

In Sudan impact of the distribution of the GSTM1 and GSTT1 genotype leukemic patients was studied in 77 leukemic patients and 107 controls by Tagelsir et al., (Submitted). The results suggest that these genotypes could play a role in the development of leukemia particularly AML. Statistical analysis showed a significant preponderance of null genotype of both genes among pooled cases [*GSTM1* OR 3.45 (95% CI, 1.65 - 7.19); $P = 0.001$] for; *GSTT1* OR 8.57 (95% CI, 3.68 -19.93); $P < 0.0001$]. Double null was also higher in patients compared to controls ($P = 0.01$). When the cases were stratified according to the disease type, AML showed the highest positive predictive value for both loci (*GSTM1* $P < 0.0001$, *GSTT1* $P < 0.0001$), ALL and CLL showed similar patterns for *GSTT1* ($P = 0.001$) while the P-values for *GSTM1* were (0.01) and (0.007) respectively. CML displayed the least positive predictive value for *GSTM1* (0.02), while for *GSTT1* the result was as same as AML ($P < 0.0001$). Double null, however, showed only association with AML ($P < 0.0001$).

When the distribution of the *GSTM1* and *GSTT1* null genotypes were compared between linguistic groups of the control subjects, different percentages were obtained and *GSTT1* null genotypes was statistically different between the Afro-Asiatic and the Nilo-Saharan groups ($P = 0.01$). Difference in frequencies between Africans population is reported; Egyptians 15-29% (Abdel-Rahman, 1996; Hamdy et al., 2003), Tunisians 29% (Hanene et al., 2007) and Zimbabweans 26% (Masimirembwa, et al., 1998). generally speaking the *GSTM1* frequency (10.3%) is close to sub-Saharan Africa range; Nigerians 22% (Zhao et al., 1994) and Zimbabweans 24% (Masimirembwa, et al., 1998). while the previously reported frequency from Sudan is 39% (Tiemersma et al., 2001) . Other African populations frequencies are; Egyptians 44-55% [Abdel-Rahman, 1996 Hamdy et al., 2003), Tunisians 50% (Hanene et al., 2007).

The Tagelsir study suggests an increased risk for leukemia associated with *GSTM1* and *GSTT1* null genotypes and highlights a potential role of genetic make up in leukaemogensis. The most statistically significant association for *GSTT1* observed for both AML and CML may highlight a possible role of GSTT1 enzyme in protection of the myeloid series. Allelic variation in the gene encoding the GST isoform theta (GSTT1) enzymes was found to modulate the rate of benzene metabolism and excretion (Rossi et al., 1999) as well as benzene-induced myelotoxicity (Wan et al., 2002; Chen et al., 2007). AML - which showed the strongest association with both genes- comprises a distinct type of leukemia with different subtypes and is shown to be to somewhat associated with environmental exposure. Epidemiological studies have shown association between AML (M2, M4, and M5) and maternal exposure to marijuana and alcohol, and maternal and paternal exposures to pesticides, (Buckley et al., 1989; Robison et al., 1989; Severson et al., 1993; Shu et al., 1996). In addition to that AML is shown to be associated with exposure to benzene and may arise as therapy related complication after treatment of other cancers (Hoffbrand & Pettit, 2001).

Paradoxically, the presence of these genes could not be excluded as a possible risk factor for leukemia as some times these enzymes are involved in bioactivation of some chemicals producing more reactive metabolites that could confer threat to the cell. An example of such risk in other cancer was found in a study on Chinese population which showed that the genotype combination of *GSTM1* and *GSTT1* double positive confers a 4.2-fold higher risk for developing esophageal cancer and a 2.6-fold for esophageal hyperplasia (Lin et al., 1998).

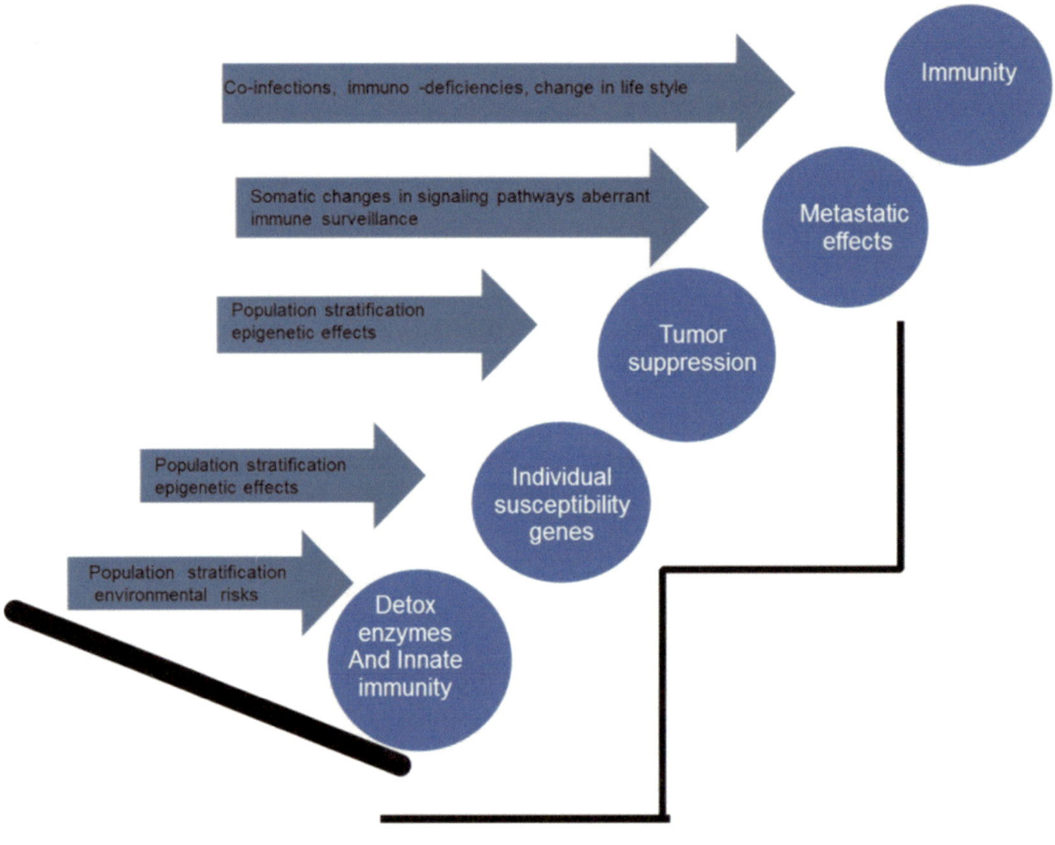

Fig. 1. The ladder and lever mechanism towards carcinogenesis. As the cancer cell struggles through multiple accumulative genetic events leading to cancer (the ladder), the cell will gain the upper hand in its surrounding tissue environment and eventually metastasize, it encounters various modifications and modulating effects that vary between individuals and communities. The variety of effects and the modifier action is expected to be greater in Africa. The up scaling of the ladder requires a lifting effect from the Environment (lever).

3.5 Epigenetics

DNA promoter methylation and histone modification are increasingly recognized as of primary importance in carcinogenesis. The two forms of aberrant methylation, hypomethylation and hypermethylation, are both well documented features of tumor cells (Hanahan and Weinberg, 2000; Jones and Baylin, 2002). The transcriptional silencing of tumor suppressor genes via promoter CpG island hypermethylation constitutes a key tumorigenic process contributing to all the typical hallmarks of a cancer cell that can result from tumor suppressor inactivation. Profiles of tumor suppressor methylation vary according to tumor type (Esteller et al., 2001) and each tumor apparently displays a distinct 'DNA hypermethylation pattern.

Recent studies revealed that specific patterns of DNA methylation characterize AML and help to distinguish AML subtypes. The contribution of this epigenetic dysregulation to leukemogenesis in AML is currently unclear. However, interactions between mutated transcription factors and epigenetic networks have already been shown to be partially responsible for leukemic transformation, for e.g. in acute promyelocytic leukemia (APL). Also, direct mutations in the epigenetic master regulators EZH2 and DNMT3A were recently identified in AML and in diseases leading to secondary leukemia (Schoofs and Muller-Tidow, 2011).

New studies reveal that 20% of individuals with AML harbor somatic mutations in DNMT3A (encoding DNA methyltransferase 3A). Although these leukemia have some gene expression and DNA methylation changes, a direct link between mutant DNMT3A, epigenetic changes and pathogenesis remains to be established.

The disruption of key protective genes through methylation is not confined to tumor suppression, it extends to other vital genes in protection /susceptibility to cancer like drug metabolizing enzymes, as been reported for the glutathione-S-transferase P1 gene silencing (Karius et al., 2011)

4. Future directions

The burden of myeloid leukemia is expected to rise as part of a global trend of increase in cancer incidence. In Africa the cost of this rise given the compound problems of health systems will be devastating. One pressing need is to challenge the preconception of cancer being a disease of the developed societies and show how this image is changing under the rapid sweep of "globalization. Even now the limited data available on leukemia indicate that the incidence of CML in some African countries may exceed those of the industrialized world. The understanding of cancer complex etiology is a prerequisite for successful management and control efforts.

Myeloid leukemia including the chronic subset that behave like a single gene disorder with the predominance of the Ph chromosome, posses complex etiology that includes multiple steps from environmental switches to inactivation of tumor suppression and other guardians of genome integrity and stability and ending with the impact of immune competence. Such complexity renders the handling of each of these potential culprits a daunting task especially in Africa. Without research into the etiology and genetic epidemiology of myeloid leukemia with all possible risk factors considered, including the genetic structure of population at risk, individual genetic effects, role of chronic and concomitant infections, and the possible trade off between infections and malignancies. For diagnosis and management an integrated genomic approach is the way forward. The vision for this approach entails an integrated and automated approach to these analyses, bringing the possibility of formulating an individualized treatment plan within days of a patient's initial presentation. With these expectations comes the hope that such an approach will lead to decreased toxicities and prolonged survival for patients (Godley et al., 2011). Such integrated approaches are expected to meet challenges pertinent to the peculiarity of African genetics.

5. Acknowledgment

The authors acknowledges financial support from the International Centre of Genetic Engineering and Biotechnology (ICGEB)

6. References

Abdel-Rahman SZ, El-zein RA, Anwar WA, Au WW. (1996). A multiplex PCR procedure for polymorphic analysis of GSTM1 and GSTT1 genes in population studies. *Cancer Lett*; 107: 229-33.

Abuidris, D.O., M.E. Ahmed, E.M. Elgaili, & R.S. Arora. (2008). Childhood cancer in Sudan: 1999-2007. *Trop Doct* 38: 208-210.

Ahmed, S.G. & U.A. Ibrahim. (2007). Significance of haemoglobin-S in the pathogenesis of hyperleucocytic syndromes in Nigerian patients with chronic myeloid leukaemia. *Eur J Haematol* 79: 174-176.

Ahuja, H., Bar-Eli, M., Advani, S.H., Benchimol, S. & Cline, M.J. (1989). Alterations in the p53 gene and the clonal evolution of the blast crisis of chronic myelocytic leukemia. Proc Natl Acad Sci U S A, 86:6783-7.

Alkhatib, M.A. (2010). Pattern of pediatric chronic myeloid leukemia in Sudan and hematological response to imatinib. *Pediatr Hematol Oncol* 28: 100-105.

Aplenc, R., T.A. Alonzo, R.B. Gerbing, F.O. Smith, S. Meshinchi, J.A. Ross, J. Perentesis, W.G. Woods, B.J. Lange & S.M. Davies. (2006). Ethnicity and survival in childhood acute myeloid leukemia: a report from the Children's Oncology Group. *Blood* 108: 74-80.

Aqundez J A (2004) Cytochrome P450 gene polymorphisms and cancer. *Curr Drug Metab* 5 (3) 211-24

Arana Trejo, R.M., Ruiz Sanchez, E., Ignacio-Ibarra, G., Baez de la Fuente, E., Garces, O., Gomez Morales, E., Castro Granados, M., Ovilla Martinez, R., Rubio-Borja, M.E., Solis Anaya, L., Herrera, P., Delgado Llamas, J. & Kofman, S. (2002). BCR/ABL p210, p190 and p230 fusion genes in 250 Mexican patients with chronic myeloid leukaemia (CML). *Clin Lab Haematol*, 24, 145-150-.

Bereir R.E.H., Mohamed1 H.S., Seielstad M, El Hassan A.M., Khalil1 E.A.G., Peacock C.S.,. Blackwell J.M & Ibrahim M.E.(2003). Allele frequency and genotype distribution of polymorphisms within disease-related genes is influenced by ethnic population sub-structuring in Sudan. *Genetica* 119: 57–63.

Bocchia, M., Wentworth, P.A., Southwood, S., Sidney, J., McGraw, K., Scheinberg, D.A., & Sette, A. (1995). Specific binding of leukemia oncogene fusion protein peptides to HLA class I molecules. *Blood*, 85, 10, 2680-2684.

Branford, S., T.P. Hughes, & Z. Rudzki. (2002). Dual transcription of b2a2 and b3a2 BCR-ABL transcripts in chronic myeloid leukaemia is confined to patients with a linked polymorphism within the BCR gene. *Br J Haematol* 117: 875-877.

Buckley JD, Robison LL, Swotinsky R, Garabrant DH, LeBeau M, Manchester P, Nesbit ME, Odom L, Peters JM, Woods WG, & Hammond GD.(1989) Occupational exposures of parents of children with acute nonlymphocytic leukemia: a report from the Children's Cancer Study Group. *Cancer Res* 49: 4030–4037.

Campbell, M.C. & S.A. Tishkoff. (2008). African genetic diversity: implications for human demographic history, modern human origins, and complex disease mapping. *Annu Rev Genomics Hum Genet* 9: 403-433.

Cavalli-Sforza, L.L. (1998). The DNA revolution in population genetics. *Trends Genet* 14: 60-65.

Chen Y, Li G, Yin S, Xu J, Ji Z, Xiu X, Liu L, & Ma D. (2007). Genetic polymorphisms involved in toxicant-metabolizing enzymes and the risk of chronic benzene poisoning in Chinese occupationally exposed populations. *Xenobiotica*; 37:103–112.

Chhaya, S.U .(2006). Human leukocyte antigens in Indian patients with chronic myeloid leukemia. *Leuk Lymphoma* 47: 291-295.Davies, J.N. & R. Owor. (1965). Chloromatous Tumours in African Children in Uganda. *Br Med J* 2: 405-407.

Davies, J.N.P. (1973) Childhood tumors. In: Templeton, A.C., ed., Tumors in a Tropical Country *(Recent Results in Cancer Research No. 41)*, Berlin, Springer Verlag

Derderian, P.M., Kantarjian, H.M., Talpaz, M., O'Brien, S., Cork, A., Estey, E., Pierce, S. & Keating, M. (1993). Chronic myelogenous leukemia in the lymphoid blastic phase: characteristics, treatment response, and prognosis. *Am J Med*, 94, 69-74.

Duy C, Hurtz C, Shojaee S, Cerchietti L, Geng H, Swaminathan S, Klemm L, Kweon SM, Nahar R, Braig M, Park E, Kim YM, Hofmann WK, Herzog S, Jumaa H, Koeffler HP, Yu JJ, Heisterkamp N, Graeber TG, Wu H, Ye BH, Melnick A & Müschen M (2011). BCL6 enables Ph+ acute lymphoblastic leukaemia cells to survive BCR-ABL1 kinase inhibition. *Nature*. 19;473(7347):384-8.

Eisenberg, A., R. Silver, L. Soper., Z. Arlin, M. Coleman, B. Bernhardt, & P. Benn.. (1988). The location of breakpoints within the breakpoint cluster region (bcr) of chromosome 22 in chronic myeloid leukemia. *Leukemia*, 2, 642–647.

Elghannam, D.M., N.K. Abousamra, D.A. Shahin, E.F. Goda, H. Azzam, E. Azmy, M.S. El-Din, and M.F. El-Refaei. (2009). Prognostic implication of N-RAS gene mutations in Egyptian adult acute myeloid leukemia. *Egypt J Immunol* 16: 9-15.

Faderl, S., Talpaz, M., Estrov, Z., O'Brien, S., Kurzrock, R. & Kantarjian, H.M. (1999) The biology of chronic myeloid leukemia. *New Engl J Med*, 341(3):164-72.]

Fleming AF (1993). Leukaemias in Africa. *Leukemia*. 7 Suppl 2:S138-41.

Ge, Y. & M.T. Elghetany. (2005). CD36: a multiligand molecule. *Lab Hematol* 11: 31-37.

Gmidene, A., H. Sennana, P. Fenaux, A. Laatiri, M. Zarrouk, H. Bouaziz, I. Harrabi, & A. Saad. (2008). Cytogenetic abnormalities in Tunisian de novo myelodysplastic syndrome: a comparison with other populations. *Leuk Res* 32: 1824-1829.

Godley LA, Cunningham J, Dolan ME, Huang RS, Gurbuxani S, McNerney ME, Larson RA, Leong H, Lussier Y, Onel K, Odenike O, Stock W, White KP & Le Beau MM (2011). An integrated genomic approach to the assessment and treatment of acute myeloid leukemia. *Semin Oncol*. 38(2):215-24.

Gordon, M.Y., S.B. Marley, J.F. Apperley, D. Marin, J. Kaeda, R. Szydlo, and J.M. Goldman. (2003). Clinical heterogeneity in chronic myeloid leukaemia reflecting biological diversity in normal persons. *Br J Haematol* 122: 424-429.

Greaves, M.F. (1993). A natural history for pediatric acute leukemia. *Blood*, 82:1043.

Greaves, M F. (1986). Differentiation-linked leukaemogenesis in lymphocytes. *Science*, 234:697.

Green, H., K. Skoglund, F. Rommel, R.A. Mirghani, & K. Lotfi. (2010) CYP3A activity influences imatinib response in patients with chronic myeloid leukemia: a pilot study on in vivo CYP3A activity. *Eur J Clin Pharmacol* 66: 383-386.

Guinn, B.A. &Mills, K.I. (1997). p53 Mutations, methylation and genomic instability in the progression of chronic myeloid leukaemia. Leuk Lymphoma, 26: 221-6.

de Haan, G., Bystrykh, L.V., Weersing, E., Dontje, B., Geiger, H., Ivanova, N., Lemischka, I., Vellenga, E. & Van Zant, G. (2002). A genetic and genomic analysis identifies a cluster of genes associated with hematopoietic cell turnover. Blood, 100, 2056–2062.

Haddock, D.R. (1967). The pattern of leukaemia in Accra, Ghana. *J Trop Med Hyg* 70: 60-62.

Hamad, H.M. (2006). Cancer initiatives in Sudan. *Ann Oncol* 17 Suppl 8: viii32-viii36.

Hamdy SI, Hiratsuka M, Narahara K, Endo N , El-Enany M , Moursi N , Ahmed MS-E & Mizugaki M. (2003). Genotype and allele frequencies of TPMT, NAT2, GST, SULT1A1 and MDR-1 in the Egyptian population. *British J Clin Pharmacol*; 55:560–569.

Hanahan D, & Weinberg RA. (2000) The Hallmarks of Cancer. *Cell* 100, 57–70.

Hanene C, Jihene L, Jamel A, Kamel H & Agnès H (2007) Association of *GST* Genes Polymorphisms with Asthma in Tunisian Children. *Mediators Inflamm* 2007:19564.

Hassan, I.B., S.I. Islam, H. Alizadeh, J. Kristensen, A. Kambal, S. Sonday, & R.M. Bernseen. (2009). Acute leukemia among the adult population of United Arab Emirates: an epidemiological study. *Leuk Lymphoma* 50: 1138-1147.

Hoffbrand AV, Pettit JE & Moss PAH (2001) Essential haematology. 4th edition, Blackwell science Inc.

Hosny, G. and S.M. Elkaffas. (2002). Patterns in the incidence of pediatric cancer in Alexandria, Egypt, from 1972 to 2001. *J Egypt Public Health Assoc* 77: 451-468.

Jacobs, P., H.S. King, and D.M. Dent. (1983). Chronic granulocytic leukaemia. A 10-year experience in the Black, Coloured and White populations of the south-western Cape Province. *S Afr Med J* 63: 879-882.

Jones SB (1999). Cancer in the developing world: a call to action. *BMJ*. 21;319(7208):505-8.

Jones PA & Baylin SB. (2002) The fundamental role of epigenetic events in cancer. *Nat Rev Genet*. 3(6):415-28..

Kang HJ, Feng Z, Sun Y, Atwal G, Murphy ME, Rebbeck TR, Rosenwaks Z, Levine AJ & Hu W (2009). Single-nucleotide polymorphisms in the p53 pathway regulate fertility in humans. *Proc Natl Acad Sci U S A*. 16;106(24):9761-6.

Kantarjian, H.M., Keating, M.J., Talpaz, M., Walters, R.S., Smith, T.L., Cork, A., McCredie, K.B. & Freireich, E.J. (1987). Chronic myelogenous leukemia in blast crisis. Analysis of 242 patients. *Am J Med*, 83, 445-454.

Kasili. E. G. (1990). Childhood Leukaemia: Is it a Problem in Tropical Africa? *Leukemia & Lymphoma*, Vol. 1, No. 3-4 , 187-193

Lee, M.S., LeMaistre, A., Kantarjian, H.M., et al. (1989). Detection of two alternative bcr/abl mRNA junctions and minimal residual disease in Philadelphia chromosome positive chronic myelogenous leukemia by polymerase chain reaction. *Blood*, 73, 2165–2170.

Lee, J.P., E. Birnstein, D. Masiello, D. Yang, & A.S. Yang. (2009). Gender and ethnic differences in chronic myelogenous leukemia prognosis and treatment response: a single-institution retrospective study. *J Hematol Oncol* 2: 30.

Leibowitz, M.R., D.P. Derman, R. Jacobson, K. Stevens, & J. Katz. (1976). Chronic myeloid leukaemia in South African blacks. *S Afr Med J* 50: 2035-2037.

Li, K., M. Yang, P.M. Yuen, K.W. Chik, C.K. Li, M.M. Shing, H.K. Lam, & T.F. Fok. (2003). Thrombospondin-1 induces apoptosis in primary leukemia and cell lines mediated by CD36 and Caspase-3. *Int J Mol Med* 12: 995-1001.

Li, Y., K.B. Moysich, M.R. Baer, J.R. Weiss, J. Brasure, S. Graham, and S.E. McCann. (2006). Intakes of selected food groups and beverages and adult acute myeloid leukemia. *Leuk Res* 30: 1507-1515.Lin D, Tang Y & Lu S. (1998) Glutathione S-transferase M1, T1 genotypes and the risk of esophageal cancer: a case-control study. *Chung Hua Liu Hsing Ping Hsueh Tsa Chih*; 19 :195–199.

Litz, C.E., Vos, J.A., Copenhaver, C.M. (1996). Aberrant methylation of the major breakpoint cluster region in chronic myeloid leukemia. *Blood* 88:2241-9.

Lowe, R.F. (1971). Chronic myelocytic leukaemia in African children. *Trans R Soc Trop Med Hyg* 65: 840-841.

Lowenthal, M.N. (1975). Chronic myeloid leukaemia in Zambians. *Trop Geogr Med* 27: 132-136.

Ma, X., Y. Park, S.T. Mayne, R. Wang, R. Sinha, A.R. Hollenbeck, A. Schatzkin & A.J. Cross (2009). Diet, lifestyle, and acute myeloid leukemia in the NIH-AARP cohort. *Am J Epidemiol* 171: 312-322.

Malinen, T., Palotie, A., Pakkala, S., Peltonen, L., Ruutu, T., Jansson, S.E. (1991). Acceleration of chronic myeloid leukemia correlates with calcitonin gene hypermethylation. *Blood* , 77, 2435-40

Majumdar, S., B.C. Mondal, M. Ghosh, S. Dey, A. Mukhopadhyay, S. Chandra, and U.B. Dasgupta. (2008). Association of cytochrome P450, glutathione S-transferase and N-acetyl transferase 2 gene polymorphisms with incidence of acute myeloid leukemia. *Eur J Cancer Prev* 17: 125-132.

Masimirembwa CM, Dandara C, Sommers DK, Snyman JR & Hasler JA. (1998) Genetic polymorphism of cytochrome P4501A1, microsomal epoxide hydrolase, and glutathione S-transferases M1 and T1 in Zimbabweans and Venda of Southern Africa. *Pharmacogenetics*; 8:83-85.

Meissner, R.V., P.M. Dias, D.T. Covas, F. Job, M. Leite, & N.B. Nardi. (1998). A polymorphism in exon b2 of the major breakpoint cluster region (M-bcr) identified in chronic myeloid leukaemia patients. *Br J Haematol* 103: 224-226.

Miao, K.R., Q.Q. Pan, M. Xue, S. Fan, X.Y. Wang, M. Pan, X.Y. Zhou, X.M. Fei, X. Zhao, and C.Y. Wang. (2007). Human leukocyte antigens in 295 Chinese patients with chronic myeloid leukemia. *Leuk Lymphoma* 48: 2152-2156.

Mitelman, F. (1993). The cytogenetic scenario of chronic myeloid leukemia. *Leuk Lymphoma*, 11, Suppl 1, 11-15.

Mondal, B.C., A. Bandyopadhyay, S. Majumdar, A. Mukhopadhyay, S. Chandra, U. Chaudhuri, P. Chakrabarti, S. Bhattacharyya, and U.B. Dasgupta. (2006). Molecular profiling of chronic myeloid leukemia in eastern India. *Am J Hematol* 81: 845-849.

Morris GJ and Mitchell EP (2008) Higher incidence pof aggressive breast cancers in African – American women; a review. *J Natl Med Assoc*. 100 (6): 698-702.

Nardi V, Azam M, Daley GQ. (2004 Jan). Mechanisms and implications of imatinib resistance mutations in BCR-ABL. *Curr Opin Hematol*.;11(1):35-43.

Nwannadi, O. Alao, G. Bazuaye, M. Nwagu & M. Borke (2011). Clinical and Laboratory Characteristics of Patients with Leukaemia in South-South Nigeria. *The Internet Journal of Oncology*.7 (2)

Obama, M.T., L. Zekeng, P.K. Ketchiozo, M.B. Owono, B.T. Kouam, & J. Mbede. (1995). Childhood leukemia is still a deadly disease in Yaounde, Cameroon: a report of 14 cases. *Pediatr Hematol Oncol* 12: 301-304.

Omoti, C.E., A.N. Olu-Eddo, & A.I. Nwannadi. (2009). Co-existence of TB and adult haematological cancers in Benin City, Nigeria. *Trop Doct* 39: 205-207.

Osman, E.A., K. Hamad, I.M. Elmula, & M.E. Ibrahim. (2010) Frequencies of BCR-ABL1 fusion transcripts among Sudanese chronic myeloid leukaemia patients. *Genet Mol Biol* 33: 229-231.

Parkin, D.M., F. Bray, J. Ferlay, and P. Pisani. (2005). Global cancer statistics, 2002. *CA Cancer J Clin* 55: 74-108.

Paz-y-Mino, C., Burgo, R., Morillo, S.A., Santos, J.C., Fiallo, B.F. & Leone, P.E. (2002). BCR-ABL rearrangement frequencies in chronic myeloid leukemia and acute lymphoblastic leukemia in Ecuador, South America. *Cancer Genet Cytogenet*, 132, 65–67.

Reich DE, Cargill M, Bolk S, Ireland J, Sabeti PC, Richter DJ, Lavery T, Kouyoumjian R, Farhadian SF, Ward R, Lander ES.(2001).Linkage disequilibrium in the human genome. *Nature*. 10;411:199-204.

Robison LL, Buckley JD, Daigle AE, Wells R, Benjamin D, Arthur DC, Hammond GD. (1989) Maternal drug use and risk of childhood nonlymphoblastic leukemia among offspring. An epidemiologic investigation implicating marijuana (a report from the Children's Cancer Study Group). *Cancer*63:1904–1911.

Rodriguez-Abreu, D., A. Bordoni, & E. Zucca. (2007). Epidemiology of hematological malignancies. *Ann Oncol* 18 Suppl 1: i3-i8.

Ross, J.A., C.M. Kasum, S.M. Davies, D.R. Jacobs, A.R. Folsom, & J.D. Potter. (2002). Diet and risk of leukemia in the Iowa Women's Health Study. *Cancer Epidemiol Biomarkers Prev* 11: 777-781.

Rossi AM, Guarnieri C, Rovesti S, Gobba F, Ghittori S, Vivoli G & Barale R. (1999). Genetic polymorphisms influence variability in benzene metabolism in humans. *Pharmacogenetics*. 9: 445–451.

Sailaja, K., D.N. Rao, D.R. Rao, & S. Vishnupriya. (2010) Analysis of CYP3A5*3 and CYP3A5*6 gene polymorphisms in Indian chronic myeloid leukemia patients. *Asian Pac J Cancer Prev* 11: 781-784.

Schoofs T & Müller-Tidow C (2011). DNA methylation as a pathogenic event and as a therapeutic target in AML Cancer Treat Rev.

Sener SF & Grey N (2005).The global burden of cancer.*J Surg Oncol*. 1;92(1):1-3.

Severson RK, Buckley JD, Woods WG, Benjamin D & Robison LL. (1993) Cigarette smoking and alcohol consumption by parents of children with acute myeloid leukemia: an analysis within morphological subgroups—a report from the Children's Cancer Group. *Cancer Epidemiol Biomark Prev*; 2: 433– 439.

Shamebo. M. (1990). Leukaemia in adult Ethiopians. *Ethiop Med J*, 28(1): 31-7

Shu XO, Ross JA, Pendergrass TW, Reaman GH, Lampkin B & Robison LL. (1996). Parental alcohol consumption, cigarette smoking, and risk of childhood leukemia: a Children's Cancer Group study. *J Natl Cancer Inst* 88: 24–31.

Siddiqui R, Nancy N, Naing WP, Ali S, Dar L, Khan BK, Padua RA & Carr R. (2010) Distribution of common genetic subgroups in childhood acute lymphoblastic leukemia in four developing countries. *Cancer Genet Cytogenet*. 200 (2):149-53.

Sill H, Goldman JM &Cross NCP. (1995). Homozygous deletions of the p16 tumor-suppressor gene are associated with lymphoid transformation of chronic myeloid leukemia. *Blood*;85:2013-6.

Stuppia L, Calabrese G, Peila R, et al. (1997). p53 Loss and point mutations are associated with suppression of apoptosis and progression of CML into myeloid blast crisis. *Cancer Genet Cytogenet*;98:28-35.

Tiemersma EW, Omer RE, Bunschoten A, Veer P, Kok FJ, Idris MO, Kadaru AMY, Fedail SS & Kampman E. (2001) Role of Genetic Polymorphism of Glutathione-*S*-Transferase *T1* and Microsomal Epoxide Hydrolase in Aflatoxin-associated Hepatocellular Carcinoma. *Can Epidemiol Biomar Preven* . 10: 785–791.

Vardiman, J.W., N.L. Harris, & R.D. Brunning. (2002). The World Health Organization (WHO) classification of the myeloid neoplasms. *Blood* 100: 2292-2302.

Voso MT, Fabiani E, D'Alo' F, Guidi F, Di Ruscio A, Sica S, Pagano L, Greco M, Hohaus S & Leone G. (2007). Increased risk of acute myeloid leukaemia due to polymorphisms in detoxification and DNA repair enzymes. *Ann Oncol*. 18(9):1523-8

Wagner TM, Hirtenlehner K, Shen P, Moeslinger R, Muhr D, Fleischmann E, Concin H, Doeller W, Haid A, Lang AH, Mayer P, Petru E, Ropp E, Langbauer G, Kubista

E, Scheiner O, Underhill P, Mountain J, Stierer M, Zielinski C & Oefner P. (1999). Global sequence diversity of BRCA2: analysis of 71 breast cancer families and 95 control individuals of worldwide populations. *Hum Mol Genet*. 8(3):413-23.

Wan J, Shi J, Hui L, Wu D, Jin X, Zhao N, Huang W, Xia Z & Hu G. (2002) Association of genetic polymorphisms in CYP2E1, MPO, NQO1, GSTM1, and GSTT1 genes with benzene poisoning. *Envirom Health Perspect* . 110: 1213–1218.

Yach D, Hawkes C, Gould CL & Hofman KJ (2004) The global burden of chronic diseases: overcoming impediments to prevention and control. *JAMA*.2;291(21):2616-22.

Zhang, M., X. Zhao, X. Zhang, & C.D. Holman. (2008). Possible protective effect of green tea intake on risk of adult leukaemia. *Br J Cancer* 98: 168-170.

Zhang J, Fackenthal JD, Huo D, Zheng Y & Olopade OI. (2010). Searching for large genomic rearrangements of the BRCA1 gene in a Nigerian population. *Breast Cancer Research and Treatment* 124, 2: 573-577.

Zhao L, Alldersea J, Fryer A, Tighe A, Oilier B, Thomson W, Jones P & Strange R (1994) Polymorphism at the glutathione S-transferase *GSTMI* locus: a study of the frequencies of the GSTMI A, B, A/B and null phenotypes in Nigerians. *Clin Chim Acta*; 225: 85-88.